ACSM's
Essentials of Exercise Oncology

Kathryn H. Schmitz, Ph.D., FACSM
Professor
Division of Hematology and Oncology
Associate Director of Population Sciences, Hillman Cancer Center
Past President, ACSM
Founder, ACSM's Moving Through Cancer Initiative
University of Pittsburgh
Pittsburgh, PA, United States of America

Anna Schwartz, Ph.D., FNP-BC, FAAN
Professor & Charlotte Peck Lienemann & Alumni Distinguished Chair in Nursing College of Nursing
Omaha Division University of Nebraska Medical Center
Omaha, NE, United States of America

President and CEO
Coleman Health LLC
Parks, AZ, United States of America

Anna Campbell, Ph.D.
Professor & Director CanRehab Ltd
School of Applied Science
Edinburgh Napier University
Edinburgh, Scotland, United Kingdom

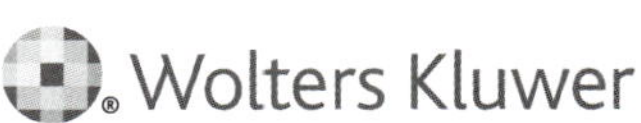

Philadelphia • Baltimore • New York • London
Buenos Aires • Hong Kong • Sydney • Tokyo

Acquisitions Editor: Lindsey Porambo
Development Editor: Amy Millholen, Robin Levin Richman (freelance)
Editorial Coordinator: Nancy Dickson
Marketing Manager: Danielle Klahr
Production Project Manager: Justin Wright
Design Coordinator: Stephen Druding
Manufacturing Coordinator: Margie Orzech
Prepress Vendor: Lumina Datamatics Ltd.
ACSM Publications Committee Chair: Karyn L. Hamilton, Ph.D., RD, FACSM
ACSM Health-Fitness Content Advisory Committee Chair: M. Allison Murphy, Ph.D., FACSM, ACSM-EP
ACSM Interim Chief Executive Officer: Katie Feltman
ACSM Director of Publishing: Angie Chastain

First Edition

9 8 7 6 5 4 3 2 1

Printed in the United States of America

Library of Congress Cataloging-in-Publication Data

ISBN-13: 978-1-9751-6743-1

Cataloging in Publication data available on request from publisher.

DISCLAIMER
Care has been taken to confirm the accuracy of the information present and to describe generally accepted practices. However, the authors, editors, and publisher are not responsible for errors or omissions or for any consequences from application of the information in this publication and make no warranty, expressed or implied, with respect to the currency, completeness, or accuracy of the contents of the publication. Application of this information in a particular situation remains the professional responsibility of the practitioner; the clinical treatments described and recommended may not be considered absolute and universal recommendations.

The authors, editors, and publisher have exerted every effort to ensure that drug selection and dosage set forth in this text are in accordance with the current recommendations and practice at the time of publication. However, in view of ongoing research, changes in government regulations, and the constant flow of information relating to drug therapy and drug reactions, the reader is urged to check the package insert for each drug for any change in indications and dosage and for added warnings and precautions. This is particularly important when the recommended agent is a new or infrequently employed drug.

Some drugs and medical devices presented in this publication have Food and Drug Administration (FDA) clearance for limited use in restricted research settings. It is the responsibility of the health care provider to ascertain the FDA status of each drug or device planned for use in their clinical practice.

To purchase additional copies of this book, call our customer service department at (800) 638-3030 or fax orders to (301) 223-2320. International customers should call (301) 223-2300.

For more information concerning the American College of Sports Medicine certification and suggested preparatory materials, call (800) 486-5643 or visit the American College of Sports Medicine Website at www.acsm.org.

shop.lww.com

SHER0524

DEDICATION

To Sara, Mack, and Tom, forever and always
-Kathryn H. Schmitz

To my tireless supporters Betsy and Okie
-Anna Schwartz

To Lucy—the light of my life
-Anna Campbell

Contributors

Kathryn H. Schmitz, Ph.D., FACSM
Professor
Division of Hematology and Oncology
Associate Director of Population Sciences, Hillman Cancer Center
Past President, ACSM
Founder, ACSM's Moving Through Cancer Initiative
University of Pittsburgh
Pittsburgh, PA, United States of America
Chapters 1, 2, 3, 6, 9, and 18

Anna Schwartz, Ph.D., FNP-BC, FAAN
Professor & Charlotte Peck Lienemann & Alumni Distinguished Chair in Nursing College of Nursing
Omaha Division University of Nebraska Medical Center
Omaha, NE, United States of America
President and CEO
Coleman Health LLC
Parks, AZ, United States of America
Chapters 4, 5, 8, 11, 13, 14, and 17

Anna Campbell, Ph.D.
Professor & Director CanRehab Ltd
School of Applied Science
Edinburgh Napier University
Edinburgh, Scotland, United Kingdom
Chapters 7, 10, 12, 15, and 16

Reviewers

Justin C. Brown, Ph.D.
Pennington Biomedical Research Center
Baton Rouge, Louisiana, United States of America

Ciaran Fairman, Ph.D., CSCS, CET
University of South Carolina
Columbia, South Carolina, United States of America

Daniel A. Galvão, Ph.D., FACSM
Edith Cowan University
Joondalup, Western Australia

Carolyn Garritt, MSc
Oomph Personal Training Ltd.
London, United Kingdom

Naomi Lynn Gerber, M.D.
Inova Health System
Falls Church, Virginia, United States of America

Katie M. Heinrich, Ph.D., FACSM
The Phoenix
Manhattan, Kansas, United States of America

Brock Thomas Jensen, Ph.D.
Slippery Rock University
Slippery Rock, Pennsylvania, United States of America

Heather J. Leach, Ph.D., FACSM
Colorado State University
Fort Collins, Colorado, United States of America

Stephen M. LoRusso, Ph.D.
St. Francis University
Loretto, Pennsylvania, United States of America

Mindy M. Mayol, Ph.D., FACSM
University of Indianapolis
Indianapolis, Indiana, United States of America

G. Stephen Morris, PT, Ph.D., FACSM
Wingate University
Wingate, North Carolina, United States of America

Karen M. Mustian, Ph.D., MPH
University of Rochester Medical Center
Rochester, New York, United States of America

Lynn B. Panton, Ph.D., FACSM
Florida State University
Tallahassee, Florida, United States of America

Madeline Paternostro-Bayles, Ph.D., FACSM
Indiana University of Pennsylvania
Indiana, Pennsylvania, United States of America

Christopher Paul Repka, Ph.D.
Northern Arizona University
Flagstaff, Arizona, United States of America

Lisa B. Sylvestri, MSPT, CLT-LANA
Oasis Physical Therapy and Wellness
San Ramon, California, United States of America

Keith Thraen-Borowski, Ph.D., FACSM
Loras College
Dubuque, Iowa, United States of America

Preface

ACSM's Essentials of Exercise Oncology is an undergraduate textbook that details the relationship between exercise and cancer prevention, and the value of exercise after a cancer diagnosis.

At present, there are 16 million cancer survivors in the United States (US), and that number is expected to grow to 20.3 million by 2026, according to the National Cancer Institute. Further, there are 1.7 million people diagnosed with cancer in the US every year, the majority of whom will live long past their treatment. Additionally, 610,000 Americans die of cancer every year, nearly the same number that die of all forms of cardiovascular disease. In short, cancer is approximately equivalent to cardiovascular disease as a cause of death in the US. Further, the burden of cancer is at least as great as cardiovascular disease, given the number and severity of long-term treatment toxicities.

This textbook will also be of interest to individuals preparing for credentialing in exercise oncology through the American College of Sports Medicine® as well as other allied health professionals, including physical and occupational therapists, nurses, nurse practitioners, physicians, and physician assistants, and anyone who specializes in working with patients with cancer.

Organization

Section 1, *Cancer Basics*, presents a scientific background for instruction on cancer epidemiology and biology, as well as cancer screening, diagnosis, treatment, survivorship, palliation, and end of life to enable the exercise oncology professional to speak with health care providers who treat cancer. Chapter 1 provides an understanding of the global burden of cancer, as well as a generalized introduction to how exercise training might be of value within this population.

Section 2, *Mechanisms Linking Exercise and Cancer Outcomes*, highlights the scientific evidence regarding the mechanisms by which exercise might have a positive effect on those living with and beyond cancer. This section explains what we know about the physiologic effects of exercise training to make clear the potential effects of exercise on cancer prevention and development.

Section 3, *Assessing and Prescribing Exercise Before, During, and After Cancer,* provides the practical knowledge base to prepare exercise oncology professionals to design and carry out high-quality, evidence-based exercise programs for people living with and beyond cancer. Described are the appropriate exercise prescriptions for an apparently healthy adult at risk for cancer, as well as an adult with varying levels of health and vitality as they go through cancer treatment and survive beyond the treatments. Clarified for the reader is how the treatment for cancer alters the ability to exercise, with appropriate adaptations that may be made for the exercise oncology professional.

Finally, chapters in **Section 4,** *Behavioral and Logistical Considerations*, cover unique issues encountered when working with patients and survivors of cancer, including behavioral and logistical considerations.

Features

Special learning features in each chapter of *ACSM's Essentials of Exercise Oncology* enrich the reader's breadth and depth of knowledge:

- **Outline and Objectives:** Each chapter begins with an outline and set of learning objectives to guide reading and study.
- **Key Terms:** They appear in bold and color at first mention, then in easily identifiable boxes within the text.
- **End-of-Chapter Features**: Every chapter closes with several practical tools to enhance the reader's comprehension and showcase real-world examples of patients and health care providers:
    - **Summaries** bring a cohesive and concise end to each chapter.
    - **Case Studies** present detailed stories about people living with and beyond cancer, and discuss approaches to develop exercise plans to accommodate their needs. Follow-up **Questions** extend the focus, with answers located in the back of the book.
    - **Meet the Expert** interviews showcase the personal trajectories for health care professionals who specialize in researching and applying exercise as a part of oncology health care.
    - **Study Questions** test the reader on the chapter information. The format varies intentionally and includes multiple-choice, true/false, and fill-in-the-blank style questions. Answers are located in the back of the book.
    - **References** reflect current evidence-based research findings and encourage further study and discussion.

Updates for the book can be found at https://www.acsm.org/education-resources/books/acsm-book-updates.

Acknowledgments

The authors would like to extend their gratitude to the scientists whose tireless work forms the basis of this volume, as well as the people living with and beyond cancer who volunteered to participate in the exercise oncology trials described herein.

Contents

Section 4: Behavioral and Logistical Considerations 239

SECTION

1 Cancer Basics

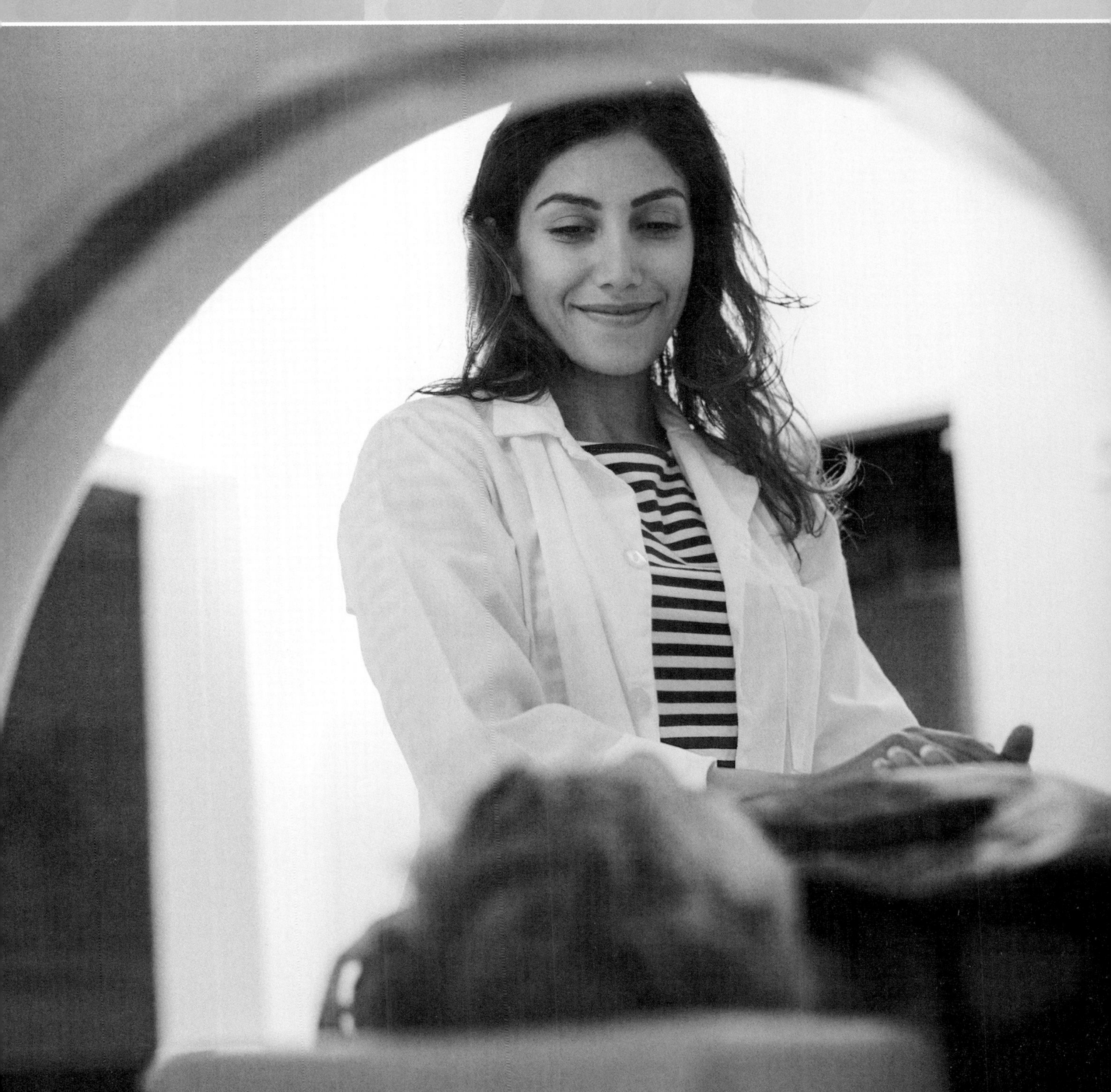

CHAPTER

1

The Burden of Cancer

OUTLINE

1. Introduction: What Is Cancer?
2. History of Cancer
3. Types of Cancer
4. Epidemiology of Cancer
    a. Occurrence of Cancer and Cancer Registries
    b. New Cases and Deaths
    c. What Types of Cancer Are Diagnosed and Where?
    d. Who Is at Risk?
    e. Who Survives?
    f. Costs of Cancer
    g. Cancer Prevention and Control
5. The Burden of Specific Common Cancers: The Role of Exercise
    a. Breast
    b. Prostate
    c. Colorectal
    d. Liver
    e. Lung
6. Summary
7. Case Study
8. Meet the Expert
9. Study Questions
10. References

OBJECTIVES

After completing review of this chapter, students will be able to:

1. Define the terms, types, and history of cancer.
2. Understand the burden of cancer in the United States and around the world.
3. Know the scientific evidence regarding the potential for exercise to alter the burden of cancer for 5 common cancers.

INTRODUCTION: WHAT IS CANCER?

Cancer is defined as a disease caused by an uncontrolled division of abnormal cells in a part of the body (1). The cells in our body are programmed to reproduce themselves continuously and eventually to die. Programmed, expected, or natural cell death is also called **apoptosis** or **cell senescence**. When the programming goes awry due to genetic mutations that occur during the replication of the cells, a genetic mutation acquired somatically (a **somatic mutation**, which is passed on in genes from parents), or through some environmental exposure that causes some other alteration of cell signaling, cells can break out of the pattern that leads to cell death. These cells achieve a kind of immortality, replicating beyond the control of the planned cell death that most of our cells experience. The biology of cancer will be explained more deeply in Chapter 2.

HISTORY OF CANCER

According to Siddhartha Mukherjee, the author of *The Emperor of All Maladies: A Biography of Cancer*, the first mention of cancer in antiquity dates back to the Edwin Smith Papyrus, from 3,000 BC, which describes 8 cases of tumors of the breast removed by cauterization (2). The writings comment that there is no treatment for the disease (Box 1.1).

The name *cancer* came from the father of medicine Hippocrates (460-370 BC), who used the terms *carcinos* and *carcinoma* to describe tumors. In Greek, these words refer to a crab, very likely applied to the disease because of the fingerlike spreading projections from a tumor called to mind the shape of a crab. The Roman physician Celsus (50-25 BC) translated the Greek term into *cancer* (the Latin word for crab). Later, Galen (130-200 AD), a Greek physician, used the word *oncos* (swelling) to describe tumors. This is the source of the term *oncologist*, a medical specialist who treats cancer.

Prior to our modern understanding that cancer is the result of an uncontrolled division of abnormal cells, there were multiple theories about the reasons and sources of the disease. Hippocrates believed that the human body had 4 humors or body fluids: blood, phlegm, yellow bile, and black bile (Figure 1.1). A balance of these humors was seen to promote health, and an excess of black bile, in particular, was thought to cause cancer (3). This theory remained unchallenged for over 1,300 years.

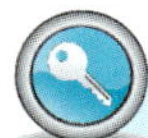

Apoptosis. Programmed cell death.

Cell senescence. Programmed cell death.

Somatic mutation. A genetic mutation that is inherited from the mother or father and is present at birth. Examples include the *BRCA1* and *BRCA2* genes that substantively increase risk for breast and ovarian cancers.

Box 1.1 Additional Recommended Reading

The Emperor of All Maladies: A Biography of Cancer, by Siddhartha Mukherjee, provides a history of cancer starting with ancient understandings of cancer, the development of chemotherapy, successes and failures in the developments of new therapies throughout the 20th century, preventive medicine, the development of the cellular focus on the nature of cancer, and a review of the current state of prevention, diagnosis, and treatment. It is highly recommended as an adjunct to the current text.

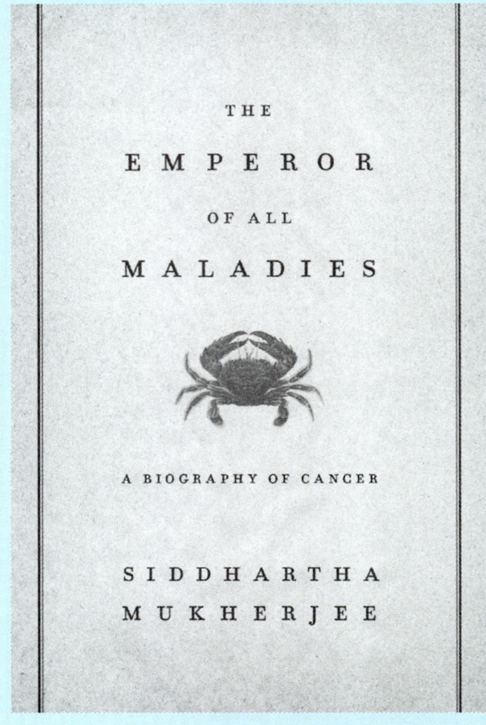

This theory was finally replaced by the lymph theory in 1695 by Stahl and Hoffman. The lymph theory posited that cancer was composed of fermenting and degenerating lymph.

The invention and improvement of microscopes allowed Muller, Virchow, and von Rokitansky to establish that cancer is a disease of cells. Karl Thiersch then documented in the 19th century that metastatic cancers arise also from the spread of malignant cells. Thus, by the 19th century, humors and lymph were dismissed as the causes of cancer, and the ancient theories of humors and lymph were replaced by the modern cellular theory of cancer.

The next questions posed by scientists concerned the etiology of cancer. Virchow posited that chronic irritation promoted cancer, whereas Hugo Ribbert thought trauma caused cancer. The development of microbiology in the 19th century

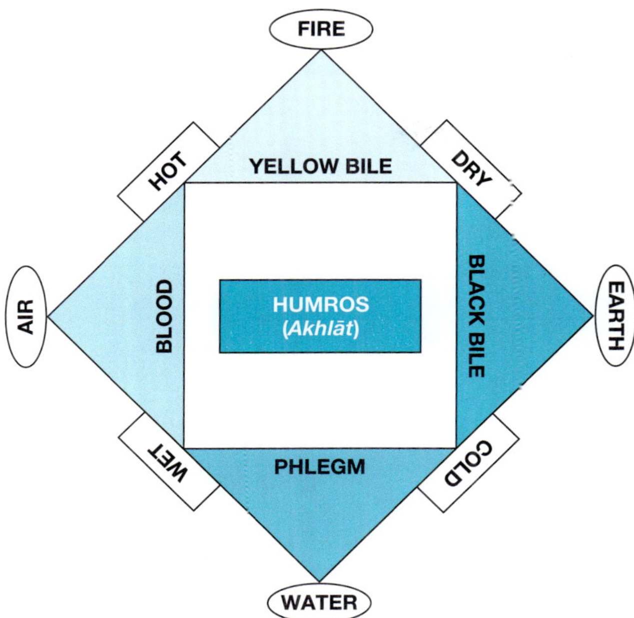

FIGURE 1.1. The 4 humors: a historic understanding of cancer. (From Husain MK, Khalid M, Penchala Pratap G, Kazmi MH. Relevance of traditional Unani (Greco-Arab) system of medicine in cancer: an update. In: Akhtar M, Swamy M, editors. *Anticancer Plants: Clinical Trials and Nanotechnology.* Singapore: Springer; 2017, pp. 273–302. https://doi.org/10.1007/978-981-10-8216-0_10.)

allowed for the accumulation of evidence that implicated infections in cancer development. There was a 50-year period during which the potential for cancer to be caused by infectious agents was dismissed. More recently, the role of viruses in the development of cancer has gained great interest.

What we understand today is that cancer is caused by accumulated damage to genes. The cause of these genetic changes might be environmental, infectious, inherited from genes of the parents, or the result of behavior choices. The substances that cause cancer are called carcinogens.

TYPES OF CANCER

There are 6 basic types of cancer as noted in Table 1.1. They are carcinoma, lymphoma, leukemia, sarcoma, melanoma, and central nervous system cancers. In what follows, we discuss each type.

Carcinoma is the most common type of cancer. It originates in the tissues that line or cover internal organs, such as the skin (basal and squamous cells), lungs, breasts, pancreas, and other organs and glands. Examples of carcinoma cancers include breast, lung, pancreatic, prostate, colorectal, kidney, bladder, endometrial, ovarian, and basal and squamous cell skin cancers. Most head and neck cancers are carcinomas that arise from squamous cells.

Lymphoma and multiple myeloma are cancers that originate in the cells of the immune system, such as the lymphocyte cells of the body. Examples of lymphoma include Hodgkin's lymphoma and non-Hodgkin's lymphoma. Non-Hodgkin's lymphoma can also occur in children. Multiple myeloma is a cancer of plasma cells that are found in the bone marrow and are an important part of the immune system.

Leukemia is cancer that starts in blood-forming tissue, such as the bone marrow, and causes large numbers of abnormal blood cells to be produced and enter the blood. It generally does not form solid tumors. There are several types of leukemia, including acute lymphocytic leukemia (ALL), acute myeloid leukemia (AML), chronic lymphocytic leukemia (CLL), chronic myeloid leukemia (CML), and chronic myelomonocytic leukemia (CMML). Several of these can occur in children.

Table 1.1 Types of Cancer

TYPE	TISSUES FROM WHICH THEY ARISE	EXAMPLES (COULD BE PICTURES)
Carcinoma	Epithelial cells	Breast, lung, pancreas, colorectal, kidney, endometrial, ovarian, head and neck
Sarcoma	Bone, muscle, fat, blood vessels, soft or connective tissue	Osteosarcoma (bone), chondrosarcoma (cartilage), angiosarcoma (blood)
Melanoma	Melanocytes (skin)	Melanoma
Lymphoma, multiple myeloma	Immune system cells	B-cell lymphoma, Hodgkin's lymphoma, mantle cell lymphoma
Leukemia	Blood-forming tissues	Acute lymphocytic leukemia, acute myeloid leukemia, chronic lymphocytic leukemia, chronic myeloid leukemia, chronic myelomonocytic leukemia
Central nervous system	Brain or spinal cord	Astrocytomas, meningiomas, medulloblastoma

Box 1.2 Cancer Epidemiology Glossary

Age adjusted: A modified statistic to eliminate the effect of different age distributions in different populations.

Attributable proportion: A measure of the public health impact of a causative factor; proportion of a disease in a group that is exposed to a particular factor that can be attributed to their exposure to that factor.

Bias: Deviation of results or inferences from the truth or processes leading to a systematic deviation. Any trend in the collection, analysis, interpretation, publication, or review of data that can lead to conclusions that are systematically different from the truth.

Case-control study: A type of observational analytic study. Enrollment into the study is based on the presence (case) or absence (control) of disease. Characteristics such as previous exposure are then compared between cases and controls.

Cohort study: A type of observational analytic study. Enrollment into the study is based on exposure characteristics or membership in a group. Disease, death, or other health-related outcomes are then ascertained and compared.

Counts: The number of cases, not defining whether they are new.

Denominator: The lower portion of a fraction used to calculate a rate or ratio. In a rate, the denominator is usually the population (or population experience, as in person-years, etc) at risk.

Incidence: New cases, often defined by a particular time period.

Incidence rate: A measure of the frequency with which an event, such as a new case of illness, occurs in a population over a period of time. The denominator is the population at risk; the numerator is the number of new cases occurring during a given time period.

Mortality rate: A measure of the frequency of occurrence of death in a defined population during a specified interval of time.

Odds ratio: A measure of association that quantifies the relationship between an exposure and a health outcome from a comparative study—also known as the cross-product ratio.

Prevalence: The number or proportion of cases or events or conditions in a given population.

Rate: An expression of the frequency with which an event occurs in a defined population. This is generally expressed in terms of the number of people with a condition PER a defined population number (often 100,000) in a particular time period (1 year, 10 years). As an example, we may say that the rate of new breast cancers in the US was 125.1 cases per 100,000 women in 2017.

Relative risk: A comparison of the risk of some health-related events, such as disease or death in 2 groups.

Risk factor: An aspect of personal behavior or lifestyle, an environmental exposure, or an inborn or inherited characteristic that is associated with an increased occurrence of disease or other health-related events or conditions.

Sarcomas arise in bone, muscle, fat, blood vessels, cartilage, or other soft or connective tissues. These are much less common than the first 3 types of cancer noted above. Osteosarcomas start in the bone. Soft-tissue sarcomas can occur in the fibrous tissue of the limbs, in the blood or lymph vessels, or in other soft tissues in the body.

Central nervous system cancers are those that begin in the tissues of the brain and spinal cord. These include gliomas, astrocytomas, oligodendrogliomas, ependymomas, meningiomas, medulloblastomas, gangliogliomas, schwannomas, and craniopharyngiomas, according to the source tissue and location of the tumor.

Finally, *melanomas* are cancers that arise in the cells that make the pigment in our skin, called melanocytes.

EPIDEMIOLOGY OF CANCER

The American Cancer Society (ACS) regularly updates epidemiologic reports on the burden of cancer (3). The text that follows draws from the most recent edition of *Global Cancer Facts and Figures 4th Edition*, freely available at www.cancer.org (3). To better understand the burden of cancer, it is important to know the terms of epidemiology. The glossary in Box 1.2 will help here and throughout this book.

Next, it is important that we understand that if we compare the burden of cancer by age, geography, gender, race, or other characteristics, then we do so using rates, not just counts. The reason for this can be illustrated with an example. In a fictitious population, there are 50,000 Hispanic people and 1,000,000 White people in 2020. If we compare the total new cases of colorectal cancer in this population, we may see that there are 250 Hispanic people and 500 White people. Does this mean that there is a lower burden of colorectal cancer in the Hispanic people? To determine this, we must determine the rate, adjusting for the size of the population. Generally, rates are expressed per 100,000 people. We can calculate that the rate is 500 per 100,000 among Hispanic people and 50 per 100,000 among White people. Despite fewer cases, the burden of colorectal cancer is 10 times larger in the Hispanic people than in the White people in our fictitious population.

Be careful to compare rates with the same denominator. In a rate, the denominator is usually the population (or population experience, as in person-years, etc) at risk.

Occurrence of Cancer and Cancer Registries

In epidemiology, the next step is to research if a cancer has occurred, the type of cancer that has occurred, and where and in whom it has occurred. A cancer registry collects and compiles detailed information about cancer patients and the initial treatments they receive, as well as deaths from cancer and other causes. With these data, we can begin to track how often cancer occurs, whether it is changing, and whether there are differences in the incidence or death from cancer by place, race, age, availability of screening and treatment, or other exposures.

In the United States (US), cancer registries begin at the hospital and communicate up to the Centers for Disease Control and Prevention (CDC). Cancer is considered a reportable disease, so if a hospital diagnoses a cancer, it must report it. A specially trained person called a cancer registrar enters information about a patient's cancer and treatment into the hospital cancer registry. Periodically, each hospital in each of the 50 states uploads their hospital registry data to a central state cancer registry. State cancer registries review the data to ensure that data are accurate and complete. Then once a year, state cancer registries send information on cancers diagnosed and deaths from cancers to the CDC, more specifically, to the National Program of Cancer Registries. These data are reviewed and added to the US Cancer Statistics database. Figure 1.2 highlights the steps of this process. Similar systems exist in other countries. The

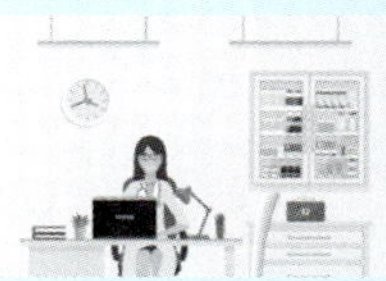

Jennifer gets a routine mammogram at her doctor's office.

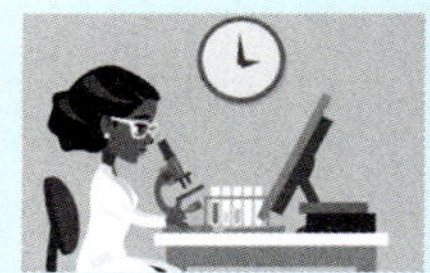

A laboratory finds that she has a tumor about the size of a large pea in her left breast.

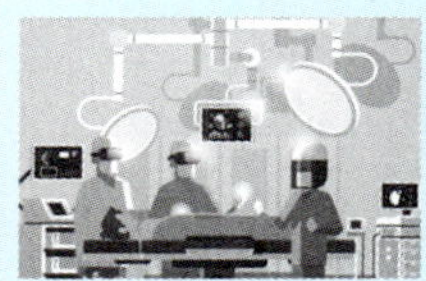

Jennifer goes to the hospital to have surgery. She gives the hospital some information about herself. Later, she gets chemotherapy to make sure that the cancer is gone.

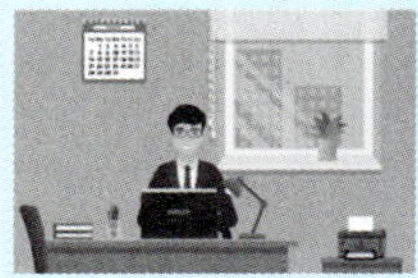

At the hospital's cancer registry, a specially trained person called a *cancer registrar* enters information about the cancer and treatment from Jennifer's medical record into a computer. The hospital registry sends this information to the central cancer registry in its state.

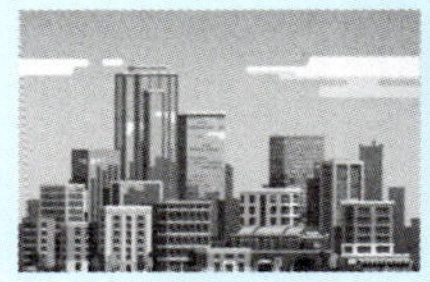

The state central cancer registry works hard to get information about all reportable cancer cases in the state. It reviews and combines the information to make sure it's complete.

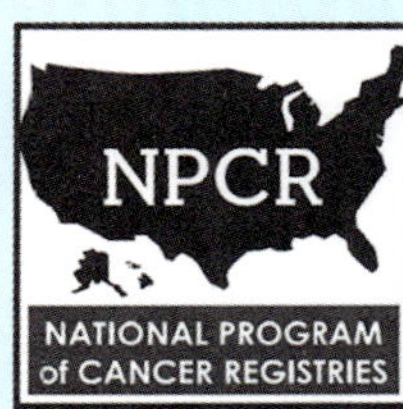

Once in a year, state central cancer registries send information on cancers diagnosed in the states to CDC.

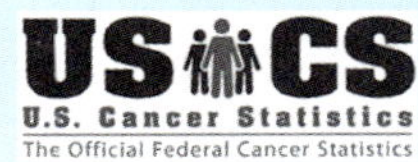

FIGURE 1.2. Example of how a cancer registry collects data about cancer patients, including treatments and deaths from cancer and other causes. The cancer information is reviewed and added to the US Cancer Statistics database. (From the National Program of Cancer Registries. https://www.cdc.gov/cancer/npcr/value/registries.htm.)

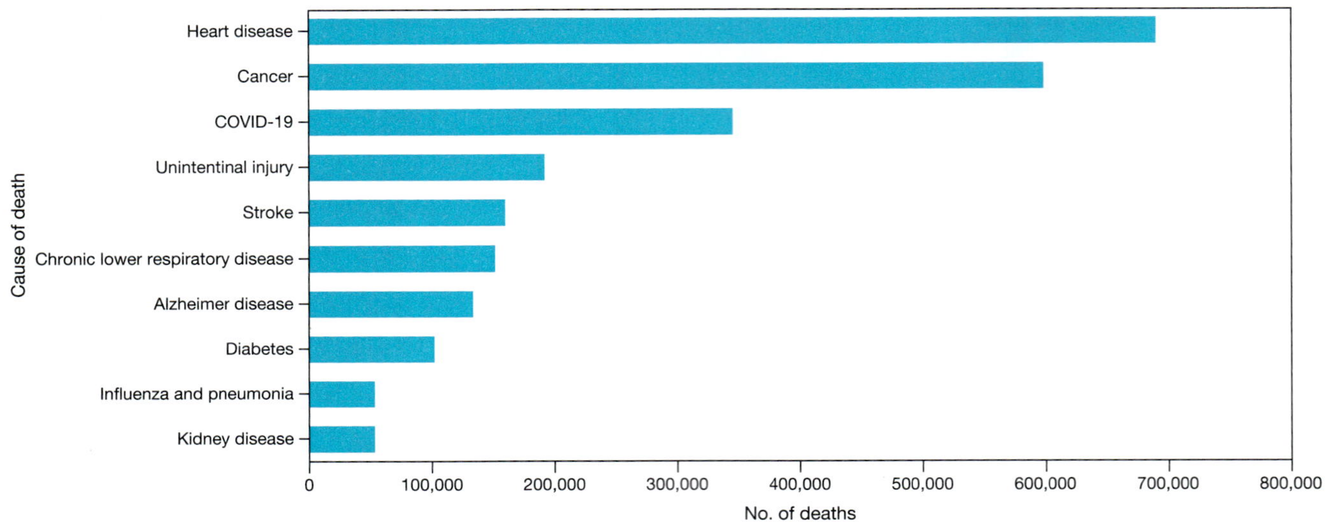

* National Vital Statistics System provisional data are incomplete. Data from December are less complete owing to reporting lags. Deaths that occurred in the United States among residents of US territories and foreign countries were excluded.

† Deaths for which COVID-19 was a contributing, but not the underlying, cause of death are not included in this figure.

FIGURE 1.3. Provisional* number of leading underlying causes of death† – National Vital statistics system, United States, 2020. (From Ahmad FB, Cisewski JA, Minino A, Anderson RN. Provisional Mortality Data—United States, 2020. MMWR *Morb Mortal Wkly Rep.* 2021; 70(14):519–22. Originally in QuickStats: number of deaths from 10 leading causes—National Vital Statistics System, United States, 2010. MMWR *Morb Mortal Wkly Rep.* 2013;62(08):155.)

infrastructure to carry out this work is intensive. As such, our ability to draw conclusions based on the cancer registry data varies according to the ability of a given country to mount the effort required. This will vary by country.

New Cases and Deaths

Cancer causes approximately 1 in every 6 deaths worldwide. This is a larger burden than AIDS, tuberculosis, and malaria combined. In many developed countries, including the US, cancer is the second leading cause of death, often following cardiovascular diseases (CVDs). Figures 1.3 and 1.4 list the top 10 causes of death in the US and globally, respectively.

It was estimated that there were 17 million new cases of cancer in 2018 and 9.5 million cancer-related deaths. By 2040, it is expected that there will be 27.5 million new cancer cases and 16.3 million cancer deaths, simply owing to the growth and aging of the global population (Figure 1.5).

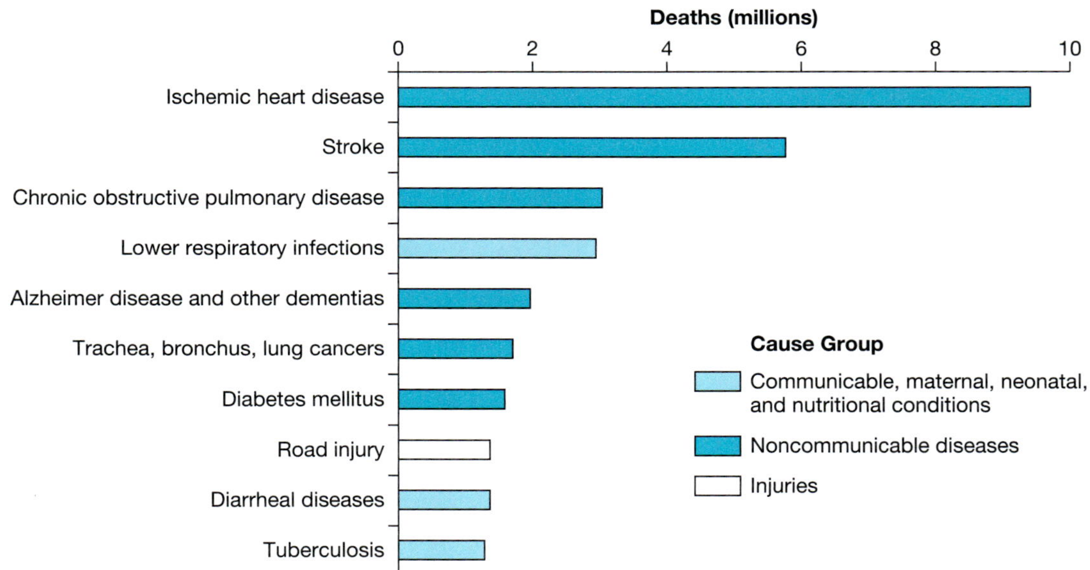

FIGURE 1.4. Top 10 causes of death worldwide. (From *Global Health Estimates 2016: Deaths by Cause, Age, Sex, by Country and by Region, 2000–2016.* Geneva: World Health Organization; 2018.)

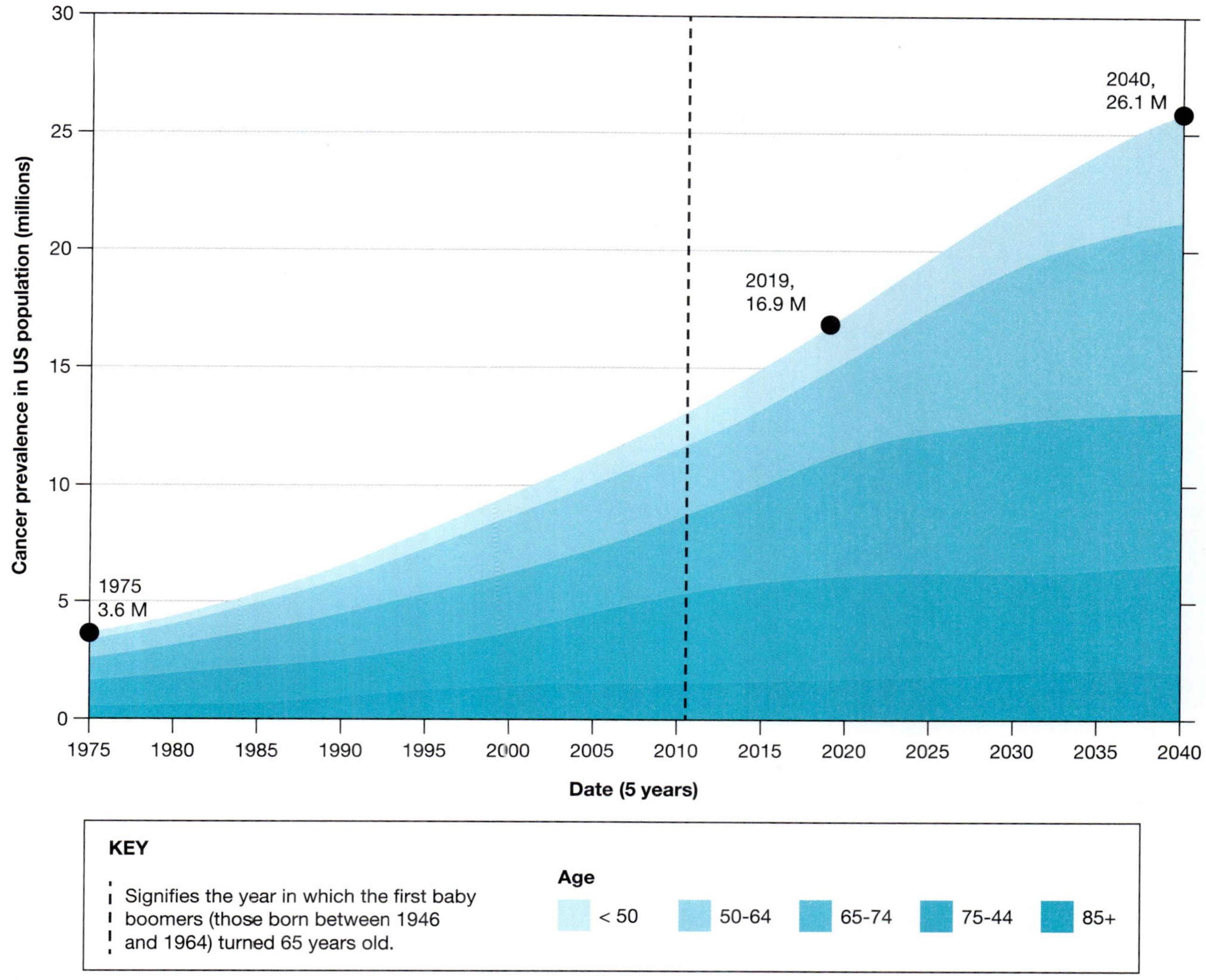

FIGURE 1.5. Cancer prevalence and projections in the US population from 1975 to 2040. (From https://guides.library.vcu.edu/cancerconsumerhealth. Originally from Bluethmann SM, Mariotto AB, Rowland JH. Anticipating the "Silver Tsunami": prevalence trajectories and co-morbidity burden among older cancer survivors in the United States. *Cancer Epidemiol Biomarkers Prev.* 2016;25(7):1029–36. https://doi.org/10.1158/1055-9965.EPI-16-0133.)

Factors expected to influence whether this estimate is accurate will include the prevalence of risk factors such as smoking, unhealthy diet, physical inactivity, and fewer pregnancies.

Figure 1.6 presents the estimated number of new cancer cases overall around the world (slightly over 17 million) by geography, as of 2018. Not surprisingly, more populated regions have more cases, including East Asia, Western Europe, and North America.

Figure 1.7 provides the number of new cases of cancer and deaths from cancer worldwide by cancer type. The most common causes of cancer in men worldwide are lung, prostate, and colon. Among women, the most common causes are breast, colon, and lung. The most common causes of cancer death are lung, liver, and stomach in men and breast, lung, and colon among women.

What Types of Cancer Are Diagnosed and Where?

The types of cancer vary around the globe according to many factors. The age distribution of a population, prevalence of risk factors, availability and use of preventive services and early detection tests, and availability of treatment all influence cancer incidence and mortality. In countries with a lower level of economic development, there is also a higher likelihood of developing a cancer related to an infectious source, such as *Helicobacter pylori* (*H. pylori*) or human papillomavirus (HPV).

In 2018, geographically, the largest number of cancer diagnoses occurred in East Asia (5.6 million), followed by North America (1.9 million). The greatest number of deaths was in Eastern Asia (3.4 million), followed by South-Central

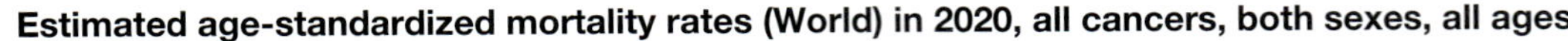

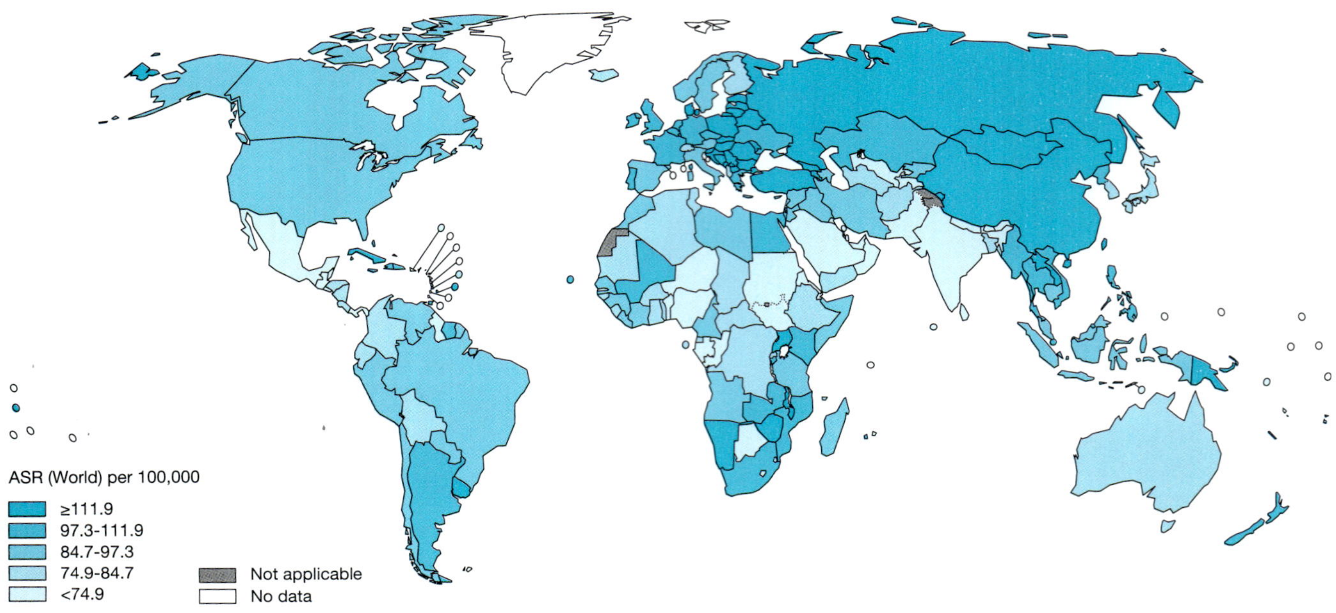

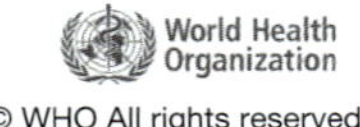

FIGURE 1.6. Worldwide cancer incidence. (From https://2016.igem.org/Team:NJU-China/Background.)

Asia (1.2 million). The number of cancer diagnoses and deaths from cancer reflects population size, cancer incidence, and survival.

Among the most developed countries, the 2 most common diagnosed cancers among men are prostate and lung cancers. Among women, the 2 most common diagnosed cancers are breast and colorectal cancers. In the least developed countries, the 2 most common diagnosed cancers among men are prostate and liver cancers, and among women, breast and cervix cancers are the 2 most common diagnosed cancers.

Lung cancer is the leading cause of cancer deaths in most places in the world, for men and women. That said, the incidence of lung cancer has been declining in a large part of the world because of tobacco control measures.

Who Is at Risk?

It is estimated that 21 out of 100 men and 18 out of 100 women around the world will develop cancer by age 75. These averages do not account for differences in genetics, environment, and health behaviors that are known to influence incidence.

Cancer is a disease of aging: Approximately 80% of all cancers are diagnosed among adults aged 50 or older. This is because the normal aging process affects many important

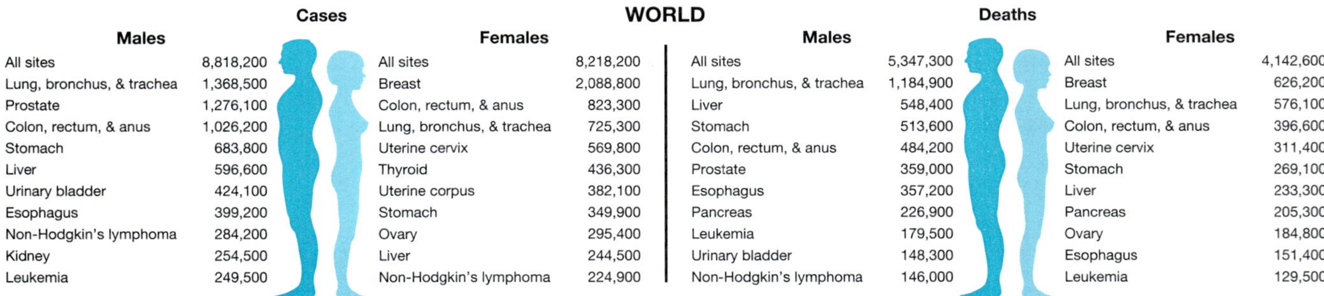

WORLD

Cases – Males		Cases – Females		Deaths – Males		Deaths – Females	
All sites	8,818,200	All sites	8,218,200	All sites	5,347,300	All sites	4,142,600
Lung, bronchus, & trachea	1,368,500	Breast	2,088,800	Lung, bronchus, & trachea	1,184,900	Breast	626,200
Prostate	1,276,100	Colon, rectum, & anus	823,300	Liver	548,400	Lung, bronchus, & trachea	576,100
Colon, rectum, & anus	1,026,200	Lung, bronchus, & trachea	725,300	Stomach	513,600	Colon, rectum, & anus	396,600
Stomach	683,800	Uterine cervix	569,800	Colon, rectum, & anus	484,200	Uterine cervix	311,400
Liver	596,600	Thyroid	436,300	Prostate	359,000	Stomach	269,100
Urinary bladder	424,100	Uterine corpus	382,100	Esophagus	357,200	Liver	233,300
Esophagus	399,200	Stomach	349,900	Pancreas	226,900	Pancreas	205,300
Non-Hodgkin's lymphoma	284,200	Ovary	295,400	Leukemia	179,500	Ovary	184,800
Kidney	254,500	Liver	244,500	Urinary bladder	148,300	Esophagus	151,400
Leukemia	249,500	Non-Hodgkin's lymphoma	224,900	Non-Hodgkin's lymphoma	146,000	Leukemia	129,500

FIGURE 1.7. Estimated new cases of cancer and cancer deaths worldwide. (From https://www.cancer.org/content/dam/cancer-org/research/cancer-facts-and-statistics/global-cancer-facts-and-figures/global-cancer-facts-and-figures-4th-edition.pdf (top section, figure 1). Data available at: https://acsjournals.onlinelibrary.wiley.com/doi/10.3322/caac.21492.)

biological processes in our bodies in a manner that results in the deterioration of proteins and DNA in our cells. The biology of cancer is discussed in detail in Chapter 2. However, to better understand why cancer is a disease of aging, it is necessary to briefly explain the relevant biologic and genetic processes. Our cells go through a consistent cycle of continuously replicating and replacing themselves. There is predictable signaling in place to instruct the cell to stop replicating, that is, to die. This process is referred to as *apoptosis* or *cellular senescence*. It is an efficient protective mechanism against cancer, forcing would-be cancer cells to stop dividing. However, sometimes this senescence process fails, allowing cancer-causing mutations to develop and accumulate. This results in the uncontrollable cell growth that can cause the formation and spread of cancer. This is more likely to occur in older individuals because the cells of an older person have had more time to reproduce and accumulate genetic mutations. In short, the longer we live, the more errors our genes accumulate (Table 1.2). Eventually, these mutations can lead to cancer. In addition, our immune system, which forms an outstanding defense against cancer, becomes less effective with age. This means that it will be less efficient at detecting and fighting diseases, including cancer.

Lifestyle factors can mitigate the development of malignant cells. There is strong research evidence that diet, exercise, and maintaining a healthy body weight can reduce the risk for cancer incidence and progression. The World Cancer Research Fund's Continuous Update Project includes a report on body fatness, weight gain, and cancer risk. Figure 1.8 summarizes how physical activity and nutrition interact with other environmental and host factors to affect the cancer process. As shown in the figure, the cancer process moves from normal cells (normal epithelium) to invasive cancer. There are 3 primary factors that contribute to this process: host factors, environmental factors, and lifestyle factors. The host factors include genetics, epigenetics, the microbiome, age, gender, metabolic state, inflammatory and immune function, among other factors. The environmental factors associate with the development of cancer and include food contaminants, viruses, ultraviolet (UV) radiation, environmental carcinogens, among other factors. The lifestyle factors include diet, energy intake, phytochemicals, alcohol, physical activity, and smoking, among other factors. These factors interact with each other in the process of a cancer developing and changes in any of them could speed or slow the process.

The most recent updated report concludes that being overweight or obesity throughout adulthood increases risks of cancers of the mouth, pharynx and larynx, esophagus, stomas, pancreas, gallbladder, liver, colorectum, breast, ovary, endometrium, prostate, and kidney (4). The magnitude of the increased risk varies by cancer type. For a 5-kg/m^2 increase in body mass index (BMI), the increased risk of incident cancer varies between 5% and 50%, depending on the site. The expert panel that led the report concluded that attaining and maintaining a healthy body weight is among the most important behavioral approaches to preventing these common cancer types. This is contrasted with evidence that nearly 2 billion adults around the world were categorized as overweight or obese in 2016. Over the past decade, there has been an increase in the proportion of adults categorized as obese. This increase has global and national economic implications, as well as having an influence on cancer risk. To address overweight and obesity, we apply principles of nutrition and exercise science. The World Cancer Research Fund conducts a review of the evidence regarding energy balance and cancer every few years in a process called the Continuous Update Project or CUP. The most recent CUP report on energy balance concluded that there is strong evidence that:

- Walking decreases the risk of weight gain, overweight, and obesity.
- Aerobic physical activity decreases the risk of weight gain, overweight, and obesity.
- Consuming foods containing dietary fiber decreases the risk of weight gain, overweight, and obesity.
- Consuming a Mediterranean-type dietary pattern decreases the risk of excess weight gain, overweight, and obesity.
- Greater screen time increases the risk of weight gain, overweight, and obesity.
- Consuming sugar-sweetened drinks increases the risk of weight gain, overweight, and obesity.
- Consuming "fast food" increases the risk of weight gain, overweight, and obesity.
- Consuming a Western-type diet increases the risk of weight gain, overweight, and obesity.

The focus of this book will largely be on exercise oncology, so we will not go into detail on nutrition topics. However, where there is published guidance regarding energy balance (the balance of energy intake with expenditure), we will include and cite brief commentary on nutrition topics so that readers may investigate further. All of the data in this section are drawn from the World Cancer Research Fund Continuous Update Project (https://www.aicr.org/research/the-continuous-update-project/).

The American College of Sports Medicine® (ACSM®) conducted a comprehensive review of the role of exercise in primary prevention of cancer and concluded, based on the review of all available scientific research studies, that there was strong evidence that regularly obtaining adequate physical activity (150 minutes per week aerobic activity) is associated with reductions of risk in 7 types of cancer, as depicted in Figure 1.9 (5).

Energy balance (obesity, diet, and physical activity) also plays a role in the risks of recurrence and death from cancer. These topics are addressed in the section on Cancer Prevention and Control.

Table 1.2 Probability of Developing Invasive Cancer by Age and Sex, United States, 2015-2017[a]

	BIRTH TO 49	50 TO 59	60 TO 69	70 AND OLDER	BIRTH TO DEATH
All sites[b]					
Male	3.5 (1 in 29)	6.2 (1 in 16)	13.6 (1 in 7)	33.2 (1 in 3)	40.5 (1 in 2)
Female	5.8 (1 in 17)	6.4 (1 in 16)	10.3 (1 in 10)	26.8 (1 in 4)	38.9 (1 in 3)
Breast					
Female	2.1 (1 in 49)	2.4 (1 in 42)	3.5 (1 in 28)	7.0 (1 in 14)	12.9 (1 in 8)
Colorectum					
Male	0.4 (1 in 254)	0.7 (1 in 143)	1.1 (1 in 92)	3.2 (1 in 32)	4.3 (1 in 23)
Female	0.4 (1 in 266)	0.5 (1 in 191)	0.8 (1 in 128)	2.9 (1 in 34)	4.0 (1 in 25)
Kidney & renal pelvis					
Male	0.2 (1 in 410)	0.4 (1 in 263)	0.7 (1 in 151)	1.4 (1 in 73)	2.2 (1 in 46)
Female	0.2 (1 in 647)	0.2 (1 in 541)	0.3 (1 in 310)	0.8 (1 in 133)	1.3 (1 in 80)
Leukemia					
Male	0.3 (1 in 391)	0.2 (1 in 549)	0.4 (1 in 255)	1.4 (1 in 69)	1.8 (1 in 55)
Female	0.2 (1 in 500)	0.1 (1 in 834)	0.2 (1 in 427)	0.9 (1 in 110)	1.3 (1 in 78)
Lung & bronchus					
Male	0.1 (1 in 776)	0.6 (1 in 163)	1.7 (1 in 58)	5.9 (1 in 17)	6.6 (1 in 15)
Female	0.1 (1 in 679)	0.6 (1 in 172)	1.4 (1 in 70)	4.9 (1 in 21)	6.0 (1 in 17)
Melanoma of the skin[c]					
Male	0.4 (1 in 230)	0.5 (1 in 198)	0.9 (1 in 109)	2.7 (1 in 37)	3.7 (1 in 27)
Female	0.6 (1 in 156)	0.4 (1 in 241)	0.5 (1 in 187)	1.2 (1 in 86)	2.5 (1 in 40)
Non-Hodgkin's lymphoma					
Male	0.3 (1 in 375)	0.3 (1 in 345)	0.6 (1 in 177)	1.9 (1 in 54)	2.4 (1 in 42)
Female	0.2 (1 in 523)	0.2 (1 in 463)	0.4 (1 in 242)	1.4 (1 in 73)	1.9 (1 in 52)
Prostate					
Male	0.2 (1 in 451)	1.8 (1 in 55)	5.0 (1 in 20)	8.7 (1 in 12)	12.1 (1 in 8)
Thyroid					
Male	0.2 (1 in 447)	0.1 (1 in 703)	0.2 (1 in 571)	0.2 (1 in 412)	0.7 (1 in 146)
Female	0.9 (1 in 114)	0.4 (1 in 258)	0.4 (1 in 283)	0.4 (1 in 263)	1.9 (1 in 53)
Uterine cervix					
Female	0.3 (1 in 362)	0.1 (1 in 837)	0.1 (1 in 916)	0.2 (1 in 590)	0.6 (1 in 158)
Uterine corpus					
Female	0.3 (1 in 322)	0.6 (1 in 157)	1.1 (1 in 94)	1.5 (1 in 67)	3.1 (1 in 32)

[a]For people free of cancer at the beginning of the age interval.
[b]All sites exclude basal cell and squamous cell skin cancers and in situ cancers except the urinary bladder.
[c]Probabilities for non-Hispanic Whites only.
From Siegel RL, Miller KD, Fuchs HE, Jemal A. Cancer statistics. *CA: Cancer J Clin.* 2021;71(1):7–33, Table 3. https://acsjournals.onlinelibrary.wiley.com/doi/10.3322/caac.21708.

Normal epithelium
Preneoplasia
Invasive cancer
CANCER PROCESS
Genetics, Epigenetics, Microbiome, Age, Gender, Metabolic state, Inflammatory state and immune function, Other host factors
Host Factors
Environmental Factors
Food contaminants, Viruses, UV radiation, Environmental carcinogens, Other environmental factors
Diet/Lifestyle Factors
Nutrients, Energy intake, Phytochemicals, Other food components, Alcohol, Physical activity, Smoking, Other lifestyle factors

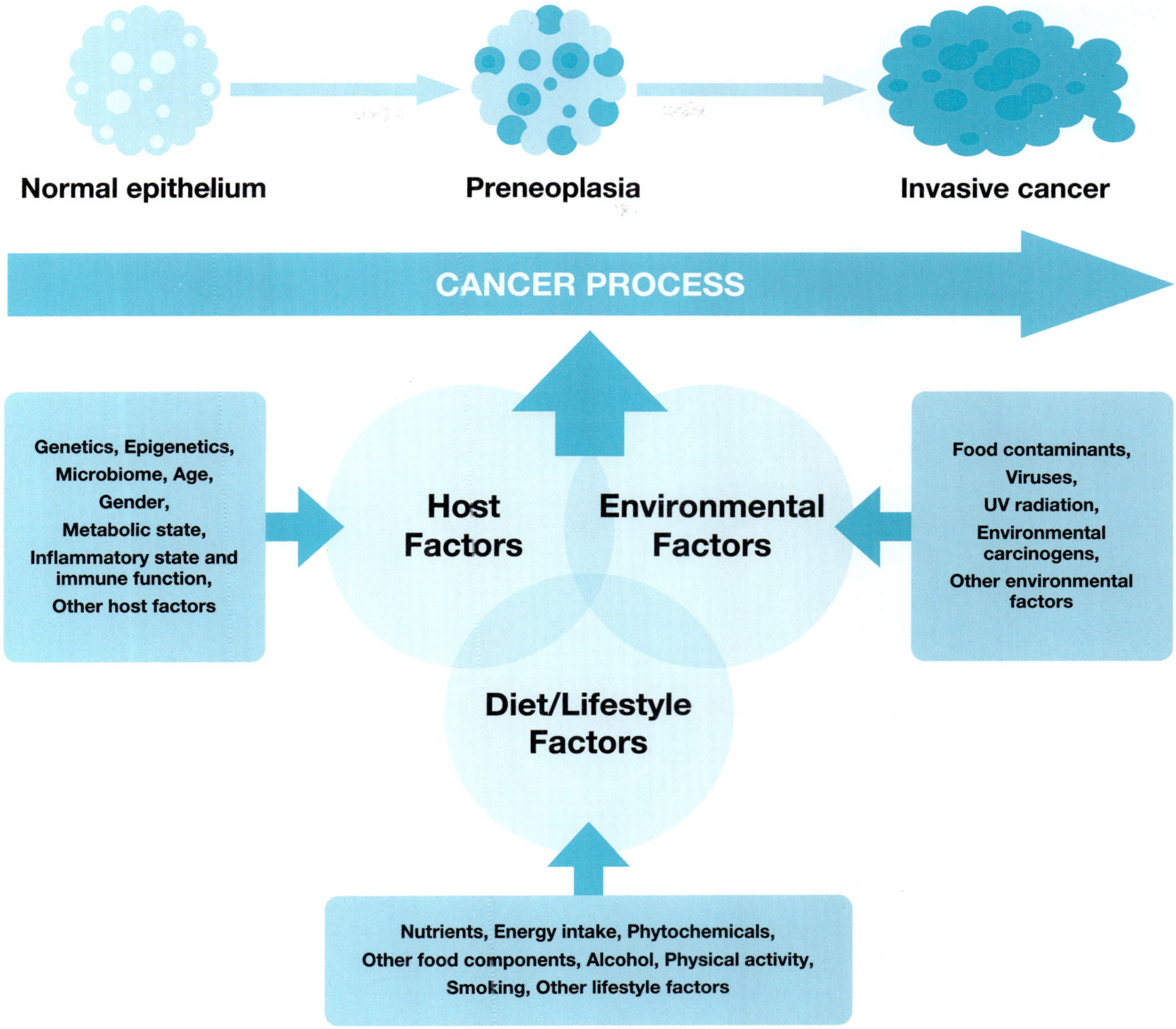

FIGURE 1.8. Diet, nutrition, and physical activity along with other environmental exposure. (From the World Cancer Research Fund International. *Diet, Nutrition, Physical Activity, and Cancer. A Global Perspective. A Summary of the Third Expert Report*, p. 21, Figure 3, 2018. https://www.wcrf.org/wp-content/uploads/2021/02/Summary-of-Third-Expert-Report-2018.pdf.)

Who Survives?

When we discuss cancer survival, it is important to note that the statistics on survival generally refer to those who are still alive 5 years after their diagnosis. As noted in the next section, this is not consistent with other common definitions used for the cancer survivor. For the purpose of counting and tracking, 5-year survival is a common, traditional way of counting and tracking who survives cancer. This figure is reported by the CDC, the ACS, and other research organizations.

Survival after cancer is influenced by the types of cancer that occur in a given population, the stage at which the cancer is diagnosed, the availability and use of early detection and screening, and the availability and use of high-quality treatments. Survival after common cancers varies across the globe according to these factors. For example, the 5-year survival rate for the patients with breast cancer in 2010 to 2014 was 90% in the US and Australia, but 65% in Malaysia. There can also be socioeconomic and racial inequalities in survival

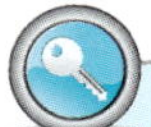

Cancer Survivor. The term survivor is defined in several ways. In the US, the National Coalition for Cancer Survivorship defines a someone as a cancer survivor from the time of diagnosis and for the balance of life. In other settings, a cancer survivor refers to someone who has completed treatment. It should be noted that some people who have had cancer prefer not to be referred to as survivors.

colon cancer
breast cancer
For all adults, exercise is important for cancer prevention and specifically lowers risk of seven common types of cancer:
stomach cancer
endometrial cancer
esophageal cancer
kidney cancer
bladder cancer

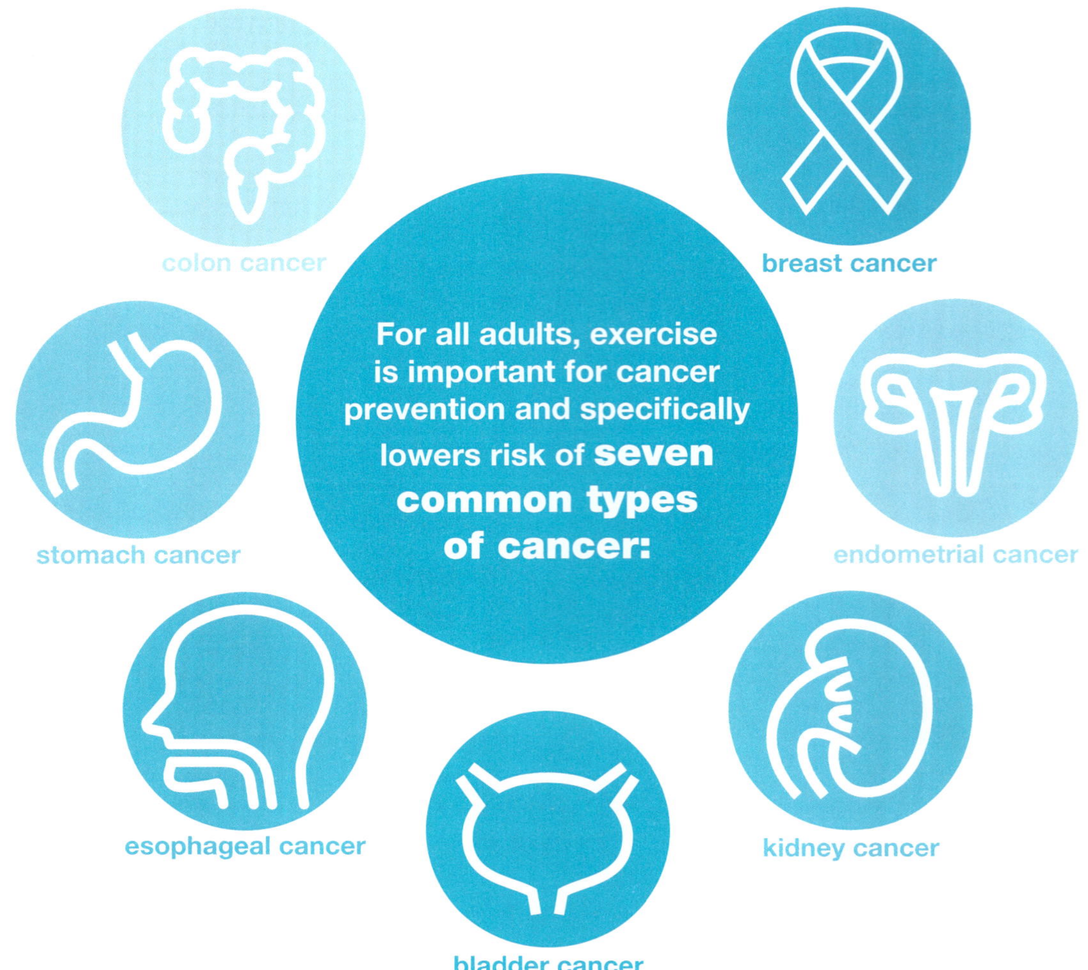

FIGURE 1.9. ACSM infographic on exercise for cancer prevention. (From Patel AV, Friedenreich CM, More SC, et al. American College of Sports Medicine Roundtable Report on physical activity, sedentary behavior, and cancer prevention and control. *Med Sci Sports Exerc.* 2019;51(11):2391–402. https://www.acsm.org/news-detail/2019/10/16/expert-panel-cancer-treatment-plans-should-include-tailored-exercise-prescriptions.)

as well. For example, in the US, survival from cervical cancer was 64% versus 56% in Whites versus African Americans, respectively. In the case of cancers for which there are no/few early detection options (liver, lung, and pancreas), survival rates tend to vary less by geography, race, or other factors because these cancers tend to be diagnosed at a later (more advanced) stage.

Also note that survival rates are only possible in the setting of high-quality cancer registries, such as the national registry system in the US described earlier. As a result, data on cancer survival are not available for many low resource countries.

Costs of Cancer

The financial burden of cancer is immense and extends far beyond the obvious direct costs (eg, medical bills) that might be more obvious to measure. These direct costs of the medical care for cancer were estimated to be 80.2 billion in the US in 2015. In Europe, the estimated annual health care expenditures for cancer in 2014 were 83 billion euros.

Beyond these costs are the indirect costs associated with the loss of work, premature death, health insurance premiums, and nonmedical expenditures (eg, transportation and child or elder care). Both direct and indirect costs of cancer are expected to rise over time, along with the number of cases and the cost of treatment.

Of particular importance in the context of exercise oncology is the recognition of the loss of function that often occurs among those living with and beyond cancer (6). At least some portion of this loss of function is unnecessary, largely the result of living a sedentary lifestyle. Some portion of this loss might be the result of adverse effects of the treatments (7). It is common to hear from the breast cancer survivors that they feel they aged a decade during the year they underwent treatment. Published evidence underscores this: Women who have undergone a year or two of breast cancer treatment typically decrease maximal fitness from treadmill testing by the same amount expected over a decade (6). There is also published evidence that these declines can largely be prevented with physical activity during and after cancer treatment (8). These functional declines have important implications in the capacity of those living with and beyond cancer to care for themselves and their families, and to work for pay. Physical activity has the potential to prevent, delay, or attenuate the commonly observed functional changes that occur during and after cancer treatments. This can have benefits far beyond the improvements in function, potentially improving the timeline to returning to work, and caring for self and family.

Cancer Prevention and Control

Risk for cancer can be reduced and diagnoses delayed. This is particularly true for cancers for which there is evidence of a connection to tobacco use, obesity, diet, physical inactivity, and infection.

It has been estimated that in 2015, 20% of cancer deaths in the world were because of tobacco use. Further, 15% to 20% of cancer diagnoses worldwide are thought to be related to excess body weight, physical inactivity, and/or poor nutrition. There are cancers caused by HPV, hepatitis B virus (HPV), hepatitis C virus (HCV), and *H. pylori*. These infectious agents are thought to cause 15% of cancers worldwide and could be prevented by vaccines, altered behavior, or treatment of the infection. Finally, many skin cancers can be prevented by avoiding excessive sun exposure and avoiding indoor tanning.

Screening is available for several common types of cancer and has been proven to result in detecting cancers earlier, presumably at a time when the tumor is more easily treated and has not spread to distant parts of the body. Screening exists now for breast, colorectal, cervical, and even lung cancer.

After a cancer diagnosis, the primary concern changes from primary prevention to the prevention of recurrence and death. Exercise has been documented to play a role in the prevention of recurrence or death for 3 major types of cancer: breast, prostate, and colon cancers. A review of scientific evidence by the ACSM® on this topic, published in 2019, concluded that patients who are regularly active during and after their treatment, doing at least 150 minutes per week of aerobic activity, may enjoy a reduction of risk for cancer-specific mortality of 31% for breast cancer, 30% for colorectal cancer, and 33% for prostate cancer (5). This was after adjustment for body weight, and thus, was independent of the effects of obesity.

THE BURDEN OF SPECIFIC COMMON CANCERS: THE ROLE OF EXERCISE

There are numerous symptoms and side effects, including fatigue, reduced quality of life, sleep disorder, poor functional status, anxiety, and depression, that are common among people living with and beyond cancer (PLWBC) for which exercise can be beneficial (9). Figure 1.10 summarizes the recommendations for exercise for people living with and beyond cance from the recent ACSM® Roundtable Exercise Guidelines for Cancer Survivors (2019).

In addition, there are tumor-specific issues that can also be addressed by exercise. There will be more detail on each of these issues in Chapters 10 to 15, which address the prescription of exercise across the time from diagnosis to the end of life. In the following sections, we provide a brief overview of the burden of several common cancers (breast, prostate, colorectal, liver, and lung) and the issues that exercise might address for each tumor type.

Breast

Breast cancer is the most common cancer diagnosed among women in the developed world, and breast cancer deaths disproportionately occur within developing countries. It is generally second to lung cancer in cancer mortality among women. According to the Susan G. Komen Foundation, the median age of a woman diagnosed with breast cancer in the US is 62 years. The risk of developing breast cancer in most developed countries is about 12.5%, meaning 1 in 8 women who live to the age of 80 can expect to be diagnosed. In developed countries, the 5-year survival rate for breast cancer is generally over 90%. Given that it is a common diagnosis and largely survivable, breast cancer is the single largest type of survivable cancer in most developed countries. The survivability of breast cancer varies across the world. For example, close to half of breast cancer deaths occur in Eastern, South Central, and Southeast Asia, even though Asia accounts for less than a third of cases (9). Breast cancer survivors are likely to be the most commonly seen cancer type of survivors that exercise oncology professionals will encounter.

From the perspective of exercise oncology, the unique burden of breast cancer starts with the location of the surgery and choices regarding reconstruction. More extensive breast surgeries, including reconstructive surgery, can significantly alter the function of the shoulder in the short and long terms. Prehabilitation, rehabilitation, and appropriate progression of exercise training are crucial to achieving the best possible function after breast surgery. In addition, many women are diagnosed with breast cancer after menopause and are prescribed hormonal therapies, such as aromatase inhibitors. These drugs can cause muscle aches and pains (called **arthralgias**) that make it more difficult for women to exercise. Research demonstrates that exercise improves the joint aches of arthralgias. There are

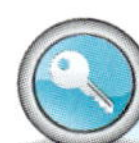

Arthralgias. Muscle aches and pains, commonly associated with treatment with aromatase inhibitors among women diagnosed with breast cancer.

MOVING THROUGH CANCER:
Exercise for people living with and beyond cancer

TO GET STARTED
Avoid inactivity; moving more and sitting less benefits nearly everyone

FOR OVERALL HEALTH
Aim to meet the current exercise guidelines for adults[1]

Moderate Aerobic Exercise
At least 150–300 mins per week
OR
Vigorous Aerobic Exercise
At least 75–150 mins per week
(or a combination of moderate/vigorous aerobic exercise)
+
Resistance Exercise
2x per week

FOR PEOPLE DURING & FOLLOWING CANCER TREATMENT
Research shows lower amounts of exercise can still help with the following cancer treatment-related symptoms:

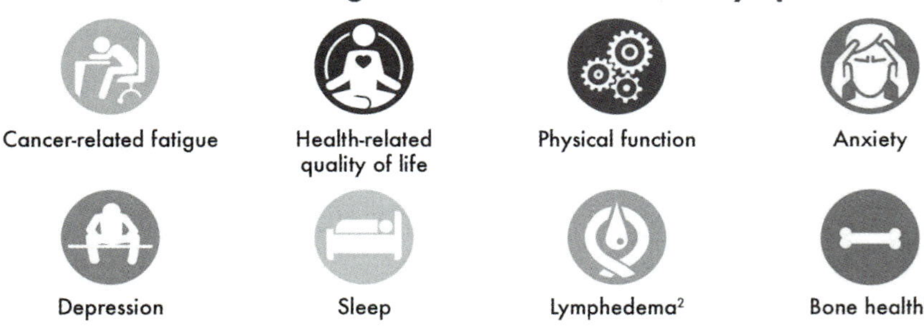

To improve these symptoms, choose an exercise plan below:

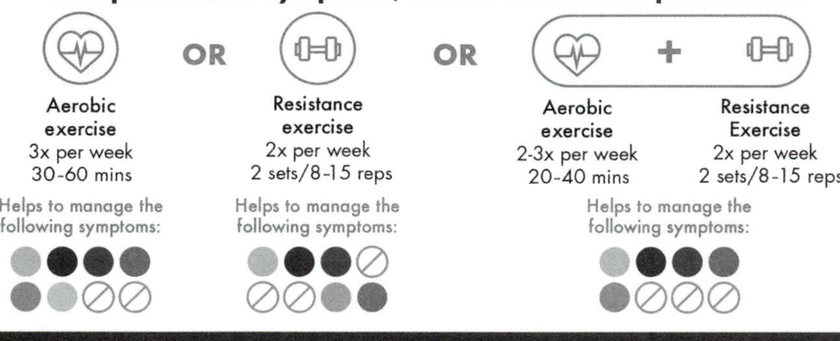

[1] Physical Activity Guidelines for Americans, 2018.
[2] Progressive supervised resistance training does not exacerbate lymphedema.
[3] At least 12-months of resistance training plus high impact training needed.

FIGURE 1.10. ACSM® infographic of exercise oncology interventions. (From Physical Activity Guidelines for Americans, 2018, v 10. https://www.exerciseismedicine.org/wp-content/uploads/2021/04/Consolidated-Infographic-for-the-ACSM-Roundtable-on-Cancer-and-Exercise.pdf.)

a number of symptoms, including fatigue, anxiety, depression, reduced quality of life, reduced physical function, sleep difficulties, and breast-cancer-related lymphedema (BCRL), breast cancer patients and survivors may experience that can be improved with regular exercise (9, 10).

Prostate

Prostate cancer is the second most common cancer diagnosed among men worldwide. It is generally second to lung cancer in terms of cancer mortality among men. According to the ACS, the median age of a man diagnosed with prostate cancer in the US is 66 years. The risk of developing prostate cancer in most developed countries is about 11%, meaning 1 in 9 men who live to the age of 80 can expect to be diagnosed with prostate cancer. In developed countries, the 5-year survival rate for prostate cancer is 98%. Given that it is a common diagnosis, prostate cancer is among the largest types of cancer survivors in most developed countries. In general, prostate cancer mortality is observed to be higher among countries with a lower human development index, a summary indicator of health, education, and income (11).

From the perspective of exercise oncology, the unique burden of prostate cancer starts with the recognition that most prostate cancers are diagnosed at an early stage. It is usually a slow growing cancer and, as such, there are questions as to the relative merits of treatment versus *active surveillance*. Active surveillance is defined as waiting to determine whether to start treatment based on ongoing surveillance of the disease. *Watchful waiting* is another term for active surveillance. There is research evidence that exercise may play a key role in the ability of men to continue with the active surveillance phase of prostate cancer treatment (12).

Once men enter active therapy, one of the key **adjuvant therapies** is androgen deprivation therapy (ADT). ADT has major effects that include reducing bone mass and rapidly reducing muscle mass and strength. These side effects have significant implications for how exercise prescriptions are developed to be maximally effective for this population. As will be discussed in later chapters, there is value to including resistance exercise in the programming for men living with and beyond prostate cancer, particularly to address bone mass, muscle mass, and strength.

Colorectal

Colorectal cancer is among the most common cancers diagnosed among men and women in the developed world. It is generally third after lung cancer and breast or prostate cancer in terms of cancer mortality among men and women. Overall, the incidence of colorectal cancer is highest among developed countries, but it is increasing in developing countries owing to the westernization of lifestyles. Incidence of colorectal cancer is inversely correlated with the human development index mentioned in an earlier section. According to the ACS, the median age of a man diagnosed with colon cancer in the US is 66 years. For women, the median age of colon cancer diagnosis is 72 years. The risk of developing colon cancer in most developed countries is about 4.6% and 4.2% in men and women, respectively, meaning 1 in 22 men and 1 in 24 women who live to the age of 80 can expect to be diagnosed with colon cancer. In developed countries, the 5-year survival rate for colorectal cancer is 80%. Given that it is a common diagnosis and largely survivable, colorectal cancer is among the largest survivable types of cancer in most developed countries.

From the perspective of exercise oncology, the unique burdens of colorectal cancer include the possibility of a reversible or irreversible stoma. A stoma is a bag outside the body that collects fecal matter, which must be emptied and cleaned regularly. Issues related to exercise with stomas include the need to ensure the proper hygiene of the site at which the stoma enters the body, the extra risk for **parastomal hernias**, the risk that the bag may get dislodged, and the embarrassment of those with a stoma for others to know about or see their stoma bag. Each of these issues can be addressed by a well-trained exercise oncology professional and will be addressed in Chapter 11. Another issue common among colon cancer patients is extensive chemotherapy-induced peripheral neuropathy (CIPN). This is a loss of feeling or a sense of numbness or tingling that is associated with taking certain types of chemotherapy. In the case of colorectal cancer, the causative agents are the platinum-based chemotherapies, such as oxaliplatin. This drug can result in loss of hearing, tinnitus, and peripheral neuropathy. Sometimes the nerve changes caused by oxaliplatin are permanent; sometimes they resolve. At present, there is insufficient evidence to discern whether exercise may improve CIPN. However, because it alters balance and the safety of exercises that require weight-bearing or balancing activities, it is an important consideration in prescribing exercise to colorectal cancer patients.

Liver

Liver cancer is the sixth most commonly diagnosed cancer and the fourth leading cause of cancer death in 2018 (13). Worldwide, over half of newly diagnosed cases occur in China. This is a cancer that is much more common in less developed countries in sub-Saharan Africa and Southeast Asia than in more developed countries. That said, liver cancer incidence rates have more than tripled since 1980, and death rates have more than doubled. As such, understanding underlying causes and the potential to alter them is worthwhile. In the case of liver cancer, there are multiple causes

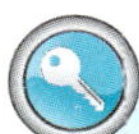

Adjuvant Therapies. Cancers are often treated with a method that is considered central to a cure if cure is the intent of treatment. For example, surgery would be central to the cure of many solid tumors. But there are other treatments that work alongside the primary treatment that may be crucial to achieving therapeutic goals. These additional treatments are termed "adjuvant therapies." Examples of adjuvant therapies include hormonal therapies for breast and prostate cancers.

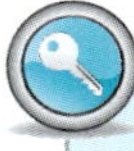

Parastomal hernia. Type of incisional hernia that allows the protrusion of abdominal contents through the abdominal wall defect created during ostomy formation.

of infectious disease, including hepatitis B and C infections. The median age of diagnosis among men and women with liver cancer in is 63 years; the disease is more common in men than women (at a ratio of 2:1). The risk of developing liver cancer varies around the world. In China, the risk is about 4% and 1.2% in men and women, respectively, meaning 1 in 25 men and 1 in 80 women can expect to be diagnosed with liver cancer. In the US, the 5-year survival rate for liver cancer is 22%. Given that it is a common diagnosis that is becoming more common, liver cancer is among the survivable types of cancer about which we need to learn more.

There is scant research on the use of exercise for people with liver cancer. That said, one of the causes of liver cancer is nonalcoholic fatty liver disease (NAFLD), for which the only known effective interventions relate to diet and physical activity (14). As such, it seems likely that exercise will also be helpful for persons with liver cancer.

Lung

Lung cancer is the second most common cancer diagnosed among men and women around the world, regardless of the level of development of a country. It is by far the leading cause of cancer mortality among men and women, accounting for 25% of all cancer deaths. The good news is that the number of cases continues to decrease, largely because of smoking cessation efforts. According to the ACS, the median age of a person diagnosed with lung cancer in the US is 65 years. The risk of developing lung cancer in most developed countries is about 6.6% and 5.9% in men and women, respectively, meaning 1 in 15 men and 1 in 17 women can expect to be diagnosed with lung cancer. In developed countries, the 5-year survival rate for lung cancer for all stages combined is 24%. Lung cancer is among the most prevalent types of cancer in most developed countries.

The specific burden of lung cancer from the perspective of exercise oncology and exercise training relates to how debilitated lung cancer patients can become after having a surgery to remove all or part of a lung. There are research studies that have documented benefits of exercise in this population, and there is value to developing and carrying out exercise programming in this unique population (15, 16). That said, the burden of disease in the lung cancer population may make exercise participation particularly challenging.

SUMMARY

The word "cancer" is somewhat of a misnomer. It denotes that cancer is a single disease. There may be common themes and biology underlying all of the hundreds of types of cancers observed in humans. However, there are many specific parameters of the specific diseases, treatments, and the physiology of a given patient that will influence the likely benefits and risks of exercise. This requires that we understand all of these elements before we proceed to design and carry out exercise programs for PLWBC. The overall burden of cancer is growing in the world as the population ages. The need for well-trained exercise oncology professionals will only increase over the coming decades. Read on!

Case Study

Mary is a 58-year-old woman who exercises 3 to 5 times a week. She has a BMI of 26 and has had a diagnosis of diabetes for the past 2 years. She reports no other chronic diseases or risk factors. Her mammogram revealed an abnormality, and she was asked to undergo an ultrasound-guided biopsy to investigate the possibility of a cancer of the breast. Her mother and sister both had breast cancer at ages 65 and 52, respectively. The biopsy results reveal invasive breast carcinoma, likely stage 1, although more medical procedures are likely to be needed to discern the exact type of breast cancer. She is angry because she feels that she eats a healthy diet, exercises regularly, follows her doctor's advice in all things, and still she was diagnosed with breast cancer. The next step for Mary is for doctors to determine whether her tumor is responsive to estrogen, progesterone, or the *HER2* gene, among other factors, so they know whether to start treatment with chemotherapy or surgery.

Questions

1. Should the exercise have prevented her breast cancer?
2. Are there any other factors that played a role in the development of cancer?
3. Did exercise likely play any role in the development of her cancer?

Meet the Expert

FEATURED PROFESSIONAL

Alpa Patel, PhD

Senior Vice Presicent, Population Science
American Cancer Society
Atlanta, GA USA
Epidemiologist

Q: "Where did you grow up?"

Ormond Beach, Florida

Q: "Where did you train? What is your training?"

I got my PhD in Epidemiology from the Keck School of Medicine at the University of Southern California.

Q: "What are you best known for?"

I think I am best known for the collective body of work I have contributed to demonstrating the link between physical activity and lower risk of several types of cancer. These epidemiologic studies have been instrumental in building physical activity guidelines for health, including cancer prevention.

Q: "What are you currently working on?"

I am currently extending my work to better understand the role of sedentary behaviors, like sitting, in relation to cancer and other health outcomes.

Q: "Anything else you want to include?"

In my 25 years in this field, I've often been asked whether there is a particular type of exercise that is the best to do. I tell people that the best exercise is the one you'll do.

Favorite Quote:

"When it comes to health and well-being, regular exercise is about as close to a magic potion as you can get."
—*Vietnamese monk, Tich Nhat Hanh*

STUDY QUESTIONS

1. Normally functioning cells undergo programmed cell death. This is called:
   a. Checkpoint inhibition
   b. Stopping rules
   c. Apoptosis
   d. Cycle inhibition
2. The term *cancer* was coined by:
   a. Hippocrates
   b. Galen
   c. Celsus
   d. Farber
3. Invasive cancer refers to a cancer that has:
   a. Remained in the original tissue from which it developed
   b. Spread to distant places in the body
   c. Properties that show it is not actually cancer
   d. Spread beyond the original tissue where it developed
4. The types of cancer described in the chapter include:
   a. Carcinoma, epithelioma, sarcoma, colorectal, and kidney
   b. Epithelial, sarcoma, melanoma, lymphoma, multiple myeloma, and central nervous system
   c. Carcinoma, sarcoma, melanoma, lymphoma, leukemia, and central nervous system
   d. Multiple myeloma, breast, colorectal, liver, and lung
5. In the example in this chapter, despite having half as many actual cases, the risk of colorectal cancer was 10 times higher in Hispanic people. This was explained by accounting for:
   a. Bias
   b. Age adjustment
   c. Counts
   d. Denominators
6. Cancer causes ____ out of _____ deaths worldwide.
7. In developing countries, most commonly diagnosed cancers in men are:
   a. Lung and liver
   b. Liver and prostate
   c. Prostate and lung
   d. Colorectal and liver

8. What percentage of cancers are diagnosed over age 50:
   a. 10
   b. 40
   c. 60
   d. 80
9. There are 7 types of cancer for which exercise has been shown to be preventive. These include:
   a. Breast, endometrial, kidney, bladder, esophageal, stomach, and colon
   b. Breast, prostate, colon, kidney, bladder, esophageal, and stomach
   c. Prostate, endometrial, kidney, bladder, esophageal, liver, and stomach
   d. Stomach, colon, rectal, liver, esophageal, ovary, and endometrial
10. Many men with prostate cancer are diagnosed at an early stage, when it is possible to delay treatment and monitor disease progression. This is called:
    a. Active anticipation
    b. Active surveillance
    c. Delayed treatment
    d. Standard of care

REFERENCES

1. Pezzella F, Kerr D, Tavassoli M. The multicellular organism and cancer. In: Pezzella F, Tavassoli M, Kerr DJ, editors. *Oxford Textbook of Cancer Biology*. Oxford (UK): Oxford University Press; 2019. Chapter 1, p. 9.
2. Mukherjee S. *Emperor of All Maladies: A Biography of Cancer*. New York (NY): Scribner Press; 2010.
3. American Cancer Society. *Global Cancer Facts and Figures*. 4th ed. Atlanta (GA): American Cancer Society; 2018.
4. World Cancer Research Fund/American Institute for Cancer Research. *Diet, Nutrition, Physical Activity and Cancer: A Global Perspective—A Summary of the Third Expert Report*. [Internet]. 2018. Available from https://www.wcrf.org/wp-content/uploads/2021/02/Summary-of-Third-Expert-Report-2018.pdf
5. Patel AV, Friedenreich CM, More SC, et al. American College of Sports Medicine Roundtable Report on physical activity, sedentary behavior, and cancer prevention and control. *Med. Sci. Sports Exerc.* 2019;51(11):2391–402.
6. Jones LW, Courneya KS, Mackey JR, et al. Cardiopulmonary function and age-related decline across the breast cancer survivorship continuum. *J Clin Oncol.* 2012;30(20):2530–7.
7. Yu AF, Flynn JR, Moskowitz CS, et al. Long-term cardiopulmonary consequences of treatment induced cardiotoxicity in survivors of ERBB2-Positive breast cancer. *JAMA Cardiol.* 2020;5(3):309–17.
8. Campbell KL, Winters-Stone KM, Wiskemann J, et al. Exercise guidelines for cancer survivors: consensus statement from international multidisciplinary roundtable. *Med. Sci. Sports Exer.* 2019;51(11): 2375–90.
9. Arnold M, Morgan E, Rumgay H, et al. Current and future burden of breast cancer: global statistics for 2020 and 2040. *The Breast.* 2022;66:15–23.
10. Irwin ML, Cartmel B, Gross CP, et al. Randomized exercise trial of aromatase inhibitor-induced arthralgia in breast cancer survivors. *J Clin Oncol.* 2015;33(10):1104–11.
11. Sharma R. The burden of prostate cancer is associated with human development index: evidence from 87 countries, 1990-2016. *EPMA.* 2019;10(2):137–52.
12. Ornish D, Weidner G, Fair WR, et al. Intensive lifestyle changes may affect the progression of prostate cancer. *J Urol.* 2005;174(3):1065–9.
13. Liu Z, Mao X, Jiang Y, et al. Changing trends in the disease burden of primary liver cancer caused by specific etiologies in China. *Cancer Med.* 2019;8(12):5787–99.
14. Romero-Gómez M, Zelber-Sagi S, Trenell M. Treatment of NAFLD with diet, physical activity and exercise. *J Hepatol.* 2017;67(4):829–46.
15. Avancini A, Sartori G, Gkountakos A, et al. Physical activity and exercise in lung cancer care: will promises be fulfilled? *Oncologist.* 2020;25(3):e555–69.
16. Himbert C, Klossner N, Coletta AM, et al. Exercise and lung cancer surgery: a systematic review of randomized-controlled trials. *Crit Rev Oncol Hematol.* 2020;156:103086.

CHAPTER

2

Cancer Biology

OUTLINE

OBJECTIVES

After completing review of this chapter, students will be able to:

1. Understand the multistep process for developing a tumor.
2. Recall the hallmarks of cancer.
3. Discuss the role of gene changes in cancer development.
4. Explain the processes by which tumors spread throughout the body.
5. Recognize the role of both the immune system and viruses in cancer development.
6. Identify the complexities of the development and spread of cancer in the body.

INTRODUCTION: THE BIOLOGY OF CANCER

In this chapter, we review the biological underpinnings of cancer. By studying this chapter, we will be better able to understand why specific treatments are prescribed for cancer. We will also gain an understanding of the complexity of the initiation, promotion, progression, and metastasis of tumors in a way that will help us when interacting with oncologists. We begin with a basic overview of cells, organelles, and genes. We then progress through a broad variety of topics relevant to the development and progression of cancer, many of which present opportunities for treatment. Where relevant, we have added text about the relevance of exercise to cancer biology.

CELLS, ORGANELLES, AND GENES: A BRIEF REVIEW

In general biology, we learn that the human body is made up of many types of cells and that these cells have predictable elements. Prior to delving into cancer biology, we provide a brief review.

Our cells have an outer phospholipid bilayer. Along that layer and inside the cell (capable of spanning the cell wall) are receptors. Ligands are attached to the receptors, and they regulate what gets into and out of the cell. They also control the growth, division, and activity of the cell. In cancer, overexpression of receptors—sometimes as a result of gene amplification—can result in overgrowth and uncontrolled replication of the cell.

Inside the cell, there are **organelles** that do specific jobs to keep the cell functioning as intended. The nucleus, at the center of the cell, is the location of deoxyribonucleic acid (DNA). DNA carries all the genetic information for the body in the form of chromosomes. A gradual accumulation of errors in the DNA is at the center of understanding cancer biology. Errors in DNA come in many forms and can be present at birth or occur because of an exposure to a carcinogen. Carcinogens are substances such as viruses, smoke, chemicals, and UV rays from the sun. Ribonucleic acid (RNA) can be found in the cytoplasm (the liquid inside the cell) and acts as a messenger carrying instructions from the DNA for the control and synthesis of proteins. As shown in Figure 2.1, common cellular organelles include the ribosomes, Golgi apparatus, endoplasmic reticulum, lysosomes, and mitochondria, among others. Cells have a cycle of replication and growth that continues until their signals, inherent in the DNA of the cell, tell them to stop.

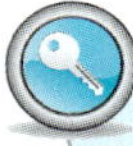

Organelles. Specialized structures within a cell.

The **cell cycle** is a predictable series of events that takes place as the cell grows and divides. As shown in Figure 2.2, the phases of a cell cycle are G1, S, G2, and M (mitosis). The period during which the cell grows and copies its DNA before moving into mitosis is called interphase. Interphase includes G1 (Gap 1), the stage when the cell is preparing to divide. It also includes the S (synthesis), the stage when all of the DNA molecules are copied. Once there is an extra set of the genetic material, the cell organizes and condenses the genetic material. This is called the G2 (Gap 2) phase. Finally, the cell enters the mitosis (M) phase. During the mitosis phase, the cell partitions the 2 copies of the genetic material into 2 daughter cells. The subpart of mitosis includes prophase, metaphase, anaphase, and telophase. After the M stage, there are 2 new cells, and the cycle can begin again. If further cell division is needed, the cell reenters G1. If there is no need for further division, the cell enters the G0 or resting phase. Alterations in the **cell signaling** that control entry into and exit from the cell cycle, as well as the actions expected for progressing through the cell cycle, are central to the development of cancer. There are checkpoints along the cell cycle progression to determine whether there have been any errors in the cell's genome. The function of cell cycle checkpoints can be altered in cancer.

Cancer cell development is thought to have multiple steps, including initiation, promotion, progression, and malignancy (1). In 1971, Dr. Alfred Knudson hypothesized that cancer required "two hits" resulting from both the activation of mutations and loss of tumor suppression activity. Since then, we have come to recognize that there are likely more than 2 hits needed, and the multiple step model has been endorsed. The following explains the multistep process (Figure 2.3).

Damage to the DNA

Initiation refers to the process by which a normal cell starts down the path toward becoming a cancer. The initiation phase refers to DNA alterations as a result of exposure to a carcinogen. **Carcinogens** are substances or exposures that can cause cancer in a living tissue. They range from exposure to the sun to other exposures, such as asbestos, pesticides, viruses (such as HPV, Epstein-Barr virus [EBV]), and particulates in the air (environmental factors). Not all carcinogens

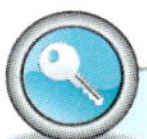

Cell cycle. A 4-step process by which a cell grows and divides.

Cell signaling. Ability of a cell to receive, process, and transmit signals within its environment and with itself.

Initiation. An event associated with the occurrence of a series of DNA mutations that starts the cellular process toward the development of cancer.

Carcinogens. Substances capable of causing cancer.

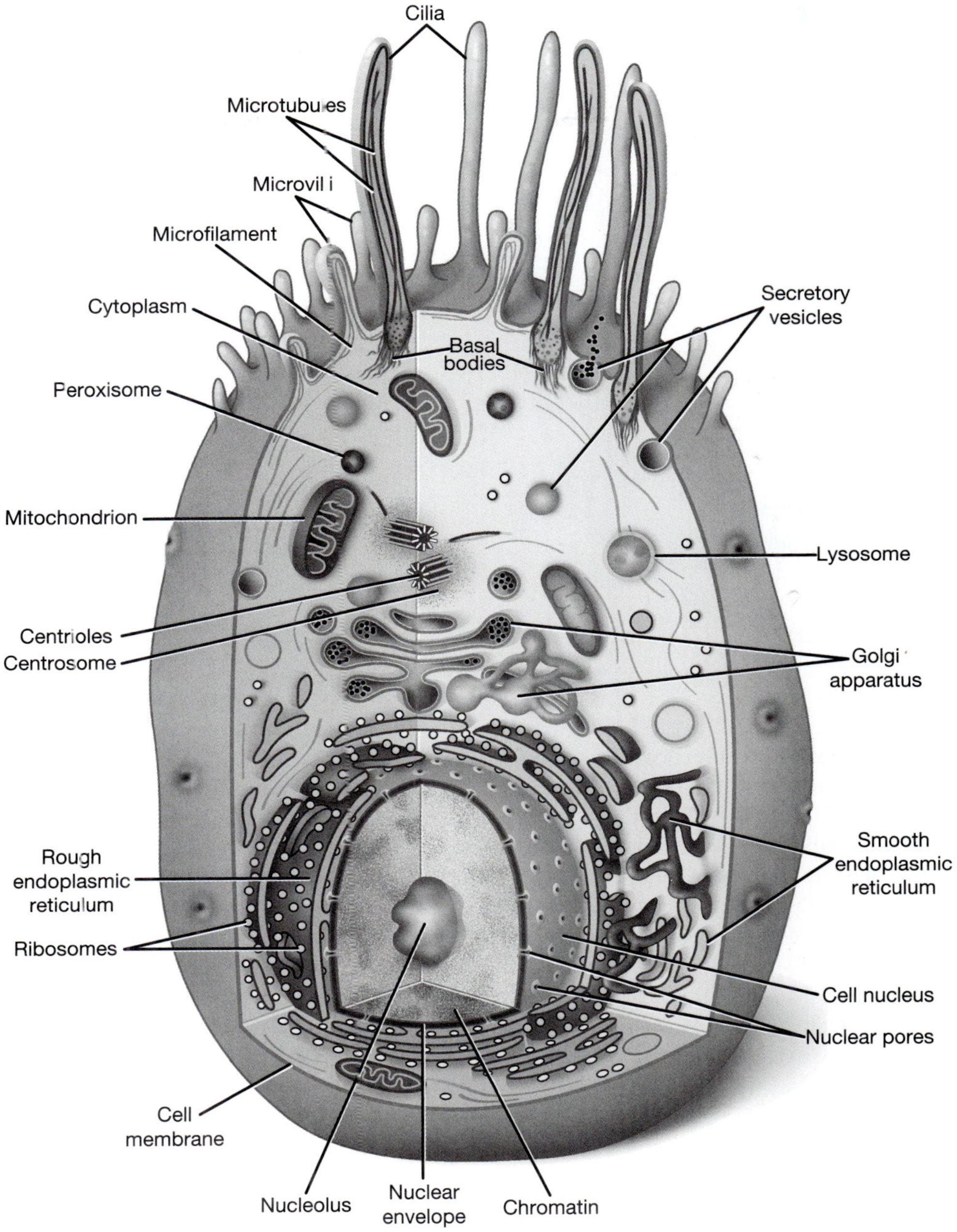

FIGURE 2.1. Review of the structure and organelles of a normal cell. (From Eroschenko VP. *Atlas of Histology with Functional Correlations.* Philadelphia (PA): LWW; 2017. Chapter 2, Figure 1.)

cause cancer upon exposure because most have varying levels of cancer-causing potential. To complicate this further, the extent of exposure is also critical. Taken together, the likelihood that a particular carcinogen will cause cancer depends on how long the exposure has been and how many carcinogens are present, the genetic backdrop in the individual, and the microenvironment at the time of the exposure. Ultimately, a carcinogen can alter the DNA of a cell, initiating the process of cancer. In some cases, DNA repair mechanisms can reverse that process. Lack of exercise has not been implicated as an initiating factor for cancer.

The Error Is Passed On

The next step in the multistep carcinogenesis model is **promotion**, which refers to the expansion and replication of the initiated cells. At this point, there are factors that promote the process, speeding the replication of the damaged

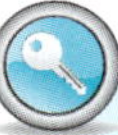

Promotion. Process by which additional mutations occur within cells, contributing to the development of cancer.

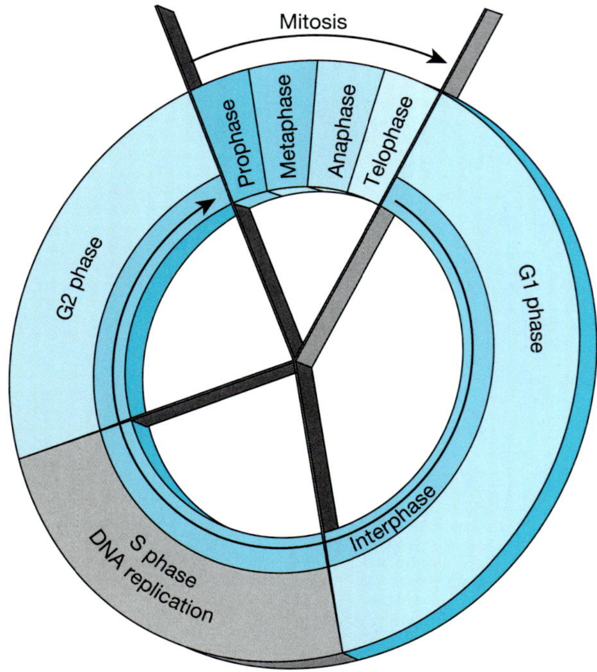

FIGURE 2.2. Cell cycle phases. (Courtesy: National Human Genome Research Institute.)

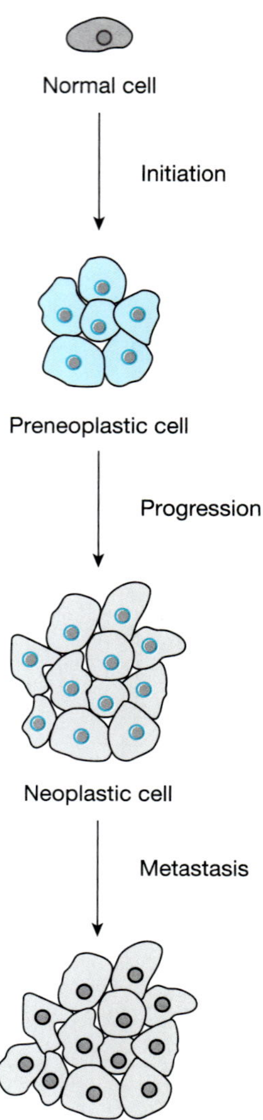

FIGURE 2.3. Example of the multistep processes of developing a tumor: the multiple-hit hypothesis.

cell. Common tumor promoters include alcohol, smoking, elevated estrogen, dietary fat, UV light, and chemicals like dioxin and polychlorinated biphenyls (PCBs). There is some evidence that antioxidant activity can help block the action of promoters if the mode of action is to damage DNA by oxidation. Oxidative stress is a bodily condition that occurs when there is an excess of highly reactive oxygen species (ROS) (called free radicals) in comparison with natural antioxidant defenses (see Figure 2.11, later in the chapter). Exercise has been shown to reduce oxidative stress in multiple studies; this may be one way exercise prevents cancer (2).

Latency and Progression

Finally, in the stages of progression and malignancy, there is the conversion of a preneoplastic cell into one that expresses the malignant phenotype. The development of cancer is the result of the accumulation of multiple mutations. Many factors within the tumor microenvironment (TME) (described later in the chapter) can influence **cell proliferation**, resulting in heterogeneous metabolic activity. The conversion rate is increased by the repeated exposure of preneoplastic cells to DNA-damaging agents and by the activation of genes involved in normal cell growth (called proto-oncogenes) and inactivation of tumor suppression genes (described in the section "Proto-Oncogenes and Tumor Suppressor Genes"). Tumor progression is the expression of a **malignancy** phenotype and tendency for these cells to become more aggressive over time.

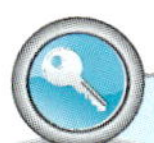

Cell proliferation. Rapid increase in the number of cells.
Malignancy. Term used to define cancer. Malignant cells grow in an uncontrolled manner, can invade nearby tissues, and spread to other parts of the body.

Hallmarks of Cancer

After the preceding steps, cells express the following hallmarks of cancer, listed below and in Figure 2.4 (3-5):

- Cancer cells are able to enter the cell cycle without growth factor.
- Cancer cells can evade growth suppressors.
- Cancer cells can divide indefinitely.
- Cancer cells show increased genetic instability.
- Cancer cells can resist programmed cell death.
- Cancer cells can sustain angiogenesis.

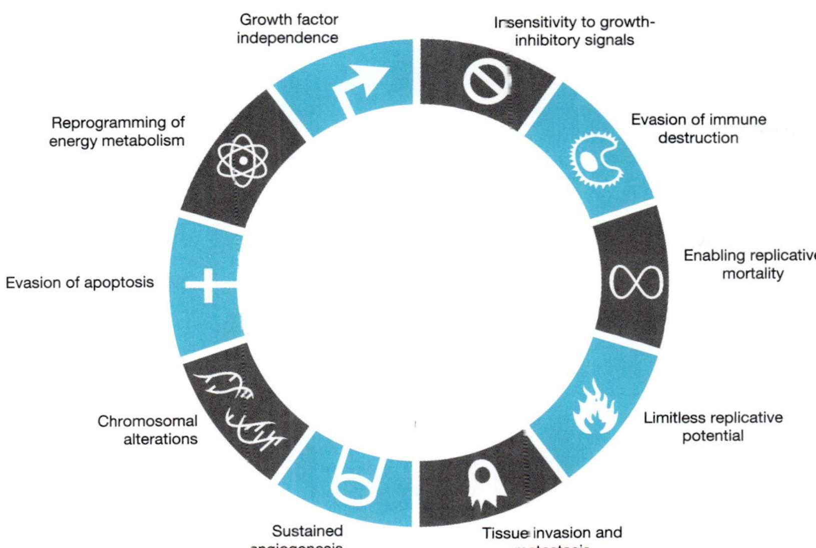

FIGURE 2.4. Hallmarks of cancer. (From Rassy E, Assi T, Pavlidis N. Exploring the biological hallmarks of cancer of unknown primary: where do we stand today?. *Br J Cancer.* 2020;122(8):1124–32. https://doi.org/10.1038/s41416-019-0723-z.)

- Cancer cells exhibit deregulated metabolism.
- Cancer cells exhibit the capacity for invasion and metastasis.
- Cancer cells have the ability to evade immune clearance.
- Cancer cells stimulate tumor-promoting inflammation.

One other common feature of tumor cells is that they consume glucose at a surprisingly higher rate than normal cells, and the glucose is converted to lactate rather than being fully oxidized. This phenomenon is known as the Warburg effect (6) and will be described more fully in the section "Metabolism and Tumor Growth."

PROTO-ONCOGENES AND TUMOR SUPPRESSOR GENES

The discovery of genetic changes that promote cancer, or proto-oncogenes changing to oncogenes, started with the studies of birds. The first altered version of normal cellular genes (proto-oncogenes) was called *v-src*; it was shown to be nearly identical to a gene in normal avian DNA. This discovery fueled research to determine whether there were proto-oncogenes in humans. The first one identified in humans is known as the Philadelphia chromosome (7). It is called ABL and is a translocation **mutation** that results in an aberrant protein of larger molecular weight and enhanced tyrosine activity. It is a defining feature associated with chronic myelogenous leukemia. The identification of many other proto-oncogenes followed, as noted in Table 2.1. Tumor initiation, expansion, and metastasis are driven by a combination of oncogene gain-of-function and tumor suppressor loss-of-function mutagenic events, which confer neoplastic properties on the population of cancer cells. These aberrations may occur at the genetic, epigenetic, transcriptomic, proteomic, or metabolic levels. Well-characterized oncogenes and tumor suppressors are listed, along with the tumors they are commonly associated with, as well as relevant diagnostic tests and approved targeted therapies.

Mutations leading to proto-oncogenes are sometimes called gain-of-function mutations. At the same time, scientists were also keenly aware of the potential for genetic mutations to result in a change in a gene that could result in the loss of normal, expected cellular functions that would suppress tumors. The early work on this topic focused on inherited and sporadic cases of a particular form of cancer called retinoblastoma. It was noticed that individuals with a single inherited mutation only required one more mutation to develop the disease, while individuals without the inherited mutation required 2 somatic mutations to develop the disease. The inherited disease was found to be because of a loss of a functional gene, specifically focused at a tumor suppressor locus. This could be termed a recessively acting gene and mutations in **tumor suppressor genes** are sometimes called a loss-of-function mutation.

It has been through the functional characterization of the proteins that result from the oncogenes and tumor suppressor genes that we have learned more about the process of **tumorigenesis**. Figure 2.5 provides a visual depiction of the nonhereditary and hereditary versions of cancer development.

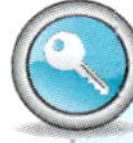

Mutation. Changing of the structure of a gene, resulting in a variation that may be transmitted.

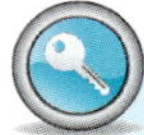

Tumor suppressor gene. Encodes a protein that acts to regulate cell division, keeping it in check.

Tumorigenesis. Initial formation of a tumor in the body. Tumorigenesis occurs when a mutation results in an altered protein that functions differently than normal.

Table 2.1 Oncogenes and Tumor Suppressor Genes

ONCOGENE	CANCER	DIAGNOSTIC	TARGETED THERAPY
p110α	Breast, prostate, endometrial, colorectal, cervical, head and neck, gastric, lung	PCR, sequencing	
EGFR	Lung, glioma, colorectal, ovarian, breast	PCR, FISH, IHC	gefitinib, erlotinib, cetuximab
ERBB2 (HER2)	Breast, gastric, ovarian, bladder	PCR, sequencing	trastuzumab, lapatinib
B-RAF	Melanoma, thyroid, colorectal, ovarian	PCR, sequencing	vemurafenib
K-RAS	Pancreatic, lung, colorectal, endometrial, ovarian	PCR, sequencing	
H-RAS	Bladder	PCR, sequencing	
N-RAS	Melanoma, AML	PCR, sequencing	
MYC	Lymphomas, colorectal, breast, prostate, melanoma, neuroblastoma, ovarian	FISH, IHC	
BCR-ABL	CML, ALL, AML	FISH, PCR	imatinib, dasatinib, nilotinib
IDH1	Glioblastoma, AML	PCR, sequencing	
IDH2	Glioblastoma, AML	PCR, sequencing	
JAK2	CML, ALL	FISH	
KIT	Gastrointestinal stromal tumors, AML, melanoma	IHC, flow cytometry	
MET	Kidney, gastric, lung, head and neck, colorectal		
FLT-3	AML	PCR	
p53	Lung, colorectal, bladder, ovarian, head and neck, gastric, breast, prostate	IHC, PCR, sequencing	
PTEN	Glioblastoma, melanoma, prostate, breast, endometrial, thyroid, lung, colorectal, AML, CLL	IHC, PCR, sequencing	
$p16^{INK4A}$	Melanoma, pancreatic, lung, bladder, head and neck, colorectal, breast	IHC, PCR, sequencing	
$p14^{ARF}$	Lung, bladder, head and neck, colorectal, breast	IHC, PCR, sequencing	
BRCA1	Breast, ovarian	PCR, sequencing	
BRCA2	Breast, ovarian	PCR, sequencing	
LKB1	Lung, gastrointestinal, pancreatic, cervical, melanoma	PCR, sequencing	
VHL	Kidney, adrenal, hemangioblastoma	PCR, sequencing	
APC	Colorectal, gastric	PCR, sequencing	
FBXW7	ALL, bile duct, colorectal, gastric, endometrial, lung, pancreatic, prostate, ovarian	PCR, sequencing	
Rb	Retinoblastoma, lung, bladder, esophageal, osteosarcoma, glioma, liver, CML, prostate, breast	IHC, PCR, sequencing	
NF1	Neurofibroma, neuroblastoma, glioma, colorectal	PCR, sequencing	
NF2	Meningioma, schwannoma, glioma	PCR, sequencing	

ALL, acute lymphoblastic leukemia; AML, acute myelogenous leukemia; CML, chronic myeloid leukemia; FISH, fluorescent in situ hybridization; IHC, immunohistochemistry; PCR, polymerase chain reaction.
From Harrington L, Tannock IF, Hill R, Cescon D. *The Basic Science of Oncology*, 8th ed. New York (NY): McGraw-Hill Education; 2021.

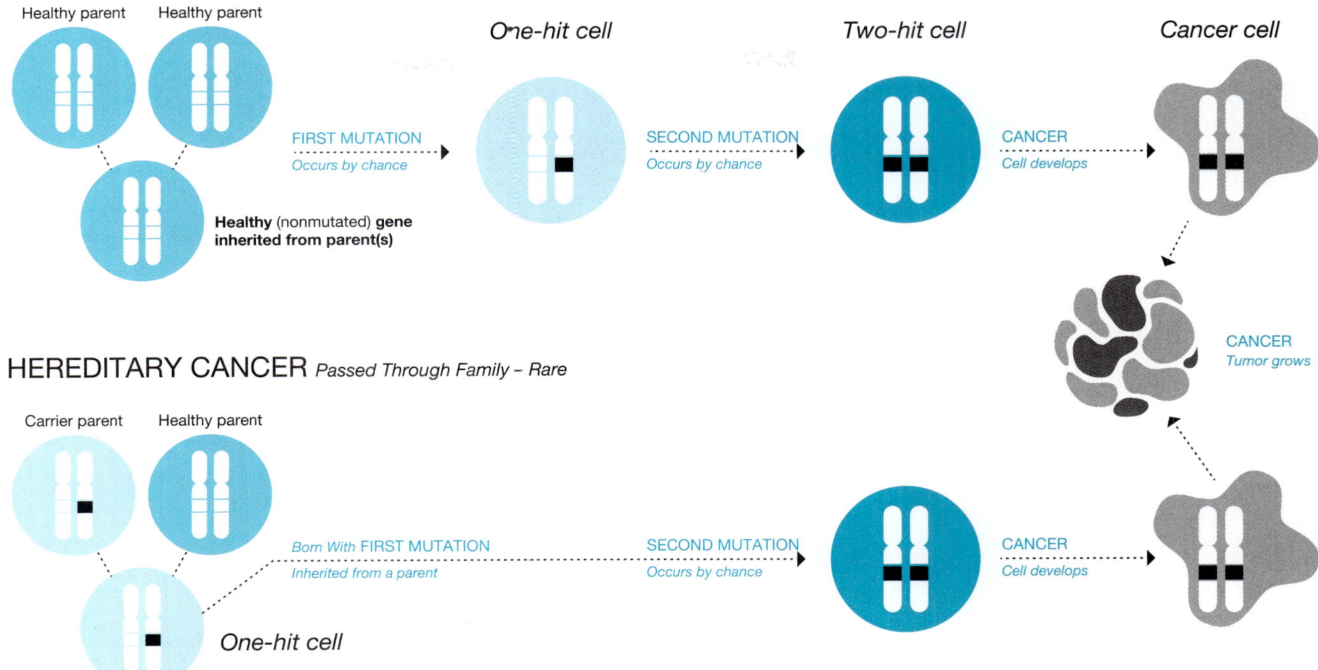

FIGURE 2.5. The two-hit model of carcinogenesis. (Redrawn from Nowsheen S, Georgakilas AG, Yang ES. Staying a step ahead of cancer. In: Georgakilas A, editor. *Cancer Prevention: From Mechanisms to Translational Benefits*. Figure 2, p. 65. © 2012 Licensee IntechOpen. This chapter is distributed under the terms of the Creative Commons Attribution 3.0 License, which permits unrestricted use, distribution, and reproduction in any medium, provided the original work is properly cited.)

In the process of learning about tumorigenesis, it has been crucial to understand the tight control of cellular processes in the body without cancer. Very specific cell signaling and growth pathways govern cell function and reproduction. Tumorigenesis occurs when a mutation results in an altered protein that functions differently than normal. There are redundant systems in the body to prevent those mutations from continuing to alter cell signaling, function, and reproduction. For example, multiple additional mutations are required for the process of cancer to proceed, and there are many proto-oncogenes and tumor suppressor genes (see Table 2.1). Here we describe one of each, in detail, as examples.

Proto-oncogene: RAS and RAF

Rat sarcoma virus (RAS) family genes are among the most commonly mutated in human cancer (8). There are 3 RAS genes; the most commonly that mutates is *K-RAS*. This mutation is particularly relevant to pancreatic, lung, colon, and endometrial cancers. In contrast, mutations of *N-RAS* are seen in melanoma, and mutations of *H-RAS* are seen in cancers of the thymus and adrenal glands. As shown in Figure 2.6, RAS binds to the inside of the biphospholipid layer of the cell wall and acts as a switch, eventually leading to alterations in cell survival, migration, proliferation, and growth. The most common version of the mutation is to turn the switch permanently on, resulting in the upregulation of 3 RAF kinases. There are a number of specific subtypes of the mutation, and drug targets have been developed for some. For example, vemurafenib is a drug that improves outcomes for patients with a particular subtype of mutation of RAF.

Tumor Suppressor Gene: *p53*

Tumor suppressor gene *p53* is the most studied tumor suppressor gene, and it is commonly called the guardian of the genome (9). As shown in Figure 2.7, the expression of hundreds of genes is directly regulated by *p53*, resulting in many important and varied effects of *p53*. This gene makes a protein that is found inside the nucleus of cells. It plays a key role in controlling cell division and cell death. Levels of *p53* are normally kept very low by an E3 ubiquitin ligase called mouse double minute 2 (MDM2). E3 ubiquitin ligase catalyzes the transfer of ubiquitin to the target protein (*p53*, in this case). In response to an oncologic cell stress, a normally functioning *p53* gene will be upregulated to allow it to take action to downregulate cell proliferation or even induce cell death. Loss of *p53* results in aberrant cell division and alters the maturation of microRNAs with growth suppressive functions (10). Mutation of the *p53* gene is present in 40% to 50% of human cancers, though the percentages will vary by type of cancer (eg, 90% in ovarian cancer, 10% in some leukemias). An inherited condition (Li-Fraumeni syndrome) includes an inborn mutation of *p53* that is associated with multiple types of cancer.

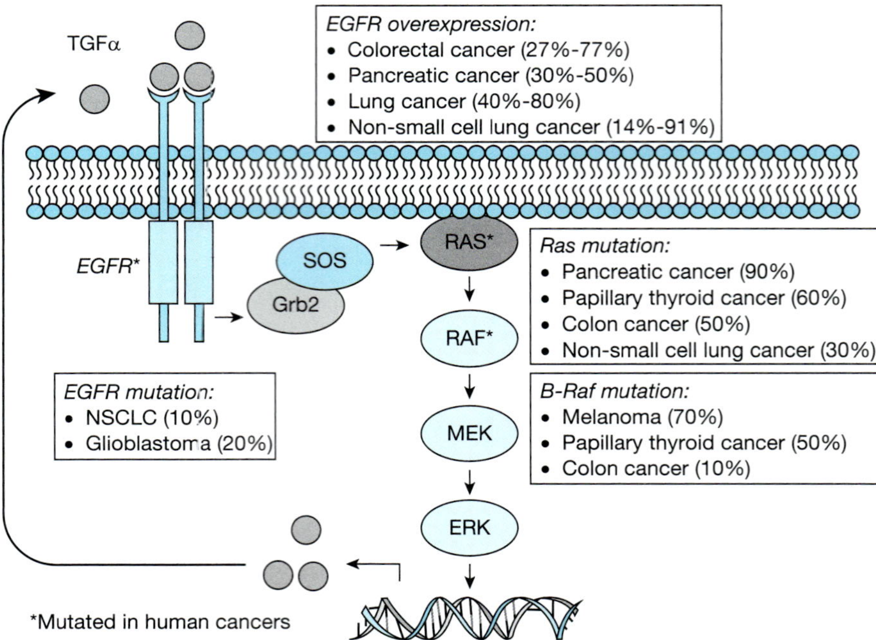

FIGURE 2.6. RAS as a proto-oncogene. By mutating, RAS binds to the inside of the biphsopholipid layer of the cell wall and acts like a switch, eventually leading to alterations in cell survival, migration, proliferation, and growth. Abbreviations: RAS, rat sarcoma virus; ERK, extracellular signal-related kinase. (From Roberts PJ, Der CJ. Targeting the Raf-MEK-ERK mitogen-activated protein kinase cascade for the treatment of cancer. *Oncogene.* 2007;26(22):3291–310. doi:10.1038/sj.onc.1210422.)

There are many ways genes and resulting cellular function can be altered. One unifying framework posited by Kinzler and Vogelstein refers to gatekeeper, caretaker, and landscaper mutations (11-14). The idea is that there are genes that encode different types of activities and, as a result, the importance to tumor development will vary. The landscaper mutations alter encoding for products that create the TME conducive to unregulated cell growth. An example of

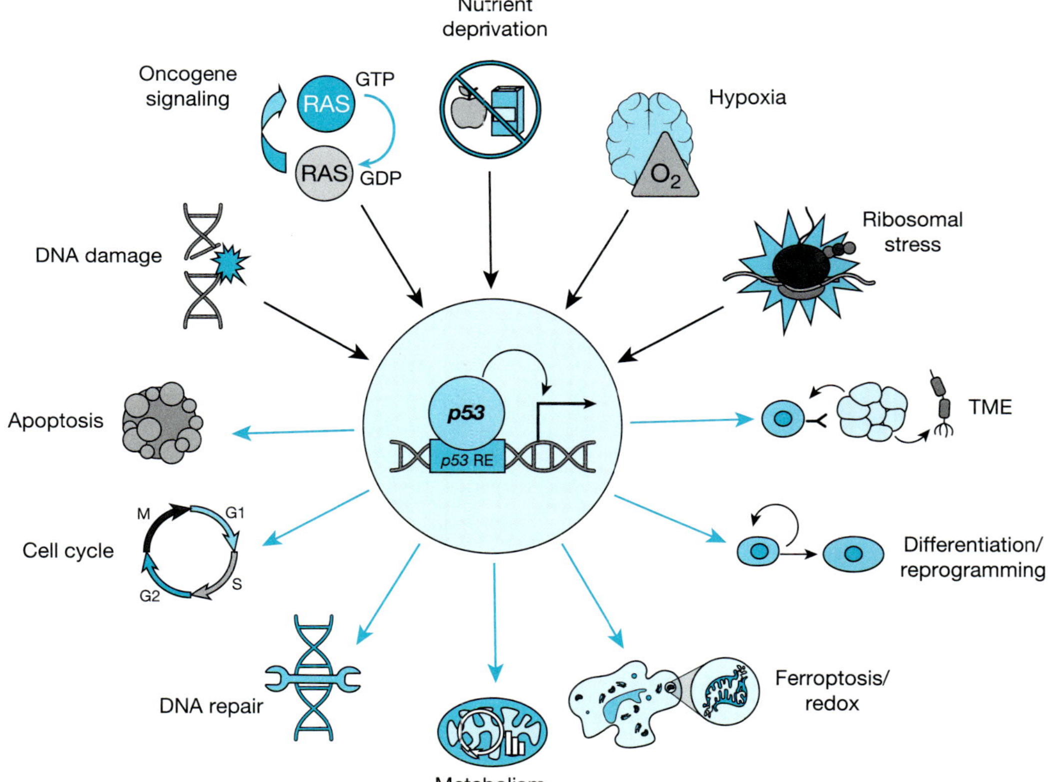

FIGURE 2.7. Tumor suppressor gene. This "guardian of the genome" has broad reaching effects protecting the body from DNA damage, controlling oncogene signaling, nutrient deprivation, hypoxia, and ribosomal stress, among other effects. Abbreviations: RAS, rat sarcoma virus; TME, tumor microenvironment. (From Boutelle AM, Attardi LD. *P53* and tumor suppression: it takes a network. *Trends in Cell Biol.* 2021;31(4):298–310.)

this type of gene is *PTEN*, which makes an enzyme found in almost all tissues of the body. The enzyme acts as a tumor suppressor, so a mutation in *PTEN* alters this function. This type of mutation is seen as having low importance for the initiation of cancer as compared with the other 2 types. The gatekeeper genes encode proteins that regulate cell proliferation. A mutation in these genes increases the likelihood of the development of a tumor much more than the landscaper gene mutation. One example of a gatekeeper gene is *p53*. The caretaker genes maintain the integrity of the genome. Mutations in these genes can result in genomic instability and specific types of genetic mutations. An example of this type of gene would be *BRCA* mutation responsible for high risk of breast and ovarian cancers.

There are a variety of ways that genes can become altered in a manner that contributes to tumorigenesis. Mutations can be the result of genetic inheritance (germline) or exposure to environmental factors (somatic). Further, the manner in which DNA is mutated varies. There are point mutations that can alter amino acid sequences in the encoded proteins, as well as gene amplification, deletions, insertions, and chromosomal translocations. Further, the expression level of genes can be epigenetically modified as a result of methylation activity. In addition, only 1% to 2% of DNA encodes for proteins. The nonencoding DNA leads to nonencoding RNA, and the activity of one particular type of nonencoding RNA, microRNA, has been studied to understand its role in cancer development. MicroRNA controls many cellular processes and regulates at least one-third of all human genes, making them key modulators in the development of cancer. This is relevant to the discussion of proto-oncogenes and tumor suppressor genes because those genes encode for microRNA as much as for encoding RNA. For example, mutations in the BCL2 protein have been found to be associated with alterations in microRNA observed in CLL. To conclude, there are a broad variety of ways that genes might become altered in a manner that results in the development of a tumor.

TUMOR GROWTH, MICROENVIRONMENT, AND METABOLISM

Tumor Growth

The rate at which tumors grow is known from 2 methods: observation (external measurements or imaging) and studies using advanced flow cytometry techniques. Observation of humans allows us to draw the conclusion that the time for a tumor to double in volume remains constant. This implies exponential growth. Doubling time for human tumors has been observed to range from 27 to 83 days (15). This applies to going from 0.01 to 0.02 cm^3 as well as going from 5 to 10 cm^3. We notice the doubling much more when the tumor is larger, but the rate of doubling does not change. Figure 2.8 presents a chart of the changes in the size of a breast tumor with a 100-day doubling time. Note that it takes 9 years to get to a 0.5-cm diameter but grows to 16-cm diameter by 13 years, without a change in the doubling rate (16).

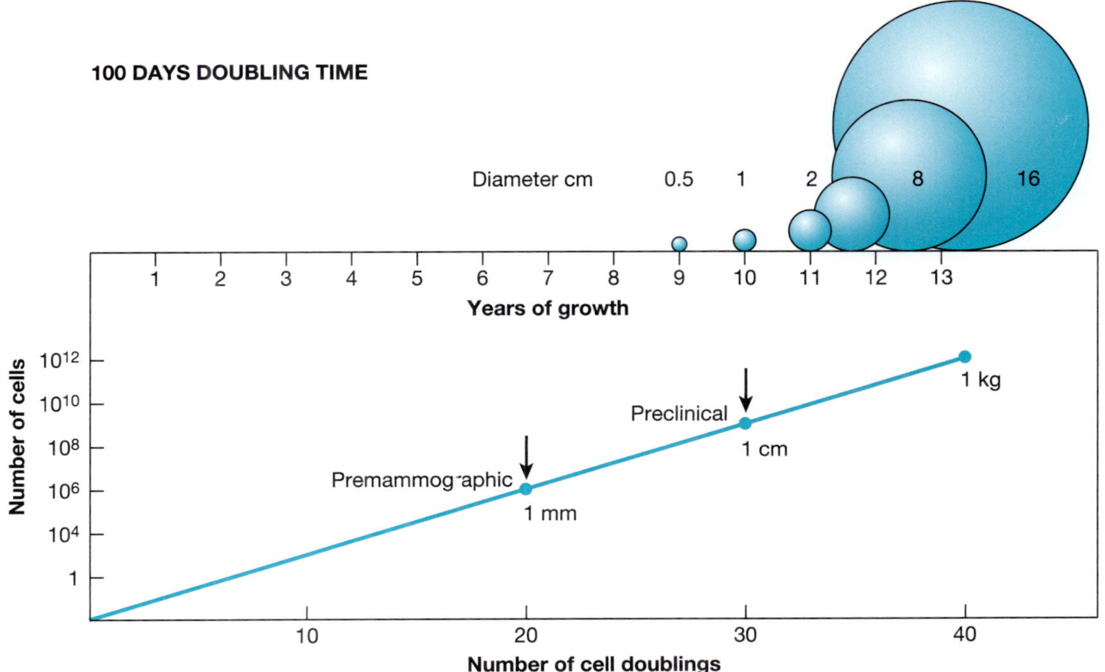

FIGURE 2.8. Effect of a 100-day doubling time on the growth of a tumor. The primary message from this figure is to note that the time from undetectable to preclinical is 10 years, and the time from preclinical to large tumor is less than 3 years. (From Gullino P. Natural history of breast cancer: progression from hyperplasia to neoplasia as predicted by angiogenesis. *Cancer*. 1977;39(suppl 6):2697–703.)

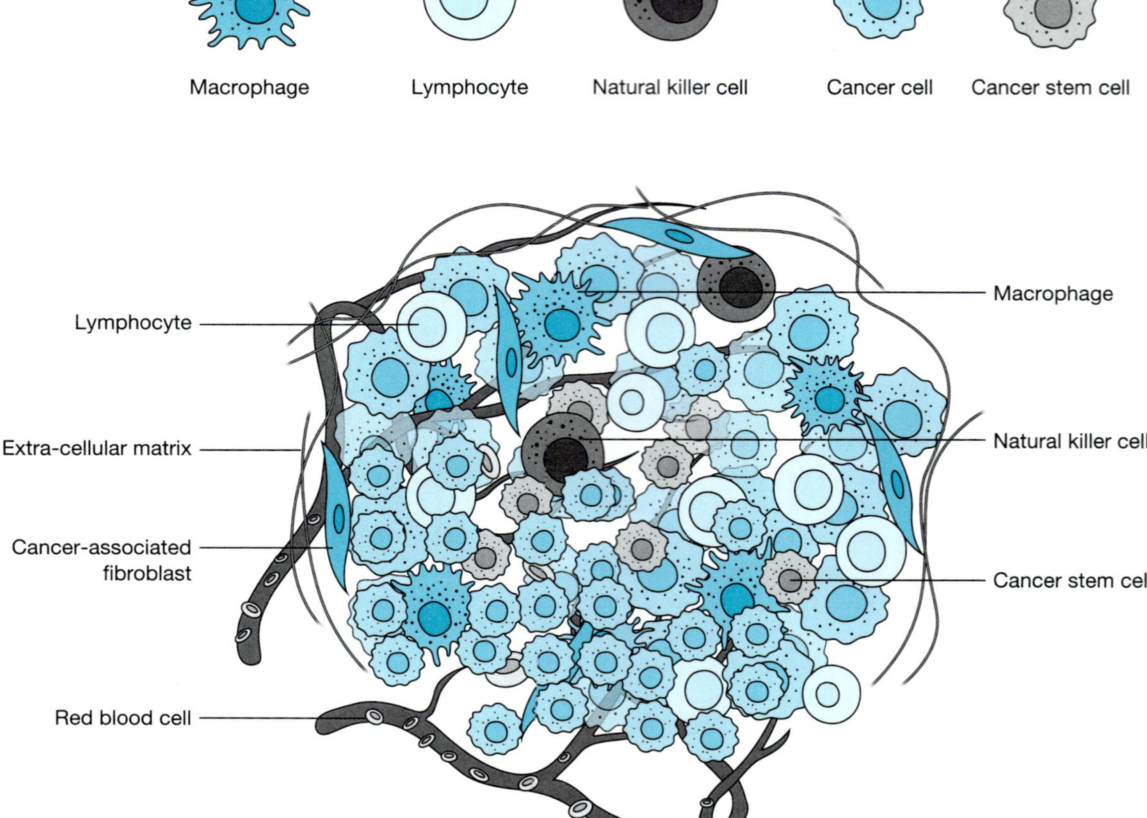

FIGURE 2.9. The tumor microenvironment includes immune cells, blood cells, blood vessels, and extracellular matrix. (From Hassan G, Seno M. Blood and cancer: cancer stem cells as origin of hematopoietic cells in solid tumor microenvironments. *Cells*. 2020;9(5):1293. https://doi.org/10.3390/cells9051293; redrawn from *Cells*. 2020;9(5):1293. https://doi.org/10.3390/cells9051293.)

Applying flow cytometry to a sample, cells can be tagged with fluorescent markers to discern the proportion of cells in each of the 4 cell cycle phases described earlier. Tumor cells are more likely to be in the G1 phase than normal cells. Further, the protein Ki67 can be used as a marker of cell proliferation, allowing for the determination of the proportion of cells that are currently proliferating. The proliferation rate is important because many treatments are more toxic to proliferating cells.

All cells in the body proliferate, and the rate at which they do so varies by tissue type. For example, bone marrow, gastrointestinal mucosa, ovarian, testis, and hair follicles all proliferate rapidly. By the time you finish reading this sentence, 50 million of your cells will have died and been replaced by others. Red blood cells (RBCs) live for about 4 months, while white blood cells live on average more than a year. Skin cells live about 2 or 3 weeks. Colon cells die off after about 4 days. Sperm cells have a life span of only about 3 days, while brain cells typically last an entire lifetime (neurons in the cerebral cortex, eg, are not replaced when they die). This explains why some tissues are so adversely affected by chemotherapy and is the basis for many chemotherapy side effects. Within tumor cells, the rate of cell proliferation is probably not what would be expected: There is a high rate of loss or cell death in the process of tumor proliferation. In short, tumor cells are more heterogeneous and less reliably able to reproduce.

Tumor Microenvironment

The **tumor microenvironment** refers to the ecosystem that surrounds the tumor in the body. As shown in Figure 2.9 (17), the TME includes immune system constituents (lymphocytes, natural killer cells [NK cells], and macrophages), cancer cells, cancer stem cells, the extracellular matrix, vasculature and blood cells, among other elements that may potentiate or fight the tumor, depending on many factors.

The behavior of the TME can contribute to or inhibit the development and progress of a tumor and the likelihood of progress to metastasis. The elements of the TME include cells, the extracellular matrix, and blood vessels. The types of cells

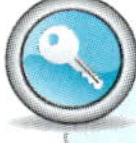

Tumor microenvironment. Normal cells, molecules, and blood vessels that surround and feed a tumor cell.

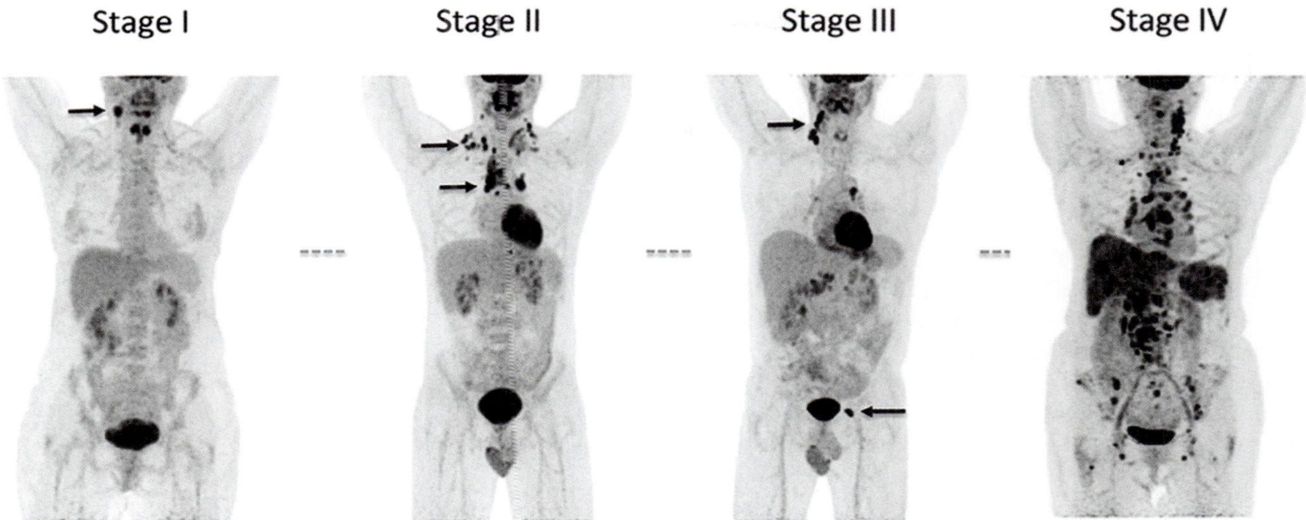

FIGURE 2.10. The tumors show as dark spots other than the heart or bladder. Stage 1 patient at the left has 1 dark spot, denoting 1 tumor. The number of dark spots (tumors) increases with stage. The tumors show up as dark spots because the tumors use so much glucose. (From Cheson BD. PET/CT in lymphoma: current overview and future directions. *Semin Nucl Med.* 2018;48(1):76–81. doi:10.1053/j.semnuclmed.2017.09.007.)

typically found in the TME include cancer-associated fibroblasts, immune cells, endothelial cells, and vascular cells (see Chapter 8). Cancer cells have 3 basic needs, all of which are provided by the surrounding microenvironment: 1. rapid generation of energy, 2. biosynthesis of the macromolecular building blocks for daughter cells, and 3. maintenance of the balance of cellular reduction oxidation status (called "redox"). Tumors typically have poor oxygen perfusion, owing to immature vasculature, so. As such, regions of tumor beds are often hypoxic. There are multiple elements of the TME that might be targets for exercise as therapy, including the resolution of hypoxia, which is a major factor in treatment resistance (18).

Metabolism and Tumor Growth

One way tumors achieve the 3 basic needs noted above is through the activity of **tumor-derived exosomes**. Tumor cells actively produce, release, and utilize exosomes (cell-derived extracellular vesicles) to promote growth. These tumor-derived exosomes interact with the TME to regulate metabolic and inflammatory activities toward the goal of tumor growth. Research is ongoing to find ways to harness tumor-derived exosomes for cancer therapeutic purposes.

The TME contributes to the metabolic activity of the tumor. Tumor metabolism is of great interest to cancer researchers as a potential target for therapies. Multiple compounds, such as gemcitabine, enasidenib, and 5-fluorouracil, have already been tested for the inhibition of tumor metabolism, and new approaches are being developed targeting the metabolism of TME elements such as stromal or immune cells. One cardinal element of tumor metabolism is the use of glycolysis rather than mitochondrial oxidative **phosphorylation**. This selective and inefficient use of glucose for fuel by the tumor is as yet unexplained. It is called the Warburg effect after the scientist who observed it first. There does not seem to be dysfunction in mitochondria to explain this reliance on glycolysis; therefore, one explanation could be that this approach combines the need for energy with the need for macromolecule building blocks and redox. By taking the mitochondria out of energy production, the tricarboxylic acid cycle can act as a hub for biosynthesis of important macromolecules. The overreliance on glucose contributes to our ability to image cancer in the body. Scans called fluorodeoxyglucose-positron emission tomography (FDG-PET) imaging employ a radioactive glucose analog that can be taken up in the cells with glucose but cannot be metabolized. Because the glucose analog is trapped in the cells, it can be imaged to detect places in the body with high glucose uptake. This approach is used to identify and monitor many cancer types (19). Figure 2.10 shows 4 PET scans with stages 1, 2, 3, and 4 lymphoma (20). The dark spots outside the heart and bladder are cancer.

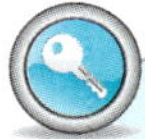

Tumor-derived exosomes. Small extracellular vesicles that are involved in cancer development, tumor progression, metastasis, and disease progression.

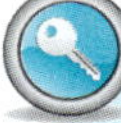

Phosphorylation. Attachment of phosphates to a cell, often resulting in a change in function.

There are a number of pathways that contribute to the regulation of tumor metabolism, including adenosine monophosphate-activated protein kinase (AMPK) and *p53*.

Adenosine Monophosphate-Activated Protein Kinase

Adenosine monophosphate-activated protein kinase functions as a metabolic checkpoint, regulating cellular response to available metabolic energy. It is responsible for shifting cells to an oxidative metabolic phenotype and inhibiting cell proliferation. To proliferate, tumor cells must overcome this pathway. Mutations in signaling pathways can suppress AMPK activity, allowing tumor cells to grow unchecked, even in less-than-ideal nutrient conditions. Loss of AMPK signaling supports a shift toward glycolytic metabolism (the Warburg effect). There is interest in the development of AMPK agonists as therapeutic agents. Recent evidence indicates that a myokine called *irisin*, released following exercise, may upregulate AMPK and inhibit pancreatic cancer cell growth (21).

Tumor Suppressor Gene p53

The tumor suppressor gene *p53* is an important regulator of metabolism by inhibiting the glycolytic pathway. It does this through the direct repression of the transcription of glucose transporters 1 and 4 (GLUT 1 and 4) (2 receptors that transport glucose into the cell). *p53* also supports the expression of *PTEN*, which, in turn, suppresses glycolysis. The loss of *p53* may be a major driver of the Warburg effect. It has been hypothesized that because aerobic exercise increases mitochondrial function and lactate clearance capacity, it may have an anti-Warburg effect. Further, exercise increases fat oxidation and decreases glycolysis. It is hypothesized that one of the mechanisms underlying the observed epidemiologic effects of exercise on cancer incidence, recurrence, and mortality may be a reversal of the metabolic switch to glycolytic metabolism in cancer cells. This may also create epigenetic responses that might help restore oxidative phenotypes (22).

Redox Status

For cells to proliferate and survive, there must be a balance of ROS (such as superoxide, hydroxyl radical, and singlet oxygen) to antioxidants in the cell (such as superoxide dismutase, catalase, glutathione, and thioredoxin reductase) (Figure 2.11). The disorganized nature of the TME tends to push toward greater ROS, a condition referred to as **oxidative distress** (see Figure 2.11), endangering the survival of the tumor. To fight this, tumor cells upregulate antioxidant systems to restore equilibrium. This balance changes during the life of the tumor. Early on, tumors tend to be more acidic. This can promote migration, invasion, and metastasis.

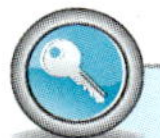

Oxidative distress. Caused by an imbalance of production and accumulation of ROS and the ability of tissues to neutralize these toxic products.

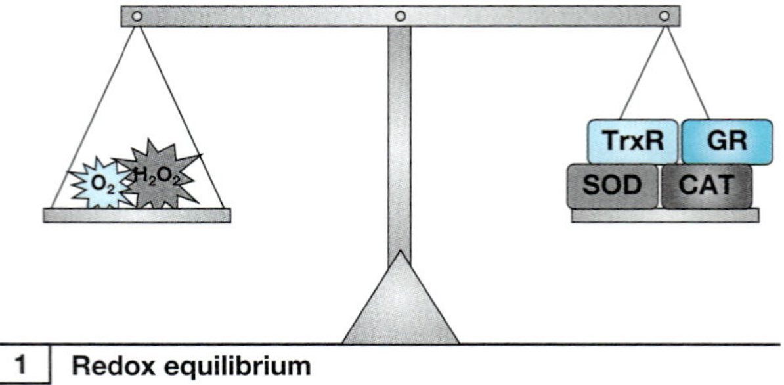

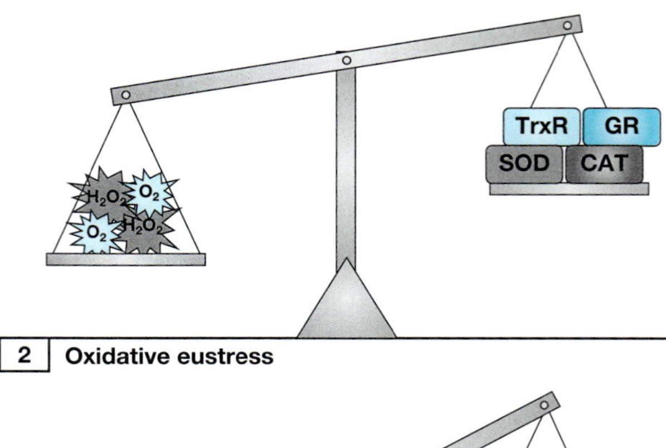

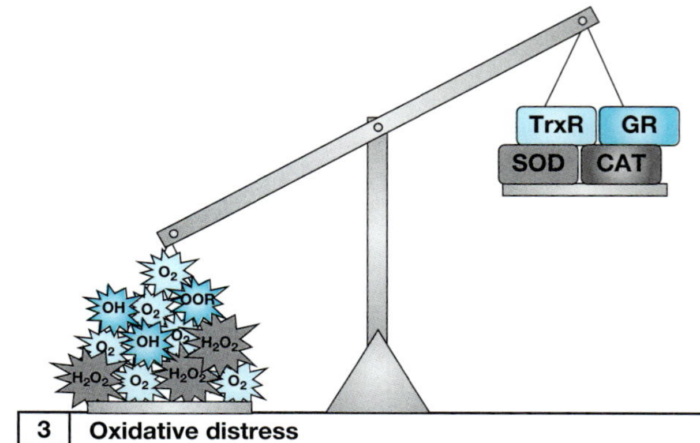

FIGURE 2.11. Redox equilibrium, oxidative eustress, and oxidative distress. The body seeks a balance between the production of free radicals (depicted on the left side of the scales in the figure) and the endogenous antioxidant systems in the body (depicted by the "bricks" on the right of the scales). The situation of free radicals overwhelming antioxidant defenses is called oxidative stress and contributes to carcinogenesis. (From Herb M, Schramm M. Functions of ROS in macrophages and antimicrobial immunity. *Antioxidants*. 2021;10(2):313. https://doi.org/10.3390/antiox10020313.)

TUMOR PROMOTERS AND GROWTH FACTORS

Tumor promotion is defined as a process in which existing tumors are stimulated to grow. Tumor promoters cannot cause tumors to form. However, these agents act to speed

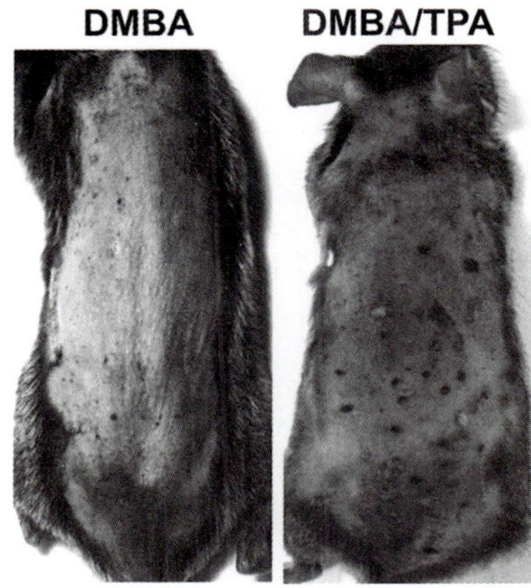

FIGURE 2.12. Imaging of mice that have been exposed to a carcinogen called DMBA (left) versus exposure to DMBA and a tumor promotor called TPA. The dark spots are tumors. (From Nasti TH, Cochran JB, Tsuruta Y, et al. A murine model for the development of melanocytic nevi and their progression to melanoma. *Mol Carcinog.* 2016;55(5):646–58, Figure 1.)

things along. There are a variety of chemicals well established to act as tumor promoters, including tetradecanoyl phorbol acetate (TPA) and phenobarbital. TPA, a compound isolated from croton oil, which is also used as an antineoplastic agent, acts to induce oxidative stress, increase inflammation by activation of tumor necrosis factor-alpha (TNF-α) (a pro-inflammatory cytokine), and increase proliferation. Experiments using TPA demonstrate the role of tumor promoters. Application of the carcinogen DMBA acts synergistically with TPA in promoting tumors in mice, as shown in Figure 2.12. The dark spots on the mice in the figure are melanoma tumors.

Phenobarbital is a drug used to control seizures and also influences cell proliferation and apoptosis. It does this by altering patterns of DNA methylation, thus modifying epigenetic control of gene expression. Chronic inflammation induced by pro-inflammatory cytokines and chemokines has long been accepted as a common mechanism for tumor promotion. This is relevant to exercise training, as exercise decreases chronic inflammation (23) (see Chapter 8).

There are also multiple classes of growth factors and associated receptors relevant to tumor progression. Growth factors in the extracellular matrix around the tumor (part of the TME) regulate receptor kinases, and related receptors play a central role in cell proliferation and migration, promoting tumor growth and metastasis (see Chapter 7). Through their interactions with receptors, growth factors mediate a diverse set of biologic responses, including proliferation, differentiation, migration, and survival of tumor cells. A common type of receptor to which these growth factors bind is receptor tyrosine kinase (RTK). There are many subtypes of RTKs, and activity is generally tightly regulated and controlled. Mutations in the genes that encode these proteins can result in overexpression of these RTKs or functional changes. This results in alterations in cell activity, contributing to tumor progression. As an example, there is a family of receptors (ErbB) that includes the epidermal growth factor receptor (EGFR). This receptor is found in multiple types of tissues in the body (cardiac, epithelial, mesenchymal) and is involved in proliferation, survival, angiogenesis, and metastasis. Mutations in EGFR and other ErbB family receptors are noted in epithelial tumors. These ErbB receptors play an important role in cancer development. The ErbB family has also been the focus of research as a therapeutic target for decades. There are several drugs available that inhibit ErbB receptor activation, including cetuximab, lapatinib, and gefitinib. Aerobic exercise has positive effects on EGFR therapy, including improved circulation and vascular development, improved oxidative stress, improved endogenous antioxidant enzymes, and facilitation of degradation of hypoxia-inducible factor 1 in tumor tissues. In a recent preclinical trial, aerobic exercise was demonstrated to potentiate the effect of gefitinib in mice with lung cancer who had acquired gefitinib resistance (24). The effects were observed to be largely related to the effects of the exercise on oxidative stress and improved cell signaling. See Chapter 7 for more on growth factors.

CELL SIGNALING

Cell signaling occurs in a complex network of pathways. Cells receive information from multiple ligands attached to multiple receptors at the cell wall and integrate this information to regulate a diversity of cell activities, such as protein synthesis, cell growth, motility, cell architecture, differentiation, and programmed cell death. Signaling molecules play different roles according to timing, location, and combination of current activities and present constituents, as well as within different cell types. Context is important in understanding cell signaling. This is also true in cancer cells that contain multiple aberrations in cell signaling activity. The backdrop of cell signaling in a cancer cell is gene mutation and **genetic instability**. It could be that a mutation causes the activation of a cell signaling pathway, which is then blocked by an inhibitory signaling pathway, which the tumor cell then evades by activating yet another signaling pathway. Inhibition of signaling pathways is a therapeutic target, particularly for early cancers, but for more advanced cancers, there is likely a need for therapy that addresses multiple pathways at one time, given that there are accumulated genetic mutations and greater instability. It is not possible in the context of this text to review all of the cell signaling pathways relevant to cancer. We review 2 as examples: mitogen-activated protein kinase (MAPK) and Int/wingless (WNT).

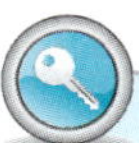

Genetic instability (heterogeneity). The increased tendency for genetic changes to occur during cell division, caused by defects in processes that control the way cells divide.

Mitogen-Activated Protein Kinase

Like many signaling pathways, the MAPK pathway is activated by a particular pattern of phosphorylation (Figure 2.13) (25). Upstream activation of RTK and phosphorylation and activation of other proteins and factors (Grb2, SOS, and RAS) precede the phosphorylation of MAP3K, MAP2K, and MAPK, which all lead to alterations in cytosolic and nuclear substrates and, in turn, alter protein transcription. In the case of MAPK, the phosphorylation activity is achieved by a group called MEKs or MKKs (MAPK-kinase). MEK stands for mitogen-activated protein (MAP)/extracellular signal-related kinase (ERK). All of these pathways are tightly controlled and respond to very distinct stimuli, such as a gene mutation or stress. Downstream of this signaling are scaffold molecules that link specific steps on the pathway. There are multiple MAPK signaling pathways that have been described and that regulate cell activities, including cell migration, proliferation, and differentiation. Dysregulation of the MAPK signaling pathways is strongly implicated in malignant development and transformation. The gene associated with this dysregulation, discussed in the section "Proto-oncogene: RAS and RAF", is RAS. Mutations in the RAS-MAPK signaling pathways are found in 80% of melanomas and 55% of colon/rectal cancers.

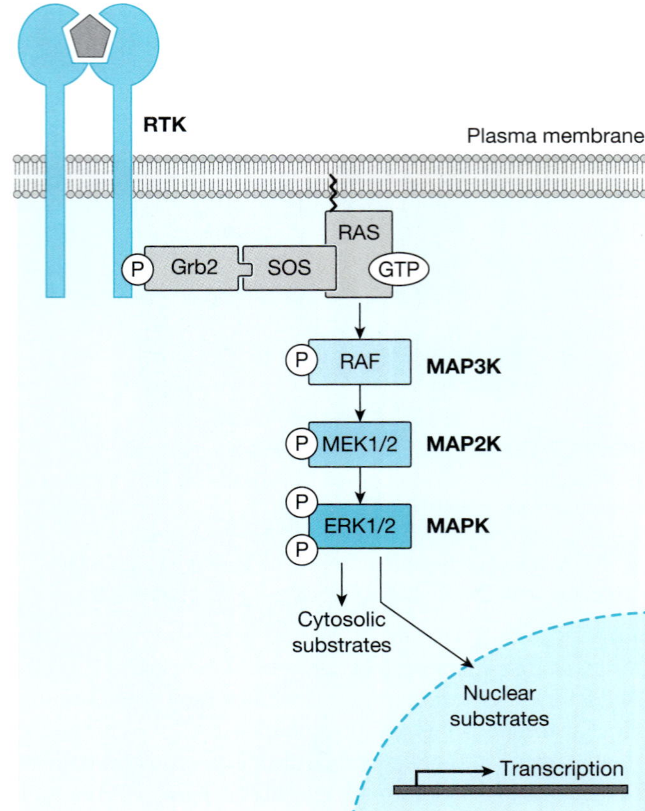

FIGURE 2.13. Mitogen-activated protein kinase activity. In this figure, we show that RAS has attached to the inside of the cell wall that leads to a cascade effect. MAPK acts to phosphorylate Raf, MEK, and ERK, leading downstream to altered protein transcription, cell migration, and differentiation. Abbreviations: RTK, receptor tyrosine kinase; RAS, rat sarcoma virus; ERK, extracellular signal-related kinase; MAPK, mitogen-activated protein kinase. (From Meister I, Tomasovic A, Banning A, Tikkanen, R. Mitogen-activated protein [MAP] kinase scaffolding proteins: a recount. *Int J Mol Sci.* 2013;14(3):4854–84; doi:10.3390/ijms14034854.)

Int/Wingless

Int/Wingless (WNT) is a growth stimulatory protein that is one of several developmental signals to indicate that the human body is developing. It assists with the crucial task of the body diversifying cell types in order to create all functioning organs and systems, particularly in the development of the heart. In normal adult cells, the WNT pathway is inactive (Figure 2.14) (26). In this state, a compound called beta-catenin is bound to glycogen synthase kinase 3beta (GSK-3beta), Axin, adenomatous polyposis coli (APC), and casein kinase-1 (CK-1) act to limit gene expression. When

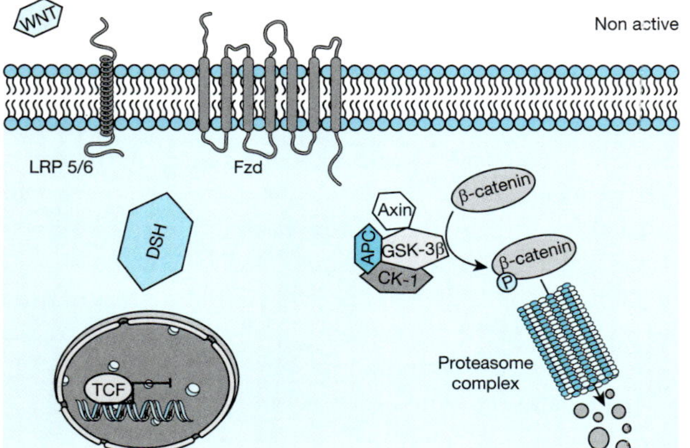

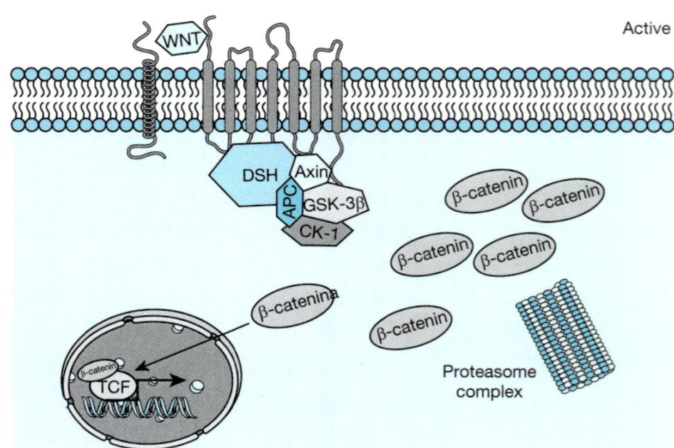

FIGURE 2.14. WNT activity. As shown in the figure, when WNT is not bound to the receptor at the cell membrane (left), beta-catenin is bound and does not act. When WNT binds to the receptor on the cell wall, it sets off a cascade effects leading to unbound beta-catenin, in turn leading to the upregulation of gene transcription. Abbreviations: WNT, Int/Wingless; APC, adenomatous polyposis coli; GSK-3beta, glycogen synthase kinase 3beta; CK-1, casein kinase-1. (From Manukjan N, Ahmed Z, Fulton D, Blankesteijn WM, Foulquier S. A systematic review of WNT signaling in endothelial cell oligodendrocyte interactions: potential relevance to cerebral small vessel disease. *Cells.* 2020;9(6):1545. doi:10.3390/cells9061545.)

WNT is bound at the cell wall to FZD (Frizzled) and coreceptor LRP5, a cascade of events in the cell leads to unbound beta-catenin (Figure 2.14, right side), which leads to the upregulation of gene transcription. Genes specifically transcribed as a result of this pathway include c-myc and Cyclin D1. In tumor cells, beta-catenin can be activated without the WNT pathway, leading to excess gene transcription. This can increase growth, proliferation, and development. In the setting of a particular mutation called APC, beta-catenin is not bound to inhibitors, and gene transcription is upregulated. This gene mutation is associated with colorectal cancer, observed in 50% of sporadic cases. In a recent pilot study, exercise was shown to decrease beta-catenin levels in breast cancer survivors (27). Further research is needed to better understand the potential for exercise to alter the WNT pathway in a manner relevant to cancer development.

DNA REPAIR IN NORMAL AND CANCER CELLS AND GENE INSTABILITY

Every day the genetic material in our cells, DNA, gets damaged 10,000+ times (28-30). This intrinsic damage can come in multiple forms (Figure 2.15) (31): nucleotides get damaged, matched up incorrectly, deleted, or added. The cells have repair pathways to deal with these errors. For example, there are redundant systems that ensure that the DNA base pairs are correct in all but 1 in 10 billion examples. Mutations to DNA can also occur because of extrinsic exposure to mutagens, including common chemicals, viruses, and environmental exposures. Some of these exposures are so common that there are specific enzymes in the body's cells to repair the damage caused by these mutations. Other exposures cause more extensive damage. For example, UV light exposure requires removal and replacement of a long strand of nucleotides, a system called nucleotide excision repair. Other exposures, such as exposure to heavy metals (cadmium, arsenic, or nickel) sever one or both strands of DNA. These repairs require the use of "sister" DNA (nearby DNA) to rebuild the DNA. The body has a variety of mechanisms to respond to intrinsic and extrinsic DNA damage intended to maintain genomic stability. These include mismatch repair, base excision repair, nucleotide excision repair, direct reversal, and the 2 types of response to double strand breaks: homologous recombination and nonhomologous end-joining. In normal tissues, these systems work to prevent extrinsic or intrinsic mutations from replicating.

One key characteristic of cancer cells is their capacity to evade or alter the DNA repair mechanisms and to develop increasing genetic instability or heterogeneity. Mutations in the genome of somatic cells lead to the activation of growth-promoting oncogenes and/or inactivation of tumor suppressor genes. This, in turn, leads to the expression of altered gene expression and loss of the normal regulatory processes in cells. If a tumor cell expands and adds more mutations, then it develops increasing heterogeneity. This can make it more difficult to treat, because multiple avenues would be needed to halt or reverse growth. In addition to the mutations noted above, genetic instability can be enhanced

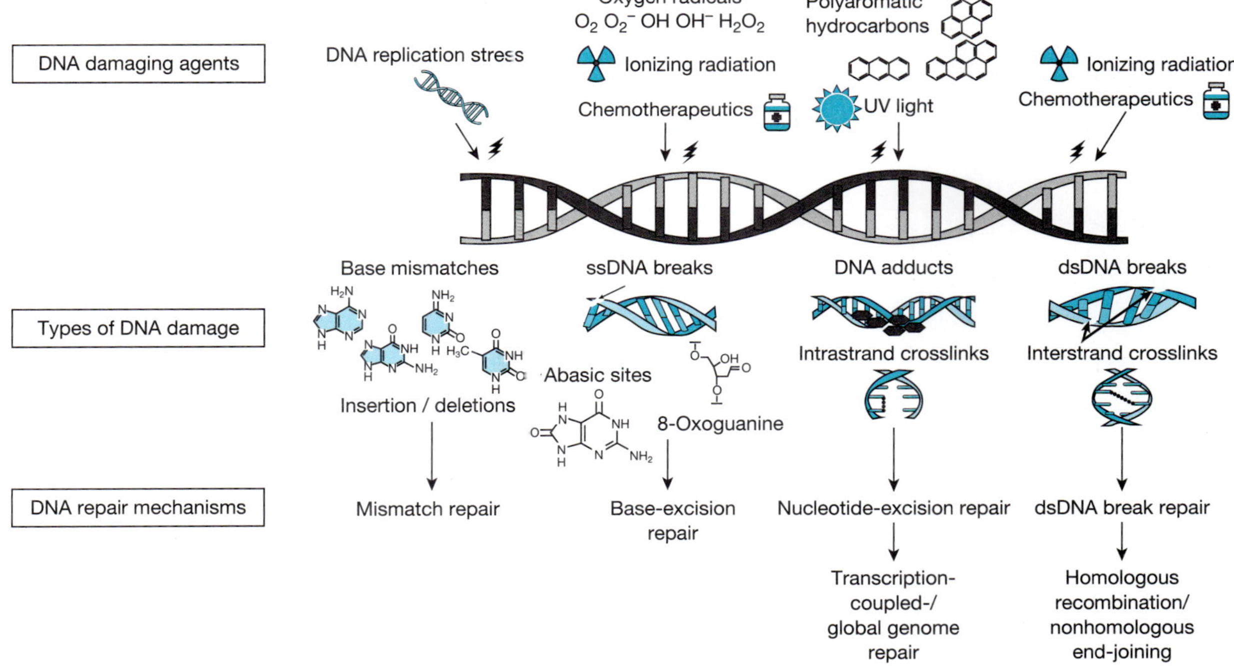

FIGURE 2.15. Types of DNA damaging agents, DNA damage, and DNA repair mechanisms. (From Helena JM, Joubert AM, Grobbelaar S, et al. Deoxyribonucleic acid damage and repair: capitalizing on our understanding of the mechanisms of maintaining genomic integrity for therapeutic purposes. *Int J Mol Sci.* 2018;19(4):1148, Figure 3. doi:10.3390/ijms19041148.)

by gene amplification, gene methylation, and acetylation. *Amplification* refers to gene expression that is enhanced above levels required for homeostasis. *Methylation* may control gene expression and cellular differentiation, altering cell cycle control, transcription, and altering the behavior of tumor suppressor genes. *Acetylation* induces proproliferative cell signaling through altered gene expression.

A number of treatments have been developed that take advantage of specific DNA repair damage from specific mutations e,g, the poly-ADP ribose polymerase or PARP inhibitors. PARP1 plays an important role in base excision repair within tumor cells. In cancer patients with a *BRCA* mutation, PARP inhibitors are effective treatments to stop tumors from repairing themselves by inhibiting base excision repair activity. Talazoparib and rucaparib are examples of PARP inhibitor drugs used for people living with breast cancer who have an altered *BRCA* gene.

ANGIOGENESIS

Angiogenesis is defined as the development of new blood vessels. All cells in the human body must be within 100 to 180 µm from the nearest functional blood vessel (capillary) in order to be viable. Capillaries deliver oxygen, nutrients, growth factors, and metabolites essential for cell survival. Cancer cells need a blood supply as much as normal cells. Cancer cells maintain access to the blood stream by growing around existing vessels (vascular cooption) or by developing their own blood vessels. The process by which tumors develop and maintain their blood supply has been a subject of study since the 1970s when Dr. Jonah Folkman (32) proposed the concept of targeting angiogenesis for therapeutic purposes. Antiangiogenic therapies target naturally occurring angiogenesis inhibitory pathways. One example is bevacizumab, a monoclonal antibody that works against angiogenic ligands or their receptors. Another example is trastuzumab that is used in the treatment of breast cancer that expresses the *HER2* gene. Trastuzumab works indirectly to promote antiangiogenic activity to block cancer growth.

One recent line of research in angiogenesis relevant to exercise oncology is the observation, in an animal model, that aerobic exercise normalizes the immature vasculature of a tumor, allowing chemotherapy to be delivered more efficiently and resulting in more reduction of tumor size than in animals treated with chemotherapy alone (33) (Figure 2.16).

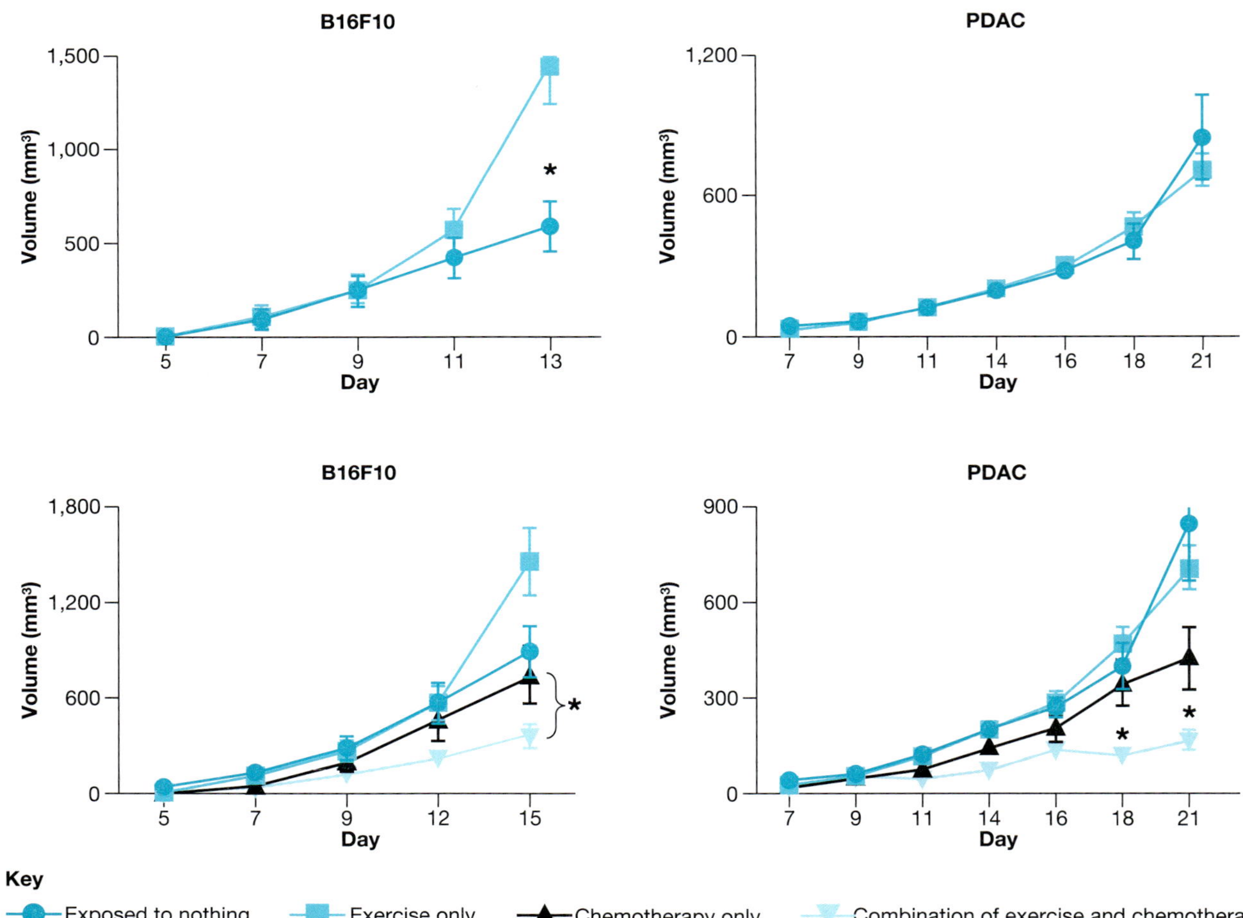

FIGURE 2.16. Exercise-induced shear stress increase chemotherapy efficacy. (From Schadler KL, Thomas NJ, Galie PA, et al. Tumor vessel normalization after aerobic exercise enhances chemotherapeutic efficacy. *Oncotarget*. 2016;7(40):65429–40. doi:10.18632/oncotarget.11748.)

It has been hypothesized that exercise would improve efficacy of chemotherapy; these data provide a possible mechanism for that hypothesis.

ESCAPING MORTALITY/ APOPTOSIS

As will be discussed in greater detail in the section "Tumor Heterogeneity," tumors are heterogeneous. In addition to cancerous cells, there are normal cells within tumors, as well as cancer stem cells. The number and variety of cancer stem cells are thought to explain both the amount of heterogeneity of tumors and the likelihood that they will evade normal programmed cell death, also called apoptosis. **Apoptosis** is defined as the process by which a cell commits to following a specific set of steps that ultimately destroys the cell. The signaling pathways that lead to apoptosis are well conserved across all animal species, an indication of their importance. There are 3 crucial purposes for apoptosis: growth, immune surveillance, and cancer prevention. The classic example given for the role of apoptosis in human growth and development is the programmed death of the cells that form the webbing between the fingers of an in utero developing fetus. In addition, apoptosis will eliminate T-cells that are immunologically deficient, to avoid auto-immunity. Cancer cells are among several types of cells killed off through apoptosis to protect the body from harm. We also destroy infected and damaged cells that are not cancerous.

There are predictable steps to the process of apoptosis. The breakdown of the cell starts with the extrinsic or intrinsic activation of proteins called caspases. Extrinsic activation can be caused by T-lymphocytes. Intrinsic activation is regulated by a balance of anti- and proapoptotic proteins in the mitochondria.

In the intrinsic pathway, a protein called BCL-2 is expressed on the membrane of the mitochondria that inhibits apoptosis from taking place. However, if there is damage to the cell, another protein called Bax moves to the mitochondria to block BCL-2, also poking a hole in the mitochondria, allowing cytochrome c to be released into the cytoplasm. This causes the activation of caspases, which cleave and breakdown the DNA and other internal structures within the cell, eventually killing the cell (34). A diagram of apoptosis is presented in Figure 2.17.

In the extrinsic pathway, the process originates outside the cell but eventually results in the caspase activation, leading to the same mechanism for cell death. The extrinsic pathway is started because there is a receptor on the outside of the cell that signals some kind of immune cell (perhaps a T cell) to bind to it, setting off the same cascade leading to the caspase cascade and cell death.

In addition, there is one other mechanism for apoptosis; it is the initiation of the apoptosis-initiating factor. If the cell is damaged in some way, this molecule is released, moves into the nucleus, and destroys the DNA of the cell.

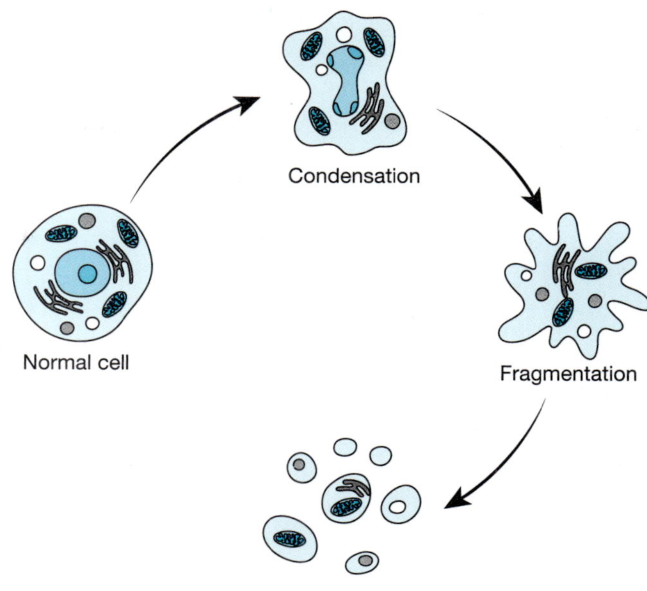

FIGURE 2.17. Apoptosis.

The discovery of specific antiapoptosis oncogenes led to a focus on developing therapeutic targets for this important cellular function. There are a limited number of approved anticancer drugs that directly target apoptotic pathways. These drugs are designed to inhibit antiapoptotic BCL-2 family members. Examples include venetoclax, a selective BCL-2 inhibitor approved for use in leukemias and lymphomas. Resistance to BCL-2 targeting therapies develops as a result of the modulation of expression and ongoing mutations.

CELL CYCLE CLOCK

Cells need to know when to grow and when to stop growing. The process by which this is regulated is a "clock" of sorts. The fate of individual cells throughout the body is dictated by the signals received from surroundings. Normal cells will not proliferate without some mitogenic growth factors. Some signaling may convince cells to enter a postmitotic state, the G0 phase, continuing to metabolize and contribute to body functions, but not growing or proliferating. The signals that help cells decide whether to enter the cell cycle are collected by the distinct cell surface receptors, funneled into a complex signal-processing circuitry in the cell cytoplasm. These signals lead to a decision to enter or not enter the cell cycle. The term **cell cycle clock** refers to the molecular circuitry operating in the cell nucleus that processes signals

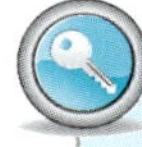

Apoptosis. Planned cell death.
Cell cycle clock. The process of cell division can be described as a clock, given a predictable sequence of events that comprise it measure times under particular circumstances.

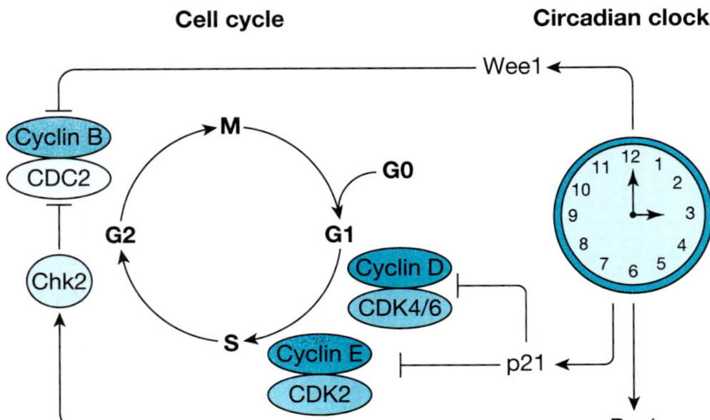

FIGURE 2.18. Cell cycle clock. Control by cyclins, phosphorylation to progress through the cell cycle. (From Aline Gréchez-Cassiau A, Rayet B, Guillaumond F, Teboul M, Delaunay F. The circadian clock component BMAL1 is a critical regulator of p21WAF1/CIP1 expression and hepatocyte proliferation. *J Biol Chem.* 2008;283(8): 4535–42, Figure 6.)

from outside and inside the cell, leading to the decision to proliferate or not. We have previously described the cell cycle phases of G1, S, G2, and M, as well as the quiescent state of G0.

Growth factors and external and internal factors influence the clock, which are essentially a series of interacting proteins. Most oncogenes and tumor suppressor genes can be explained in terms of their effect on the cell cycle clock. There are important checkpoints in the cell cycle that impose quality control to ensure that a cell has properly completed all the requisite steps of one phase of the cell cycle before it is allowed to advance into the next phase. The operation of these checkpoints influences the formation of tumors, with a particular focus on the process of deciding to enter the G1 phase or late in G1, the restriction point, when the cell is given license to make decisions. For example, during the G1 phase, cells are responsive to mitogenic growth factors. Toward the end of G1, there is a restriction point. Entrance to the S phase is blocked if there is evidence of genome damage. Deregulation of the restriction point decision-making machinery is associated with the formation of most types of cancer cells. If the process proceeds into the S phase and genome damage is noted, DNA replication is halted. During G2, DNA replication completion is required for entrance into the M phase.

As shown in Figure 2.18 (35), the cell cycle clock is controlled by cyclins and cyclin-dependent kinases (CDKs). Phosphorylation of these cyclins by CDKs plays an important role in the progress through the cell cycle. For example, phosphorylation of proteins prior to the S phase enables DNA replication sites along the chromosomes to be activated. CDKs are rational targets for cancer therapy because their expression is often altered in tumor cells. Their inhibition can result in tumor death. Inhibitors of CDKs can also block transcription. One example of a CDK inhibitor is ribociclib, a CDK 4/6 inhibitor approved for use in metastatic breast cancer.

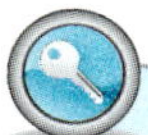

Invasion. Direct extension and penetration by cancer cells into neighboring tissues.

Metastasis. Spread of cancer cells from where they first formed to another part of the body.

INVASION AND METASTASIS

Invasion

Invasion is defined as the direct extension and penetration by tumor cells into neighboring tissues (36). For this to occur, tumors need to undergo a loss of contact inhibition (Figure 2.19). This means a loss of normal cessation of cellular movement, growth, and division upon contact with other cells. Contact inhibition enables noncancerous cells to cease proliferation and growth when they contact each other. This characteristic is lost when cells undergo malignant transformation. This loss of contact inhibition contributes to uncontrolled proliferation and solid tumor formation.

Metastasis and the Metastatic Cascade

Metastasis

Metastasis is defined as the spread of a tumor to sites that are physically discontinuous with the primary tumor (eg, metastasis to the lung from a primary breast tumor). Metastasis marks a tumor as being malignant, as benign tumors are incapable of spreading to distant sites. Approximately 30% of cancers are present as metastatic tumors. The likelihood of

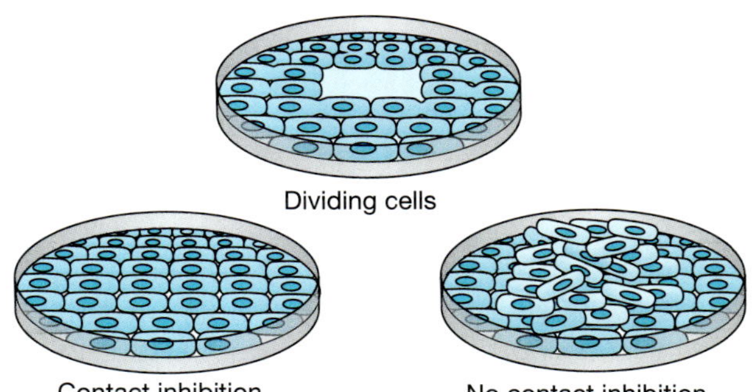

FIGURE 2.19. Contact inhibition. Normal cells, when given space to grow, stop at a natural barrier, such as the edge of a petri dish. Cancer cells exhibit a loss of contact inhibition and continue to divide, piling on top of each other.

metastasis correlates with the lack of differentiation, aggressive local invasion, rapid growth, and large size, although there are always exceptions. Metastasis is a complex and unpredictable process that is typically described as having 5 major steps: 1. invasion, 2. intravasation, 3. survival in the circulation, 4. extravasation, and 5. establishment of a new growth. For metastasis, tumor cells must accumulate a metastatic phenotype, including complementary genetic and epigenetic alterations, as well as a conducive TME. This process is called the *metastatic cascade*.

Metastatic Cascade

The metastatic cascade starts with the invasion of the extracellular matrix, followed by vascular dissemination, tissue homing (eg, the selective preference of tumor tissues for certain organs as sites of metastasis), and colonization. To invade the extracellular matrix, first tumor cells have to experience mutations that lead to the loss of glycoproteins that cause tumor cell adhesion. There is some evidence for a process called the epithelial-mesenchymal transition in metastasis. In this transition, a tumor cell loses properties of epithelial cells and gains markers of mesenchymal cells, which then favors the development of a promigratory cell phenotype. Not all metastatic tumors undergo this full transition, but it is included here to illustrate the complexities of the metastatic process. There are specific transcriptional factors that promote the metastatic transition. When one or more tumor cells has made this transition, the basement membrane of the primary site undergoes remodeling to allow the invasion of the tumor cell into the extracellular matrix. Simultaneously, chemotactic, angiogenic, and growth factors are released that promote the movement of the tumor cells out of the primary site.

Next, the cells experience locomotion, which is a multistep process promoting the movement of the tumor cells from the extracellular matrix into the bloodstream. The factors involved in this step include chemokines and growth factors released by the tumor cells, which act as autocrine motility factors, as well as alterations to the extracellular matrix, and paracrine factors from stromal cells. As shown in Figure 2.20 (37), the tumor penetrates blood vessels by intravasation through the basement membrane of the blood vessel, after which they travel to distant sites. While traveling through the bloodstream, tumor cells undergo changes that allow them to survive and evade the immune system, including coagulation factors and attachment to platelets. Tumor cells migrate as multicellular aggregates (groups), and some of the tumor cells will have the properties of stem cells, which helps them grow in a new site. One theory of metastasis posits that primary tumors do not need as many mutations as originally thought if cancer stem cells are present that guide the process of metastasis.

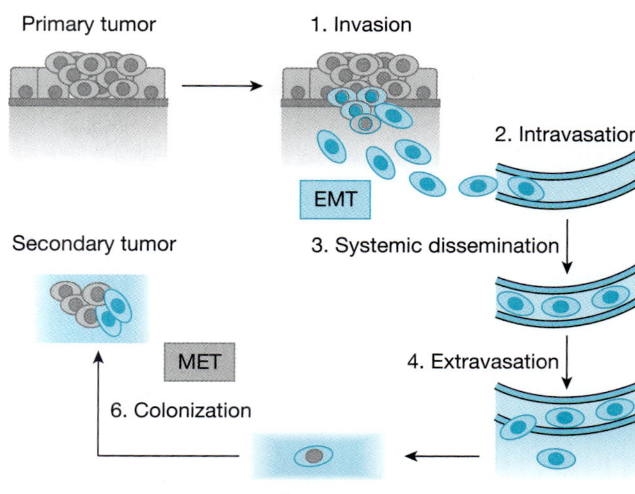

FIGURE 2.20. Steps by which tumors become metastatic. The first step is the invasion of the basement membrane to leave the tissue where the primary tumor started. Step 2 is intravasation, meaning the cells enter the bloodstream. In Step 3, the cells disseminate throughout the body. The cancer cells have preference for specific tissues bed and escape the bloodstream at those sites (often lung, liver, and bone), at which time the cancer cells may become dormant but, at some point in the future, may colonize the new site, causing a secondary tumor. (From Scheel C, Weinberg RA. Cancer stem cells and epithelial mesenchymal transition: concepts and molecular links. *Semi Cancer Biol.* 2012;22(5e6):396e403.)

Extravasation from the blood stream and vascular remodeling to allow other tumor cells to join the secondary tumor site require many of the same factors required to leave the primary site. The 3 factors determine the site of exit from the bloodstream:

- First, the location and vascular drainage of the primary tumor (the nearest organ—eg, lung is the nearest organ for the breast).
- Second, tumor cells express adhesion molecules whose ligands are found preferentially on the endothelial cells of a particular organ. This fits with Paget's "seed and soil" hypothesis that posits that tumor cells interact with host organs to favor or hinder metastases.
- Third, there is the hypothesis of escape from tumor dormancy. This refers to the possibility that metastatic cells exit the bloodstream and fail to grow in the secondary site, and so they become dormant. But factors can change and cause the tumor to come out of dormancy and start to grow again, sometimes a decade later. Once the tumor cell group reaches the location favorable for the growth of a secondary tumor, it will egress through the basement membrane of the blood vessel by the action of adhesion molecules, proteolytic enzymes, and chemokines. Tumor cells secrete growth factors and cytokines that act on stromal cells that work to make the metastatic site habitable.

The most common routes through which tumor cells travel through the body to secondary sites are the lymph system, the blood system, and direct seeding of body cavities or surfaces.

Once tumor cells reach the site of possible metastasis, most of them die because of the selective pressure of the new environment. Those that survive are likely to modify their environment to support growth, a step called **colonization**. They might secrete or inhibit peptides to create space for the growth of metastases. Metastatic growth requires successful recruitment of several cell types. At this point in tumor growth, the immune system places an outsized role in stopping the growth of the secondary tumor.

TUMOR IMMUNOLOGY

How the Immune System Fights Cancer

Our immune systems work to prevent and fight cancer, and the elements of the immune system can be used to develop special treatments called immunotherapy. One of the hallmarks of cancer cells is that they can evade the immune system. Therefore, some researchers (38) have noted that the TME is the site of an ongoing battle between the immune system, which seeks to eliminate cancer when it arises, and the tumor, which acts to adapt and evade immune system efforts. As shown in Figure 2.21, there are 3 stages in the immune surveillance against cancer: elimination, equilibrium, and escape.

Elimination is the earliest stage during which the immune system works to recognize and destroy developing tumors before they become clinically apparent. At this stage, innate and adaptive immunity works to prevent cancer progression.

Equilibrium describes the phase when there are residual tumor cells not destroyed in the elimination phase, but which have not evaded the immune system yet. At this phase, there is increasing genetic instability and immune selection. During both elimination and equilibrium, our immune cells work to kill tumor cells. For example, NK cells sense a damaged or stressed tissue, such as tumor cells, and destroy them. Dendritic cells will activate cytotoxic T cells, which then bind to tumor cells as well. Once bound to the tumor cells, the NK cells and cytotoxic T cells release chemokines and some inflammatory factors that poke holes in the tumor cells, causing them to undergo apoptosis. Helper T cells help the dendritic cells and release cytokines that contribute to the cell-mediated immune response to tumors, by recruiting and activating more cytotoxic T cells and NK cells.

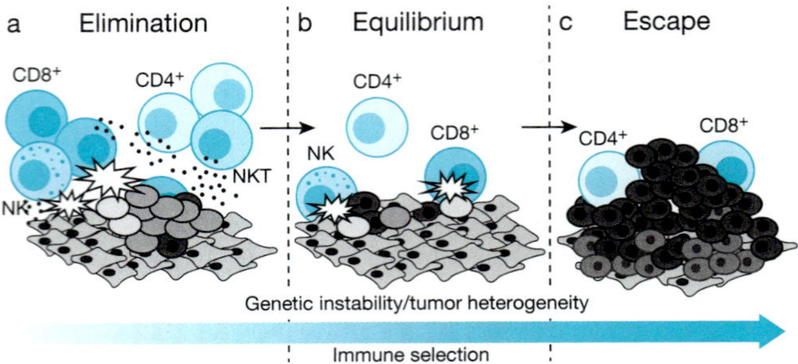

FIGURE 2.21. Tumor immunology stages: elimination, equilibrium, escape.

The third phase of immune surveillance against cancer is called *escape*. During the escape phase in the battle between the immune system and the tumor, genetic changes occur within a tumor, which allow the tumor to evade the immune response just described. This can occur because tumors fail to express the factors that are recognized by the immune cells, or express the factors that kill the immune cell, or act to suppress the immune cells. There are many accelerators and brakes in the TME that can also alter the effectiveness of the immune response to a tumor. The entire immune system is a balance of stimulatory (accelerator) and inhibitory (brakes) activities, and the balance of these factors strongly influences the likelihood of the development and progression of a tumor. An example of the inhibitory action of the immune system is a T regulatory cell that can kill the cytotoxic T cells and NK cells if conditions promote this activity. Over time, the only tumor cells left are the ones that cannot be recognized by the immune system, a process known as immunoediting. Tumor cells can also express specific inhibitors for immune response, such as PDL1, which then bind to PD1 on the cytotoxic T cell, inactivating it. This is called an immune checkpoint. Tumors can also attract certain types of immunosuppressive cells that inhibit the activity of NK cells and cytotoxic T cells, promoting tumor growth.

Boosting the Body's Immune Response

Recent advances have allowed for the use of the immune system to boost the body's response to a tumor, using some of the checks and balances inherent in the immune system. For example, T cells can be taken from the patient, the best killers isolated and then reinjected into the patient. This is called chimeric antigen receptor T-cell (CAR-T) therapy. Patients can also be treated with cytokines, such as interferon (INF) and other factors intended to boost the immune response. Alternatively, the immune checkpoints can be targeted. For example, an antibody can block PDL1 expressed on the tumor, preventing binding with PD1 and allowing the cytotoxic T cell to destroy

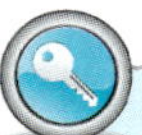

Colonization. Final biological events required for cancer cells to form a clinically relevant metastasis at a distant site in the body.

the tumor cell. This is called an immune checkpoint inhibitor. These approaches can be combined with chemotherapy to improve treatment response. That said, when we activate the immune system, adverse effects can occur, such as skin reactions, flu-like symptoms, muscle aches, shortness of breath, and hormone changes, among others.

There is a robust evidence base in the field of exercise immunology that suggests that exercise may play an important role in the success of immunotherapy. For example, moderate exercise increases NK cells and their activities. However, there have been no human studies, to date, that have tested the potential for exercise to improve outcomes for cancer patients receiving immunotherapy.

VIRUSES AND CANCER

We generally think of cancers as being primarily caused by smoking and other lifestyle factors, UV radiation exposure, air pollution, and other common exposures. However, viruses contribute to about 20% of all cancer incidence worldwide (39, 40). Viruses act at a variety of stages of tumorigenesis and in a multitude of ways. Some work as direct carcinogens, contributing to the transformation of cancer cells. Others work as indirect carcinogens, acting through chronic infection and inflammation that, in turn, leads to carcinogenic mutations. Yet others work in completely different ways and do not fit into the direct or indirect category. In general, tumors associated with immunosuppression are more likely to be caused by a virus. The viruses associated with cancer are noted in Table 2.2. Immunosuppression may occur as a result of underlying disease (hepatitis B, HIV), use of drugs to avoid organ rejection after transplant, or aging.

There is a common paradox in the relationship of viruses and cancer that has complicated the ability of scientists to establish a causal link between viruses and cancer. For several of the viruses that are known to cause cancer, a large proportion of the population is infected (eg, 80% of the population is infected with HPV at some point), but a very small proportion of the infected population develops cancer. The reasons for this are many, including the observation that there are over 200 types of HPVs, but only a small number of these are carcinogenic. A common feature of tumorigenic viruses is their ability to evade the immune system by turning off proteins that might be sensed by cell-mediated immune factors. Common targets for the role of tumorigenesis for viruses include *p53*, WNT, P13K, AKT, mTOR, and beta-catenin, some of which have been discussed earlier in the sections "Tumor Suppressor Gene *p53*" and "Int/Wingless." Viruses can also target cell cycle checkpoints and antiapoptotic mechanisms and might contribute to genomic instability, all of which may contribute to carcinogenesis. Overall, viruses compound the acquired genetic mutations in infected cells, contributing to tumorigenesis.

The first virus recognized to cause cancer was observed by Dr. Peyton Rous and is called the Rous sarcoma virus

Table 2.2 Viruses Associated With Cancers

VIRUS	CANCER
Epstein-Barr virus	• 40% of Hodgkin's lymphoma • >95% of endemic Burkitt lymphoma • 10% gastric carcinoma • Most (types II and III) nasopharyngeal carcinoma • Kaposi sarcoma • Other lymphomas
Hepatitis B virus	• 53% of hepatocellular carcinoma
Human T-lymphotropic virus 1	• >99% of adult T cell leukemia
Human papillomavirus	• >95% of cervical carcinoma • 70% of oropharyngeal carcinoma • Other anogenital carcinomas
Hepatitis C virus	• 25% of hepatocellular carcinoma • Non-Hodgkin's B cell lymphomas
Kaposi sarcoma-associated herpesvirus	• >99% of Kaposi sarcoma • >99% of primary effusion lymphoma
Merkel cell polyomavirus	• 80% of Merkel cell carcinoma

Adapted from Krump NA, You J. Molecular mechanisms of viral oncogenesis in humans. *Nat Rev Microbiol*. 2018;16(11):684–98. https://doi.org/10.1038/s41579-018-0064-6.

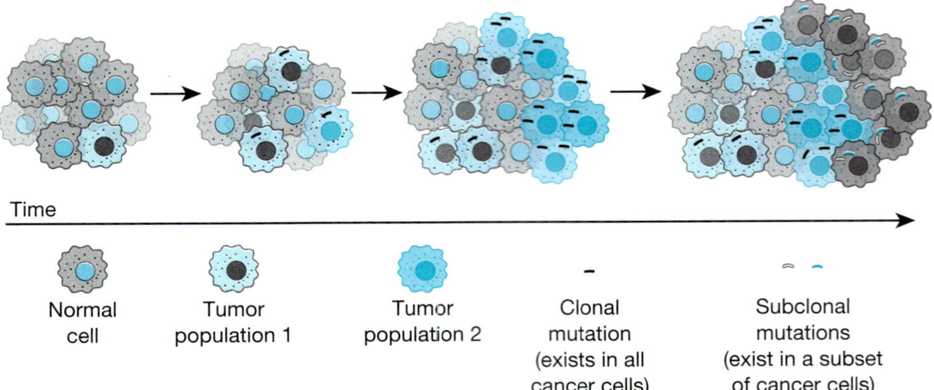

FIGURE 2.22. Tumor heterogeneity. The concept is that the normal cells develop mutations leading to cancer, but additional mutations develop over time, meaning that while the tumor started as just the lightest blue type of cells shown below, eventually the darker blue type of cancer cells develop. The challenge in this situation is that the drugs developed to treat this cancer may kill the light blue cancer cells and do nothing to the darker blue cancer cells, allowing them to grow unchecked, untreated. (From El-Sayes N, Vito A, Mossman K. Tumor heterogeneity: a great barrier in the age of cancer immunotherapy. *Cancers*. 2021;13(4):806. https://doi.org/10.3390/cancers13040806.)

(RSV), a retrovirus that causes sarcomas in chickens (41). The RSV virus results in the mutation of the *src* gene, which has important roles in growth signaling, angiogenesis, survival, proliferation, and motility or invasion. It does so through altering pathways discussed earlier, including *p53*, WNT, MAPK, and others. The first human virus identified to be an oncovirus was the EBV. EBV targets the B lymphocyte, causing latent infection and, under the right conditions, might contribute to tumorigenesis. EBV acts through an indirect pathway of carcinogenesis. These viruses can be transmitted between humans and can establish chronic infections that can sometimes last years, sometimes without any symptoms, and very few result in the development of cancer.

TUMOR HETEROGENEITY

One challenge of treating cancer is that cancers vary between patients (interpatient) and within patients (intrapatient). **Tumor heterogeneity** is defined as the differences between and within tumors in gene expression, pathophysiology, and molecular features that are associated with variations in tumor phenotypes, such as tumor aggressiveness and sensitivity to treatment, as shown in Figure 2.22. This is supposed to result from a concept called clonal evolution that assumes that we acquire cumulative mutations as cancer develops, leading to multiple subclonal populations. Contributors to this heterogeneity include genetic mutations, epigenetic factors (such as microRNA), and the TME. As a cancer develops, mutations add up; some are more important to the further development of the cancer, whereas others come along for the ride, becoming important only if particular conditions are present. Treatment targets tend to focus on the more important mutations, but the likelihood of treatment success might relate to both the number and types of mutations.

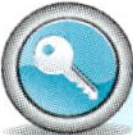

Tumor heterogeneity. Differences between tumors of the same type in different patients, the differences between cancer cells in a single tumor, or differences between cells in a primary versus and secondary (metastatic) site.

Clinicians may respond to this by testing the genetic signature of a tumor or series of tumor samples to understand what specific mutations are present, so that they know which treatments will work the best to treat the cancer. As an example, genomic signatures can predict responses of metastatic melanoma to immune checkpoint blockade therapies (42-46). This is called personalized medicine and is described further in Figure 2.23.

Tumor heterogeneity explains why treatments fail in some patients. The concept of personalized medicine could be important to targeting exercise as an adjunct to cancer therapies, as exercise might be more helpful for targeting particular genetic profiles. For example, it could be hypothesized that exercise would be particularly useful in the setting of an RAS mutation, given downstream effects on metabolism for that pathway. Research has only just started to understand whether exercise might be of particular value in some subsets of patients. Until we know otherwise, the recommendation is to prescribe exercise to all patients undergoing treatment, with a focus on the benefits of addressing the side effects and symptoms of treatment (see Chapter 8).

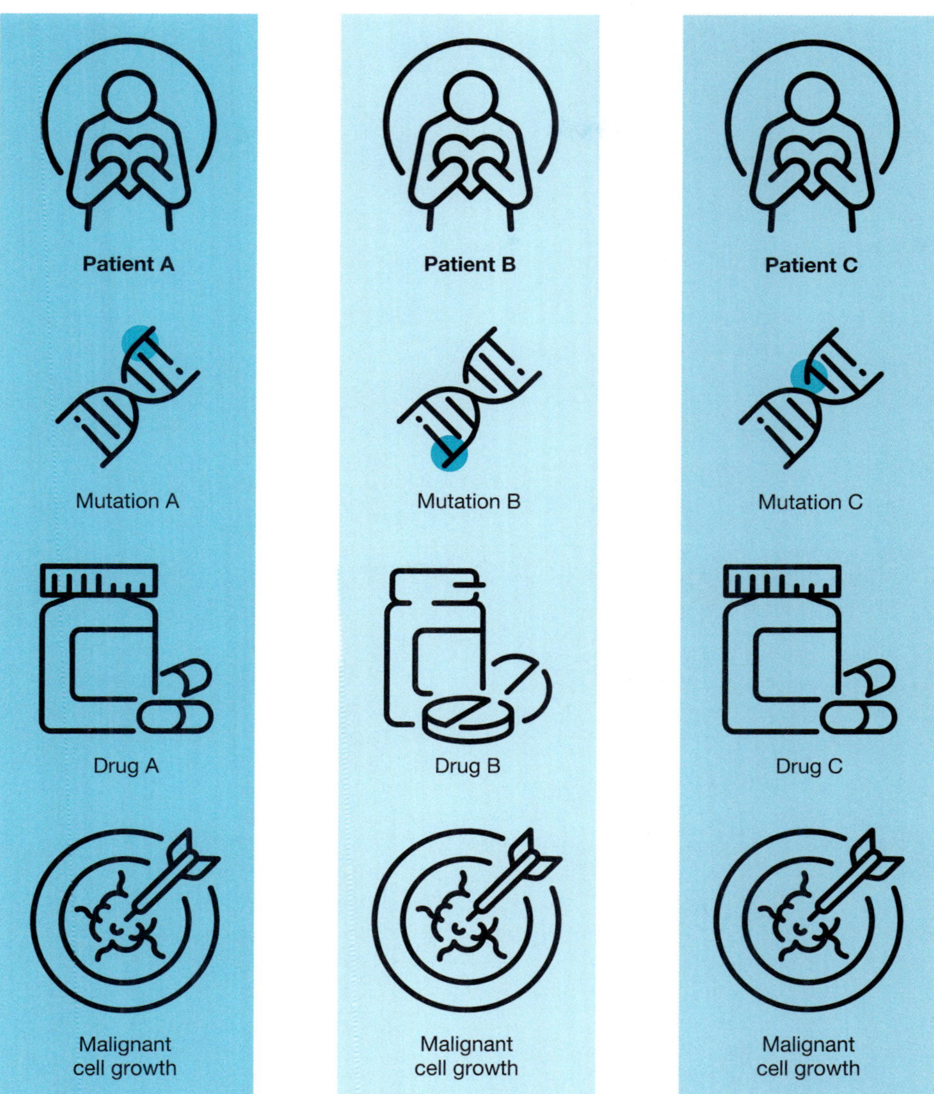

FIGURE 2.23. Personalized medicine. Patients are tested for specific mutations and treated with the drugs that are specific to their mutation for best treatment outcomes.

SUMMARY

The development of cancer is a complex biological process. By better understanding this process, scientists have uncovered several opportunities for treatment. These treatments, while lifesaving, exert a pressure in the form of symptoms, side effects, and long-term effects discussed elsewhere in this book. Exercise has the capacity to interrupt the process of developing cancer, as well as to address the symptoms and side effects of treatment. Ongoing research is exploring the biological underpinnings of the purported link between physical inactivity and cancer risk. Much of this research will take place in animal model studies. Until we have more complete data regarding the biological effects of exercise on tumor development, we prescribe exercise to address treatment symptoms and side effects.

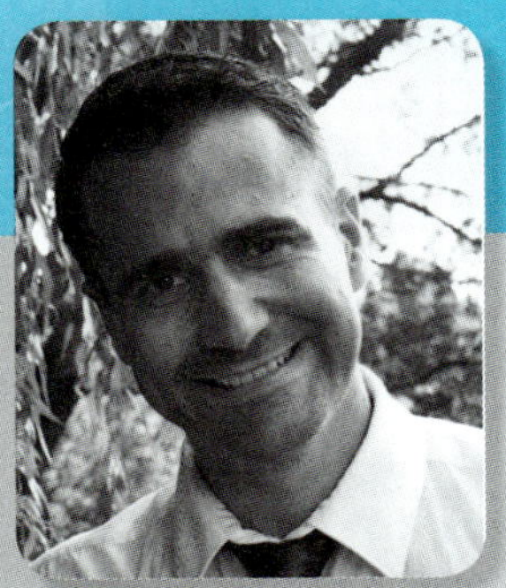

Meet the Expert

FEATURED PROFESSIONAL

Jesper Frank Christensen, MSc, PhD

Senior Researcher, Center for Physical Activity Research, Rigshospitalet, Denmark
Associate Professor in Exercise as Medicine, University of Southern Denmark

Q: "Where did you grow up?"

In Uvelse, a small village 30 kilometers outside of Copenhagen, Denmark.

Q: "Where did you train? What is your training?"

I did my master's degree in Human Physiology at the Department of Nutrition and Exercise Science, Copenhagen University. Almost by coincidence, I then stumbled onto a position as a research assistant, which led to a PhD position within the Body and Cancer program at the Department of Oncology, Rigshospitalet, Copenhagen University Hospital.

Q: "What are you best known for?"

My PhD project—the Progressive Resistance Training and Cancer Tests (PROTRACT) study—was the first exercise trial to collect muscle biopsies in patients undergoing chemotherapy, gaining some of the very first molecular data on muscle adaptation to exercise during toxic systemic therapy. In continuation, I have largely focused on mechanistic and integrative physiological experiments conducted within the specialized (and diverse) settings of modern clinical oncology in patients with esophageal-gastric, colorectal, pancreatic, and prostate cancer.

Q: "What are you currently working on?"

In parallel with research into the clinical application of exercise training, I am recently drawn to more explorative work into the role of "integrative pathophysiology" in cancer. Specifically, if, how, and why patients' general physiological (dys)function, for example, homeostatic control, immune function, interorgan crosstalk, etc, influences tumor pathogenesis, treatment response/tolerability, and late effects.

Favorite Quote:

"It's not the will to win, that matters—everyone has that. It is the will to prepare to win, that matters."
—*Paul "Bear" Bryant*

STUDY QUESTIONS

1. The term for programmed cell death is ____________________.
2. In the classic model of tumor development, there are 3 phases:
   a. Promotion, progression, and metastasis
   b. Initiation, promotion, and progression
   c. DNA damage, loss of contact inhibition, and metastasis
   d. Oxidative damage, cell cycle changes, and metastasis
3. Name 3 of the hallmarks of cancer cells.
4. A proto-oncogene is:
   a. A gene that has not yet been mutated in a way that causes cancer
   b. A gene that has been mutated in a way that increases the function of a protein
   c. A gene that has been mutated in a way that leads to the loss of the function of a protein
5. A gatekeeper gene refers to a gene that:
   a. Controls the tumor microenvironment
   b. Maintains the integrity of the genome
   c. Encode proteins that regulate cell proliferation
6. The doubling time of human tumors ranges from:
   a. 1 to 5 days
   b. 10 to 1,000 days
   c. 27 to 83 days
   d. 3 to 9 months
7. The tumor microenvironment refers to:
   a. The hormonal levels in the tissue around a tumor
   b. The ecosystem that surrounds the tumor in the body
   c. The microtubules that feed the tumor
   d. The way the environment of the tumor appears in a microscope
8. True or false. Loss of AMP-activated protein kinase signaling supports a shift toward glycolytic metabolism in tumors and surrounding tissue.

9. Reversal of the Warburg effect is a possible mechanism through which exercise may prevent cancer. This means that:
   a. Exercise increases aerobic fitness and decreases body fat
   b. Exercise improves symptoms during cancer treatment
   c. Exercise increases genomic stability
   d. Exercise increases mitochondrial function and lactate clearance capacity
10. True or false. Tumor promoters cause tumors to form.
11. Mutations in the genes that encode receptor tyrosine kinase can result in:
   a. Altered growth factor signaling
   b. Overexpression of receptor tyrosine kinase
   c. Altered function of receptor tyrosine kinase
   d. All of the above
12. Understanding cell signaling in a cancer cell is made more complex because of the backdrop of:
   a. The tumor microenvironment
   b. Gene mutations and genetic instability
   c. Hypoxic environment
   d. The Warburg effect
13. The genetic material in our cells, called DNA, gets damaged ______ times per day, even without cancer.
   a. 10
   b. 100
   c. 1,000
   d. 10,000
   e. 1 million
14. There are multiple ways the body has to repair DNA damage and, in turn, prevent cancer. Name 3.
15. Trastuzumab is a drug used to treat breast cancer. It works by:
   a. Preventing the growth of blood vessels
   b. Repairing DNA through mismatch repair
   c. Reducing oxidative stress
   d. Blocking mutations to growth factor receptors
16. What are the 3 crucial purposes for apoptosis?
17. The cell cycle clock refers to:
   a. The loss of function that occurs in cells with cancer with respect to time
   b. The process by which cells know when to grow and when to stop
   c. The way we know when to wake up
   d. The way cells speed up and slow down activities according to the intake of ketones
18. The loss of normal cessation of cellular movement, growth, and division upon contact with other cells is a definition of:
   a. Loss of contact inhibition
   b. Tumor microenvironment inhibition
   c. Cyclin B mutation history
   d. The Warburg effect
19. The 3 stages in immune surveillance against cancer are:
   a. Mitochondrial transition, ketogenic monitoring, and growth factor mutations
   b. Watchful waiting, active treatment, and survivorship
   c. Elimination, equilibrium, and escape
   d. Escape, mutation, and release
20. Viruses such as Epstein-Barr, HPV, and HIV contribute to ___ % of cancers worldwide.
   a. 2
   b. 90
   c. 50
   d. 20
21. Tumor heterogeneity:
   a. Refers to the variety of ways a tumor expresses mutations when examining one patient versus another
   b. Is one of the reasons treatments fail
   c. Explains why exercise won't work for some patients
   d. a and b
   e. b and c
   f. All of the above

REFERENCES

1. Genetics Glossary. *Cell Cycle*. [Internet]. 2023. Available from www.genome.gov/genetics-glossary/cell-cycle
2. Leaf DA, Kleinman MT, Hamilton M, Deitrick RW. The exercise-induced oxidative stress paradox: the effects of physical exercise training. *Am J Med Sci*. 999;317(5):295–300. doi:10.1097/00000441-199905000-00005
3. Hanahan D, Weinberg RA. The hallmarks of cancer. *Cell*. 2000; 100(1):57–70. doi:10.1016/s0092-8674(00)81683-9
4. Hanahan D, Weinberg RA. Hallmarks of cancer: the next generation. *Cell*. 2011;144(5):646–74. doi:10.1016/j.cell.2011.02.013
5. Rassy E, Assi T, Pavlidis N. Exploring the biological hallmarks of cancer of unknown primary: where do we stand today? *Br J Cancer*. 2020;122(8):1124–32. doi:10.1038/s41416-019-0723-z
6. DeBerardinis RJ, Lum JJ, Hatzivassiliou G, Thompson CB. The biology of cancer: metabolic reprogramming fuels cell growth and proliferation. *Cell Metab*. 2008;7(1):11–20. doi:10.1016/j.cmet.2007.10.002
7. Feldman SR, Yaar M. Oncogenes: the growth control genes. *Arch Dermatol*. 1991;127(5):707–11. doi:10.1001/archderm.127.5.707
8. Goodsell DS. The molecular perspective: the RAS oncogene. *Stem Cells*. 1999;17(4):235–6. doi:10.1002/stem.170235

9. Boutelle AM, Attardi LD. P53 and tumor suppression: it takes a network. *Trends Cell Biol.* 2021;31(4):298–310. doi:10.1016/j.tcb.2020.12.011
10. Lee EY, Muller WJ. Oncogenes and tumor suppressor genes. *Cold Spring Harb Perspect Biol.* 2010;2(10):a003236. doi:10.1101/cshperspect.a003236
11. Weinberg RS. Goal setting and performance in sport and exercise settings: a synthesis and critique. *Med Sci Sports Exerc.* 1994;26(4):469–77.
12. Deininger P. Genetic instability in cancer: caretaker and gatekeeper genes. *Ochsner J.* 1999;1(4):206–9.
13. Macleod K. Tumor suppressor genes. *Curr Opin Genet Dev.* 2000; 10(1):81–93. doi:10.1016/s0959-437x(99)00041-6
14. Milinkovic V, Bankovic J, Rakic M, et al. Genomic instability and p53 alterations in patients with malignant glioma. *Exp Mol Pathol.* 2012;93(2):200–6. doi:10.1016/j.yexmp.2012.05.010
15. Tubiana M. Tumor cell proliferation kinetics and tumor growth rate. *Acta Oncol.* 1989;28(1):113–21. doi:10.3109/02841868909111193
16. Wertheimer MD, Costanza ME, Dodson TF, D'Orsi C, Pastides H, Zapka JG. Increasing the effort toward breast cancer detection. *JAMA.* 1986;255(10):1311–15.
17. Hassan G, Seno M. Blood and cancer: cancer stem cells as origin of hematopoietic cells in solid tumor microenvironments. *Cells.* 2020;9(5):1293. doi:10.3390/cells9051293
18. Wiggins JM, Opoku-Acheampong AB, Baumfalk DR, Siemann DW, Behnke BJ. Exercise and the tumor microenvironment: potential therapeutic implications. *Exerc Sport Sci Rev.* 2018;46(1):56–64. doi:10.1249/JES.0000000000000137
19. Jadvar H, Alavi A, Gambhir SS. 18F-FDG uptake in lung, breast, and colon cancers: molecular biology correlates and disease characterization. *J Nucl Med.* 2009;50(11):1820–7. doi:10.2967/jnumed.108.054098
20. El-Galaly TC, Gormsen LC, Hutchings M. PET/CT for staging; past, present, and future. *Semin Nucl Med.* 2018;48(1):4–16. doi:10.1053/j.semnuclmed.2017.09.001
21. Liu J, Song N, Huang Y, Chen Y. Irisin inhibits pancreatic cancer cell growth via the AMPK-mTOR pathway. *Sci Rep.* 2018;8(1):15247. doi:10.1038/s41598-018-33229-w
22. San-Millan I, Brooks GA. Reexamining cancer metabolism: lactate production for carcinogenesis could be the purpose and explanation of the Warburg effect. *Carcinogenesis.* 2017;38(2):119–33. doi:10.1093/carcin/bgw127
23. Fujiki H, Sueoka E, Suganuma M. Tumor promoters: from chemicals to inflammatory proteins. *J Cancer Res Clin Oncol.* 2013;139(10):1603–14. doi:10.1007/s00432-013-1455-8
24. Yang H, Liu Y, Kong J. Effect of aerobic exercise on acquired gefitinib resistance in lung adenocarcinoma. *Transl Oncol.* 2021;14(11):101204. doi:10.1016/j.tranon.2021.101204
25. Meister M, Tomasovic A, Banning A, Tikkanen R. Mitogen-activated protein (MAP) kinase scaffolding proteins: a recount. *Int J Mol Sci.* 2013;14(3):4854–84. doi:10.3390/ijms14034854
26. Manukjan N, Ahmed Z, Fulton D, Blankesteijn WM, Foulquier S. A systematic review of WNT signaling in endothelial cell oligodendrocyte interactions: potential relevance to cerebral small vessel disease. *Cells.* 2020;9(6):1545. doi:10.3390/cells9061545
27. Chang JS, Kim TH, Kong ID. Exercise intervention lowers aberrant serum WISP-1 levels with insulin resistance in breast cancer survivors: a randomized controlled trial. *Sci Rep.* 2020;10(1):10898. doi:10.1038/s41598-020-67794-w
28. Lord CJ, Ashworth A. The DNA damage response and cancer therapy. *Nature.* 2012;481(7381):287–94. doi:10.1038/nature10760
29. Kalimutho M, Nones K, Srihari S, Duijf PHG, Waddell N, Khanna KK. Patterns of genomic instability in breast cancer. *Trends Pharmacol Sci.* 2019;40(3):198–211. doi:10.1016/j.tips.2019.01.005
30. Klinakis A, Karagiannis D, Rampias T. Targeting DNA repair in cancer: current state and novel approaches. *Cell Mol Life Sci.* 2020;77(4):677–703. doi:10.1007/s00018-019-03299-8
31. Helena JM, Joubert AM, Grobbelaar S, et al. Deoxyribonucleic acid damage and repair: capitalizing on our understanding of the mechanisms of maintaining genomic integrity for therapeutic purposes. *Int J Mol Sci.* 2018;19(4):1148. doi:10.3390/ijms19041148
32. Folkman J. Tumor angiogenesis: therapeutic implications. *N Engl J Med.* 1971;285(21):1182–6. doi:10.1056/NEJM197111182852108
33. Schadler KL, Thomas NJ, Galie PA, et al. Tumor vessel normalization after aerobic exercise enhances chemotherapeutic efficacy. *Oncotarget.* 2016;7(40):65429–40. doi:10.18632/oncotarget.11748
34. Genetics Glossary. *Apoptosis.* [Internet]. 2024. Available from https://www.genome.gov/genetics-glossary/apoptosis
35. Grechez-Cassiau A, Rayet B, Guillaumond F, Teboul M, Delaunay F. The circadian clock component BMAL1 is a critical regulator of p21WAF1/CIP1 expression and hepatocyte proliferation. *J Biol Chem.* 2008;283(8):4535–42. doi:10.1074/jbc.M705576200
36. Friedl P, Alexander S. Cancer invasion and the microenvironment: plasticity and reciprocity. *Cell.* 2011;147(5):992–1009. doi:10.1016/j.cell.2011.11.016
37. Beuran M, Negoi I, Paun S, et al. The epithelial to mesenchymal transition in pancreatic cancer: a systematic review. *Pancreatology.* 2015;15(3):217–25. doi:10.1016/j.pan.2015.02.011
38. Chew V, Toh HC, Abastado JP. Immune microenvironment in tumor progression: characteristics and challenges for therapy. *J Oncol.* 2012; 2012:608406. doi:10.1155/2012/608406
39. Moore PS, Chang Y. Why do viruses cause cancer? Highlights of the first century of human tumour virology. *Nat Rev Cancer.* 2010; 10(12):878–89. doi:10.1038/nrc2961
40. Krump NA, You J. Molecular mechanisms of viral oncogenesis in humans. *Nat Rev Microbiol.* 2018;16(11):684–98. doi:10.1038/s41579-018-0064-6
41. Weiss RA, Vogt PK. 100 years of Rous sarcoma virus. *J Exp Med.* 2011;208(12):2351–5. doi:10.1084/jem.20112160
42. Snyder A, Makarov V, Merghoub T, et al. Genetic basis for clinical response to CTLA-4 blockade in melanoma. *N Engl J Med.* 2014; 371(23):2189–99. doi:10.1056/NEJMoa1406498
43. Van Allen EM, Miao D, Schilling B, et al. Genomic correlates of response to CTLA-4 blockade in metastatic melanoma. *Science.* 2015; 350(6257):207–11. doi:10.1126/science.aad0095
44. Hugo W, Zaretsky JM, Sun L, et al. Genomic and transcriptomic features of response to anti-PD-1 therapy in metastatic melanoma. *Cell.* 2016;165(1):35–44. doi:10.1016/j.cell.2016.02.065
45. Chen PL, Roh W, Reuben A, et al. Analysis of immune signatures in longitudinal tumor samples yields insight into biomarkers of response and mechanisms of resistance to immune checkpoint blockade. *Cancer Discov.* 2016;6(8):827–37. doi:10.1158/2159-8290
46. Meacham CE, Morrison SJ. Tumour heterogeneity and cancer cell plasticity. *Nature.* 2013;501(7467):328–37. doi:10.1038/nature12624

CHAPTER

3

Cancer Risk Reduction: Screening and Health Behaviors

OUTLINE

1. Introduction: Cancer Risk Reduction Strategies
2. Cancer Risk Reduction
   a. Achieve and Maintain a Healthy Weight
   b. Be Physically Active
   c. Follow a Healthy Eating Pattern
   d. Breastfeed, If Possible
   e. Avoid Smoking/Smoking Cessation/e-Cigarettes
   f. Avoid Secondhand Smoke
   g. Protection From the Sun
   h. Get Vaccinated for Human Papillomavirus and Hepatitis B Virus
   i. Get Tested for Hepatitis C
   j. Myths About Causes of Risks for Cancer
   k. Attributable Risks: Relative Merits of the Cancer Risk Reduction Strategies
3. Finding It Early: Evidence-Based Cancer Screening Strategies
   a. Breast Cancer Screening
   b. Cervical Cancer Screening
   c. Colorectal Cancer Screening
   d. Lung Cancer Screening
   e. Cancers for Which Screenings Are Not Recommended
4. Summary
5. Case Study
6. Meet the Expert
7. Study Questions
8. References

OBJECTIVES

After completing review of this chapter, students will be able to:

1. Understand the behaviors that have the potential to substantively reduce the burden of cancer (risk reduction and screening).
2. Recognize all of the cancer risk reduction strategies currently recommended by scientific evidence.
3. Know cancer screening guidelines for breast, cervical, colon, and lung cancers.

INTRODUCTION: CANCER RISK REDUCTION STRATEGIES

There are approximately 1.8 million cancers diagnosed in the US each year. It is estimated that if the cancer risk reduction approaches outlined in this chapter were all followed, it would prevent 30% to 50% of diagnoses per year. As such, cancer risk reduction strategies offer the most cost-effective long-term strategy for the control of cancer.

Although cancer screening does not prevent cancer, it does allow diagnosis at an earlier stage, presumably when it is easier to treat the cancer. Screening has helped lower the cervical cancer death rate by more than 50% over the past 30 years. It is estimated that mammograms prevent around 12,000 deaths per year. And if colorectal cancer screening guidelines were followed, it is estimated that about 33,000 lives would be saved each year.

The objective of this chapter is to review the cancer risk reduction and screening guidelines. The primary sources for this chapter are the ACS, the CDC, and the U.S. Preventive Services Task Force (USPSTF).

It is crucial for the exercise oncology professional to understand evidence-based cancer risk reduction and screening guidelines for several reasons. First, people living with and beyond cancer will assume the exercise oncology professional has knowledge of cancer from risk reduction, to screening, to treatment, and to survivorship. Second, while working with people living with and beyond cancer (and their caregivers), the exercise professional will have opportunities to guide people toward evidence-based primary and secondary risk reduction and screening strategies. Patients and survivors will ask for advice regarding risk reduction and screening strategies. In such cases, the advice given should be based on the scientific evidence reviewed below.

CANCER RISK REDUCTION

Studies show that certain lifestyle factors can have an impact on the risk of developing cancer. In this section, we review each of these in turn, including:

- achieving and maintaining a healthy body weight
- regular physical activity
- eating a healthy diet
- avoiding alcohol consumption
- avoiding smoking
- avoiding secondhand smoke
- protecting oneself from the sun
- getting several specific vaccines, and
- getting tested for hepatitis C.

Finally, we also include a brief section about **cancer prevention** myths that may be heard during work as an exercise oncology professional. Note that we use the phrase *cancer risk reduction* rather than *cancer prevention*. This is because, as discussed in Chapter 2, the development of cancer is complex. It is completely possible for someone to be a healthy weight, exercise regularly, eat a healthy diet, avoid alcohol consumption, avoid smoking, and all of the other risk reduction strategies discussed, and still s/he be diagnosed with cancer. It is important to understand that the language around risk reduction should not blame patients for their cancer diagnoses. It is very likely that the healthy person who follows all the guidance was diagnosed later than what would have happened without the healthy behaviors, at a lower stage, and will tolerate treatment better than if they had not been so healthy. For using the term *prevention*, there needs to be evidence that carrying out a behavior/action could actually result in a cancer not occurring that would have occurred otherwise. That may be true for some of the health behaviors for some people but not for 100% of people in 100% of cases. As a result, the phrase **cancer risk reduction** is preferred. It may be useful to preferentially use this phrase when working with survivors, as it is less likely to result in a conversation about attributing blame for a cancer diagnosis.

How do we know the information about cancer risk reduction? For the most part, the scientific evidence that the noted health behaviors reduce cancer risk comes from large epidemiologic observational studies. These studies are generally either **cohort studies** or **case control studies**. Cohort studies often enroll a large group of people and follow them prospectively over time to see who develops and dies from cancer. Retrospective cohort studies enroll a large group of people and look backward to see what their behaviors were, to discern whether exposures like obesity or physical activity alter cancer incidence or mortality risk. Finally, case control studies start at the end of follow-up, like retrospective cohort studies. In a case control study, the researchers identify a group of people who already have a

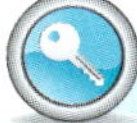

Cancer prevention. Actions taken to lower the risk of cancer.

Cancer risk reduction. Actions taken to lower the risk of cancer with further acknowledgment that all efforts to prevent cancer are imperfect and that there are aspects of cancer risk beyond the control of individual behavior choices, such as exercise and nutrition.

Cohort studies. Observational studies that follow participants over time. These studies can follow participants forward in time (prospective) or look backward through time (retrospective). The comparison group within a cohort study can be within the original study group or may be external.

Case control studies. Observational studies that start with the comparison of participants according to the outcome of interest (eg, incident cancer vs no incident cancer) to compare exposures between these groups.

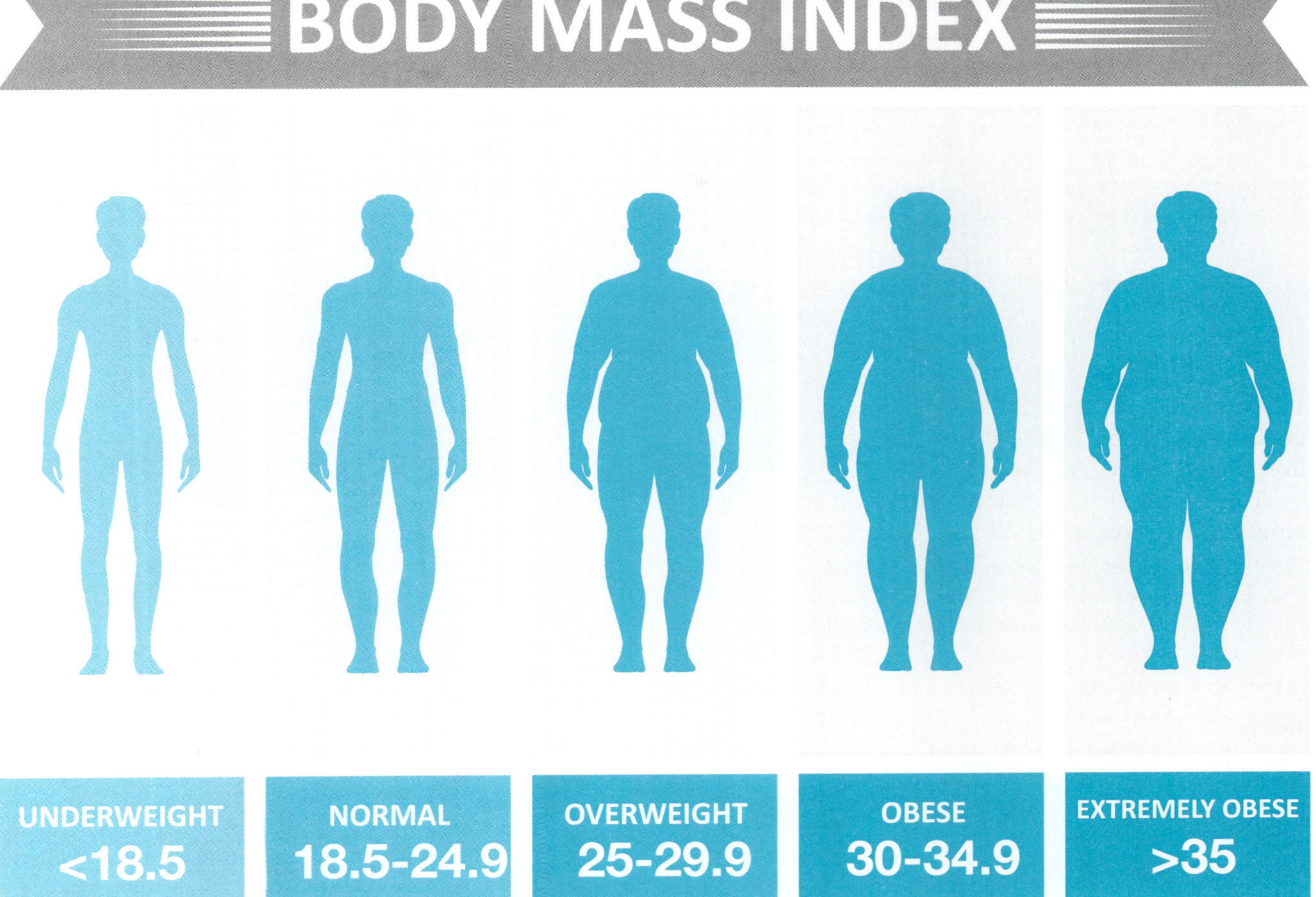

FIGURE 3.1. Body mass index (BMI) categories from the World Health Organization. BMI is calculated as weight in kilograms divided by height in meters squared (kg/m^2). (From the Centers for Disease Control and Prevention. *About Adult BMI, Source: Division of Nutrition, Physical Activity, and Obesity, National Center for Chronic Disease Prevention and Health Promotion*. [Internet]. 2022. Available from https://www.cdc.gov/healthyweight/assessing/bmi/adult_bmi/index.html.)

disease (like cancer), and then identify a comparison group (called controls), ascertain past exposures, and discern effects on disease incidence and mortality. For the most part, there are no gold standard randomized controlled trials (RCTs) in the field of cancer risk reduction, because it typically takes so long for cancers to develop, and follow-up also takes a longer time.

Achieve and Maintain a Healthy Weight

Recommendation

Advice from the ACS and the American Institute for Cancer Research suggests that achieving and maintaining an adult body weight in the healthy range is associated with reduced risk for several types of cancer. Healthy body weight is generally expressed as BMI in weight (in kilograms) divided by height (in meters squared) The healthy range is from 18.5 to 24.9 kg/m^2. Figure 3.1 shows the BMI categories as defined by the WHO and the CDC (1).

Risk Reduction for Specific Cancers

Convincing evidence from the Third Expert Report from the World Cancer Research Fund suggests that being overweight or obese is associated with the incidence of 13 types of cancer, including breast, colorectal, endometrial, esophageal, gallbladder, kidney, liver, oral, ovarian, pancreatic, prostate, certain types of brain cancers, and stomach cancers, as shown in Figure 3.2 (2).

Physiologic Mechanisms Linking Obesity With Cancer Risk

Carrying excess weight can increase chronic inflammation. As discussed in Chapter 2, a state of chronic inflammation means that there are more opportunities for cancer to both occur and grow. In addition, excess body weight can cause

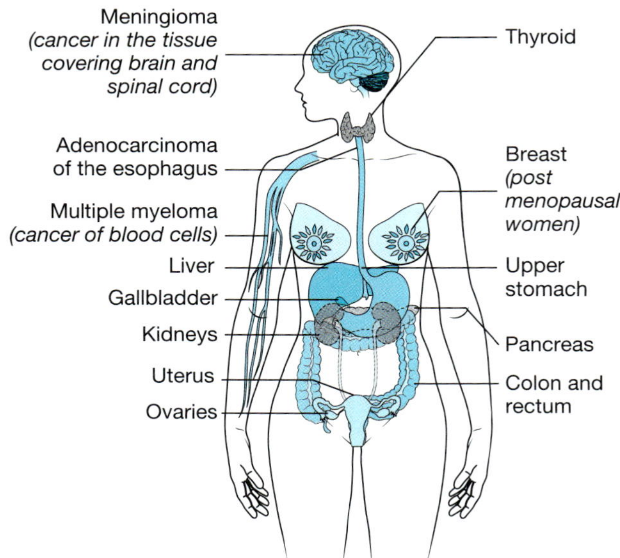

FIGURE 3.2. Cancers associated with being overweight or obese. (From the Centers for Disease Control and Prevention, Division of Cancer Prevention and Control. *About Obesity and Cancer.* [Internet]. 2023. Available from https://www.cdc.gov/cancer/obesity/index.htm.)

the body to produce too much estrogen, which can contribute to the excess risk of both breast and endometrial cancers. Further, being overweight can cause high levels of insulin and other hormones that can then contribute to the growth of cancer cells. Finally, excess fat in the center of the belly, called visceral fat, alters hormones and insulin exposure in a manner that leads to growth in cancer cells.

Guidelines for Achieving a Healthy Body Weight

There are many approaches to weight loss and health maintenance that can be recommended to prevent cancer and prevent recurrence of cancer. The primary methods recommended by the American Institute for Cancer Research are to eat a plant-rich diet, avoid sugary drinks and alcohol, be mindful of portions and proportions, be physically active, move more and sit less, and to maintain these behaviors for the long term.

Be Physically Active

Recommendations

Adults should get 150 to 300 minutes of moderate intensity or 75 to 150 minutes of vigorous intensity activity each week (or a combination of these). Getting to or exceeding the upper limit of 300 minutes is ideal. It is also recommended that we limit sedentary behavior, such as sitting, lying down, watching television, or other forms of screen-based activities. Finally, it is also recommended that adults get 2 to 3 times weekly resistance exercise. These recommendations are outlined in an infographic from the WHO (see Figure 3.3).

Reduction of Cancer Risk Associated With Physical Activity

There have been hundreds of epidemiologic, observational studies that have examined whether being more physically active is associated with a reduced risk of cancer. As an

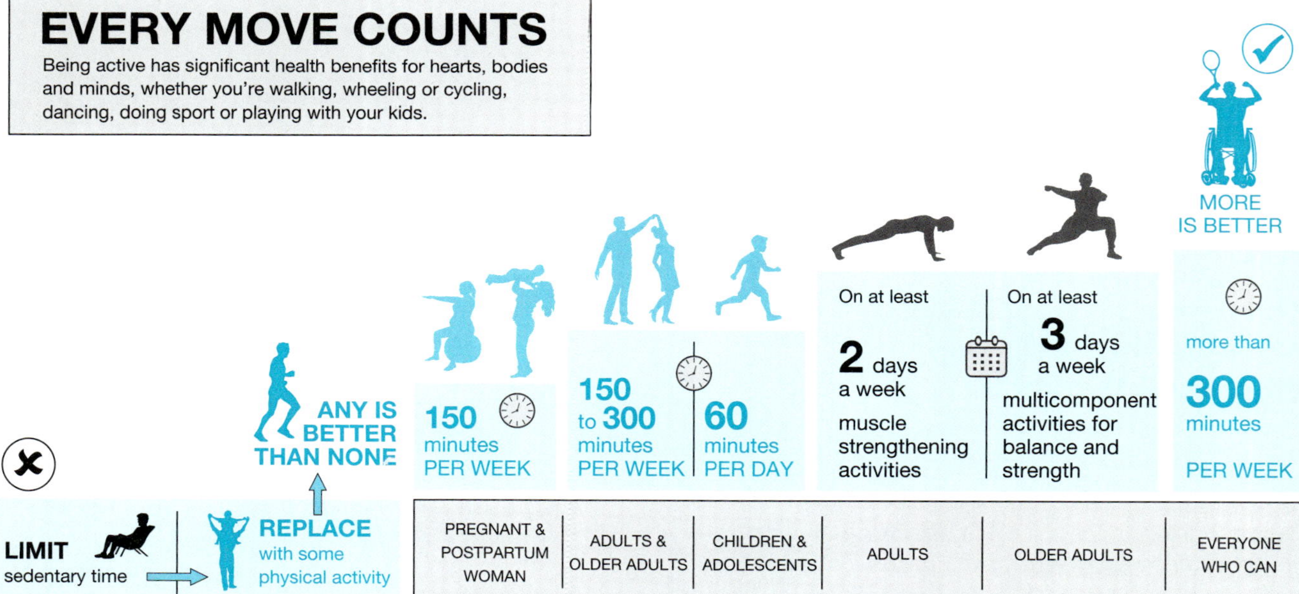

FIGURE 3.3. World Health Organization infographic depicting all of the current public health physical activity recommendations for health, including cancer risk reduction. (From World Health Organization. *Global Recommendations on Physical Activity for Health.* [Internet]. 2010. Available from https://www.who.int/publications/i/item/9789241599979.)

Box 3.1 Types of Physical Activity

Most epidemiologic studies on physical activity and cancer risk focus on 1 particular type of physical activity: leisure time physical activity. Below are the 3 most common types of physical activity:

- **Leisure time:** These activities refer to what we do when we are not working or taking care of ourselves or others. Examples include swimming, running, group fitness classes, hiking, lifting weights, high-intensity interval training, and walking. Although resistance exercise is included in leisure time physical activity, the focus of the self-report instruments used in epidemiologic studies is on leisure time aerobic activities.
- **Occupational:** These activities refer what we do during employment. This could include lifting and carrying boxes, lifting children and carrying them, carrying trays of food and delivering them, walking to and from meetings across a work campus, or, in many cases, sitting at a desk most of the day.
- **Household:** These activities refer to what we do to care for the places which we live. This could include raking leaves, washing clothes and dishes, vacuuming, cleaning bathrooms, or sweeping.

example, Dr. Steve Moore from the National Cancer Institute (NCI) put together data from 12 prospective cohorts from the US and Europe, totaling 1.44 million people, and examined whether leisure time physical activity was associated with incidence of 26 types of cancer (3). High versus low levels of leisure time physical activity (Box 3.1), defined by **metabolic equivalent (MET)** hours per week (Box 3.2 about MET hours per week) resulted in lower risk of 10 cancers, after adjustment for body size: esophageal adenocarcinoma, lung, kidney, myeloid leukemia, myeloma, colon, head and neck, rectal, bladder, and breast.

Two other publications reviewed the literature on this topic, including slightly different studies each time. Both McTiernan et al (4) and Patel et al (5) concluded that there was evidence that physical activity reduces risk for breast, colon, endometrial, kidney, bladder, esophageal, and stomach cancers. Patel also observed that minimizing time spent in sedentary activities could reduce risk of endometrial, colon, and lung cancers. The differences in the conclusions

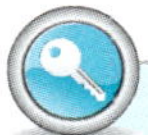

Metabolic equivalent (MET). Intensity of energy needed to accomplish a given task. For example, 1 MET is required to sit in a chair, and 5 METs are required to walk 4 miles per hour.

Box 3.2 Describing Physical Activity Intensity: The Compendium of Physical Activity and Metabolic Equivalent for Task (MET) Minutes (or Hours) Per Week

Most of the research that has been done to link physical activity with reduced risk for disease, including cancer, has asked people about their leisure time physical activity. Understanding the dose of physical activity needed to reduce risk requires that we understand the frequency, intensity, time, and type of activities performed.

Researchers have developed a metric for aerobic leisure time physical activity (a type of activity) that allows a single value to communicate frequency, intensity, and time. For all activities (leisure time, occupational, and household), there is a corresponding intensity level called a MET. This metric to describe activity volume is called MET minutes or MET hours per week. A crucial component of this metric are METs that denote the intensity of activities. The intensity of the exercise (in METs) is then combined with the time spent exercising, in minutes or hours, to express the dose of exercise in a way that includes both intensity and time (MET-hours or MET-minutes). The Compendium of Physical Activities (6), originally developed by Dr. Barbara Ainsworth and colleagues, is regularly updated now and available online for review here: https://sites.google.com/site/compendiumofphysicalactivities/home?authuser=0.

from Moore et al (3) versus the other 2 reviews (4, 5) likely result from the inclusion of different epidemiologic cohorts and research methodology.

Table 3.1 provides a small sample of the compendium of physical activities, including the unique code for each entry, the MET level, the major headings (which often repeat, as in this sample), and the specific activity description. An MET level of 1 denotes an intensity equivalent to sitting quietly. An activity with an MET level of 3 has an intensity that is 3 times greater than sitting quietly. Examples of activities with an MET level of 3 include walking briskly, bowling, or walking and carrying a child weighing 15 pounds or more. Examples of activities with an MET level of 6 include jogging 4 miles an hour, vigorous scrubbing of floors on hands and knees, sawing hardwood, competitive skateboarding, and competitive volleyball. The published physical activity guidelines recommend that we get 150 to 300 minutes of "moderate to vigorous" physical activity. Moderate-intensity physical activity is defined as an MET level of 3.00 to 5.99. Vigorous intensity activity is defined as an MET level of 6.0 or greater.

Epidemiologists quantify the overall activity level by combining the intensity of an activity done in METs with the amount of time spent doing the activity. The combination

Table 3.1 Sample of the 2011 Compendium of Physical Activities

CLASSIFICATION OF THE INTENSITY LEVEL OF THOUSANDS OF ACTIVITIES			
CODE	METS	MAJOR HEADING	SPECIFIC ACTIVITIES
01003	14.0	Bicycling	Bicycling, mountain, uphill, vigorous
01004	16.0	Bicycling	Bicycling, mountain, competitive, racing
01008	8.5	Bicycling	Bicycling, BMX
01009	8.5	Bicycling	Bicycling, mountain, general
01010	4.0	Bicycling	Bicycling, <10 mph, leisure, to work or for pleasure (Taylor Code 115)
01011	6.8	Bicycling	Bicycling, to/from work, self selected pace
01013	5.8	Bicycling	Bicycling, on dirt or farm road, moderate pace
01015	7.5	Bicycling	Bicycling, general
01018	3.5	Bicycling	Bicycling, leisure, 5.5 mph
01019	5.8	Bicycling	Bicycling, leisure, 9.4 mph
01020	6.8	Bicycling	Bicycling, 10-11.9 mph, leisure, slow, light effort
01030	8.0	Bicycling	Bicycling, 12-13.9 mph, leisure, moderate effort
01040	10.0	Bicycling	Bicycling, 14-15.9 mph, racing or leisure, fast, vigorous effort
01050	12.0	Bicycling	Bicycling, 16-19 mph, racing/not drafting or >19 mph drafting, very fast, racing general
01060	15.8	Bicycling	Bicycling, >20 mph, racing, not drafting
01065	8.5	Bicycling	Bicycling, 12 mph, seated, hands on brake hoods or bar drops, 80 rpm
01066	9.0	Bicycling	Bicycling, 12 mph, standing, hands on brake hoods, 60 rpm
01070	5.0	Bicycling	Unicycling

Data from the Compendium of Physical Activities, Arizona State University, Healthy Lifestyles Research Center, School of Nutrition and Health Promotion, Phoenix, AZ. Available from https://sites.google.com/site/compendiumofphysicalactivities/home?authuser=0.

is called **MET minutes per week** (or MET hours per week). This defines a combination of intensity (in METs) with the time spent being active. As an example, someone who runs 5 miles per hour (8.3 METs), for a total time of 224 minutes per week, would net 1,859 MET minutes per week. However, that person probably does note run that much every week. The MET minutes per week used in epidemiologic studies is an average per week over time (often a year). If our sample person performed the above-described activity half of the weeks per year and did nothing the other weeks, the average MET minutes per week would be 930. The current recommendations to perform 150 minutes of activity between 3 and 5.99 METs of weekly activity translate into minimum of 450 MET minutes per week. Some researchers use MET hours per week rather than MET minutes per week as the metric. These are equally good ways of expressing activity intensity and time in 1 value. Both values are used; so if 2 sources are being compared, determine whether the metric used in both sources is in minutes or in hours.

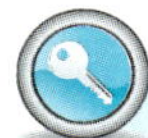

MET minutes per week. An expression of the intensity and time of physical activity performed over the course of a week. This is generally used to express the total volume of leisure time physical activity. For example, if a person performs walking at 4 miles per hour for 5 hours over the course of the week, s/he will have performed 1,500 MET minutes per week (5 METs × 300 min per week = 1,500 MET min × week).

Physiologic Mechanisms of Physical Activity to Reduce Cancer Risk

Physical activity has systemic effects on a variety of endogenous factors that can either contribute to or reduce risk for cancer. These include insulin and glucose metabolism, immune function, inflammation, sex hormones, oxidative stress, genomic instability, and myokines. As shown in Figure 3.4 (7, 8), the

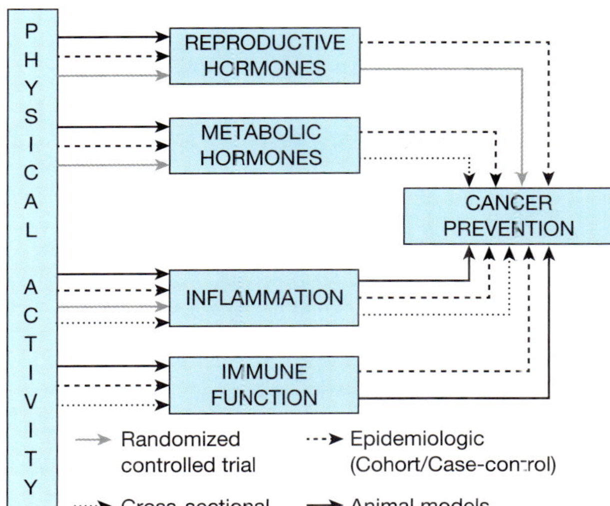

FIGURE 3.4. Mechanisms through which physical activity may reduce risk for cancer, emphasizing the types of evidence available for each category of mechanism (eg, randomized controlled trials, cross-sectional studies, epidemiologic studies, or animal model studies). (From Brown JC, Winters-Stone K, Lee A, Schmitz KH. Cancer, physical activity, and exercise. *Compr Physiol*. 2012;2(4):2775–809. doi:10.1002/cphy.c120005, Figure 6.)

source of the data supporting the various mechanisms through which physical activity reduces cancer risk includes RCTs, cross-sectional studies, epidemiologic observational studies, and animal model studies.

Research on the mechanisms underlying the role of physical activity in cancer risk reduction is ongoing and includes human and animal model studies. By better understanding the mechanisms, we can perhaps clarify the modes, intensity, frequency, and duration of exercise prescription that will reduce risk.

Public Health Guidelines for Achieving Physical Activity Recommendations

There are numerous public health efforts to improve the physical activity levels of the general public. At present, it is estimated that 53.3% of Americans meet the current Physical Activity Guidelines for Americans for aerobic activities (9). This number drops to 23.2% when we consider the proportion of Americans meeting both the aerobic and resistance exercise guidelines.

Efforts to increase physical activity levels include a focus on all types of activities, as noted in Figure 3.5 (10). The

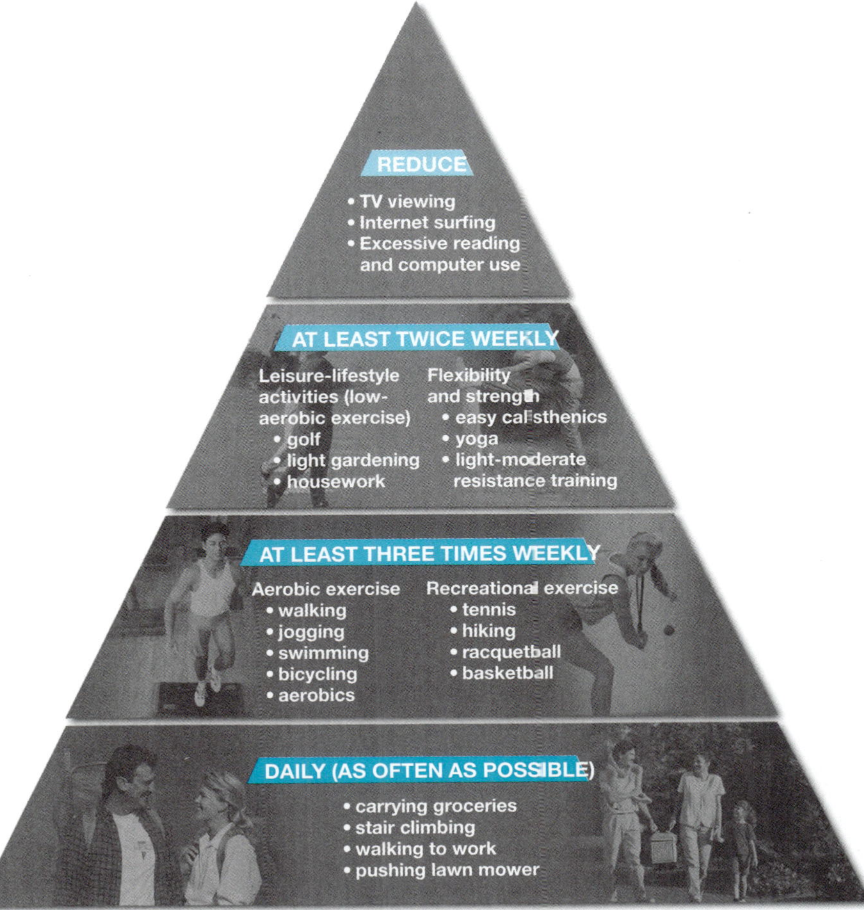

FIGURE 3.5. The physical activity pyramid. Public health guidelines as to how to meet the physical activity recommendations for cancer risk reduction. (From VonArx, R. *Brochure Post #5: What Is Your Level of Physical Activity?* [Blog Post]. Pennsylvania State University; 2015. Available from https://sites.psu.edu/rvonarxnutrition/2015/11/08/where-do-you-fit-on-the-physical-activity-pyramid/.)

FOLLOW A HEALTHY EATING PATTERN

MORE FRUITS AND VEGGIES ... LESS JUNK

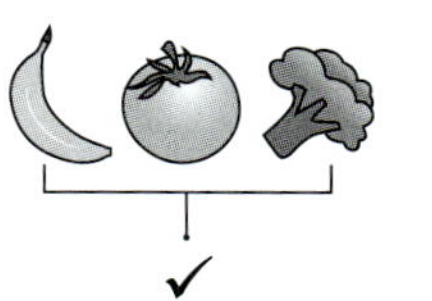

✓

- **Foods high in vitamins, minerals, and other nutrients** in amounts that help you get to and stay at a healthy body weight
- **A colorful variety of vegetables** - dark green, red, and orange
- **Fiber-rich** beans and peas
- **A colorful variety of whole fruits**
- **Whole grains,** like whole wheat bread and brown rice

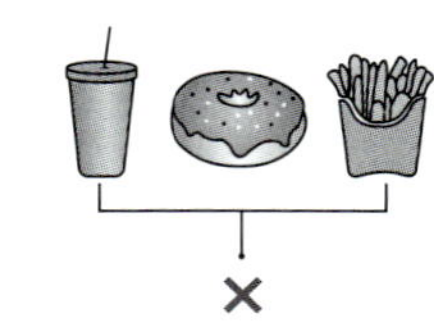

✕

- **Red meats** such as beef, pork, and lamb and **processed meats** such as bacon, sausage, deli meats, and hot dogs
- **Sugar-sweetened beverages**
- **Highly processed foods** and refined grain products

IT IS BEST NOT TO DRINK ALCOHOL

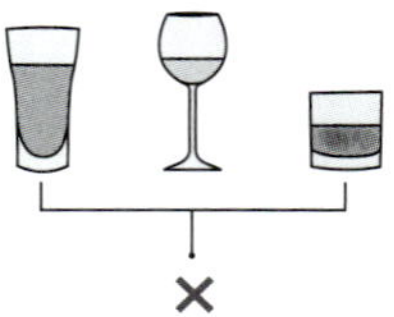

✕

- If you do choose to drink alcohol, **women** should have **no more than one drink per day** and **men** should have **no more than two drinks per day.**
- A drink is 12 ounces of regular beer, 5 ounces of wine, or 1.5 ounces of 80-proof distilled spirits.

FIGURE 3.6. Following a healthy eating pattern. (© 2023 American Cancer Society, Inc. Available from https://www.cancer.org/healthy/eat-healthy-get-active/acs-guidelines-nutrition-physical-activity-cancer-prevention/infographic.html.)

pyramid approach shown in the figure parallels a similar approach to explaining dietary recommendations, with the goal of recommending the limitation of sedentary behavior and providing examples of ways to be more active in all levels of the pyramid.

Another approach being taken in several health systems across the US is the adoption of the Physical Activity Vital Sign and the use of an **SBIRT**: screening, behavioral intervention, and referral to treatment approach. This approach is consistent with the ACSM's Exercise is Medicine® program (11). The Physical Activity Vital Sign approach is to add a screening about physical activity to the process of rooming patients in primary care, along with the other vital signs (eg, temperature, weight, and blood pressure). By doing so, a signal is sent to the patient that physical activity is important, but also it is revealed whether the patient is meeting current physical activity guidelines. If not, a brief intervention can be applied, advising the patient that being regularly physically active has important health benefits (including reducing the risk of cancer). This can be followed by a referral to physical activity programming. One health system that has fully adopted this approach is Prisma Health in Greenville, SC, US (12).

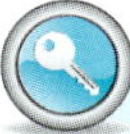

SBIRT. Screening, behavioral intervention, and referral to treatment. This is a well-documented approach to promoting physical activity.

Follow a Healthy Eating Pattern

Recommendations

According to the ACS, a healthy eating pattern that reduces cancer risk includes foods that are high in nutrients in amounts that help you get to and stay at a healthy body weight: a variety of vegetables—dark green, red, and orange, fiber-rich legumes (beans and peas), and others; fruits, especially whole fruits in a variety of colors; and whole grains. Further, a healthy eating pattern limits or does not include alcohol consumption, red and processed meats, sugar-sweetened beverages, or highly processed foods and refined grain products. These tips are summarized in the Figure 3.6 (13).

Cancer Risk Reduction Associated With Healthy Eating

Studies on this topic have been summarized by experts from the ACS and others (Figure 3.7) (14, 15).

An expert panel from the ACS lists the following food patterns to reduce the risk of cancer:

- **Breast cancer** risk is reduced by following a dietary pattern rich in plant foods and low in animal products and refined carbohydrates.
- **Colorectal cancer** risk may be reduced by a healthy eating pattern of whole grains, higher fiber, and less added sugar, consuming nonstarchy vegetables and whole fruits, consuming calcium-rich dairy foods, avoiding processed meat intake, and limiting red meat.

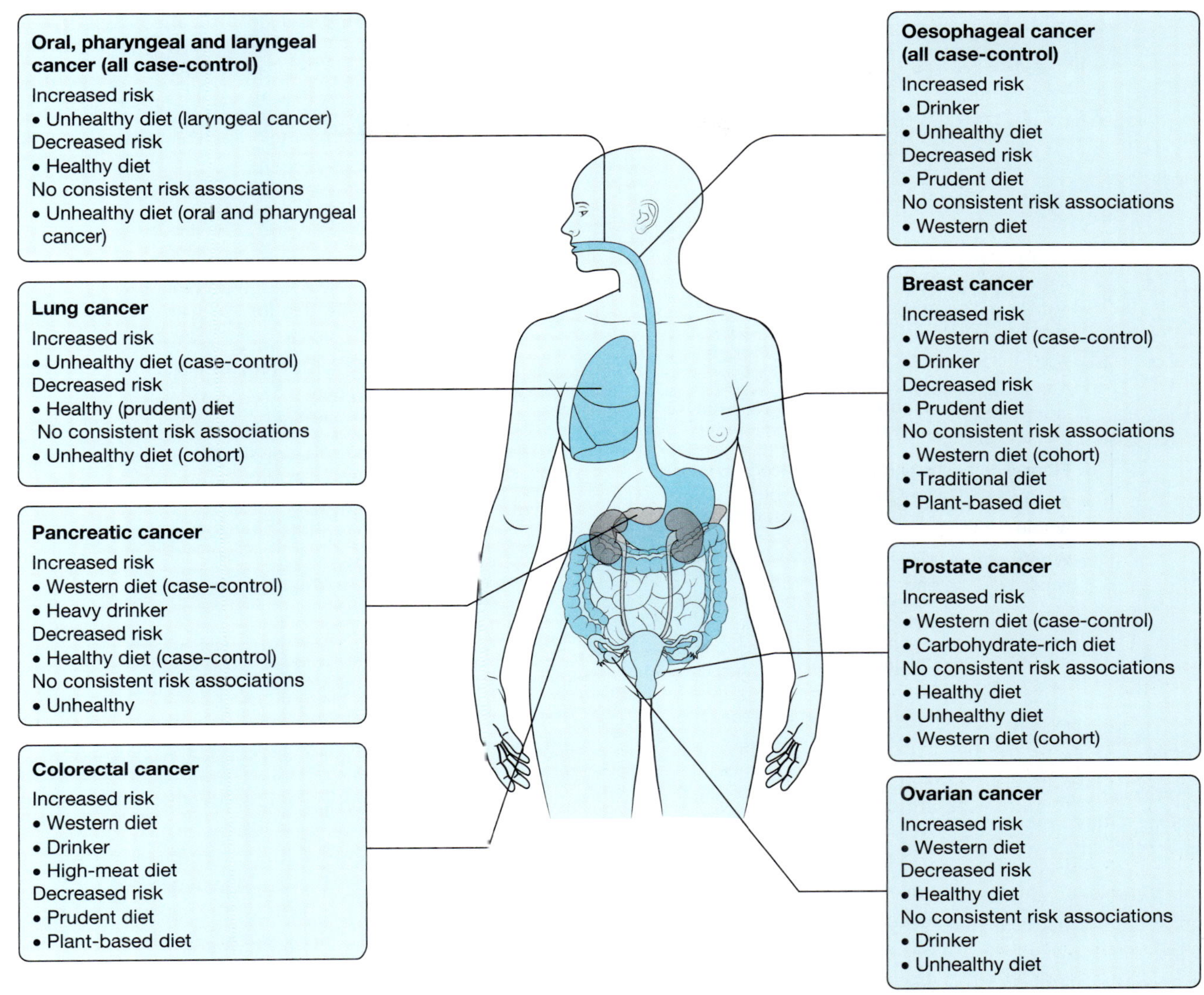

FIGURE 3.7. Cancers for which healthy dietary pattern is associated with incidence. (From Steck SE, Murphy EA. Dietary patterns and cancer risk. *Nat Rev Cancer*. 2020;20(2):125–38. https://doi.org/10.1038/s41568-019-0227-4.)

- **Endometrial cancer** risk may be reduced by avoiding sweets, high-sugar/low-fiber foods, and sweetened beverages.
- **Liver cancer** risk may be reduced by increased consumption of fish.
- **Lung cancer** risk may be reduced by consuming nonstarchy vegetables and whole fruits, including those high in vitamin C, and avoiding processed foods and red meat, while adding beta-carotene supplementation.
- **Pancreatic cancer** risk may be reduced by avoiding processed and red meats, saturated fats, and sugar-sweetened beverages.
- **Prostate cancer** risk is reduced by a higher consumption of dairy products and calcium.
- **Gastric cancer** risk is reduced by the regular intake of nonstarchy vegetables and whole fruits, particularly citrus fruits, as well as avoiding the intake of processed, grilled, or charcoaled meats.
- **Upper aerodigestive (lips, mouth, tongue, nose, throat, vocal cords, and esophagus)** risk is reduced by the consumption of nonstarchy vegetables and whole fruits.
- **Alcohol consumption** may increase risk for breast, colorectal, liver, stomach, head and neck, and esophageal cancers (16). The recommendation from the ACS and the World Cancer Research Fund is not to drink alcohol at all. If you do drink, the advice is not to have more than 1 drink per day (Figure 3.8).

Physiologic Mechanisms of a Healthy Diet to Reduce Cancer Risk

As with physical activity, the factors that result in the development of an invasive cancer are complex and involve many processes that are not related to dietary or physical activity patterns. That said, there are physiologic effects of our

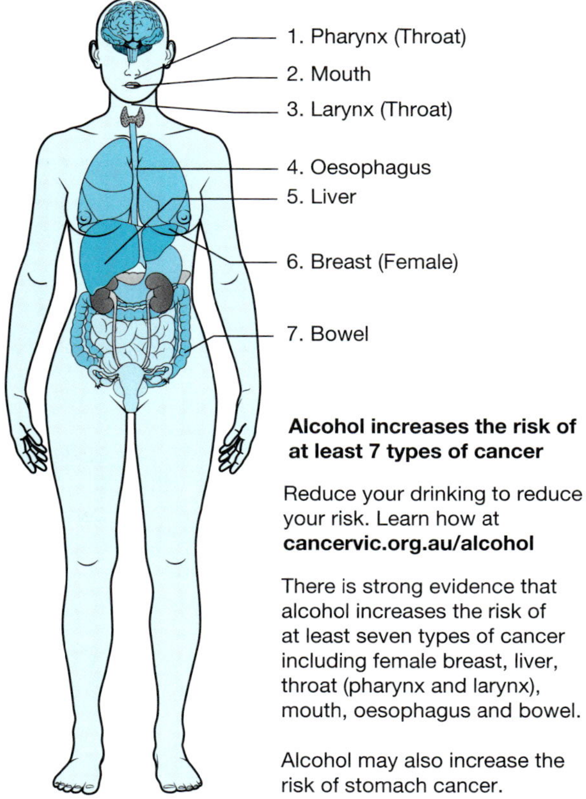

FIGURE 3.8. Alcohol is associated with 7 types of cancer. (From Cancer Council, Melbourne, Victoria, 3004, Australia. Available from https://www.cancervic.org.au/preventing-cancer/limit-alcohol/reduce-your-drinking.)

regular dietary patterns that can shift endogenous processes toward versus away from cancer development. As shown in Figure 3.9 (15), these processes include alterations in the bacteria in the gut (gut dysbiosis), alterations in immune function and inflammation, metabolic and hormonal disturbances, elimination or detoxification of elements that could cause DNA damage, repairing DNA damage, and ensuring that cells with DNA damage do not survive. Our dietary patterns can also up- or down-regulate endogenous factors that reduce oxidative stress and alter the effectiveness of our endogenous systems that fight oxidative stressors. There are also dietary compounds that influence pathways by which carcinogens are metabolized. Diet can influence epigenetic changes in cells, and alcohol intake increases the production of metabolites that are carcinogenic.

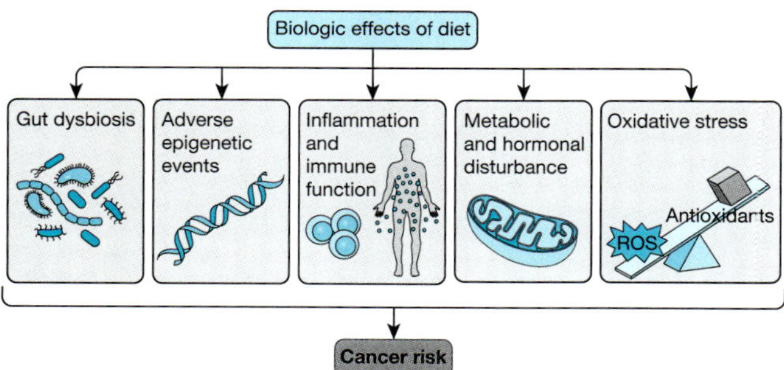

FIGURE 3.9. Biologic effects of diet on cancer risk. (From Steck SE, Murphy EA. Dietary patterns and cancer risk. *Nat Rev Cancer*. 2020;20(2):125–38, Figure 6. https://doi.org/10.1038/s41568-019-0227-4.)

Guidelines for Following a Healthy Eating Pattern

The ACS recommends that people:

- fill most of our plates with colorful vegetables and fruits, beans, and whole grains;
- choose fish, poultry, or beans as main sources of protein instead of red meat or processed meats;
- if eating red or processed meats, eat smaller portions; and
- avoid alcohol consumption.

Breastfeed, If Possible

Recommendations

The American Institute for Cancer Research and the World Cancer Research Fund recommend that mothers breastfeed their babies if they can. The American Academy of Pediatrics recommends that babies be exclusively breastfed for the first 6 months of life, with continued breastfeeding along with the introduction of solid foods for 1 year.

Reduction in Risk for Specific Cancers From Breastfeeding

Breastfeeding reduces risk of breast and ovarian cancer for the mother and reduces risk of obesity in babies. This, in turn, may reduce the risk for obesity-related cancers in the baby.

Physiologic Mechanisms by Which Breastfeeding May Reduce Cancer Risk

Research on this topic is ongoing. However, 1 mechanism by which breastfeeding may alter breast and ovarian cancer risk in the mother is the hormonal changes that delay the return of menstrual periods. This reduces lifetime exposure to estrogen, which is linked to increased risk for breast and ovarian cancer.

Guidelines for Breastfeeding

The CDC in the US has a multipronged strategy to promote breastfeeding in the community (17). The strategies include promoting practices to support breastfeeding while mother and baby are still in the hospital, education of health care professionals (HCPs) regarding the importance of breastfeeding, ensuring access of the mother to appropriate supports from HCPs (eg, lactation specialists), creating and disseminating peer support programs, ensuring support for breastfeeding in the workplace, ensuring support for breastfeeding in daycare and early education, access to breastfeeding education and information, social marketing, and addressing the marketing of infant formula.

Avoid Smoking/Smoking Cessation/ e-Cigarettes

Recommendations

People who successfully avoid or quit smoking can add as much as a decade of life expectancy and reduce their risk of many types of cancer. Smoking cessation at the time of a cancer diagnosis can also improve outcomes for cancer survivors who are current smokers. Avoiding smoking is often referred to as the most important cancer risk reduction strategy (18). With regard to e-cigarettes, they have not been around long enough for scientists to know whether their use causes cancer. However, it is important to know that the vapor from an e-cigarette contains cancer-causing chemicals, although in lower amounts than in cigarette smoke. The ACS has recommended that no one should begin using any tobacco product, including e-cigarettes, and that anyone who uses any tobacco product of any kind, including e-cigarettes, should stop.

Reduction in Risk for Specific Cancers by Not Smoking

As shown in Figure 3.10, quitting smoking reduces the risk of 12 different types of cancer, including lung, larynx, oral cavity and pharynx, esophagus, pancreas, bladder, stomach, colon and rectum, liver, cervix, kidney, and AML (19). Smoking cessation improves prognosis in people with cancer and may improve all-cause mortality in patients with cancer.

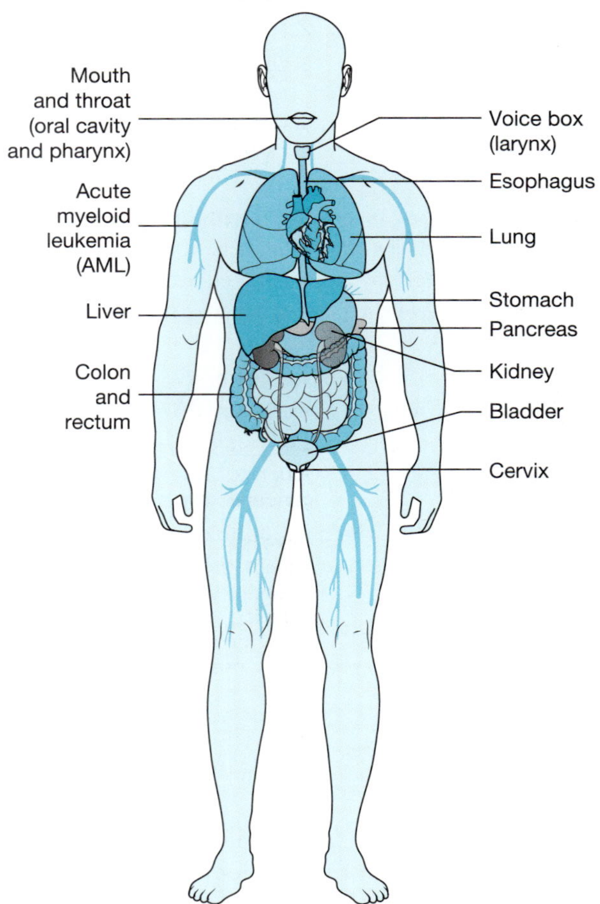

FIGURE 3.10. Quitting smoking decreases risk of 12 different cancers. (From Office on Smoking and Health, National Center for Chronic Disease Prevention and Health Promotion. CDC, U.S. Department of Health & Human Services. Available from https://www.cdc.gov/tobacco/quit_smoking/how_to_quit/benefits/index.htm#cancer-related-benefits.)

Physiologic Mechanisms by Which Smoking May Increase Cancer Risk

Smoking causes a wide range of diseases and cancer types. As such, it is likely that there are multiple biological mechanisms at play (20). Over 7,000 chemicals have been identified in cigarette smoke, including arsenic (a poison), benzene (a toxin), and formaldehyde (a preservative for dead bodies). Many of these have been classified as carcinogens in rigorous reviews of the literature. Tobacco smoking is also responsible for DNA mutations and DNA methylation that may lead to important changes in the function of *p53* (see Chapter 2 for the importance of *p53*).

Guidelines for Smoking Cessation

According to the ACS, quitting smoking successfully usually requires multiple attempts (21). Food and Drug Administration (FDA)-approved cessation medications, including nicotine replacement therapy (NRT), prescription medications (eg, bupropion and varenicline), and behavioral counseling (individual, group, or telephone), improve the chances of long-term cessation among adults, especially when used together. The ACS very specifically recommends that e-cigarettes not be used to assist in quitting smoking.

Avoid Secondhand Smoke

Recommendations

The ACS recommends avoiding secondhand smoke (22). There is no safe level of exposure to secondhand smoke, which is defined as being a mixture of 2 forms of smoke that come from burning tobacco: 1. mainstream smoke that is the smoke exhaled by a person who smokes and 2. sidestream smoke that is the smoke from the lighted end of a cigarette, pipe, cigar, or tobacco burning in a hookah. This type of smoke has higher concentrations of nicotine and carcinogens than mainstream smoke. This exposure is sometimes also called passive smoking.

Reduction in Risk for Specific Cancers From Avoiding Exposure to Secondhand Smoke

Secondhand smoking is associated with lung cancer, even in people who have never smoked. There is also evidence that secondhand smoke may be associated with multiple other cancers, including larynx, nasopharynx, nasal sinuses, and breast cancer (22).

Physiologic Mechanisms by Which Secondhand Smoke May Increase Cancer Risk

The mechanisms by which secondhand smoke increases cancer risk are similar to those observed in smokers, including the repeated exposure of lungs to DNA damaging material that leads to multiple genetic and epigenetic changes, which may ultimately culminate in the development of cancer (23).

Guidelines for Avoiding Secondhand Smoke

In the US there are now federal laws that help preventing smoking in many indoor and outdoor public places, including work places, retail, restaurants, and bars, and sporting arenas. To the extent that adherence to these laws is high, exposure to secondhand smoke in the public setting is relatively low as compared with exposure before these laws. That leaves exposure in the home and other private settings (such as in the car) as the only places without smoke-free policies. The CDC recommends insisting on a smoke-free home to reduce further exposure. Reasons one can give for a smoke-free home include protecting pregnant women, children, other nonsmoking family members, pets, and guests. This becomes more important if there are members of the family with health conditions exacerbated by secondhand smoke exposure (eg, asthma). Further, a smoke-free home and car environment can help smokers cut down on cigarette consumption, which may help them quit (or maintain quitting). There are also esthetic, hygienic, economic, and safety considerations, including eliminating odors, eliminating cigarette burns on personal property, and eliminating the risk of fires caused by discarded cigarettes (24).

Protection From the Sun

Recommendations

The CDC notes that being outside can be healthy, including getting more physical activity, but recommends avoiding too much exposure to UV light from sun exposure by following a few guidelines (Figure 3.11) (25):

- Reduce risk for sun damage and skin cancer by staying in the shade when outdoors.
- Wear long-sleeved shirts and long pants to provide an extra layer of protection from UV rays.
- Wear a hat with a brim all the way around to protect your face and shoulders.
- Sunglasses can protect your eyes from UV rays and reduce the risk of developing cataracts (a clouding of the normally clear lens of the eye that can cause blurry vision).
- Wear a broad spectrum sunscreen that blocks both types of UV light (UVA and UVB), with a sun protection factor (SPF) of 15 or higher. Reapply sunscreen if you stay outside for more than 2 hours.
- Do not use tanning beds.

Reduction in Risk for Specific Cancers From Following Sun Safety Practices

Most skin cancers are the result of exposure to the UV rays in sunlight. There are 2 common types of skin cancer (basal cell and squamous cell) that are often found on exposed parts of the body, and their occurrence tends to be associated with lifetime exposure. The risk of melanoma is also related to sun exposure (26).

Physiologic Mechanisms by Which Exposure to Ultraviolet Light May Increase Cancer Risk

UV light damages DNA integrity and causes the modification of expression of a plethora of genes. There is also evidence of immune system suppression from UV exposure. Mutations to the important genome guardian *p53* gene result from UV light exposure. One of the common mutations observed in melanoma is to the *BRAF* gene (from the RAF family discussed in Chapter 2). Intermittent overexposure to the sun is particularly associated with *BRAF* mutations leading to melanoma.

Guidelines for Avoiding Overexposure to the Sun

The ACS (27) reminds us that people do not have to avoid the sun completely. In fact, a small amount of sun exposure is needed to replenish the body's supply of vitamin D. The most obvious first step in avoiding overexposure is to avoid tanning beds. Beyond this, the ACS urges paying attention to factors that affect UV light exposure, such as time of day (rays are strongest midday), season of the year (rays are strongest in summer), distance from the equator (rays are stronger near the equator), altitude (rays are stronger at

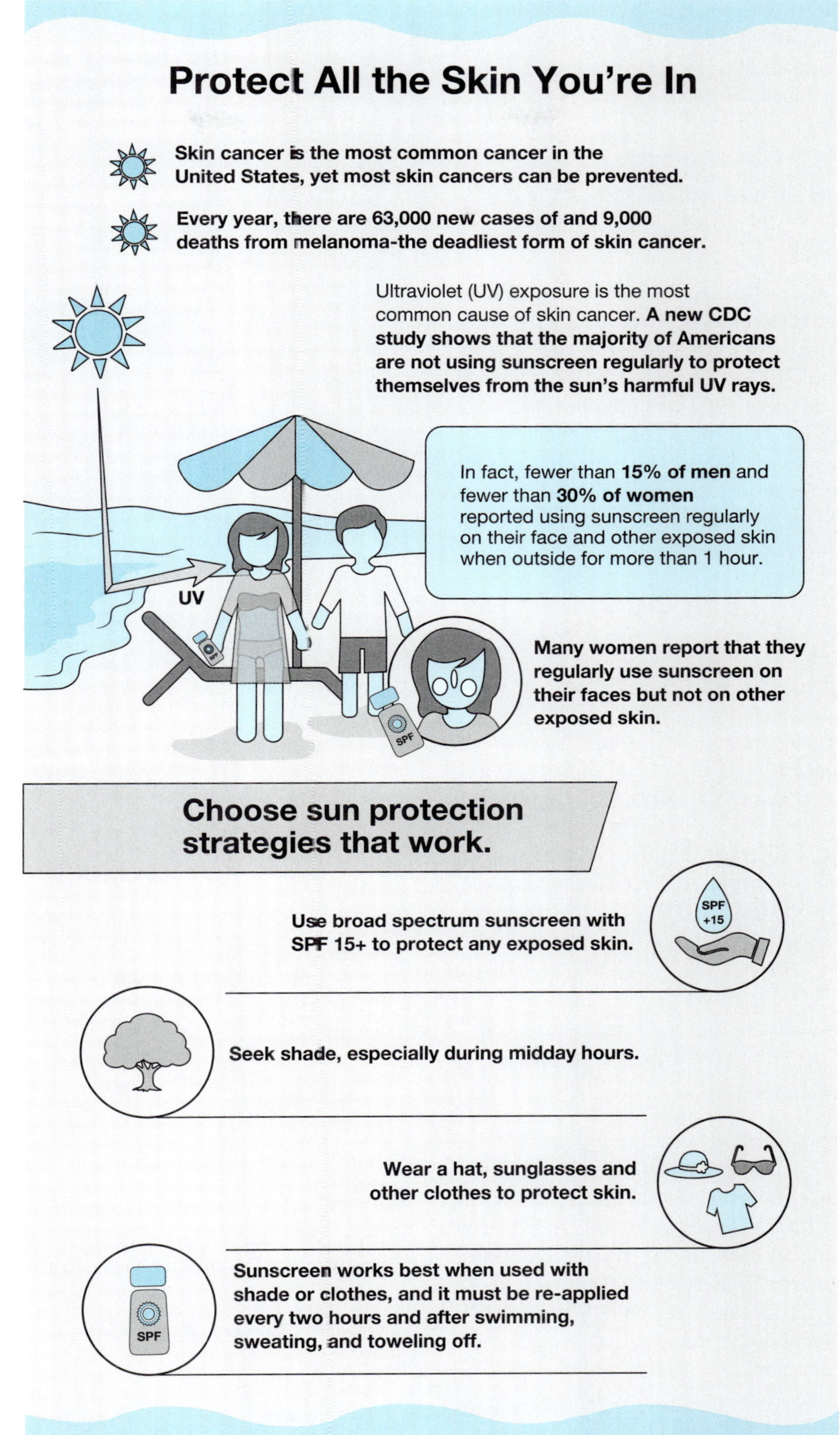

FIGURE 3.11. Guidelines for sun safety from the CDC. Abbreviation: CDC, Centers for Disease Control and Prevention. (From CDC, U.S. Department of Health & Human Services. Available from https://www.cdc.gov/cancer/skin/basic_info/sun-safety.htm.)

higher altitude), cloud cover (surprisingly, rays pass through clouds), and reflection off of surfaces (water, sand, and snow). Choose to be outside at times that minimize UV rays and/or follow the steps noted earlier.

Get Vaccinated for Human Papillomavirus and Hepatitis B Virus

Recommendations

The U.S. CDC recommends that children aged 11 to 12 years should get 2 doses of HPV vaccine, given 6 to 12 months apart. HPV vaccines can be given starting at age 9 years. Children who start the HPV vaccine series on or after their 15th birthday need 3 doses, given over 6 months (28).

The hepatitis B (HBV) vaccine is recommended for all infants and children up to age 18 years by the WHO and the CDC. The CDC also recommends that adults in high-risk groups be vaccinated (owing to sexual exposure or exposure by blood) (29).

Reduction in Risk for Specific Cancers Associated With Hepatitis B Virus Infection

Figure 3.12 (30) provides an infographic from the CDC with an overview of the cancers associated with HPV infection that can be largely prevented through vaccination. HPV is thought to cause 90% of all cervical cancers, as well as cancers of the back of the throat, anus, vulva, penis, and vagina (30, 31).

HBV is associated with hepatocellular carcinoma (liver cancer). As discussed in Chapter 1, liver cancer is one of the 5 major cancers worldwide. HBV is thought to be the most important etiologic agent of liver cancer around the world (32).

Physiologic Mechanisms by Which Human Papillomavirus or Hepatitis B Virus May Increase Cancer Risk

There are multiple types of HPV. Most are low risk and will never cause a cancer (33). The likelihood that an HPV infection will lead to a cancer depends on the interaction of the immune system and the HPV infection. Several high-risk HPV viruses cause inactivation of *p53* tumor suppressor pathways, leading to a broad variety of dysregulation in cell signaling (see Chapter 2 for more on *p53*). Overall, HPV infection can lead to genomic instability that promotes the likelihood of the development of a cancer.

HBV contributes to liver cancer through direct and indirect mechanisms (34). Integration of HBV into the host genome leads to genomic instability and direct mutation of multiple important genes. The virus leads to the dysregulation of cell transcription and proliferation control. It also alters liver cell sensitivity to carcinogenic factors. Epigenetic changes also occur as a result of HBV infection. HBV-related

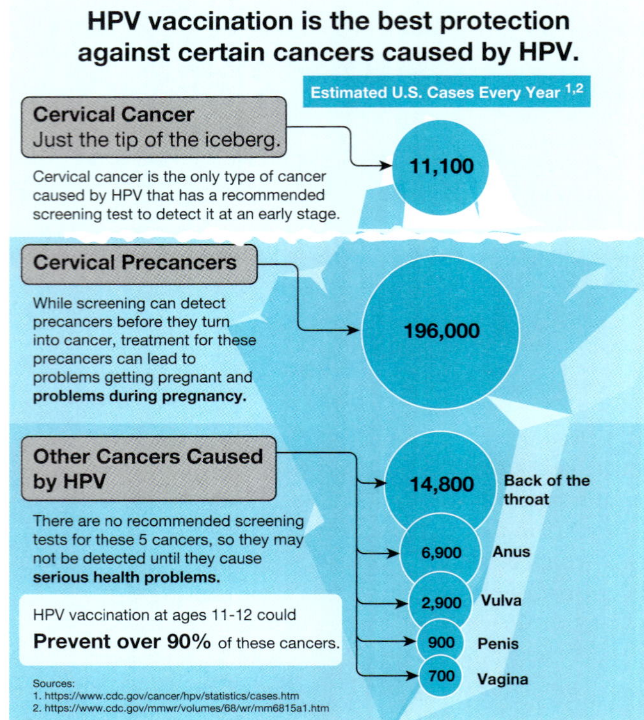

FIGURE 3.12. Cancers prevented by HPV vaccine. CDC Infographic. Abbreviations: HPV, human papilloma virus. (From the Centers for Disease Control and Prevention. Available from https://www.cdc.gov/hpv/hcp/hpv-important/infographic-hpv-screening-508.pdf; https://www.cdc.gov/cancer/hpv/statistics/cases.htm; https://www.cdc.gov/mmwr/volumes/68/wr/mm6815a1.htm.)

tumors often have the dysregulation of *p53*, and the WNT/beta-catenin pathway (discussed in Chapter 2) is often activated as well. The host immune system function likely plays a role in susceptibility of the host infected by HBV to develop liver cancer.

Guidelines for Avoiding Human Papillomavirus and Hepatitis B Virus Infections

The CDC recommends vaccination of infants up to age 18 against HBV and advices that HPV vaccines (a set of 2) be administered to 11- and 12-year-old children.

Get Tested for Hepatitis C

Recommendations

The USPSTF recommends screening for HCV infection in all adults aged 18 to 79 years (35). There is a further recommendation that screening also occurs in individuals younger than 18 years of age who are at high risk for infection (such as those who have a history of injection drug use). This is a 1-time screening for most adults, with repeated screening recommended for those at elevated risk. Getting tested is important because, when found early, treatments can cure most people with HCV in 8 to 12 weeks.

Reduction in Risk for Specific Cancers Associated With Hepatitis C Virus

HCV infection is mostly associated with liver cancer. However, it is also associated with lymphoma and CLL (36).

Physiologic Mechanisms by Which Hepatitis C May Increase Cancer Risk

In a person with a normal functioning liver, liver cancer starts with an increase in fatty tissue in the liver, chronic inflammation of the liver, cirrhosis (degeneration of liver cells, inflammation, and fibrous thickening of liver tissue), which eventually leads to liver cancer. The molecular mechanisms through which this occurs include alterations in blood flow, chronic inflammation, oxidative stress, genome instability, dysregulated lipid metabolism, alterations in apoptosis, and alterations in cellular proliferation pathways (37).

Guidelines for Avoiding Hepatitis C Infection

The primary risk reduction strategy is to not inject drugs. Health care workers at risk for finger sticks are urged to follow universal precautions and to wear appropriate personal protective equipment. Further, get tested for HCV, given that treatment to clear the infection is available and prevents the liver damage from continuing in the direction toward liver cancer.

Myths About Causes of Risks for Cancer

Myth: Using Antiperspirants or Deodorants

There is no evidence that use of products with aluminum compounds or parabens can be absorbed through the skin and or enter the body through nicks caused by shaving underarms. No clinical studies have shown any adverse effect of using these products on breast cancer risk. That said, if someone is worried about this, there are plenty of antiperspirant/deodorant products on the market without these ingredients.

Myth: Microwaving Food in Plastic Containers and Wraps Releases Harmful, Cancer-Causing Substances

Plastic containers and wraps labeled as safe for microwave use do not pose a threat. That said, use of containers NOT intended for microwave use could melt the plastic, leaking chemicals into food. Check to see that the container you use in a microwave is labeled as microwave safe.

Myth: People Who Have Cancer Should Avoid Sugar Because It Makes Cancer Grow Faster

Giving sugar to cancer cells does not make them grow faster. Depriving tumors of sugar does not make them grow slower.

Myth: Cancer Is Contagious

There is no need to avoid someone with cancer. It is NOT contagious, and it is safe to touch and spend time with someone with cancer. In fact, supporting someone with cancer may be invaluable. There are, however, cancers that are spread by viruses. Examples include HPV and HBV or HCV. There are vaccines for HPV and HBV. If you have possibly been exposed to HCV (through sexual intercourse or use of infected intravenous [IV] needles or exposure to infection as a health care worker), it is recommended that you be tested. Hepatitis B and C both cause liver cancer.

Attributable Risks: Relative Merits of the Cancer Risk Reduction Strategies

Of the preceding risk reduction strategies, which are most important? One way to express the relative importance of each of the risks is by population. For this approach, the prevalence of the risk (15% of the population smokes, ~50% of the population is insufficiently active) is combined with the likelihood of the risk causing cancer (25 times increased risk of lung cancer from smoking, 40% to 60% increased risk of cancer from being sedentary). We can combine these values to express the proportion of cancer risk attributable to a given risk factor (called the **attributable risk**). Figure 3.13 provides the attributable risk for some, but not all, of the risks reviewed in this section (38). The figure shows that if you were to choose 1 thing to do to reduce your cancer risk, it should be to avoid smoking. It is important for exercise professionals to recognize the relative importance of smoking compared with physical inactivity when considering cancer risk reduction.

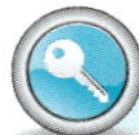

Attributable risk. The proportion of a health outcome in exposed individuals, which can be attributed to the exposure.

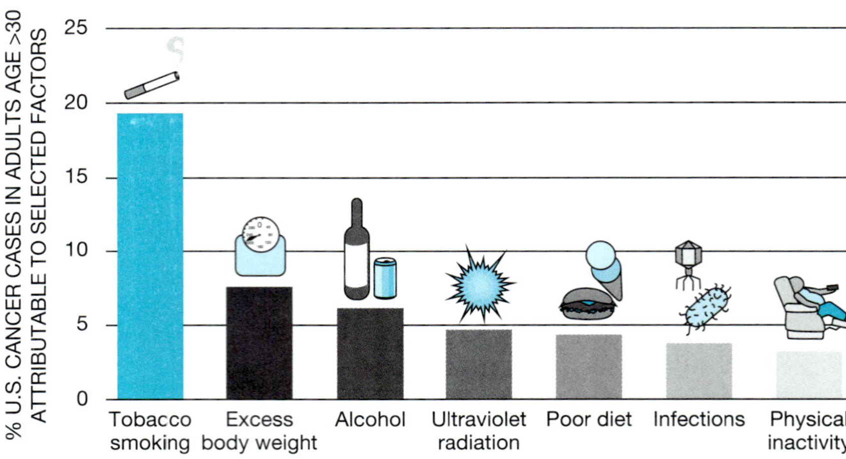

FIGURE 3.13. Attributable risks associated with the exposures reviewed in this chapter. (From the American Association of Cancer Research. *AACR Cancer Progress Report*, 2019. Preventing Cancer: Identifying Risk Factors, Figure 2. Philadelphia (PA). Available from: https://cancerprogressreport.aacr.org/progress/cpr19-contents/cpr19-preventing-cancer.)

FINDING IT EARLY: EVIDENCE-BASED CANCER SCREENING STRATEGIES

Cancer screening is an important strategy to reduce the burden of cancer. Theoretically, a screening-detected cancer should be at an earlier stage, easier to treat, and less likely to lead to a cancer death. The morbidity associated with treatment of earlier stage cancers should also be more favorable, meaning that treatments would be less toxic, and thus, side effects may be less disabling. That said, cancer screening does not prevent cancer or reduce cancer risk. Cancer screening detects cancer. Cancer screening is best used in a situation in which:

- The test is inexpensive (since it will be used in large populations).
- The test is easy to administer.
- The screening test is acceptable to the population to be screened.
- The test is reliable (gives the same results on repeated tests).
- The test is valid (distinguishes diseased and not diseased people).
- Cancers caught earlier, because of screening, can be treated in a way that results in a more favorable symptom burden and mortality outcome.
- The test has low false positives (tests that indicate that there is cancer when there is no cancer).
- The test has low false negatives (tests that indicate there is no cancer when there is a cancer).

In the US there are several not-for-profit organizations that make recommendations for cancer screening, including the ACS, the National Comprehensive Cancer Network (NCCN), and the American Medical Association. At the federal level, the organization that reviews the scientific evidence regarding the safety, efficacy, and logistical characteristics of cancer screening tests, toward the goal of making recommendations, is the USPSTF. In this section, we focus on USPSTF guidelines. The guidelines for other organizations can be easily found online. As shown in Table 3.2, the USPSTF grades the quality of the scientific evidence from A to D, with an additional option of "I" for insufficient (39).

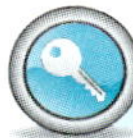

Cancer screening. Looking for cancer before symptoms appear. The goal is to find cancers when they are easier to treat.

Breast Cancer Screening

The screening test used most widely for breast cancer is called a **mammogram**. This test uses x-ray images to review the breast tissue and find cancers. The USPSTF recommends with a grade of C that women aged 40 to 49 years should decide on an individual basis whether the merits of screening outweigh the risks. For women aged 50 to 74 years, the recommendation is to screen every 2 years, with a grade of B. For women aged 75 years or older, there is insufficient evidence to make a recommendation for mammography. There are also additional types of screening tests available for women at high risk of breast cancer, including magnetic resonance imaging and ultrasound, but these also receive a grade of I for insufficient evidence (40). Figure 3.14 presents the image of a woman receiving a mammogram screening, as well as images of 2 breasts screened by mammography, in which one of the breasts shows a cancerous lesion (41, 42).

Cervical Cancer Screening

The most common test used for cervical cancer screening is called the **Pap smear**, where "Pap" is short for the name of the developer of this test, Dr. George Papanicolaou. A Pap

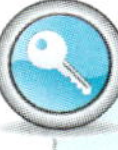

Mammogram. An x-ray image of the breast, taken for the purpose of cancer screening.

Pap smear. A test carried out on a sample of cells from the cervix to screen for cervical cancer.

Table 3.2 U.S. Preventive Services Task Force Definitions for Grading of Evidence

GRADE	DEFINITION	SUGGESTIONS FOR PRACTICE
A	The USPSTF recommends the service. There is high certainty that the net benefit is substantial.	Offer or provide this service.
B	The USPSTF recommends the service. There is high certainty that the net benefit is moderate or there is moderate certainty that the net benefit is moderate to substantial.	Offer or provide this service.
C	The USPSTF recommends selectively offering or providing this service to individual patients based on professional judgment and patient preferences. There is at least moderate certainty that the net benefit is small.	Offer or provide this service for selected patients depending on individual circumstances.
D	The USPSTF recommends against the service. There is moderate or high certainty that the service has no net benefit or that the harms outweigh the benefits.	Discourage the use of this service.
I	The USPSTF concludes that the current evidence is insufficient to assess the balance of benefits and harms of the service. Evidence is lacking, of poor quality, or conflicting, and the balance of benefits and harms cannot be determined.	Read the clinical considerations section of USPSTF Recommendation statement: If the service is offered, patients should understand the uncertainty about the balance of benefits and harms.

From https://www.uspreventiveservicestaskforce.org/uspstf/about-uspstf/methods-and-processes/grade-definitions, October 2018.

smear is a procedure in which a small brush is used to gently remove cells from the surface of the cervix so that they can be checked under a microscope for cervical cancer or cellular changes consistent with developing cervical cancer. Figure 3.15 shows what would be seen in the microscope if there were cervical cancer cells found in a Pap smear test (43). The USPSTF recommends, with a grade of A, that all women aged 21 to 65 years should receive a Pap smear every 3 years, with additional testing for HPV in combination with the Pap smear every 5 years. The USPSTF recommends against screening for cervical cancer among women younger than 21 years, women who have had a hysterectomy, or women who are older than 65 years, with a grade of D for all 3 populations.

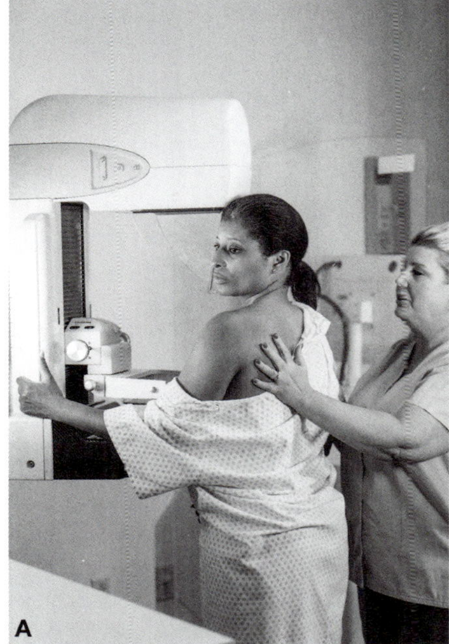

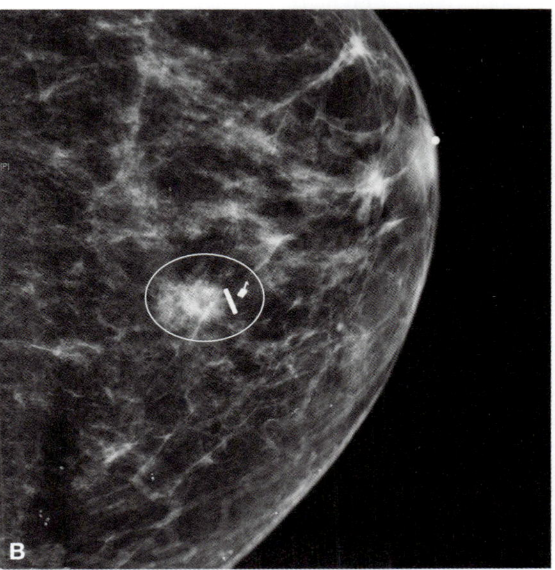

FIGURE 3.14. (A) Woman receiving a mammogram and (B) mammogram showing a nonpalpable tumor in the central lower region of the breast (in white circle). (Panel A from iStock/kali9. Panel B reprinted from Hoda SA, Rosen PP, Brogi E, Koerner FC. *Rosen's Breast Pathology*. 11th ed. Wolters-Kluwer; 2021.)

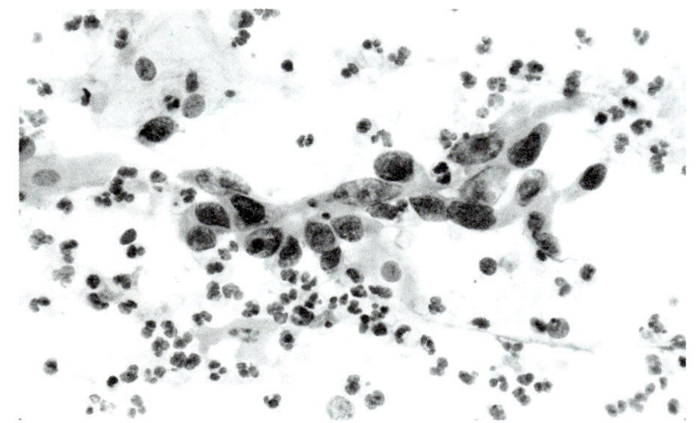

FIGURE 3.15. Image from a microscope examining cervical cells from a Pap smear. The dark cells are cancerous. (From the National Cancer Institute. Available from https://visualsonline.cancer.gov/details.cfm?imageid=2578.)

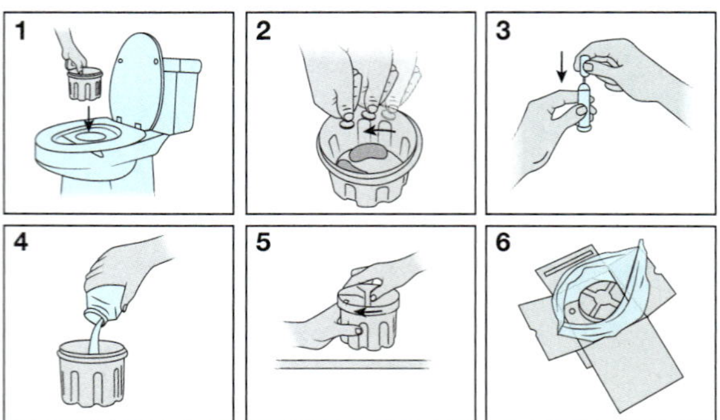

FIGURE 3.16. Six steps for the collection of fecal sample for a Cologuard® Stool DNA test. (From Prince M, Lester L, Chiniwala R, Berger B. Multitarget stool DNA tests increases colorectal cancer screening among previously noncompliant Medicare patients. *World J Gastroenterol.* 2017;23(3):464–71, Figure 1.)

Colorectal Cancer Screening

The USPSTF recommends that adults aged 50 to 75 years undergo colorectal cancer screening with a grade of A. For adults aged 45 to 49 years, the recommendation is the same, but with a grade of B. There are numerous colorectal cancer screening methods. One category of screening tests is stool based, including the fecal immunochemical test (FIT) and a stool DNA test. The FIT test detects blood in the stool; the stool DNA test detects DNA biomarkers for cancer in cells shed from the lining of the colon and rectum in the stool. A combination of FIT and the stool DNA test every 1 to 3 years is recommended. Figure 3.16 describes the process patients undergo to complete the sample collection for a version of the stool DNA test, Cologuard® (44, 45).

Lung Cancer Screening

The USPSTF recommends annual screening for lung cancer with low-dose computed tomography (CT) in adults aged 50 to 80 years who have a 20-pack-year smoking history (equivalent to a pack a day for the past 20 years) and currently smoke or have quit smoking in the past 15 years. The grade level for this recommendation is B. At the beginning of this section on screening, we noted that a criterion of a successful screening test was the ability to detect disease at an earlier stage when curative treatment might be possible. Figure 3.17 shows an image of an early-stage lung cancer detected by low-dose CT scan that was not detected on x-ray (43). Without this screening test, this early-stage tumor would have grown and possibly spread before clinical detection.

Cancers for Which Screenings Are Not Recommended

The USPSTF recommends against screening for the following cancers, based on the current levels of evidence: melanoma, bladder, oral cancers, ovarian, pancreatic, and testicular.

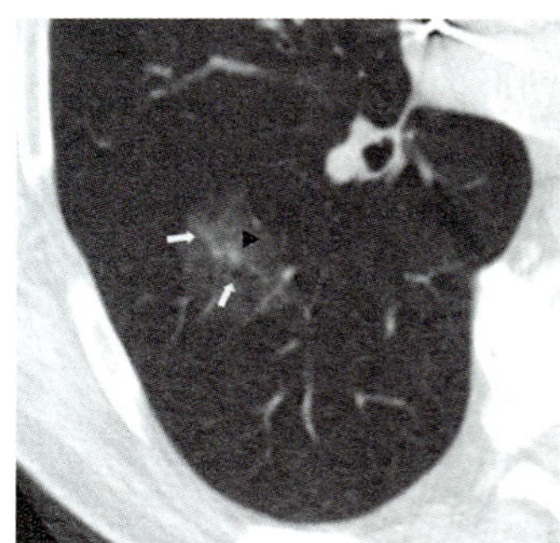

FIGURE 3.17. Low dose CT scan shows a 25-mm part-solid nodule of the right lower lobe. This nodule is characterized by a 3-mm central solid component (arrowhead) surrounded by a pure ground-glass opacity. The vessels and a small peripheral airway (arrow) can be clearly depicted within the ground-glass opacity. (From Rampinelli C, Calloni SF, Minotti M, et al. Spectrum of early lung cancer presentation in low-dose screening CT: a pictorial review. *Insights Imaging.* 2016;7(3):449–59.)

SUMMARY

The health potential for the population to reduce the burden of cancer through applying the cancer risk reduction strategies and screening guidelines described in this chapter is enormous. The strategies outlined herein represent the few things within our control with regard to cancer incidence and mortality. The challenge is that cancer is complex, and it is not possible to provide guarantees to anyone that following all the recommendations will prevent cancer from occurring. What can be said, with tremendous support from scientific evidence, is that if a cancer is diagnosed in someone who follows all guidelines in this chapter, it is likely to be an earlier stage, less aggressive, and—as a result—less likely to be deadly. Prevention and screening are sometimes a hard sell because when we succeed, nothing happens. Promoting cancer risk reduction and screening may be easier among those who are at high risk or who have already had cancer, in whom all of the strategies described are still of value.

Case Study

George is a 59-year-old teacher at a local high school. His BMI is 33, he takes his lunch at fast-food places for most days, and he drinks a 6 pack of beer about 3 nights a week. He quit smoking 2 years ago (after smoking a pack a day for 30 years). George is not regularly physically active, although he loves to go to the beach. In high school, he injected illegal drugs for about 3 months.

Questions:

1. What are his cancer risk factors that could be altered to reduce his cancer risk?
2. What are your recommendations regarding his weight?
3. What are your recommendations regarding his diet?
4. George drinks 18 beers a week. If he reduced his alcohol intake, which cancers would he be at reduced risk for?
5. What would you recommend regarding George's smoking habits?
6. What would you recommend regarding George's physical activity?
7. Are there cancer screenings you would recommend for George?

Meet the Expert

FEATURED PROFESSIONAL

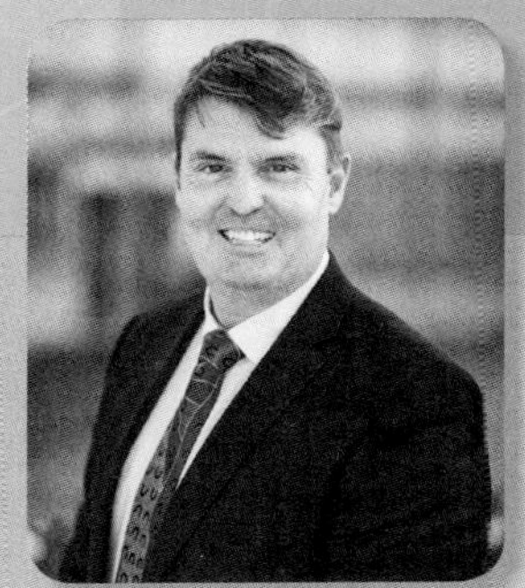

Rob Newton, PhD, DSc, AEP, CSCS*D, FACSM, ESSAF, FNSCA

Vice-Chancellor's Professorial Research Fellow
Professor of Exercise Medicine, Exercise Medicine Research Institute
Edith Cowan University, Western Australia

Q: "Where did you grow up?"

Lismore, on the east coast of Australia. Most people would know the area for what is now one of our most famous towns, which is Byron Bay (Chris Hemsworth [Thor] and his family live there).

Q: "Where did you train? What is your training?"

I completed my bachelor's degree and master's in Exercise Physiology at the University of Queensland and then my PhD in Biomechanics at Southern Cross University on the east coast of Australia. In 2021, I was awarded a higher doctorate (DSc) in Exercise Oncology from the University of Queensland.

Q: "What are you best known for?"

The first 20 years of my career I was a researcher and practitioner in the exercise sciences, predominantly focusing on strength and power assessment and development in athletes and became quite well known and had an opportunity to work with many famous organizations, including the Chicago Bulls and Nike. In 1994, during a sabbatical at Penn State University, I became increasingly interested in using advanced training methodologies with healthy elderly people and patient populations, principally people with cancer. I am probably best known for translating advanced strength and conditioning methods for exercise medicine in people with cancer. I introduced periodization, autoregulation, and targeted exercise prescription to address critical discrepancies in patients. These are all concepts well established in athlete training but not previously used with patients.

Q: "What are you currently working on?"

It is well established that there is a relationship between physical activity and cancer survival, but we do not have a complete understanding of the mechanisms by which exercise actually alters tumor biology. My current work is directed toward expanding our knowledge of the 10 to 12 mechanisms by which exercise suppresses cancer growth with particular emphasis on body composition, cytokines, and the immune system.

Q: "Anything else you want to include?"

I find great reward in research and clinical practice of exercise oncology. The benefits for patients are substantial with no side effects. This is a fantastic field for aspiring exercise professionals and the opportunities will only increase, and we can have a profound positive impact on the lives of people with cancer.

Favorite Quote:

"Beyond mainstream cancer treatments, exercise medicine has the greatest potential to improve both quality and quantity of life for people with cancer and must be included as a critical component in patient care."

—*Rob Newton*

STUDY QUESTIONS

1. What is the most important of the cancer risk reduction strategies discussed?
2. Define a healthy body weight?
3. What are the recommendations for being adequately physically active?
4. Elements of a healthy eating pattern include:
   a. Alcohol, cheeseburgers, ice cream, and coffee
   b. Fruits, vegetables, fiber, and dairy
   c. Fiber, fruit, avoiding alcohol, and avocados
   d. Fruits, vegetables, avoiding alcohol, and limiting red meat
5. Breastfeeding reduces risks for what types of cancer in the mother?
6. What is the primary remaining setting in which someone might be exposed to secondhand smoke?
7. There are 6 recommended behaviors to limit your exposure to UV light. Name 3.
8. HPV vaccination reduces risk of 6 cancers. Name 3.
9. Hepatitis B vaccine is recommended in what age range?
   a. 10 to 11 years
   b. Infants to 18 years
   c. 50 to 75 years
   d. Only in intravenous drug users older than 50
10. Why is screening for hepatitis C virus important?
    a. Because it shows whether you are likely to develop lung cancer
    b. Because it is treatable in most people in 8 to 12 weeks
    c. Because it is associated with the development of liver cancer
    d. a and b
    e. b and c
    f. All of the above
11. Which of the following is a myth?
    a. Cancer is contagious
    b. Antiperspirant can cause cancer
    c. People with cancer shouldn't eat sugar
    d. All of the above
    e. a and c
12. There are 8 characteristics of a good screening test. Name 4.
13. The name of the organization that provides federal recommendations for cancer screening in the US?
14. True or false. The USPSTF recommends ultrasound as a screening test for breast cancer.
15. The cervical cancer screening test is called a Pap smear. It is recommended every 3 years for women in what age range?
    a. 11 to 18 years
    b. 18 to 50 years
    c. 50 to 75 years
    d. 21 to 65 years
16. Colorectal cancer screening test options include:
    a. Colonoscopy
    b. Fecal immunochemical tests
    c. Stool DNA tests
    d. Bristol stool tests
    e. a and d
    f. a–c
    g. All of the above
17. Low-dose computed tomography (CT) is recommended for lung cancer screening for what population?
    a. All adults of 21 to 65 years
    b. Current smokers who are of 50 to 80 years of age
    c. Former smokers of 50 to 80 years of age who quit smoking within the past 15 years
    d. All of the above
    e. b and c only
    f. a and b only
18. What is the hypothesized mechanism by which breastfeeding reduces risk for breast and ovarian cancer?
19. Name one of the hypothesized mechanisms by which physical inactivity may increase risk for cancer.
20. Name 2 of the hypothesized mechanisms by which excess weight may increase risk for cancer.

REFERENCES

1. Centers for Disease Control and Prevention. *Healthy Weight, Nutrition, and Physical Activity: About Adult BMI.* [Internet]. 2023. Available from https://www.cdc.gov/healthyweight/assessing/bmi/adult_bmi/index.html
2. Centers for Disease Control and Prevention. *Obesity and Cancer.* [Internet]. 2023. Available from https://www.cdc.gov/cancer/obesity/index.htm
3. Moore SC, Lee IM, Weiderpass E, et al. Association of leisure-time physical activity with risk of 26 types of cancer in 1.44 million adults. *JAMA Intern Med.* 2016;176(6):816–25. doi:10.1001/jamainternmed.2016.1548
4. McTiernan A, Friedenreich CM, Katzmarzyk PT, et al. Physical activity in cancer prevention and survival: a systematic review. *Med Sci Sports Exerc.* 2019;51(6):1252–61. doi:10.1249/MSS.0000000000001937
5. Patel AV, Friedenreich CM, Moore SC, et al. American College of Sports Medicine® roundtable report on physical activity, sedentary behavior, and cancer prevention and control. *Med Sci Sports Exerc.* 2019;51(11):2391–402. doi:10.1249/MSS.0000000000002117

6. Ainsworth BE, Haskell WL, Whitt MC, et al. Compendium of physical activities: an update of activity codes and MET intensities. *Med Sci Sports Exerc.* 2000;32(9 Suppl):S498–504.
7. Chen PL, Roh W, Reuben A, et al. Analysis of immune signatures in longitudinal tumor samples yields insight into biomarkers of response and mechanisms of resistance to immune checkpoint blockade. *Cancer Discov.* 2016;6(8):827–37. doi:10.1158/2159-8290.CD-15-1545
8. Brown JC, Winters-Stone K, Lee A, Schmitz KH. Cancer, physical activity, and exercise. *Compr Physiol.* 2012;2(4):2775–809. doi:10.1002/cphy.c120005
9. Statistics NCfH. *National Health Interview Survey: Early Release of Selected Estimates Based on Data from the 2018 National Health Interview Survey.* [Internet]. 2023. Available from https://www.cdc.gov/nchs/nhis/releases/released201905.htm#7a
10. University PS. *Brochure Post #5: What Is Your Level of Physical Activity?* [Internet]. 2023. Available from https://sites.psu.edu/rvonarxnutrition/2015/11/08/where-do-you-fit-on-the-physical-activity-pyramid/
11. Medicine ACoS. *Exercise Is Medicine®*. [Internet]. 2023. Available from https://www.exerciseismedicine.org/
12. Trilk JL, Phillips EM. Incorporating "Exercise is Medicine®" into the University of South Carolina School of Medicine Greenville and Greenville Health System. *Br J Sports Med.* 2014;48(3):165–7. doi:10.1136/bjsports-2013-093157
13. American Cancer Society. *Infographi: Diet and Activity Guidelines to Reduce Cancer Risk.* [Internet]. 2023. Available from https://www.cancer.org/healthy/eat-healthy-get-active/acs-guidelines-nutrition-physical-activity-cancer-prevention/infographic.html
14. Rock CL, Thomson C, Gansler T, et al. American Cancer Society guideline for diet and physical activity for cancer prevention. *CA Cancer J Clin.* 2020;70(4):245–71. doi:10.3322/caac.21591
15. Steck SE, Murphy EA. Dietary patterns and cancer risk. *Nat Rev Cancer.* 2020;20(2):125–38. doi:10.1038/s41568-019-0227-4
16. Victoria CC. *Alcohol Causes at least 7 Types of Cancer.* [Internet]. 2023. Available from https://www.cancervic.org.au/preventing-cancer/limit-alcohol/reduce-your-drinking
17. National Center for Chronic Disease Prevention and Health Prom. *Strategies to Prevent Obesity and Other Chronic Diseases: The CDC Guide to Strategies to Support Breastfeeding Mothers and Babies.* [Internet]. 2013. Available from http://www.cdc.gov/breastfeeding
18. Centers for Disease Control and Prevention. *Smoking and Tobacco Use: Cancer Care Settings and Smoking Cessation.* [Internet]. 2023. Available from https://www.cdc.gov/tobacco/patient-care/care-settings/cancer/index.htm
19. Centers for Disease Control and Prevention. *Smoking and Tobacco Use: Benefits of Quitting.* [Internet]. 2023. Available from https://www.cdc.gov/tobacco/quit_smoking/how_to_quit/benefits/index.htm#cancer-related-benefits
20. Jha P. The hazards of smoking and the benefits of cessation: a critical summation of the epidemiological evidence in high-income countries. *eLife.* 2020;9:e49979. doi:10.7554/eLife.49979
21. American Cancer Society. *How to Quit Smoking.* [Internet]. 2023. Available from https://www.cancer.org/latest-news/how-to-quit-smoking.html
22. American Cancer Society. *Health Risks of Secondhand Smoke.* [Internet]. 2023. Available from https://www.cancer.org/healthy/stay-away-from-tobacco/health-risks-of-tobacco/secondhand-smoke.html
23. Besaratinia A, Pfeifer GP. Second-hand smoke and human lung cancer. *Lancet Oncol.* 2008;9(7):657–66. doi:10.1016/S1470-2045(08)70172-4
24. U.S. Department of Health and Human Services. *The Health Consequences of Involuntary Exposure to Tobacco Smoke: A Report of the Surgeon General.* Atlanta (GA): U.S. Department of Health and Human Services, Centers for Disease Control and Prevention, Coordinating Center for Health Promotion, National Center for Chronic Disease Prevention and Health Promotion, Office on Smoking and Health, 2006, pp. 1–727.
25. Centers for Disease Control and Prevention. *Skin Cancer: Sun Safety.* [Internet]. 2023. Available from https://www.cdc.gov/cancer/skin/basic_info/sun-safety.htm
26. American Cancer Society. *Ultraviolet Radiation.* [Internet]. 2023. Available from https://www.cancer.org/cancer/cancer-causes/radiation-exposure/uv-radiation.html
27. American Cancer Society. *How Do I Protect Myself from Ultraviolet (UV) Rays?* [Internet]. 2023. Available from https://www.cancer.org/healthy/be-safe-in-sun/uv-protection.html
28. Centers for Disease Control and Prevention. *Human Papillomavirus (HPV): HPV Vaccine.* [Internet]. 2023. Available from https://www.cdc.gov/hpv/parents/vaccine-for-hpv.html
29. Heptitis B Foundation. *Vaccine for Hepatitis B.* [Internet]. 2023. Available from https://www.hepb.org/prevention-and-diagnosis/vaccination/
30. Centers for Disease Control and Prevention. *HPV Vaccination Is the Best Protection Against Certain Cancers Caused by HPV.* [Internet]. 2023. Available from https://www.cdc.gov/hpv/hcp/hpv-important/infographic-hpv-screening-508.pdf
31. Centers for Disease Control and Prevention. *Cancers Caused by HPV.* [Internet]. 2023. Available from https://www.cdc.gov/hpv/parents/cancer.html
32. Chang MH. Hepatitis B virus and cancer prevention. *Recent Results Cancer Res.* 2011;188:75–84. doi:10.1007/978-3-642-10858-7_6
33. Munger K, Baldwin A, Edwards KM, et al. Mechanisms of human papillomavirus-induced oncogenesis. *J Virol.* 2004;78(21):11451–60. doi:10.1128/JVI.78.21.11451-11460.2004.
34. Levrero M, Zucman-Rossi J. Mechanisms of HBV-induced hepatocellular carcinoma. *J Hepatol.* 2016;64(suppl 1):S84–101. doi:10.1016/j.jhep.2016.02.021
35. US Preventive Services Task Force; Owens DK, Davidson KW, et al. Screening for hepatitis C virus infection in adolescents and adults: US Preventive Services Task Force Recommendation Statement. *JAMA.* 2020;323(10):970–5. doi:10.1001/jama.2020.1123
36. Liu B, Zhang Y, Li J, Zhang W. Hepatitis C virus and risk of extra-hepatic malignancies: a case-control study. *Sci Rep.* 2019;9(1):19444. doi:10.1038/s41598-019-55249-w
37. Vescovo T, Refolo G, Vitagliano G, Fimia GM, Piacentini M. Molecular mechanisms of hepatitis C virus-induced hepatocellular carcinoma. *Clin Microbiol Infect.* 2016;22(10):853–61. doi:10.1016/j.cmi.2016.07.019
38. American Association for Cancer Research. *Preventing Cancer: Identifying Risk Factors.* [Internet]. 2023. Available from https://cancerprogressreport.aacr.org/progress/cpr19-contents/cpr19-preventing-cancer/
39. US Preventive Services Task Force. *Grade Definitions.* [Internet]. 2023. Available from https://www.uspreventiveservicestaskforce.org/uspstf/about-uspstf/methods-and-processes/grade-definitions
40. US Preventive Services Task Force. *Final Recommendation Statement Breast Cancer Screening 2016.* [Internet]. 2023. Available from https://www.uspreventiveservicestaskforce.org/uspstf/recommendation/breast-cancer-screening
41. Breast360.org. *Beneath the Surface: A Guide to Breast Imaging.* [Internet]. 2023. Available from https://breast360.org/topic/2017/01/01/beneath-surface-guide-breast-imaging/
42. Centers for Disease Control and Prevention. *Breast Cancer: What Is Breast Cancer Screening?* [Internet]. 2023. Available from https://www.cdc.gov/cancer/breast/basic_info/screening.htm
43. National Cancer Institute. *Cytological Specimen Showing Cervical Cancer.* [Internet]. 2023. Available from https://visualsonline.cancer.gov/details.cfm?imageid=2578
44. Hirsch FR, Franklin WA, Gazdar AF, Bunn PA, Jr. Early detection of lung cancer: clinical perspectives of recent advances in biology and radiology. *Clin Cancer Res.* 2001;7(1):5–22.
45. Prince M, Lester L, Chiniwala R, Berger B. Multitarget stool DNA tests increases colorectal cancer screening among previously noncompliant Medicare patients. *World J Gastroenterol.* 2017;23(3):464–71. doi:10.3748/wjg.v23.i3.464

CHAPTER

4

Diagnosis and Treatment

OUTLINE

1. Introduction: Diagnosis and Treatment
2. Diagnosis
   a. Imaging
   b. Endoscopy
   c. Biopsy
   d. Cancer Staging
3. Treatment
   a. Surgery
   b. Radiation Therapy
   c. Chemotherapy
   d. Immunotherapies and Targeted Therapies
   e. Vaccine Therapies
   f. Cytokine Treatments
   g. Administration of Chemotherapy and Immunotherapy
   h. Duration of Treatments
   i. Nadir
   j. Hormonal Therapy
   k. CAR-T Cell Therapy
   l. Blood and Marrow Transplant
4. Side Effects of Cancer and Its Treatments
   a. Acute Effects
5. Summary
6. Case Study
7. Meet the Expert
8. Study Questions
9. References

OBJECTIVES

After completing review of this chapter, students will be able to:

1. Describe the steps in diagnosis.
2. Know the different stages of cancer.
3. Explain different ways in which radiation therapy can be delivered.
4. Define chimeric antigen receptor therapy (CAR-T).

INTRODUCTION: DIAGNOSIS AND TREATMENT

There are more than a hundred different types of cancer. However, there is no single test to diagnose cancer. Some early-stage cancers may not have any symptoms or findings on routine physical examination or serological measures, whereas others have common, relatively easily identifiable presenting signs and symptoms. Common signs and symptoms of cancer are unintentional weight loss, pain, fatigue, headache, fever, cough, night sweats, hoarseness, changes in voice, appetite, bowel habits, unusual bleeding, bruising, skin changes, and enlarged lymph node(s) (Box 4.1). As a cancerous tumor grows, it may press on a nerve or other organ and cause pain, weakness, or nausea, which may be a presenting symptom. Cancerous tumors are malignant. The cells grow uncontrollably and invade nearby tissues and can spread into other areas of the body. There are many different tests that may be required to diagnose each type of cancer. We present a broad overview of diagnostics available but cannot provide the detail needed to identify and diagnose all cancers.

Box 4.1 Common Signs and Symptoms of Cancer

Fatigue or extreme tiredness that does not get better with rest.

- Weight loss or gain of 10 pounds or more for no known reason.
- Eating problems such as not feeling hungry, feeling full with minimal intake, trouble swallowing, belly pain, or nausea and vomiting.
- Swelling or lumps anywhere in the body.
- Thickening or lump in the breast or other part of the body.
- Pain, especially new or with no known reason, which does not go away or gets worse.
- Skin changes such as a lump that bleeds or turns scaly, a new mole or a change in a mole, a sore that does not heal, or a yellowish color to the skin or eyes (jaundice).
- Cough or hoarseness that does not go away.
- Unusual bleeding, for example, in stools or gums, or bruising for no known reason.
- Change in bowel habits, such as constipation or diarrhea, which does not go away or a change in the appearance of stools.
- Bladder changes such as pain when passing urine, blood in the urine, or needing to pass urine more or less often.
- Fever or nights sweats.
- Headache.
- Vision or hearing problems.
- Mouth changes such as sores, bleeding, pain, or numbness.

Data from American Cancer Society. *Signs and Symptoms of Cancer: American Cancer Society.* [Internet]. 2021. Available from https://www.cancer.org/cancer/cancer-basics/signs-and-symptoms-of-cancer.

DIAGNOSIS

Diagnosis usually begins with a history, physical examination and diagnostic testing that may include laboratory tests, imaging (x-rays, CT scans, magnetic resonance imaging [MRI], nuclear scan, bone scan, positron emission tomography [PET] scan, endoscopic exams), genetic testing, and biopsies.

Laboratory tests, such as complete blood count (CBC), complete metabolic panel, urinalysis, and tumor markers can detect different chemicals in blood and urine that may indicate malignant growth. A CBC is used in diagnosing leukemia and lymphoma, in addition to many other health conditions. A complete metabolic panel can provide information on fluid and electrolyte balance, blood sugar, kidney and liver function, and protein levels. Urine tests can be used to detect some bladder cancers and multiple myeloma.

Tumor markers are released by cancer cells into the blood or urine and reflect tumor and disease activity. They can be used in diagnosis, staging disease, determining prognosis, predicting response to treatment, determining optimal targeted treatment, and monitoring response to treatment. Not all cancers have a specific tumor marker. Common tumor markers used to diagnose and monitor response to treatment are: prostate-specific antigen (PSA), CA 125, carcinoembryonic antigen (CEA), alpha-fetoprotein (AFP), human chorionic gonadotropin (HCG), CA 19-9, CA 15-3, and lactate dehydrogenase (LDH) (Table 4.1). Tumor markers can also be used to determine targeted treatments. For example, the *BRC-ABL* fusion gene (Philadelphia chromosome), *BCL2* gene re-arrangement, *BRAF* V600 mutations are 2 mutations that indicate if a specific treatment will work for chronic myelogenous leukemia, colorectal cancer and melanoma. A useful resource can be found on the NCI website, which also provides links to guidelines for markers used for cancer screening (https://www.cancer.gov/about-cancer/diagnosis-staging/diagnosis/tumor-markers-fact-sheet).

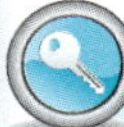

Tumor markers. Cancer cells release them into the blood or urine, where they reflect tumor and disease activities. Tumor markers are used in diagnosis, staging disease, determining prognosis, predicting response to treatment, determining optimal targeted treatment, and monitoring response to treatment.

Table 4.1 Common Tumor Markers

	WHAT IS ANALYZED	TYPE OF CANCER	PURPOSE
ALK gene rearrangements and overexpression	Tumor	Non–small-cell lung cancer, anaplastic large cell lymphoma	Treatment and prognosis
Alfa-fetoprotein	Blood	Liver, germ line tumors (eg, testicular)	Diagnose, stage, determine prognosis and assess response to treatment
B-cell immunoglobulin gene rearrangement	Blood, bone marrow	B-cell lymphoma	Diagnosis, assess response to treatment, check for recurrence
Beta-2 microglobulin	Blood, urine	Multiple myeloma, chronic lymphocytic leukemia, some lymphomas	Prognosis and response to treatment
BRCA1 and *BRCA2* gene mutations	Blood or tumor	Breast and ovarian cancers	Determine treatment
BCR-ABL fusion gene (Philadelphia chromosome)	Blood or bone marrow	Chronic myeloid leukemia, acute lymphoblastic and myelogenous leukemia	Confirm diagnosis, predict response to treatment, determine treatment, monitor disease
BRAF V600 mutations	Tumor	Melanoma, colorectal cancer, non–small-cell lung cancer	Determine treatment
CA-125	Blood	Ovarian cancer	Diagnose, assess response to treatment and evaluate recurrence
Carcinoembryonic antigen	Blood	Colorectal and some other cancers	Track treatment and recurrence
CD20	Blood	Non-Hodgkin's lymphoma	Determine treatment
Lactate dehydrogenase	Blood	Germ cell tumors, lymphoma, leukemia, melanoma, neuroblastoma	Assess stage, prognosis and response to treatment
Prostate-specific antigen	Blood	Prostate cancer	Diagnosis, response to treatment, recurrence

Data from National Cancer Institute. *Tumor Markers in Common Use: National Cancer Institute.* [Internet]. 2021. Available from https://www.cancer.gov/about-cancer/diagnosis-staging/diagnosis/tumor-markers-list.

Imaging

Diagnostic imaging is used to pinpoint the location and extent of a tumor. Imaging can also be used to guide a precise biopsy. Diagnostic scanning can determine the size of the tumor and if it has spread beyond the site of origin (metastasized). Cancers commonly metastasize to the liver, lungs, bones, and brain, and imaging is used for diagnosis to determine if the cancer is confined to one area or has spread to other organs. During and after treatment, imaging is used to assess response to treatment and determine if a patient is responding to treatment, in remission, or has distant spread of disease (metastasis). There are 3 types of diagnostic imaging used in cancer diagnosis and follow-up: transmission, reflection, and emission imaging.

Transmission imaging uses a beam of high-energy photons that are passed through the body part being examined. The beam passes through blood, fat, and water leaving a dark image on the x-ray, while muscle, ligaments, tendons, and cartilage appear gray, and bones appear white. Transmission imaging includes x-rays, CT scans, bone scans, mammograms, and fluoroscopy (Figure 4.1).

Reflection imaging uses high-frequency sound waves that produce an image based on the density of the tissue. A solid tumor will appear as a lighter colored image because the sound waves will bounce off the tumor. Ultrasounds uses this technology to image blood vessels, tissues, and organs.

Emission imaging uses nuclear particles or magnetic energy to produce an image. Nuclear medicine records the amount of nuclear material discharged into the body part being examined. Areas with higher uptake indicate greater metabolic activity, which generally reflects malignant disease. MRI uses radio waves that create a strong magnetic field and ultimately an image. MRI is used instead of CT scan when a study is needed to only examine organs, nerves and other soft tissue, but not bones.

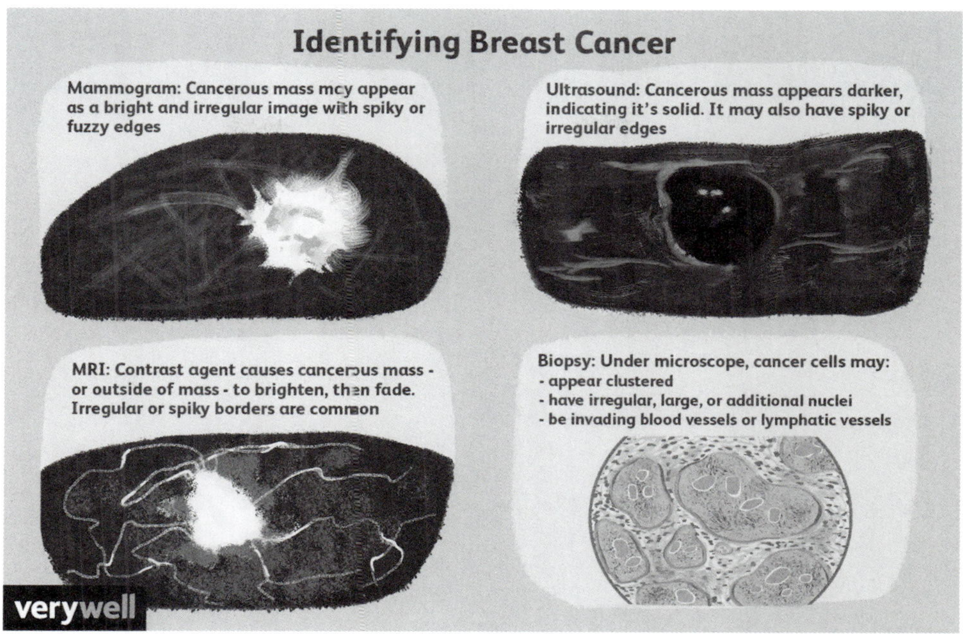

FIGURE 4.1. Identifying breast cancer with mammogram, ultrasound, MRI and biopsy. (From Stephan P, illustration by Olah J. *Very Well Health. Distinguishing Breast Cancer Tumors from Benign Masses.* [Internet]. 2021. Available from https://www.verywellhealth.com/breast-cancer-tumors-or-benign-masses-430277.)

PET scan is another imaging technique that uses radioactive tracers to visualize abnormal metabolic uptake of the tracer. The tracer is injected into a vein and will collect in an area of high metabolic uptake or biochemical activity. PET scans combine CT and MRI technology and can pinpoint areas of higher metabolic activity. Cancer cells show up as bright spots on PET scans because they have higher metabolic rates than normal cells; cancer cells divide faster. These scans are sometimes called PET-CT of PET-MRI.

Endoscopy

Endoscopic examinations use an instrument with a small fiberscope or magnifying lens to view the interior of a canal or interior of an organ (stomach, esophagus, bronchi, colon, rectum, bladder, etc). Colonoscopy is performed to examine the rectum, sigmoid colon, anal verge, and the entire colon. Polyps or suspicious tissue can be sampled for pathologic evaluation. Bronchoscopy is a way to visualize the bronchi of the lungs. The scope may be passed through the oral or nasal passage. Laparoscopy is used to examine the abdomen or reproductive system. Endoscopic examinations are methods to obtain tissue samples for pathologic review and diagnosis.

Biopsy

A biopsy is a small sample of tissue taken from a suspicious site that is then examined in the laboratory. A biopsy specimen is the most accurate means of diagnosing cancer. Biopsies include endoscopic biopsies from sites such as the colon, rectum, bladder wall, lung, or bronchus; skin biopsies to obtain cells to diagnose melanoma or other cancers; and bone marrow biopsy to examine cell development and reproduction.

There are different types of skin biopsies. A shave biopsy takes a thin layer of the surface of skin; a punch biopsy removes a small section of a deeper layer of skin; an incisional biopsy removes a small area of skin; and an excisional biopsy removes a larger area of abnormal skin or a lump and usually requires stitches to close the skin. Surgical biopsies are necessary when the suspicious area cannot be reached by other means, or the other biopsies are inconclusive.

Needle biopsies are often combined with imaging to collect cells from a suspicious lymph node or area, such as a breast lump. Needle biopsy procedures include fine needle aspiration, core needle biopsy, vacuum-assisted biopsy, and image-guided biopsy.

Bone marrow biopsy is obtained if leukemia, lymphoma, or multiple myeloma are suspected. In this procedure, a needle is used to draw bone marrow out of the posterior pelvic bone. The bone marrow sample provides detailed information about cell development and numbers.

After a biopsy is obtained, it is sent to the laboratory for pathology review. The sample is sectioned into thin slices, placed on slides, stained to enhance the material, and examined under a microscope. The pathologist reviews the characteristics of the cells and determines the type of cancer and its aggressiveness, and then the grade. Cells are graded from Grade 1, slow growing and less aggressive cells, to Grade 4,

Table 4.2 Stages of Cancer

STAGE	WHAT IT MEANS
Stage 0: Carcinoma in situ	Abnormal cells present but have not spread to nearby tissue. Also called carcinoma in situ or CIS. CIS is not cancer, but it may become cancer.
Stage 1: Early stage	Small invasive mass. No spread to lymph nodes or other tissues.
Stage 2: Localized	Larger mass that is affecting nearby tissue and may have spread to lymph nodes.
Stage 3: Regional spread	Mass is large and affects more surrounding tissues and spread to distant lymph nodes away from mass.
Stage 4: Distant spread	Cancer has spread to other tissues or organs beyond the region it originated. Also called metastatic cancer.
In situ	Abnormal cells are present but have not spread to nearby tissue.
Localized	Cancer is limited to the place where it started, with no sign that it has spread.
Regional	Cancer has spread to nearby lymph nodes, tissues, or organs.
Distant	Cancer has spread to distant parts of the body.
Unknown	There is not enough information to figure out the stage.

Data from National Cancer Institute. *Cancer Staging*. [Internet]. 2021. Available from https://www.cancer.gov/about-cancer/diagnosis-staging/staging.

fast growing (high grade) and more aggressive cells. The pathology report provides details about the biopsy and the characteristics of the tumor.

Cancer Staging

Cancer staging is a way to describe the extent of cancer, including how large the tumor is and if it has spread. There are different staging systems, but most commonly diseases are classified by the TNM system, where T is the size and extent of the tumor, N refers to the number of lymph nodes involved, and M indicates whether the cancer has metastasized. Table 4.2 explains the different stages of cancer.

Often clinicians will talk about cancer being in situ, localized, regional, distant, or unknown (Box 4.2). It is good to be familiar with these terms because they give a quick understanding of the extent of disease a patient has and help make decisions regarding an exercise prescription.

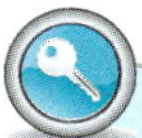

Cancer staging. Describes the size of the tumor (T), the number of lymph nodes involved (N), and if the tumor has metastasized (M).

TREATMENT

Cancer treatment may be delivered in different ways depending on the person's physical and medical condition. Treatment generally includes a combination of surgery,

Box 4.2 Terminology Related to Extent of Disease

In situ—Abnormal cells are present but have not spread to nearby tissue.

- Localized—Cancer is limited to the place where it started, with no sign that it has spread.
- Regional—Cancer has spread to nearby lymph nodes, tissues, or organs.
- Distant—Cancer has spread to distant parts of the body.
- Unknown—There is not enough information to figure out the stage.

Data from the National Cancer Institute. *Cancer Staging: National Cancer Institute*. [Internet]. 2021. Available from https://www.cancer.gov/about-cancer/diagnosis-staging/staging.

chemotherapy, biologic or immunotherapy, hormonal therapy, radiation therapy, and blood and marrow transplant (BMT). The order of treatment is often determined by the type and size of the tumor. Adjuvant therapy is given after the primary treatment (surgery or radiation therapy) to reduce the risk of recurrence. *Neoadjuvant chemotherapy* is a term used to describe a treatment plan that includes chemotherapy or biologic therapy administered before surgery with the goal of reducing the tumor size to make surgical excision more effective. For example, a woman with a large breast tumor (Stage 3) might receive several cycles of neoadjuvant therapy: a combination of different chemotherapy drugs every 2 to 3 weeks, followed by surgery, ample recovery time, and then the resumption of chemotherapy.

A tumor board is a multidisciplinary team that usually includes medical oncologist(s), oncology nurse(s), radiation oncologist(s), radiation oncology nurse(s), radiation dosimetrist(s), and surgeons of a variety of specialties (eg, breast, gastrointestinal [GI], orthopedic, neurology, plastic, and reconstructive). Rehabilitation professionals (physiatrists and occupational and physical therapists) participate when appropriate to plan for managing the functional impact of the disease and its treatment. As a team, they meet to review a patient's history, disease presentation, radiological images, and pathology and discuss optimal treatment plans that include issues of morbidity, mortality, and function. The treatment plans are usually based on recommendations of the NCCN Guidelines. The team may discuss participation in possible **clinical trials** in which the patient may be eligible to enroll. The NCCN Guidelines are continuously updated evidence-based guidelines for the treatment of cancer by type of cancer, stage of disease, and recurrence to support decision-making. The NCCN is considered the authoritative reference for oncology treatment. The tumor board discusses the case and then often meets with the patient to present their recommendations and discuss treatment options with the patient.

Surgery

The goal of surgery for cancer treatment is to remove as much as possible, if not all, of the cancer without unduly compromising the health and function of the patient. Surgery can be done for a variety of purposes:

- Diagnostic surgery: to remove the tissue sample for biopsy.
- Staging surgery: to determine the extent of cancer.
- Debulking surgery: to remove part of the tumor when removing the entire tumor would cause excessive damage to an organ. Chemotherapy or radiation therapy is used afterward to further shrink the tumor.
- Palliative surgery: to treat advanced cancer to relieve discomfort; not for a cure.
- Supportive surgery: to help deliver a treatment.
- Restorative or reconstructive surgery: used after treatments to restore one's appearance. Examples are breast reconstruction after breast cancer, facial reconstruction after oral cancer, or a nose prosthesis after a nasal melanoma.

Radiation Therapy

Radiation therapy is used to prevent the spread of cancer or relieve symptoms caused by advanced cancer. Radiation therapy can be delivered externally or internally. External beam radiation uses high-energy radiation that is delivered from a machine externally from the body (Figure 4.2). The beam precisely targets the treatment to the site of the cancer. Internal radiation therapy is also called brachytherapy. An implant (tube, catheter, or applicator) is placed in the body near the tumor and the radiation is delivered directly to the tumor. Both types of radiation deliver treatment directly to the site of the cancer and are painless. External radiation is usually delivered 5 days a week for 3 to 9 weeks, depending on the type of cancer, extent of disease, and treatment plan. Sometimes a mold of a body part is made to prevent movement and ensures treatment is delivered precisely to the affected area. Small ink marks are placed on the body (radiation tattoos) or on the mask to use when lining up the radiation machine before each treatment. These marks ensure that the treatment is delivered to the same area each time.

The side effects of radiation therapy develop gradually over time. Fatigue, loss of appetite, and skin irritation (**radiation dermatitis**) at the treated site are the most common side effects. Fatigue can make engaging in daily activities and work difficult. If radiation is directed to the head and neck, it may make swallowing and eating difficult. Skin irritation may necessitate wearing loose-fitting clothing, protecting the skin from the sun, avoiding shaving lotions, creams, powders, and ointments that may contain alcohol. The long-term impact on soft tissues often causes debilitating consequences, including muscle fibrosis, GI tract strictures, abdominal adhesions, boney necrosis, and joint contractures. Treatments for these problems, for example, pentoxifylline, pirfenidone, and other antifibrotic agents, are available and people have some improvements in symptoms with these medications.

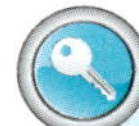

Clinical trials. Controlled studies with human participants to discover a new drug or treatment, dose or efficacy that help determine if it is better than the current standard of care.

Radiation dermatitis. Erythema (redness) that appears on the skin from exposure to radiation. The skin can blister and become irritated and painful.

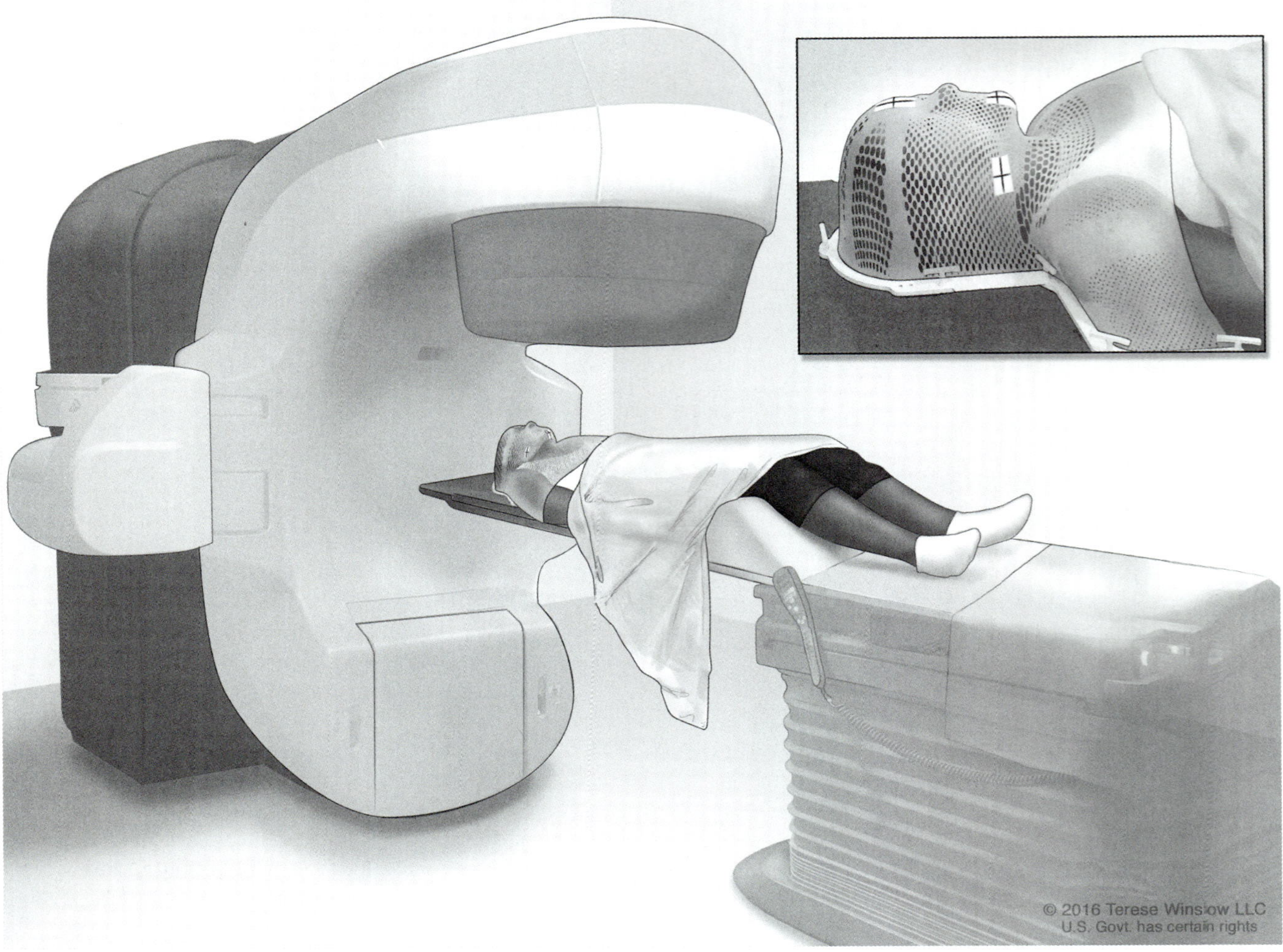

FIGURE 4.2. External beam radiation of the head and neck with radiation immobilizer. (Reprinted from National Cancer Institute. *External radiation therapy: National Cancer Institute.* [Internet]. 2021. Available from https://www.cancer.gov/publications/dictionaries/cancer-terms/def/external-radiation-therapy.)

Chemotherapy

Chemotherapy includes a wide range of drugs that stop cancer cells from growing, dividing, and spreading. These drugs affect the whole body, and because of their systemic effects, the side effects damage healthy cells. The goals of chemotherapy depend on the type and stage of cancer. Sometimes the goal is to cure the cancer, and other times, the goal is to put the disease into remission or delay further growth. Table 4.3 lists common chemotherapy drugs, some of the diseases each drug treats and common side effects.

Chemotherapy is often given as a combination of drugs because the medications often work in different ways on the cell cycle. There are 5 groups of chemotherapy drugs. They are as follows:

- **Alkylating agents:** Most active when cells are in the resting phase.
- **Plant alkaloids:** These are specific to the cell cycle and attack the cells during specific phases of division. These drugs are derived from plants. For example, vinca alkaloids are made from the periwinkle plant, taxanes are from the Pacific Yew tree.
- **Antitumor antibiotics:** specific to the cell cycle and interrupt the G2 phase.
- **Antimetabolites:** disrupt cell cycle and cell division and interfere with folate metabolism.
- **Topoisomerase inhibitors:** block cell division in the late S-G2 phase.

While these drugs interrupt the malignant cell cycle, they also affect rapidly dividing healthy cells. Some common side effects of systemic chemotherapy include alopecia (hair loss), stomatitis (mouth sores), fatigue, peripheral neuropathy (decreased sensation in fingers and toes), neutropenia (low white blood count), anemia (low red blood cell count), and thrombocytopenia (low platelet count), which increases

Table 4.3 Common Chemotherapy Drugs, Diseases Treated and Common Side Effects

DRUG	DISEASE TREATED	SIDE EFFECTS
Bleomycin	Hodgkin's lymphoma, non-Hodgkin's lymphoma, testicular cancer	Mild myelosuppression, dose limiting lung toxicity, fatigue, weakness
Busulfan	Chronic myelogenous leukemia	Pulmonary fibrosis, hyperpigmentation, seizures, hepatic occlusive disease, nausea, vomiting, thrombocytopenia
Carboplatin	Ovarian, breast, lung, brain, head and neck cancer, neuroblastoma	Myelosuppression, nephrotoxicity nausea, vomiting, fatigue, weakness
Capecitabine	Breast, gastric, colorectal cancer	Abdominal pain, nausea, vomiting, diarrhea, weakness, rashes, cardiomyopathy, myelosuppression, hand-foot syndrome, fatigue, weakness
Cisplatin	Testicular, ovarian, cervical, breast, bladder, esophageal, lung, brain, head and neck cancers, neuroblastoma	Nephrotoxicity, neurotoxicity, hearing loss, nausea, vomiting, fatigue, weakness
Cyclophosphamide	Non-Hodgkin's lymphoma, leukemias, multiple myeloma, breast, ovarian cancer	Bone marrow suppression, increased risk of infection, nausea, vomiting, alopecia, fatigue, weakness, secondary malignancies
Cytarabine	Leukemias, non-Hodgkin's lymphoma	Myelosuppression, stomatitis, pneumonitis, hand-foot syndrome, peripheral neuropathy, fatigue
Daunorubicin	Leukemias	Bone marrow suppression, stomatitis, cardio toxicity, fatigue, weakness
Docetaxel	Breast, head and neck, stomach, prostate, non–small-cell lung cancers	Cytopenia, pneumonitis, myalgias
Doxorubicin	Breast and bladder cancer, sarcoma, lymphoma, acute lymphocytic leukemia	Alopecia, stomatitis, bone marrow suppression, myelosuppression, nausea, vomiting, fatigue, weakness, cardiac toxicity
Etoposide	Testicular, colorectal cancer, small-cell lung cancers	Severe myelosuppression, diarrhea, bone marrow suppression, fatigue, weakness, liver function abnormalities, hemorrhagic cystitis
5-Fluorouracil (5-FU)	Colorectal, esophageal, stomach, pancreatic, breast, cervical cancers.	Myelosuppression, stomatitis, alopecia, fatigue, weakness, hand-foot syndrome
Gemcitabine	Breast, testicular, ovarian, non–small-cell lung cancer, pancreatic and bladder cancer	Bone marrow suppression, nausea, rash, alopecia, liver and kidney impairment, fatigue, weakness
Hydroxyurea	Chronic myelogenous leukemia, cervical cancer	Myelosuppression, shortness of breath, diarrhea, fatigue, weakness
Irinotecan	Colorectal cancer	Myelosuppression, diarrhea, hemorrhagic cystitis, bone marrow suppression, liver function abnormalities, fatigue, weakness
Melphalan	Multiple myeloma, ovarian cancer	Myelosuppression, pulmonary fibrosis, interstitial pneumonitis, nausea, alopecia, fatigue, weakness, cardiac arrest
Methotrexate	Acute lymphocytic leukemia, Burkitt's lymphoma, breast, head and neck tumors, osteogenic sarcoma. Noncancer uses psoriasis, rheumatoid arthritis	Myelosuppression, increased risk of infection, hepatotoxicity, ulcerative stomatitis, leukopenia, nausea, fatigue, weakness
Oxaliplatin	Colorectal cancer	Chemotherapy induced peripheral neuropathy, nausea, diarrhea, myelosuppression, fatigue, weakness
Paclitaxel	Breast, lung, ovarian, pancreatic and cervical cancer	Chemotherapy induced peripheral neuropathy, nausea, diarrhea, myelosuppression, pulmonary inflammation, fatigue, weakness
Vincristine	Acute lymphocytic leukemia, acute myeloid leukemia, Hodgkin's lymphoma, neuroblastoma, small-cell lung cancer	Chemotherapy induced peripheral neuropathy, foot drop, hearing loss, neutropenia, thrombocytopenia, fatigue, weakness
Vinblastine	Hodgkin's lymphoma, non–small-cell lung cancer, bladder, brain, testicular cancer and melanoma	Constipation, myelosuppression, shortness of breath, fatigue, weakness

Data from Chu E. Cancer chemotherapy. In: Katzung BG, Vanderah TW, editors. *Basic & Clinical Pharmacology*. 15th ed. New York (NY): McGraw-Hill; 2021.

Box 4.3 Side Effects of Chemotherapy

The following are the side effects of chemotherapy:

Alopecia: Hair loss caused from chemotherapy and sometimes from radiation if directed to scalp.

Anemia: Low RBCs sometimes requiring transfusion of RBCs. Can cause shortness of breath, dizziness, rapid heart rate, and fatigue. Caused from many cancer treatments.

Bone marrow suppression: Occurs when bone marrow does not produce adequate amounts of RBCs, white blood cells, or platelets. May be caused by cancer treatments or be a symptom of some cancers, such as myeloma or leukemia.

Cardiomyopathy: May develop as a late effect of treatment and manifest as arrythmia, arterial stenosis, conduction disorders, and valvular disease. Causes shortness of breath, fatigue, and swelling in the legs.

Chemotherapy-induced peripheral neuropathy (CIPN): Occurs during treatment with chemotherapy drugs (paclitaxel and oxaliplatin). Causes decreased sensation, burning, and pain in fingers, toes, hands, feet, and can extend to forearm and lower legs. This side effect often does not resolve.

Foot drop: From nerve damage and prevents flexion of the foot.

Hand-foot syndrome: Palms of hands and bottom of feet become red when the drug leaks out of the capillaries into surrounding tissues. The condition is painful and can lead to blisters and ulcers. Makes walking and using hands difficult and may require dose reduction or cessation. Hand-foot syndrome can erase fingerprints, but this is rare.

Myelosuppression: Bone marrow suppression caused by cancer treatments.

Neutropenia: Low neutrophils, a type of white blood cells that are critical in fighting infection. Neutrophils are commonly suppressed with many chemotherapy treatments. Granulocyte colony-stimulating factors (G-CSF) are routinely given to prevent febrile neutropenia (profound neutropenia) that often requires hospitalization.

Pneumonitis: Inflammation of the alveoli in the lungs. Can cause lifelong changes.

Pulmonary fibrosis: Lungs become scarred and stiff. May develop from pneumonitis.

Stomatitis: Inflammation of the mucosa of the mouth, throat, and esophagus that causes painful red sores in the mouth, gums, and throat. The lesions (sores) may be severe enough to cause inability to eat. Also called mucositis.

Thrombocytopenia: Low platelet count. Can increase risk for bleeding. May require platelet transfusion if critically low.

the risk for infection, anemia, and bleeding, respectively. See Box 4.3 for additional side effects and descriptions. The side effects of treatment are monitored closely during active treatment and may lead to treatment delays or dose reductions to make the treatment regimen tolerable.

Immunotherapies and Targeted Therapies

Targeted therapy increases the body's ability to fight disease and includes nonspecific immunomodulating agents, INF, interleukin (IL), colony-stimulating factors, monoclonal antibodies (MABs), and vaccines. Targeted therapy identifies key features of a cancer cell, which differentiate the cancer cell from a normal cell, and then the therapy uses a targeted approach to interfere with the cancer cell's growth (Figure 4.3). MABs and antiangiogenesis drugs are the 2 main categories of drugs. MABs target specific receptors. Antiangiogenesis drugs stop the blood supply to the cells. Thalidomide and interferon-alpha are 2 antiangiogenesis drugs. More research is needed in the field of antiangiogenesis. Table 4.4 includes common targeted therapy drugs and identifies some of the diseases they treat and what the drugs target (1).

Rituximab is a monoclonal antibody that specifically targets CD20 expression in patients with diffuse large B-cell

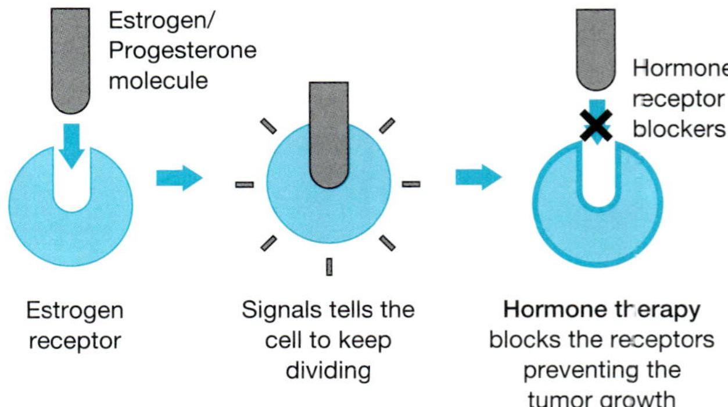

FIGURE 4.3. Hormone positive breast cancer signals the cell to divide; antiestrogen therapy (eg, tamoxifen and exemestane) block cell division and tumor growth. (Reprinted from Jotwani A. Demystifying breast cancer and its treatment. *Onco.com*. [Internet]. 2020. Available from https://onco.com/blog/demystifying-breast-cancer-and-its-treatment/.)

Table 4.4 Common Targeted Therapy Drugs, Diseases and Targets

TYPE	DRUG NAME	DISEASES: TARGETS
Monoclonal antibodies	Alemtuzumab	B-cell lymphocytic leukemia, chronic lymphocytic leukemia: targets CD52
	Gemtuzumab	Acute myeloid leukemia: targets CD33
	Rituximab	Non-Hodgkin's lymphoma, chronic lymphocytic leukemia: targets CD20
Targeted therapies	Cetuximab	Colorectal cancer, head and neck cancer: inhibits the growth factor receptor only in tumors with negative KRAS mutation
	Trastuzumab	Breast and stomach cancer: HER2 receptor positive
	Lapatinib	Breast and other solid tumors: breaks the HER2/neu and epidermal growth factor receptor pathway
Colony-stimulating factors	Pegfilgrastim	Stimulates white cells: prevents neutropenia
	Filgrastim	Stimulates white cells: prevents neutropenia
	Erythropoietin	Stimulates red cells: prevents anemia
	Romiplostim	Stimulates platelets: prevents thrombocytopenia
Bisphosphonate	Denosumab	nhibit osteoclasts cells that break down bone tissue
	Zoledronic acid	inhibit osteoclasts cells that break down bone tissue

Data from Chu E. Cancer chemotherapy. In: Katzung BG, Vanderah TW, editors. *Basic & Clinical Pharmacology.* 15th ed. New York (NY): McGraw-Hill; 2021.

lymphoma (DLBCL). It is a form of personalized precision medicine—selecting the best available drug to achieve the maximum benefit. Tafasitamab is an antibody that targets the CD19 antigen on the surface of B lymphocytes that can also be used to treated DLBCL. Some antibodies work in conjunction with a chemotherapy drug they are attached to. Polatuzumab is an anti-CD79b antibody that finds lymphoma cells and attaches to the protein CD79b. Once attached, it goes into the lymphoma cell where the chemotherapy is released and kills the cell. Biologic therapy is the forefront of cancer treatment and is rapidly evolving.

Colony-stimulating factors are the growth factors that stimulate specific cell lines to grow: white blood cells (G-CSF), RBCs (erythropoietin), and platelets (romiplostim). These drugs stimulate the stem cells to produce more cells specific to the cell line that they stimulate. This enables the body to tolerate ongoing chemotherapy treatments and reduces risks of infection

Vaccine Therapies

Vaccine therapies are treatments to help the body's immune system recognize and react to cancer cells. The vaccines contain a tumor-associated antigen that is not present in normal cells or is present in extremely low levels. Vaccine therapy is used to treat metastatic prostate cancer in men who have few symptoms and whose cancer does not respond to hormone therapy and in patients with melanoma that returns after surgery and cannot be removed with further surgery.

Cytokine Treatments

Cytokines are substances made by immune cells to help the body fight cancer infection and other diseases. Cytokine therapies include a broad and diverse category of treatments. An example of cytokines are growth factors that simulate white blood cells to grow to reduce the risk of infection. These are discussed in greater in the "Nadir" section. CAR-T cell therapy is a form of cancer treatment used primarily for blood cancers (eg, leukemia, lymphoma, and multiple myeloma). This is also described in greater in the "CAR-T Cell Therapy" section.

Administration of Chemotherapy and Immunotherapy

Chemotherapy and immunotherapy, depending on the drug, can be given by intravenous (IV) infusion, intramuscular injection, or by mouth. When the drugs are given by IV administration, they are usually given through a **central line catheter**, such as a Port-a-Cath®, Broviac®, Groshong®, or Hickman® (Figure 4.4).

Central line catheter. Also called a central venous access device (CVAD) or central venous catheter (CVC). This type of catheter is one that is inserted into a vein that leads to the heart.

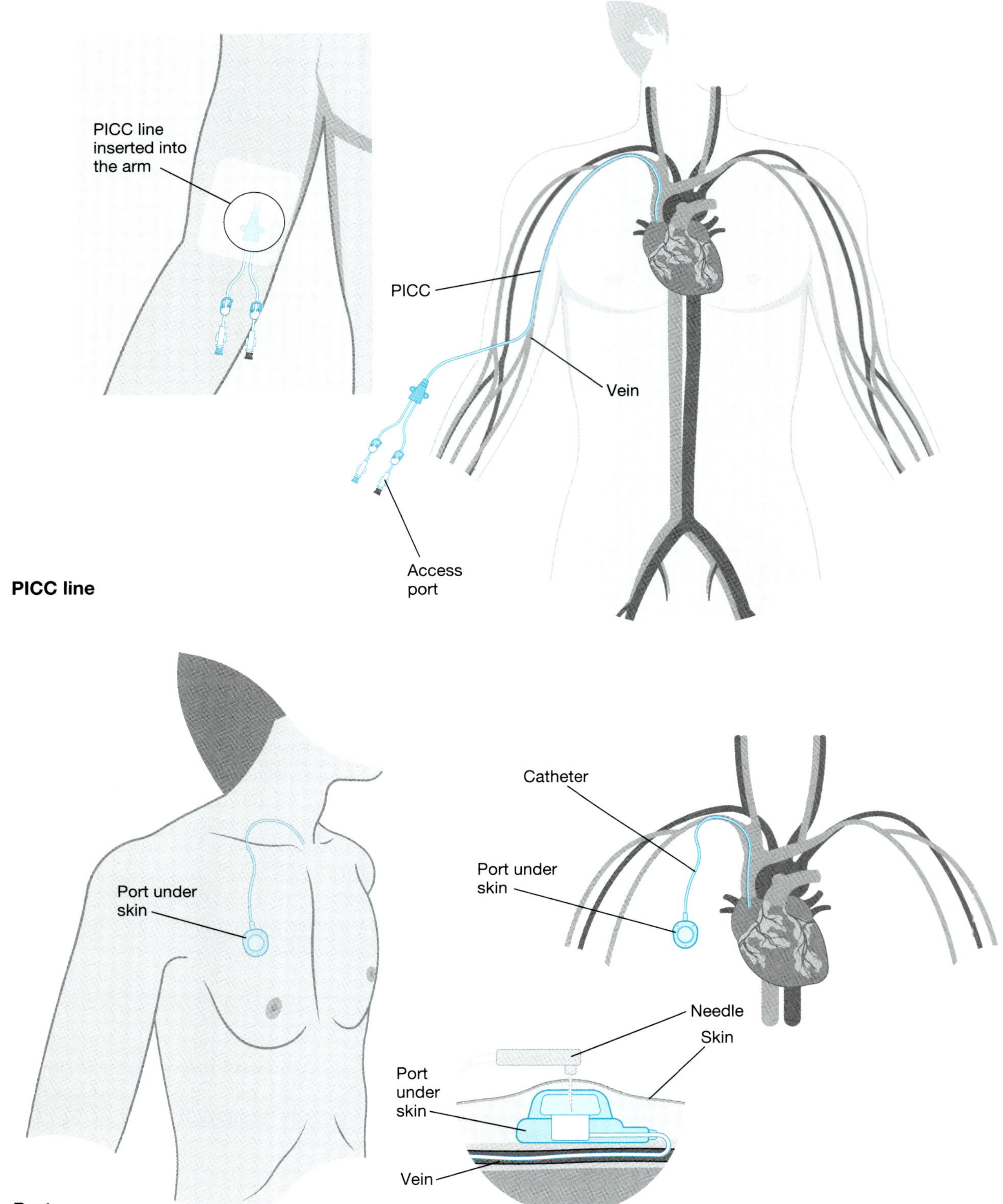

FIGURE 4.4. Central line indwelling catheters (PICC line, Port-a-Cath, Broviac, Groshong, angiocatheter) and Port-a-Cath. The tip, end, of these catheters all sit in the vena cava. Abbreviation: PICC, peripherally inserted central catheter. (From Rumruay. Port-a-Cath. *Shutterstock*. [Internet]. 2021. Available from https://www.shutterstock.com/image-illustration/peripherally-inserted-central-catheter-172528925; https://www.shutterstock.com/image-vector/picc-line-insert-neck-tube-vein-2160899489.)

A Port-a-Cath is inserted into the superior vena cave at the entrance of the right atrium of the heart. Ports are placed in the operating room, and with proper care can be functional for many years. Patients who are getting a BMT and who need to have several IV access lines available at once may have a catheter that is tunneled through the skin into the middle of the chest into the superior vena cava vessel at the entrance to the right atrium. The catheters are called Broviac®, Groshong®, and Hickman® catheters, according to their brand names. Chemotherapy and immunotherapy can also be given through an angiocatheter into a vein but there is a risk that the drugs may move out of the vein, which can compromise the surrounding tissues and cause serious problems. The administration of chemotherapy requires special handling and training.

Most drugs do not cross the blood-brain barrier, making it difficult to adequately treat some leukemias and brain tumors. There are 2 ways to get drugs to reach the cerebrospinal fluid (CSF). Intrathecal or lumbar puncture is a way to deliver small quantities of chemotherapy directly into the CSF. The other way is through an Ommaya reservoir, which is a device that is placed in the subcutaneous tissue between the scalp and the skull and threaded into the lateral ventricle of the brain (Figure 4.5) (2). This allows regular administration of chemotherapy into the Ommaya reservoir, directly into the central nervous system.

Chemotherapy can also be instilled in other cavities. Intrapleural chemotherapy can be given into the pleural lining of the lung to control malignant pleural effusions, an accumulation of fluid in the pleural space in the lungs that can make breathing difficult and cause the lungs to collapse. Intravesical chemotherapy can be instilled into the bladder through a urinary catheter and clamped closed so that the medication remains in the bladder. The patient is rolled from side to side to help the medications reach all the areas of the bladder wall.

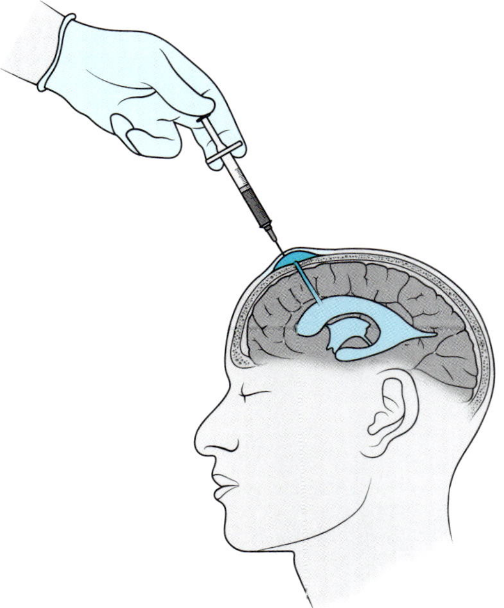

FIGURE 4.5. Instilling medication into an Ommaya reservoir.

Duration of Treatments

The length of chemotherapy and immunotherapy treatments is determined by the type of cancer and the stage of disease. Treatment regimens are determined through rigorous clinical trial studies that compare the best treatments we have today with what we think, scientifically, might be better. That means a higher rate of cure, a more tolerable treatment regimen or one with fewer side effect or that helps people to live longer.

Cancer treatments are usually given in cycles of varying lengths. For some breast cancer treatments, a cycle is every 2 weeks, whereas for some lymphoma treatments, a cycle is every 3 weeks but may include several days of treatment during that week. The length of a cycle varies by the treatment protocol. Cycle length allows the body's healthy normal cells time to recover before the next cycle of treatment.

The number of cycles and the length of treatment are determined to a great extent by research and the intent of the treatment. If the treatment intent is to achieve a cure, the patient receives adjuvant chemotherapy (therapy after surgery). Adjuvant chemotherapy is common for breast, colon, and testicular cancers, and their treatments may last 4 to 6 months. Adjuvant chemotherapy for Hodgkin's and non-Hodgkin's lymphoma and leukemias may extend up to a year. When there is persistent disease, the length of treatment is variable. If the disease disappears completely, treatment usually continues for 1 to 2 cycles beyond the last scan to optimize the response to treatment and kill any microscopic residual disease. If the tumor shrinks but does not disappear, treatment will continue as long as it is tolerated, and the disease does not grow. However, if the tumor grows, the treatment will be stopped, and alternative options will be explored, for example, different drugs, or changing focus to palliative care.

Nadir

Chemotherapy affects rapidly dividing cells, such as the blood cell (red and white cells and platelets), hair, and the cells that line the intestinal tract and the mouth. The stem cells, which make blood cells, are particularly sensitive to chemotherapy. When the stem cells are not reproduced quickly enough, there are insufficient numbers of mature cells. When the mature cells reach the end of their life span, the circulating number of the cells in the blood count decreases. The **nadir** period is when the white blood cells, red RBCs, and platelets are at their lowest point. This is a time when

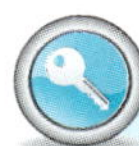

Nadir. The period during cancer treatment when white blood cells, red blood cells, and platelets are at their lowest point and risk for infection is greatest.

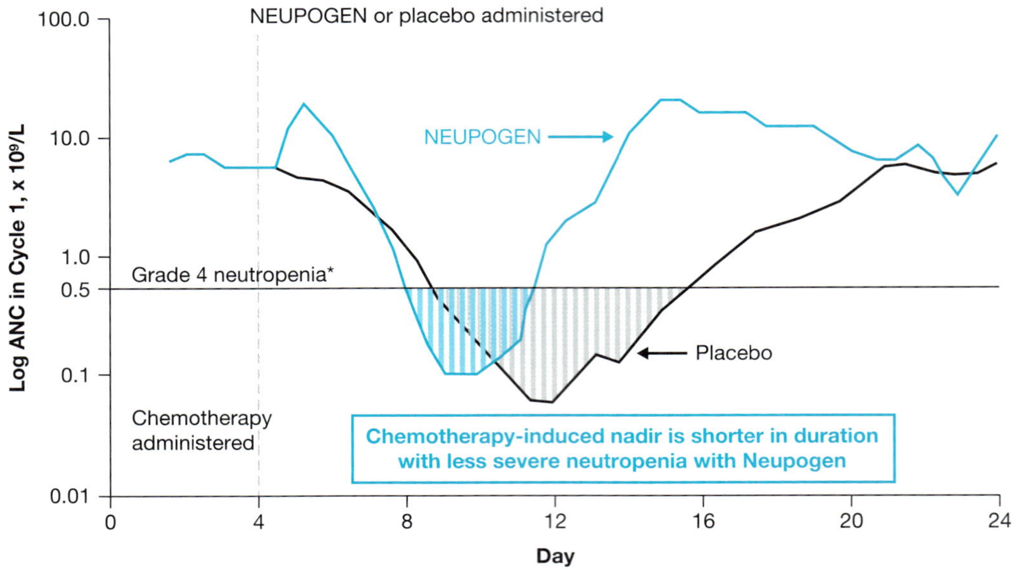

FIGURE 4.6. Pattern of neutropenia with and without pegfilgrastim (Neulasta). Note that the nadir is not as profound or as long with pegfilgrastim. Note: *Grade 4 Neutropenia is defined as neutrophil count <500/microL of blood. (From Crawford J, Ozer H, Stoller R, et al. Reduction by granulocyte colony-stimulating factor of fever and neutropenia induced by chemotherapy in patients with small-cell lung cancer. *N Engl J Med.* 1991;325(3):164–70.)

a patient is at the greatest risk for infection, bleeding, or shortness of breath and fatigue related to anemia. The nadir period, for many treatments, is about 10 days after treatment (Figure 4.6). Some chemotherapies affect specific cell line more than others. For example, gemcitabine causes a decrease in all blood cells but particularly affects platelet cells. Nadir counts are important to consider when working with patients who are exercising during cancer treatment, even if they are receiving growth factors, such as, pegfilgrastim or erythropoietin. Growth factors, such as pegfilgrastim, reduce the length and severity of neutropenia, which decreases the risks of infection.

Hormonal Therapy

Hormonal therapy is used to block endogenous hormones that stimulate certain cancers, such as breast, prostate, endometrial, and ovarian cancers. In these hormonally modulated cancers, hormones are taken that block the action of the endogenous hormones. For example, if a woman has an estrogen receptor positive breast cancer, she may be given an antiestrogen drug to block her body's estrogen. Antiestrogen therapy can cause hot flashes, fatigue, bone loss, and muscle aches. This same principle is used in treatment of prostate cancer. Men receive androgen blockade drugs, ADT, which stop the production and action of testosterone that stops tumor growth. ADT causes hot flashes, fatigue, loss of bone, and muscle mass. Table 4.5 lists common antiestrogen and androgen ablation drugs.

In contrast, hormone replacement therapy is necessary for thyroid cancer patient who had a thyroidectomy. Their body no longer makes thyroid hormone, and it must be replaced for the person to maintain the normal function, feel well, and function optimally. Replacement hormone therapy, if given in the appropriate dosage, does not cause untoward side effects.

Table 4.5 Common Antiestrogen, Aromatase Inhibitors, and Androgen Ablation Drugs

TYPE	DRUG NAME
Antiestrogen	Tamoxifen
	Raloxifene
Aromatase Inhibitors	Anastrozole
	Exemestane
	Letrozole
Androgen ablation	Bicalutamide
	Flutamide
	Nilutamide
	Leuprolide

Data from Chu E. Cancer chemotherapy. In: Katzung BG, Vanderah TW, editors. *Basic & Clinical Pharmacology.* 15th ed. New York (NY): McGraw-Hill; 2021.

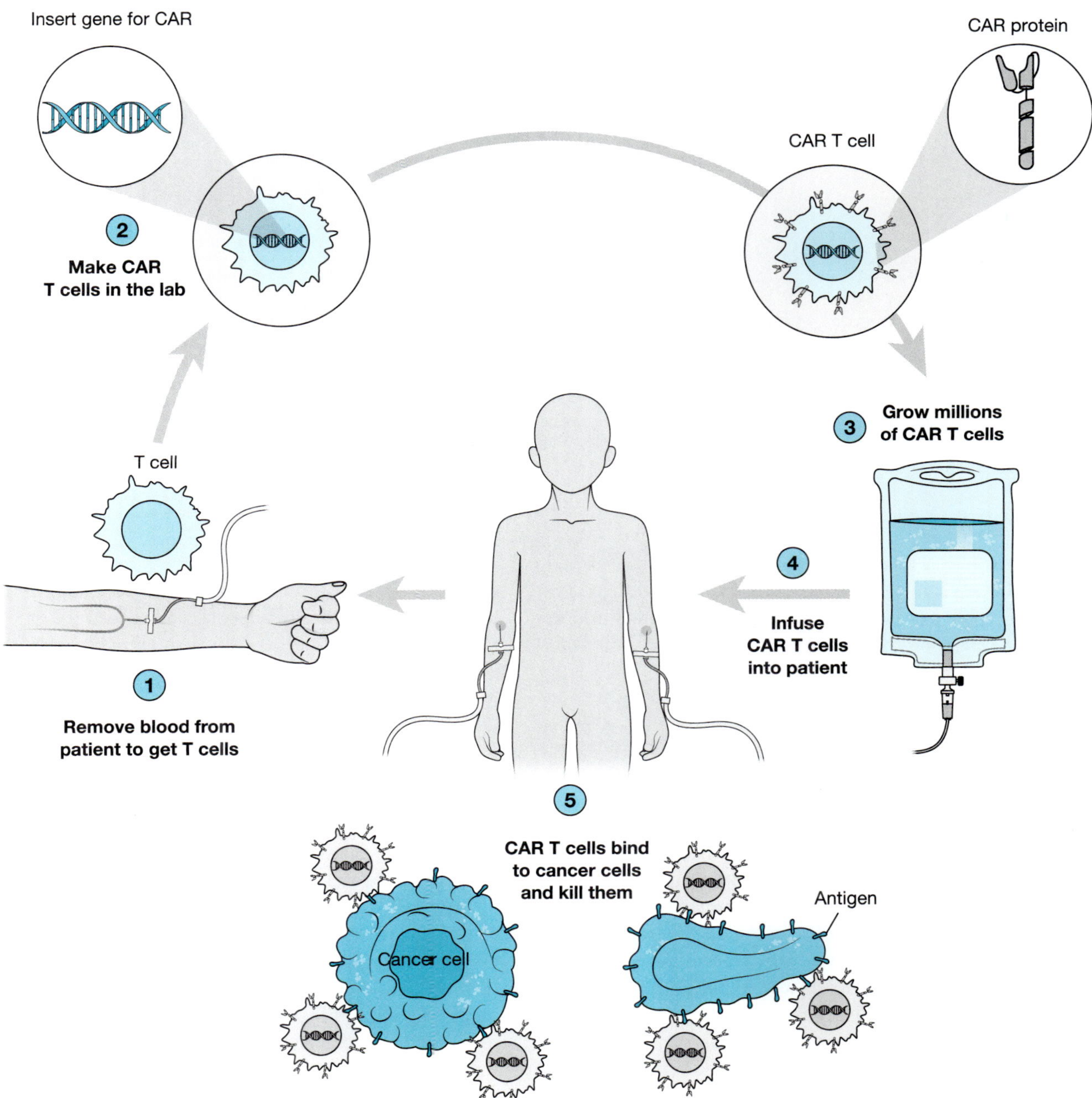

FIGURE 4.7. Steps in CAR-T cell therapy. Abbreviation: CAR, chimeric antigen receptor. (From National Cancer Institute. [Internet]. 2023. Available from https://visualsonline.cancer.gov/details.cfm?imageid=12069.)

CAR-T Cell Therapy

Chimeric antigen receptor therapy (**CAR-T cell therapy**) involves genetically modifying the patient's own T cells to active their immune system to recognize and destroy certain cancer cells (Figure 4.7). CAR-T cell therapy starts with the patient's own T cells that are genetically modified in the lab, grown, and infused into the patient (3).

> **CAR-T cell therapy.** Genetic modification of a patient's own T cells to activate the immune system to fight specific cancers.

CAR-T cell therapy is used to treat relapsed or refractory B-cell lymphoblastic leukemia, non-Hodgkin's lymphoma, mantle cell lymphoma follicular lymphoma, and multiple myeloma. CAR-T cell therapy requires that the patient stay in the hospital for an extended period of time (eg, often weeks) so that side effects can be closely monitored and managed. Common side effects include cytokine release syndrome and neurologic toxicities (Table 4.6). Like other cancer treatments,

Table 4.6 Cytokine Release Syndrome and Neurologic Side Effects From CAR-T Cell Therapy

CYTOKINE RELEASE SYNDROME	NEUROLOGIC TOXICITIES
Difficulty breathing	Altered consciousness
Fever	Delirium
Chill and shaking	Confusion
Severe nausea, vomiting, or diarrhea	Agitation
Severe muscle and joint pain	Seizures
Dizziness or lightheadedness	Difficulty speaking and understanding
Low blood pressure	Loss of balance

Data from Shimabukuro-Vornhagen A, Gödel P, Subklewe M, et al. Cytokine release syndrome. *J ImmunoTher Cancer.* 2018;6(1):56. doi:10.1186/s40425-018-0343-9; Gust J, Taraseviciute A, Turtle CJ. Neurotoxicity associated with CD19-targeted CAR-T cell therapies. *CNS Drugs.* 2018;32(12):1091–101. doi:10.1007/s40263-018-0582-9.

CAR-T therapy can cause serious infections, prolonged low blood cell counts, **hypogammaglobulinemia** (low immunoglobulin [IgGs]), and risk for developing secondary cancers.

Blood and Marrow Transplant

BMT is a procedure that is used when other treatment options have failed. BMT is used to restore blood forming stem cells in people who have diseases such as acute leukemia, chronic leukemia, Hodgkin's lymphoma, non-Hodgkin's, neuroblastoma, and multiple myeloma. Cells may be infused from one's own body (autologous transplant), a genetically related donor (allogeneic transplant), or an unrelated transplant donor. The patient receives high doses of chemotherapy and/or radiation therapy that completely depletes their bone marrow. When the marrow is depleted, it is replaced by the autologous, allogeneic, or unrelated donor transplant. The actual transplant material looks like a bag of RBCs. The transplanted cells take many days to engraft, during which time the patient is at high risk for infection. There are numerous risks and serious complications with BMT, but it can be lifesaving. BMT is a rigorous and lengthy inpatient hospital procedure that is physically and emotionally demanding.

SIDE EFFECTS OF CANCER AND ITS TREATMENTS

Side effects of cancer and/or its treatments occur at different phases in an individual's cancer journey. Side effects will be discussed as acute, immediate posttreatment, long-term, and late effects. It is critically important to be aware of an individual's exposures to different treatment regimens and potential acute, long-term, and late effects that may impact the ability to exercise and necessitate medical supervision or adaptation of an exercise depending on the severity of the side effect.

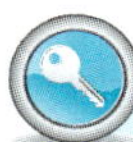

Hypogammaglobulinemia. Low IgG and loss of antibodies. Can be a lifelong side effect of CAR-T therapy and rituximab.

Acute Effects

Acute effects of treatment occur during active treatment. All forms of treatments are fraught with side effects. Side effects in all phases of cancer care are managed by the oncology team. It is particularly important to manage acute phase side effects early, before they become severe. Patients need to be well educated in symptom management so that they can learn to treat their symptoms when they are mild and manageable before they become severe and disabling and require more medication and a longer time period to get the symptom under control. Interventions may include palliation and rehabilitation in order to maintain functional independence and quality of life (QoL).

Surgical side effects most commonly are pain at the surgical site that causes limited mobility and range of motion (ROM). Pain is primarily controlled with medications some of which, like narcotics, can cause significant constipation and altered mentation (4). Immediately after surgery physical activity is encouraged (transfers from bed to chair, activities of daily living including geed and grooming and mobility, as permitted) but exercise is generally limited to range of motion exercises as directed by the surgeon and physical therapy team. An exercise program would not begin until the patient is cleared to begin exercise.

Chemotherapy, immunotherapy, hormonal therapy, and radiation have many side effects that are unique and overlap. Side effects must be managed and controlled for a patient

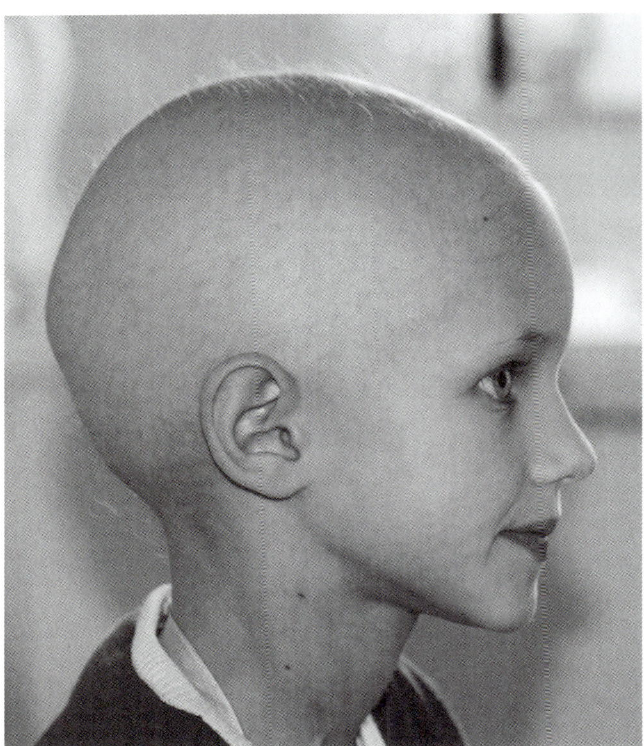

FIGURE 4.8. Child with alopecia (hair loss) due to chemotherapy. (Reprinted from 123RF, frantab01. *Caucasian Girl with Hair Loss Due to Chemotherapy Treatment for Cancer: 123RF.* [Internet]. 2021. Available from https://www.123rf.com/photo_9590090_a-caucasian-girl-with-hair-loss-due-to-chemotherapy-treatment-for-cancer.html.)

to be able to exercise successfully. The side effects that have the greatest impact on one's ability to exercise include fatigue, nausea, vomiting, diarrhea, pain, chemotherapy-induced peripheral neuropathy, neutropenia, thrombocytopenia, anemia, **lymphedema**, muscle weakness, skin rashes, radiation dermatitis, depression, anxiety, and declines in QoL (5, 6). Alopecia is hair loss (Figure 4.8). Alopecia from chemotherapy and immunotherapy is not permanent, and hair grows back, but alopecia from radiation therapy generally causes permanent hair loss. There is limited research to show that wearing a scalp cooling cap during chemotherapy helps to preserve hair and reduce alopecia (Figure 4.9) (7-9). Long term and late effects of cancer treatment will be discussed in Chapter 13.

Chemotherapy has other profound side effects (10-12). For example, it may put young women into early menopause and make young adults infertile. It may also cause cardiomyopathy and **pulmonary dysfunction** that can limit exercise tolerance (13-15). These side effects often develop insidiously and may not be noticed during treatment.

In contrast, fatigue is almost universal. It affects over 90% of patients during treatment with fatigue continuing to persist in as many as 60% of survivors after treatment ends (16). Although fatigue is the most common reason to rest, exercise is the best "medicine" to reduce feelings of fatigue. Research consistently demonstrates the benefits of exercise to reduce

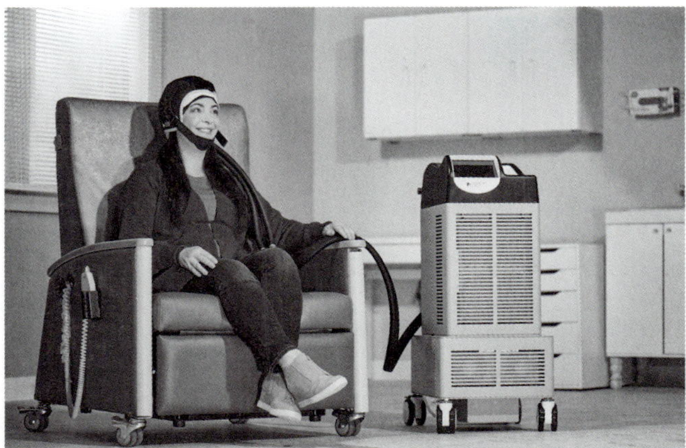

FIGURE 4.9. Scalp cooling cap to minimize hair loss. The DigniCap® Scalp Cooling System. © Diginatin, 2023.

many of the acute side effects of cancer treatment, including fatigue, muscle weakness, and risk for lymphedema.

It is important to understand that if side effects are uncontrolled, they may lead to other more significant problems. For example, a young man with colon cancer who is receiving chemotherapy and is experiencing uncontrolled diarrhea should not and probably can not exercise, not only because it may be impractical but because of the risk that exercise may further contribute to the patient's dehydration. This patient should be referred to the oncology team for symptom management. Once the patient is able to control her/his side effects, beginning or resuming exercise is reasonable. Chapter 12 will provide a greater insight into exercise prescription during treatment.

A diagnosis of cancer is life-changing, emotionally shocking, and it requires lifelong vigilance. People experience a wide variety of emotions and often feel vulnerable, anxious, depressed, and uncertain about the future. The diagnosis and treatment time is a period when people are open to changing their lifestyle. However, survivors have significant emotional concerns about exercising with others such as, risk of infection, changes in body image and limitations to their phsyical ability. An individual's emotional state must be taken into consideration when beginning an exercise program, whether that person is new to exercise, familiar with exercise, or a professional athlete.

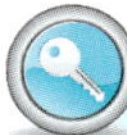

Lymphedema. Swelling caused by impaired lymphatic system drainage. Frequently seen after lymph node dissection for breast cancer. Managed with compression sleeves, wraps, elevation, and exercise.

Pulmonary dysfunction. Caused by chemotherapy with bleomycin and other drugs and mediastinal (chest) radiation and can cause pulmonary fibrosis, bronchiectasis, chronic pleural effusions, and recurrent pneumonia. Causes fatigue and decreased functional ability.

SUMMARY

Cancer is considered a chronic illness, and the diagnosis and treatment of cancer is often a long and complex process. Cancer treatments are usually given in combination (eg, surgery, chemotherapy, and radiation, or a combination of different chemotherapy drugs) to optimize the efficacy. The side effects of these different types and combinations of treatments manifest in different ways at various periods across the cancer trajectory. Commitment to activity (physical and mental) as well as exercise programming needs to be adapted to the individual needs of the person living with and beyond cancer. Future chapters will address, in depth, how treatments may impact exercise and how exercise prescription needs to be adapted for each individual during treatment, after treatment, and in patients with metastatic disease.

Case Study

Joan is a 59-year-old high school teacher who has a routine screening mammogram. A solid 2.2-cm mass is noted in her right breast. Before she leaves the radiology facility, Joan is taken in for an ultrasound to obtain a better image of the mass. Three days later her primary care provider informs her that she needs to have a breast biopsy the next day. Joan has an ultrasound-guided needle biopsy with sentinel lymph node mapping performed, and several days later she learns that the pathology is positive for intraductal carcinoma.

Joan is scheduled to see the oncology team in 10 days. The waiting creates great anxiety. Finally, the day to meet the oncology team arrives, and she waits in the examination room with her partner. The oncology team (an oncologist, a surgeon, a radiation a therapist, a chemotherapy nurse, a radiation nurse, a nurse navigator, and a social worker) comes in and introduces themselves

The surgeon reviews the pathology: a 2.2 c tumor, 1 of 3 lymph nodes positive, estrogen and progesterone positive (ER/PR+). Because the tumor is Stage 2, the surgeon talks to Joan at length about different surgical approaches (partial mastectomy with lymph node dissection or total mastectomy with lymph node dissection and then different reconstruction options). The medical oncologist then presents his opinion on optimal treatment that includes chemotherapy with 3 different drugs: 2 drugs (doxorubicin and cyclophosphamide) given every 2 weeks for a total of 4 cycles and then 1 drug (paclitaxel) given every 2 weeks for another 4 cycles. Like a well-orchestrated play, the radiation therapist then explains how radiation therapy will be focused specifically to the area where the tumor was located to kill any remaining cancer cells and that the treatment will continue Monday through Friday and last for about 5 weeks. The medical oncologist then explains that once radiation is complete, antiestrogen therapy will be started. She stresses that this part of treatment is important because the tumor is hormone-receptor positive and requires blocking the action of estrogen and progesterone to prevent any further chance of tumor growth. She explains that the medicine is a pill taken for 5 years.

The team assures Joan that the nurses and social worker will be there to help her through the journey and can answer her questions. Joan leaves the office feeling completely overwhelmed. She has a follow-up appointment with the surgeon to discuss her surgical decision and a date for surgery and is given a handful of materials to read.

Two weeks later Joan undergoes a complete mastectomy with lymph node dissection. She chooses not to have reconstruction at this time. Joan heals quickly and after 1 month, she is ready to start chemotherapy, but before starting, she gets a Port-a-Cath placed.

The first day of chemotherapy is terrifying. Joan is afraid of how she will feel during treatment and unsure if she will be able to drive home and how she will feel the next few days. The nurses spend time educating her about the drugs she is receiving, how to manage the side effects, and how she will be monitored. When the chemotherapy infusion is complete, she is given an injection of pegfilgrastim, a white blood cell growth factor, and sent home with medications to manage her nausea. Joan does not feel nauseated until the second day after treatment, takes her ANTIEMETIC (nausea) medication, and feels better. She begins to notice that she is feeling tired. By the third day, she starts to feel very tired and worn out and spends a lot of time resting on the couch. About 9 days after her treatment, she feels good again and starts to go about her usual life.

On the day of cycle 2, she gets her blood drawn, and the oncology team looks at her blood count to be sure that she has an adequate number of white cells, RBCs, and platelets to receive the next cycle of treatment. Her lab reports look great. Joan gets cycle 2 and goes home feeling confident that she can manage her side effects. This time, however, her hair starts falling out in big clumps. She feels sad and very self-conscious. The reality of this is even more shocking—first her breast and now her hair! Her hair is on her pillow and her clothing, and clogs the shower. Her partner shaves her head. Now her head is cold. Joan is depressed, tired, and spends even more time on the couch. She does not want to do anything and notices that she is feeling weak and worn out and not rebounding like she did after the first treatment.

Note: This case study reflects only the first few months in the life of a newly diagnosed person living with cancer. Cancer treatment goes on for an extended amount of time and physical and emotional fatigue accumulates. It is important for people living with cancer (PLWC) to have a support team that encourages them to exercise and engage in positive life-enhancing activities.

Questions

1. Why is the diagnosis period so long?
2. What are acute side effects?
3. List 3 side effects of doxorubicin and paclitaxel? How are they different?
4. What are some of the acute effects of treatment Joan should expect?
5. What can Joan do about her fatigue?

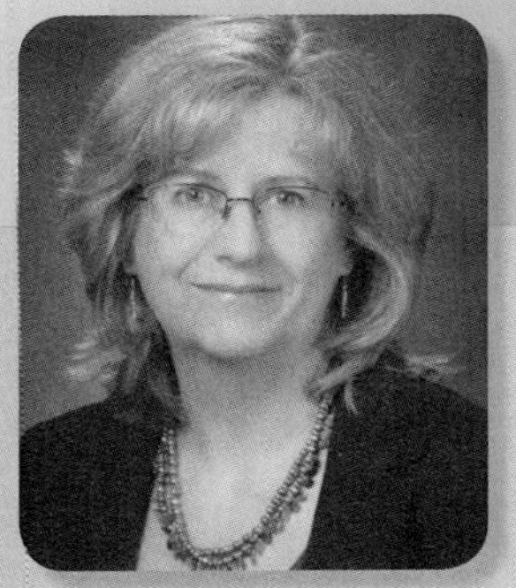

Meet the Expert

FEATURED PROFESSIONAL

Karen Basen-Engquist, PhD, MPH

Professor of Behavioral Science and the Director of the Center for Energy Balance in Cancer Prevention and Survivorship
The University of Texas, MD Anderson Cancer Center

Q: "Where did you grow up?"

Waterville, Minnesota, a small town about 60 miles south of Minneapolis, in the valley of the Jolly Green Giant!

Q: "Where did you train? What is your training?"

I received a PhD in Community Psychology from the University of Texas in Austin and did a postdoctoral fellowship and Master of Public Health (MPH) at the School of Public Health at University of Texas, Houston Health Science Center.

Q: "What are you best known for?"

Testing behavioral interventions to help cancer survivors and high-risk individuals improve their physical functioning and quality of life through increasing physical activity.

Q: "What are you currently working on?"

Dissemination and implementation of the Active Living After Cancer Program, a group-based program to help sedentary cancer survivors learn the skills they need to increase their physical activity and improve their physical functioning and quality of life. At this time, it has been provided to over 1,400 Texas cancer survivors in English and Spanish through partnerships with community organizations that reach out to minority and medically underserved survivors and provide the program. The current project is funded by the Cancer Prevention and Research Institute of Texas. We are currently testing new modifications of the program and also exploring national dissemination.

Q: "Anything else you want to include?"

As we develop exercise and physical programming, we need to take into account the needs of people who don't enjoy exercising—like me! Finding ways to encourage myself to be more active has helped me. "Walk in the shoes" of cancer survivors who don't enjoy exercise so that we can develop more responsive programming.

Favorite Quote:

"Knowing is not enough; we must apply. Willing is not enough; we must do."
—*Johann Wolfgang von Goethe*

STUDY QUESTIONS

1. Why is a biopsy needed to diagnose cancer?
2. What are tumor markers and why are they important?
3. List tumor markers for prostate and colon cancer.
4. Why is cancer staging important?
5. List 4 central lines.
6. How common is cancer-related fatigue?
7. What is the nadir count?
8. What are risks for patients during the nadir?
9. What diseases are trastuzumab (Herceptin) and Imatinib (Gleevec) used for? What do you call these kinds of drugs?
10. List 2 aromatase inhibitor and androgen ablation drugs and describe the difference between the 2 types of drugs.
11. What is CAR-T therapy?

REFERENCES

1. Phelps MA. Rituximab immunotherapy: it's getting personal. *Blood.* 2017;129(19):2595–6. doi:10.1182/blood-2017-03-772061
2. Zubair A, De Jesus O. Ommaya reservoir. In: *StatPearls* [Internet]. Treasure Island (FL): StatPearls Publishing; 2024
3. National Cancer Institute. *T-Cell Transfer Therapy.* [Internet]. 2021. Available from https://www.cancer.gov/about-cancer/treatment/types/immunotherapy/t-cell-transfer-therapy
4. Jiang C, Wang H, Wang Q, Luo Y, Sidlow R, Han X. Prevalence of chronic pain and high-impact chronic pain in cancer survivors in the United States. *JAMA Oncol.* 2019;5(8):1224–6. doi:10.1001/jamaoncol.2019.1439
5. Palesh O, Scheiber C, Kesler S, Mustian K, Koopman C, Schapira L. Management of side effects during and post-treatment in breast cancer survivors. *The Breast J.* 2018;24(2):167–75. doi:10.1111/tbj.12862
6. Schirrmacher V. From chemotherapy to biological therapy: a review of novel concepts to reduce the side effects of systemic cancer treatment. *Int J Oncol.* 2019;54(2):407–19. doi:10.3892/ijo.2018.4661
7. Komen MMC, van den Hurk CJG, Nortier JWR, van der Ploeg T, Smorenburg CH, van der Hoeven JJM. Patient-reported outcome assessment and objective evaluation of chemotherapy-induced alopecia. *Eur J Oncol Nurs.* 2018;33:49–55. doi:10.1016/j.ejon.2018.01.001
8. Williams LA, Ginex PK, Ebanks GL, Jr., et al. ONS guidelines for cancer treatment-related skin toxicity. *Oncol Nurs Forum.* 2020;47(5):539–56. doi:10.1188/20.ONF.539-556
9. Quenqua D. *A New Treatment Aims to Prevent Hair Loss in Cancer Patients: CNBC.* [Internet]. 2018. Available from https://www.cnbc.com/2018/02/01/scalp-cooling-prevents-hair-loss-in-cancer-patients.html
10. Maltaris T, Seufert R, Fischl F, et al. The effect of cancer treatment on female fertility and strategies for preserving fertility. *Eur J Obstet Gynecol Reprod Biol.* 2007;130(2):148–55. doi:10.1016/j.ejogrb.2006.08.006
11. Barcroft JF, Galazis N, Jones BP, et al. Fertility treatment and cancers: the eternal conundrum—a systematic review and meta-analysis. *Hum Reprod.* 2021;36(4):1093–107. doi:10.1093/humrep/deaa293
12. Huang Z, Berg WT. Iatrogenic effects of radical cancer surgery on male fertility. *Fertil Steril.* 2021;116(3):625–9. doi:10.1016/j.fertnstert.2021.07.1200
13. Hahn VS, Zhang KW, Sun L, Narayan V, Lenihan DJ, Ky B. Heart failure with targeted cancer therapies. *Circ Res.* 2021;128(10):1576–93. doi:10.1161/CIRCRESAHA.121.318223
14. Stone JR, Kanneganti R, Abbasi M, Akhtari M. Monitoring for chemotherapy-related cardiotoxicity in the form of left ventricular systolic dysfunction: a review of current recommendations. *JCO Oncol Pract.* 2021;17(5):228–36. doi:10.1200/op.20.00924
15. Maltser S, Cristian A, Silver JK, Morris GS, Stout NL. A focused review of safety considerations in cancer rehabilitation. *PM&R.* 2017;9(suppl 2):S415–28. doi:10.1016/j.pmrj.2017.08.403
16. Weis J. Cancer-related fatigue: prevalence, assessment and treatment strategies. *Expert Rev Pharmacoecon Outcomes Res.* 2011;11(4):441–6. doi:10.1586/erp.11.44

CHAPTER

5

Long-Term Issues: Survival, Recurrence, Palliation, and End-of-Life Issues

OUTLINE

1. Introduction: Long-Term Issues
2. Survival After Treatment
   a. Immediate Post Treatment
   b. Long-Term and Late Effects
3. Recurrence
   a. Psychological Impacts
   b. Treatment
4. Clinical Trials
5. End of Life
6. Summary
7. Case Study #1
8. Case Study #2
9. Meet the Expert
10. Study Questions
11. References

OBJECTIVES

After completing review of this chapter, students will be able to:

1. Describe survival concerns that affect PLWBC, including immediate posttreatment effects, long-term and late effects of treatment.
2. Describe cancer recurrence and its treatment and emotional impact.
3. Explain end-of-life transition and choices people with cancer and their family make, including maintaining QoL, palliative care, and hospice care.

INTRODUCTION: LONG-TERM ISSUES

Living beyond cancer presents many challenges including fear of recurrence, need to cope with ongoing side effects, and even the development of additional side effects of treatment that may develop many years after treatment ends. People living beyond cancer can have a recurrence of their cancer and even develop second cancers. Recurrences can extend beyond the primary site of the cancer. When this happens, the cancer has metastasized. This chapter will discuss the many physical and psychological challenges faced by people living beyond cancer, the impact of recurrence, and the transition to palliative care and hospice at the end of life.

SURVIVAL AFTER TREATMENT

At the conclusion of treatment, the cancer survivor enters a new phase focused on recovery and regaining control of life. While there is joy at concluding treatment, many survivors feel anxious about losing touch with their oncology team. Patients do not need to be seen as often after therapy ends, which can cause anxiety. Although regular medical appointments are taxing, they provide a feeling of security, a safety net that is removed when treatment ends. At the end of treatment, follow-up appointments with a physical examination, blood work, and possibly imaging are usually obtained at 3-month intervals to assess recovery from treatment and determine if the patient is still in remission. In the US, the follow-up schedule for diagnostic testing is determined by the survivor's condition and by the national published clinical guidelines from organizations, such as the NCCN and the American College of Surgeons Commission on Cancer (CoC) (Table 5.1) (1, 2). The following sections discuss side effects of treatment that affect survivors after treatment ends. The lingering effects are important to understand as they can directly influence how a survivor will be able to exercise.

Table 5.1 Organizations That Set Standards for Care in Oncology

National Comprehensive Cancer Network	A nonprofit alliance of leading cancer centers devoted to patient care, research, and education that continuously updates detailed cancer care recommendations
American College of Surgeons Commission on Cancer	A multidisciplinary professional organization to improve survival and quality of life for cancer patients by setting standards of care to promote cancer prevention, research, education, and monitoring of comprehensive quality care

Immediate Post Treatment

The immediate posttreatment period covers the time from the completion of treatment through the first 12 months of recovery. During this time, many of the acute side effects begin to attenuate and survivors begin to think about resuming their normal life. The immediate posttreatment is an opportune time to encourage healthy behaviors, such as exercise (3), which help survivors recover from some of the most common side effects of treatment (fatigue, muscle weakness, pain, and psychosocial distress) that occur with all types of treatments (Table 5.2). The following sections

Table 5.2 Percent of Patients Who Experience Side Effects During and After Treatment

SIDE EFFECT	% DURING TREATMENT	% AFTER TREATMENT
Cancer-related fatigue	25%-99% (4)	20%-79% (5, 6)
Pain	40%-80% (7, 8)	10%-34.5% (9, 10)
Psychosocial effects	50%-75% (11)	
Fear of recurrence	30%-70%	22%-70% (5, 12)
Chemotherapy-induced peripheral neuropathy	30%-60% (13)	27% (14, 15)
Cardiotoxic effects	1%-26% (16)	5% (17)
Pulmonary toxic effects	1%	48%-50% (18-20)

Box 5.1 Proposed Mechanisms of Fatigue

Proposed mechanisms of cancer fatigue are:

- Pro-inflammatory cytokines
- Hypothalamic-pituitary-adrenal (HPA) axis dysregulation
- Circadian rhythm desynchronization
- Skeletal muscle wasting
- Genetic dysregulation

Data from Berger AM, Mooney K, Alvarez-Perez A, et al. Cancer-related fatigue, Version 2.2015. *J Natl Compr Canc Netw.* 2015;13(8):1012–39. doi:10.6004/jnccn.2015.0122; Bower JE. Cancer-related fatigue: links with inflammation in cancer patients and survivors. *Brain Behav Immun.* 2007;21(7):863–71. doi:10.1016/j.bbi.2007.03.013; Miller AH, Ancoli-Israel S, Bower JE, Capuron L, Irwin MR. Neuroendocrine-immune mechanisms of behavioral comorbidities in patients with cancer. *J Clin Oncol.* 2008;26(6):971–82. doi:10.1200/JCO.2007.10.7805 Berger AM, Wielgus K, Hertzog M, Fischer P, Farr L. Patterns of circadian activity rhythms and their relationships with fatigue and anxiety/depression in women treated with breast cancer adjuvant chemotherapy. *Support Care Cancer.* 2009;18(1):105. doi:10.1007/s00520-009-0636-0; Al-Majid S, McCarthy DO. Cancer-induced fatigue and skeletal muscle wasting: the role of exercise. *Biol Res Nurs.* 2001;2(3):186–97. doi:10.1177/109980040100200304; Rich T. Symptom clusters in cancer patients and their relation to EGFR ligand modulation of the circadian axis. *J Support Oncol.* 2007;5(4):167–74.

provide an overview of the common side effects immediately following treatment. Exercise is beneficial for all of these side effects and will be discussed in more detail in Chapters 13 and 14.

Cancer-Related Fatigue

Cancer-related fatigue (CRF) continues to be the most common side effect for people living beyond cancer many months after treatment ends (4, 6, 21, 22). Fatigue is a complex process that is comprised of physical, mental and emotional aspects. Despite the plethora of research on fatigue, the specific pathophysiologic mechanisms involved are unknown. There are several proposed mechanisms of fatigue (Box 5.1). One is that fatigue is caused from inactivity and the accompanying cardiopulmonary deconditioning and muscle weakness that occur from extended periods of sedentary behavior. Another theory is that inflammation from cancer and different treatment modalities leads to fatigue (23).

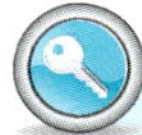

Cancer-related fatigue. The most common side effect of cancer treatment. It is an unrelenting feeling of profound fatigue that is not relieved by rest or sleep. At this time, exercise is the best treatment recommended for cancer-related fatigue.

Fatigue may also be worsened by **comorbid conditions**, such as cardiac dysfunction, untreated hypothyroid or depression, and side effects of hormonal treatment. Comorbid conditions that are not well controlled or, for example, cause a decrease in cardiac function as a result of a chemotherapy drug (eg, Adriamycin), often have a negative additive effect on physical function. Research has clearly demonstrated that both aerobic and resistance exercise reduce fatigue.

Muscle Weakness

Muscle weakness is primarily associated with inactivity and **debilitation** (24, 25). Cancer is more common in older people who, undoubtedly, already have age-related weakness and suffer from the loss of muscle mass (sometimes called **sarcopenia** and/or **cachexia**). Some treatments, particularly **androgen deprivation therapy** for prostate cancer and high-dose steroids (eg, prednisone or dexamethasone) for Hodgkin's lymphoma and non-Hodgkin's lymphoma can cause a rapid loss of muscle mass and strength. Resistance exercise is effective when muscle weakness is a result of inactivity, ADT, steroids, or is related to age. Resistance training effectively improves muscle strength for all cancer survivors (26).

Pain

Pain can result from surgery, radiation therapy, chemotherapy, biologic therapy, or immunotherapy. Pain related to surgery or radiation therapy is generally localized to the treatment area and may limit ROM because of skin, muscle, or joint involvement. Chemotherapy may cause **chemotherapy-induced peripheral neuropathy** (CIPN)

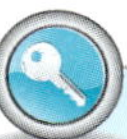

Comorbid conditions. Medical conditions that coexist with another disease.

Debilitation. Physical weakness or frailty. May be caused by illness or significant inactivity.

Sarcopenia (muscle weakness). Muscle atrophy associated with aging or immobility. It is a component of frailty and significantly increases risk for falls.

Cachexia. Wasting condition associated with the loss of muscle mass, body weight, and appetite.

Androgen deprivation therapy. Hormonal therapy used in prostate cancer to block androgens (testosterone and dihydrotestosterone) produced in the testes, the prostate, and the adrenal glands.

Chemotherapy-induced peripheral neuropathy. Results from some drugs that cause decreased sensation and numbness in the fingers, hands, toes, and feet.

that may affect the upper and lower extremities and impact functions, such as the ability to button a shirt or pick up a piece of paper, and mobility. This effect is due to the decreased sensation and numbness in the fingers, hands, toes, and feet. In extreme cases, the numbness can extend up to the forearms and lower legs. CIPN can become severe enough that the dose of the drug that is causing the neuropathy may need to be reduced to preserve function. Hormonal therapy may cause arthralgias and myalgias that may limit exercise tolerance. **Arthralgias** are joint aches and pains, and **myalgias** are muscle aches and pains. Studies have demonstrated that moderate-intensity aerobic and resistance exercise reduce joint pain and pain severity in both breast cancer survivors and head and neck cancer survivors (27, 28).

Psychosocial Distress

Psychosocial distress may be caused by depression, anxiety, and fear of recurrence (22, 29-31). Distress can be severe enough to develop into posttraumatic stress disorder. While, medications can alleviate many of these clinical symptoms, exercise can help to reduce depression and anxiety and improve mood. Fear of recurrence is common and may be triggered by a cough or a pain that a survivor may interpret as a sign of a recurrence. This fear is real and, unfortunately, may sometimes indicate a recurrence. Lingering physical side effects also impact the emotional burden of cancer affecting one's self-image, self-esteem, and even readiness to return to exercise in a group setting. Consideration of changes in the body (eg, loss of a limb or breast, or a disfiguring scar) from cancer is important to recognize when working with survivors who are beginning to exercise.

Long-Term and Late Effects

Long-term and late effects of cancer begin 1 to 2 years after treatment and may develop many years after treatment ends. At this point in survivorship, side effects such as alopecia, nausea, vomiting, neutropenia, thrombocytopenia, and anemia are already resolved, but some of the intermediate posttreatment effects may linger for years after treatment and interfere with daily function (eg, peripheral neuropathy, fatigue, depression, anxiety, and fear of recurrence). Although survivors do not see their oncology team for follow-up as often at this stage, this is when new problems that are directly related to cancer treatment may begin to appear. This section will describe some of the long-term and late effects of cancer treatment with which PLWBC may be diagnosed. Fatigue and CIPN are 2 side effects that may linger years after treatment ends.

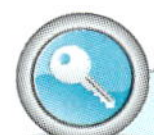

Arthralgias. Achiness and pains in joints often associated with aromatase inhibitors. Fear of cancer recurrence: distress, concern, or worry about the possibility that cancer may come back or progress.

Myalgias. Muscle soreness and achiness commonly associated with aromatase inhibitors and paclitaxel.

Fatigue

Fatigue can become a chronic and persistent problem for long-term cancer survivors, affecting as many as 30% of people living beyond cancer (6, 32) (see Table 5.2). These side effects are often worsened when survivors are coping with other side effects such as CIPN, pain, anxiety, and depression. The debilitation from a sedentary lifestyle only increases the cycle of fatigue and weakness, which contributes to anxiety and depression. An individualized structured, progressive, exercise program can break this cycle and reduce fatigue, anxiety, and depression.

Chemotherapy-Induced Peripheral Neuropathy

CIPN, unfortunately, is a side effect that may never go away (33, 34). CIPN is an additional side effect that compounds the impact of the constellation of treatment side effects. CIPN can affect the 2 types of nerve fibers: afferent (sensory) and efferent (motor). Afferent nerves project into the central nervous system, and efferent nerves extend to the periphery of the body. Efferent nerve fibers are classified into 3 types: group A, group B, and group C. Groups A and B fibers are myelinated, and group C nerve fibers are unmyelinated. Schwann cells form the myelin sheath (35). In neuropathy, the nerve signaling is disrupted in 3 ways: 1. signals are not sent normally; 2. there is inappropriate signaling when the nerve should be quiet, and 3. there is distorted signaling. Most CIPN affects motor and sensory nerves and is length dependent. This means that the neuropathy effects the nerve endings farthest from the origin of the nerve—the toes, fingers, hands, and feet first, and then gradually moves toward the body. Figure 5.1 shows where different chemotherapies damage the nerve and cause CIPN.

CIPN causes tingling, pain, feelings of fullness in the appendage, and sensitivity to vibration. Over time, CIPN can interfere with the patient's balance and fine motor function, such as buttoning a shirt, playing guitar, or picking up a piece of paper. CIPN is a dose-limiting side effect of chemotherapies, such as paclitaxel, oxaliplatin, and vincristine, which means that if CIPN gets severe, the dose of the offending drug needs to be reduced or stopped (Table 5.3). The targeted therapies also cause neuropathy that can be severe and limit the dose and duration of treatment (Table 5.4). Currently, there

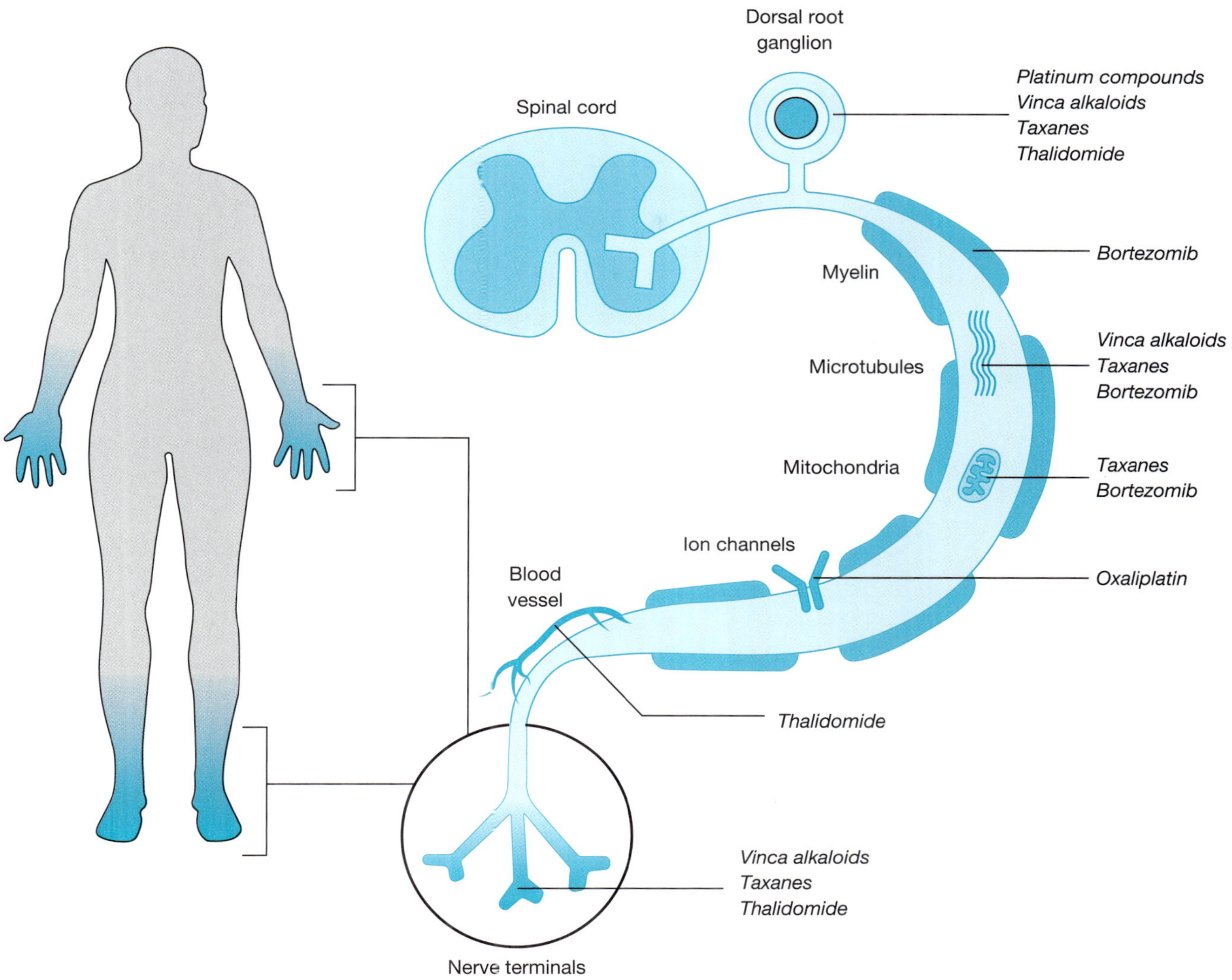

FIGURE 5.1. Depiction of glove-and-stocking distribution of CIPN from the dorsal ganglion to the axon and axonal components to the distal nerve terminals. (From Park SB, Goldstein D, Krishnan AV, et al. Chemotherapy-induced peripheral neurotoxicity: a critical analysis. *CA Cancer J Clin*. 2013;63(6):419–37. doi:10.3322/caac.21204.)

is no known antidote to CIPN except to stop the drug that is causing neuropathy.

Lymphedema

Lymphedema is swelling in an arm, leg, torso, or head caused by a blockage in the lymphatic system (36, 37). It can be caused by surgery that removes lymph nodes owing to cancer treatment, such as lymph node dissection in breast cancer surgery. The risk for lymphedema is increased with radiation therapy, excessive strain exerted on the affected limb, and airplane travel (Figure 5.2). The buildup of lymph fluid causes restricted movement, discomfort and pain. Exercise, wrapping, massage, and compression of the limb can alleviate some swelling.

Lymphedema can be an ongoing problem or a new problem that presents with a sudden onset years after treatment has ended. It may be a problem that limits physical activity and contributes to a sedentary lifestyle, if a survivor does not know how to exercise safely to reduce the risk and severity of lymphedema. Research supports the use of slowly progressive resistance exercise for preventing and attenuating the effects of breast cancer-related lymphedema (38, 39).

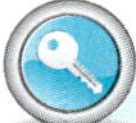

Lymphedema. Swelling in an arm or leg caused by the accumulation of lymph fluid that is unable to drain because of vessels being blocked or damaged or removed by surgery that impairs lymphatic drainage.

Table 5.3 Typical Clinical Features of Chemotherapy-Induced Peripheral Neuropathy With Common Chemotherapeutic Agents

DRUG	TYPICAL SYMPTOMS/SIGNS
Platinum	
Cisplatin	Early reduction/loss of DTR
	Distal, symmetric, upper and lower limb impairment/loss of all sensory modalities
	Sensory ataxia and gait imbalance are frequent
	Neuropathic pain can be present, but it is not frequent
	Coasting[a] phenomenon is frequent
Carboplatin	Similar to cisplatin but milder
Oxaliplatin	Acute
	Cold-induced transient paresthesia in mouth, throat, and limb extremities
	Cramps/muscle spasm in throat muscle, jaw spasm
	Chronic
	Very similar to cisplatin
Bortezomib	Reduction/loss of DTR
	Mild to moderate, distal, symmetric loss of all sensory modalities occurs. Small myelinated and unmyelinated fibers are markedly affected, leading to severe neuropathic pain.
	Mild distal weakness in lower limbs is possible
Taxanes (paclitaxel, docetaxel)	Reduction/loss of DTR
	Myalgia syndrome is frequent (as an atypical neuropathic pain?)
	Distal, symmetric, upper and lower limb impairment/loss of all sensory modalities
	Gait unsteadiness is possible because of proprioceptive loss
	Distal, symmetric weakness in lower limbs is generally mild
Epothilones (ixabepilone, sagopilone)	Signs and symptoms are similar to taxanes, but neuropathic pain is less frequent, and recovery is reportedly faster
Vinca alkaloids (vincristine, other compounds with similar but much lower neurotoxicity)	Reduction/loss of DTR
	Neuropathic pain/paresthesia at limb extremities is relatively frequent
	Distal, symmetric, upper and lower limb impairment/loss of all sensory modalities
	Distal, symmetric weakness in lower limbs progressing to foot drop
	Autonomic symptoms (eg, orthostatic hypotension, constipation) may be severe
Thalidomide	Reduction/loss of DTR
	Relatively frequent neuropathic pain at limb extremities
	Mild to moderate, distal, symmetric loss of all sensory modalities
	Weakness is rare

DTR, deep tendon reflexes.
[a]Coasting = worsening of signs/symptoms of neuropathy over months after drug withdrawal.
From Cavaletti G, Alberti P, Marmiroli P. Chemotherapy-induced peripheral neurotoxicity in cancer survivors: an underdiagnosed clinical entity? *Am Soc Clin Oncol Educ Book.* 2015(35):e553–e60. doi:10.14694/EdBook_AM.2015.35.e553.

Table 5.4 Common Targeted Treatments for and Description of Chemotherapy-Induced Peripheral Neuropathy

DRUG	REPORTED PREVIOUS NEUROTOXIC TREATMENT	DESCRIPTION OF PERIPHERAL NERVOUS SYSTEM TOXICITY
Alemtuzumab	None	Progressive peripheral sensorimotor radiculoneuropathy and/or myelitis
Brentuximab vedotin	Previous chemotherapy (undefined)	Peripheral sensory neuropathy: any grade in up to 66%; grade 3 in up to 8% Peripheral motor neuropathy: any grade in up to 11%; grade 3 in up to 7%
Carfilzomib	Lenalidomide or thalidomide	Treatment-related neuropathy: any grad in up to 17%; rarely grade 3
Ibritumomab	CVP or COP or CHOP	Paresthesia: grade 1 in up to 13%
Imatinib	Cytarabine	"Pain in limbs": any grade in up to 11%; grades 3-4 in up to 1%
Ipilimumab	Carboplatin	Guillain-Barré syndrome
Lapatinib	Taxanes, vinorelbine	"Pain in extremities": any grade in up to 13%; grade 3 in <1%
Regorafenib	Oxaliplatin	Sensory neuropathy: any grade in up to 7%; grade 3 in <1%
Rituximab	CHOP (first-line), ProMACE CytaBOM (second-line)	Guillain-Barré syndrome
	None	Guillain-Barré syndrome
Sorafenib	Previous chemotherapy (undefined)	Treatment-emergent sensory neuropathy: grades 1-2 in up to 20%
Vemurafenib	Previous chemotherapy (undefined)	Peripheral neuropathy: any grad in up to 10%; grade 3 in 1%
Vorinostat	Previous chemotherapy (undefined)	Cutaneous polyneuropathy (tingling) was reported as leading to discontinuation

CVP, cyclophosphamide, vincristine, prednisone; COP, cyclophosphamide, vincristine, prednisone; CHOP, cyclophosphamide, doxorubicin, vincristine, prednisone; ProMACE CytaBOM, cyclophosphamide, doxorubicin, etoposide cytozar, bleomycin, vincristine, methotrexate, prednisone.
From Cavaletti G, Alberti P, Marmiroli P. Chemotherapy-induced peripheral neurotoxicity in cancer survivors: an underdiagnosed clinical entity? *Am Soc Clin Oncol Educ Book.* 2015(35):e553–e60. doi:10.14694/EdBook_AM.2015.35.e553.

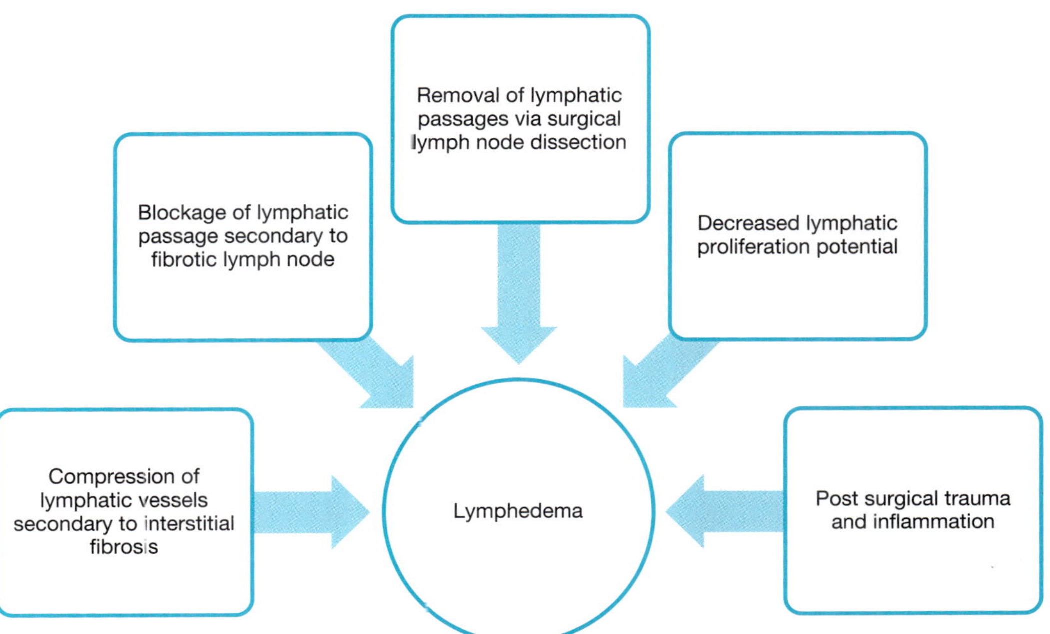

FIGURE 5.2. Radiation and surgical-induced factors leading to lymphedema. (From Allam O, Park KE, Chandler L, et al. The impact of radiation on lymphedema: a review of the literature. *Gland Surg.* 2020;9(2):596–602. doi:10.21037/gs.2020.03.20.)

Childhood Cancer Treatment
Overall 5-Year Survival 83%
10.6%
Heart failure incidence within 40 years after cardiotoxic treatment
Multivariable Risk Prediction
• Cardiotoxic exposure
• Cardiovascular risk factors
• Genetics
• Cardiac function
Radiotherapy
Mitoxantrone, anthracyclines
Coronary artery disease
Heart failure
Arrhythmia
Pericardial disease
Valvular disease
EARLY
LATE
Life-long risk
Potential Primary Prevention
• Physical activity
• Diet
• Weight control
Coronary artery disease
Heart failure
Valvular disease
Arrhythmia
0 1 2 3 4 5
All Survivors at Age 45 (%)
Cardiac Surveillance and Management
• Electrocardiograms at follow-up initiation
• Cardiovascular risk factor management

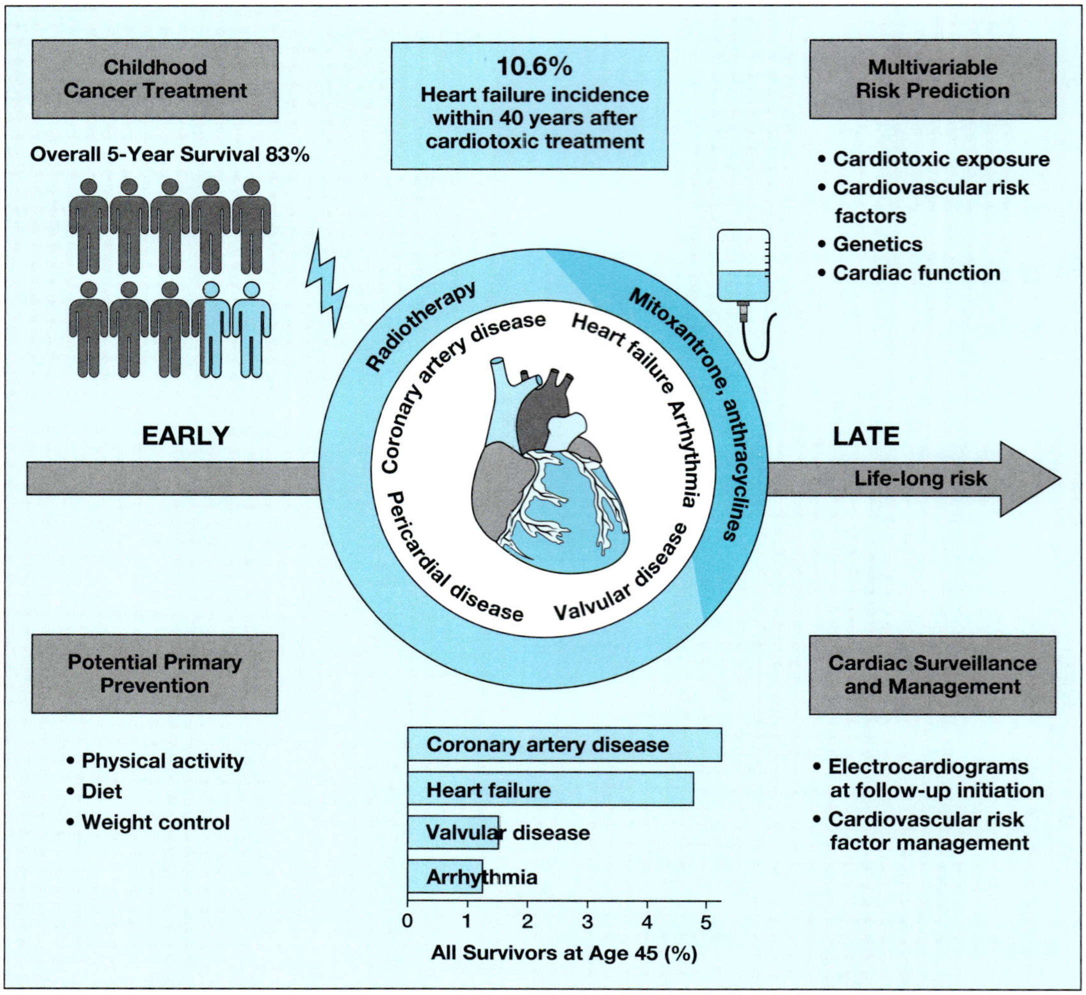

FIGURE 5.3. Overview of childhood cancer survivors at risk for cardiotoxicity. (From Leerink JM, de Baat EC, Feijen EAM, et al. Cardiac disease in childhood cancer survivors: risk prediction, prevention, and surveillance. *JACC: CardioOncology*. 2020;2(3):363–78, central figure. doi:10.1016/j.jaccao.2020.08.006.)

Cardiopulmonary Dysfunction

Cardiopulmonary dysfunction may develop many years after treatment has ended or the damage that was incurred initially can worsen over time (40, 41). Cardiopulmonary dysfunction can be caused by radiation therapy, and chemotherapy agents, for example, anthracyclines (eg, doxorubicin), antitumor antibiotics (eg, bleomycin and mitoxantrone), and targeted treatments with trastuzumab and pertuzumab (Box 5.2). These drugs can cause heart failure and **cardiomyopathy** (Figure 5.3). Hypertension is a common side effect of a class

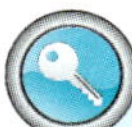

Cardiopulmonary dysfunction. A variety of different disorders and diseases that affect the heart (cardio) and lungs (pulmonary).

Cardiomyopathy. Any disorder that impairs the ability of the heart muscle to pump or causes arrhythmias (irregular heartbeats).

Box 5.2 Common Chemotherapy (Cardiotoxic) Drugs

Cardiotoxic chemotherapeutic drugs include the following:

- Anthracyclines (eg, doxorubicin)
- Antitumor antibiotics (eg, bleomycin, mitoxantrone)
- 5-FU (brand name Adrucil®)
- Taxanes (eg, docetaxel, paclitaxel)
- Vinca alkaloids (eg, vincristine, vinblastine)
- Cyclophosphamide (brand name Cytoxan®)
- Trastuzumab (brand name Herceptin®)
- Tamoxifen (brand name Nolvadex®)
- Bevacizumab (brand name Avastin®)

of drugs called tyrosine kinase inhibitors (TKIs), targets therapies for cancers with specific abnormal genes. TKIs can cause an increase in blood pressure. Radiation therapy to the chest or left breast increases the risk of coronary disease and cardiac perfusion deficits (42). Cancers that are commonly associated with cardiopulmonary dysfunction include breast cancer, non-Hodgkin's lymphoma, Hodgkin's lymphoma, and testicular cancer. These treatment-related impairments can be directly related to treatment with certain drugs or radiation therapy. That may cause **cardiotoxicities**. For example, **heart failure** is associated with doxorubicin, trastuzumab, and bleomycin. Other late effects of treatment include hypertension, hyperlipidemia, arrhythmias, **arterial stenosis**, conduction disorders, and **valvular disease.** These late effects can cause profound declines in a cancer patient's physical function, fatigue, and cardiac and pulmonary dysfunction. Exercise and a healthy lifestyle can have an important impact on the health of PLWBC (43).

Cardiovascular Risk Factors

Cardiovascular risk factors include hypertension, obesity, **dyslipidemia**, and diabetes. The cluster of these risk factors is called *metabolic syndrome* (44). Metabolic syndrome is a group of 5 conditions that can lead to heart disease, diabetes, stroke, and other health problems (Box 5.3). Three of the conditions are required for a diagnosis of metabolic syndrome. Metabolic syndrome occurs in as many as 32% of childhood cancer survivors. Hypertension is the most prevalent cardiovascular risk affecting nearly 40% of people living beyond cancer who are aged 50 years or older (45). Healthy lifestyle interventions that include physical activity, a well-balanced diet, and weight control will contribute to reduced cardiac morbidity and **mortality** (43). See Figure 5.3 to understand how cancer treatment can impact risk for CVD.

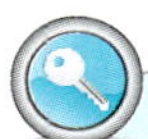

Cardiotoxicity. Damage to the heart muscle. It can be caused by drugs used to treat cancer and radiation therapy.

Heart failure/congestive heart failure. Occurs when the heart muscle does not pump blood properly. It can affect one or both sides of the heart. In cancer patients, left-sided heart failure is more common and may be caused by a reduced ejection fraction (how much blood the heart can pump from the left ventricle) because of damage from certain chemotherapy drugs or radiation.

Arterial stenosis. Narrowing down of the aortic valve opening that restricts blood flow from the left ventricle to the aorta. May also increase the pressure in the left atrium.

Valvular disease. Radiation therapy can be caused by certain drugs (eg, trastuzumab) and can cause left ventricular changes.

Dyslipidemia. Abnormal levels of lipids that pose a risk factor for atherosclerotic CVD (coronary artery disease, cerebrovascular disease, and peripheral artery disease).

Mortality. Death.

Box 5.3 Five Conditions That Lead to Metabolic Syndrome

The following 5 conditions lead to metabolic syndrome:

- High blood glucose (sugar)
- Low levels of HDL (good) cholesterol
- High triglycerides
- Large waist circumference
- High blood pressure

Endocrine Dysfunction

Endocrine dysfunction can emerge long after treatment ends (41, 46). Dysregulation of the endocrine system has far-reaching metabolic effects, including obesity, hypertension, dyslipidemia, and impaired glucose metabolism. These cardiometabolic effects increase risks for CVD, which are already increased for many people living beyond cancer because of exposures to certain chemotherapy drugs. The rate of endocrine dysfunction varies by type of treatment. ADT for the treatment of prostate cancer causes multiple endocrine complications, including osteoporosis, loss of muscle mass, sexual dysfunction, hot flashes and gynecomastia (enlargement of breast tissue in men), and decreased QoL (47). ADT is also associated with impaired glucose metabolism, insulin resistance, and metabolic syndrome (48). Radiation to the chest and neck is a well-documented cause of **hypothyroidism** (49, 50). Many of the immunotherapy drugs can severely impair the thyroid and pituitary glands. Figure 5.4 shows the incidence of thyroid and pituitary dysfunction after treatment with different types of immunotherapy drugs called immune check point inhibitors (51). In a study of a check point inhibitor, pembrolizumab, 80% of patients with non-small cell lung cancer developed thyroid antibodies that impair thyroid function and cause hypothyroidism (52). This is an irreversible side effect that requires lifelong thyroid replacement. Hypothyroidism, when it is not well managed, can cause fatigue weakness, weight gain, and mental changes (53). There is a delicate balance in the human body, and when any one element is dysregulated, the effects are far-reaching.

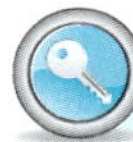

Hypothyroidism. The thyroid gland does not produce enough thyroid hormones: triiodothyronine (T3) and thyroxin (T4). Symptoms include weight gain, constipation, fatigue, and cold sensitivity.

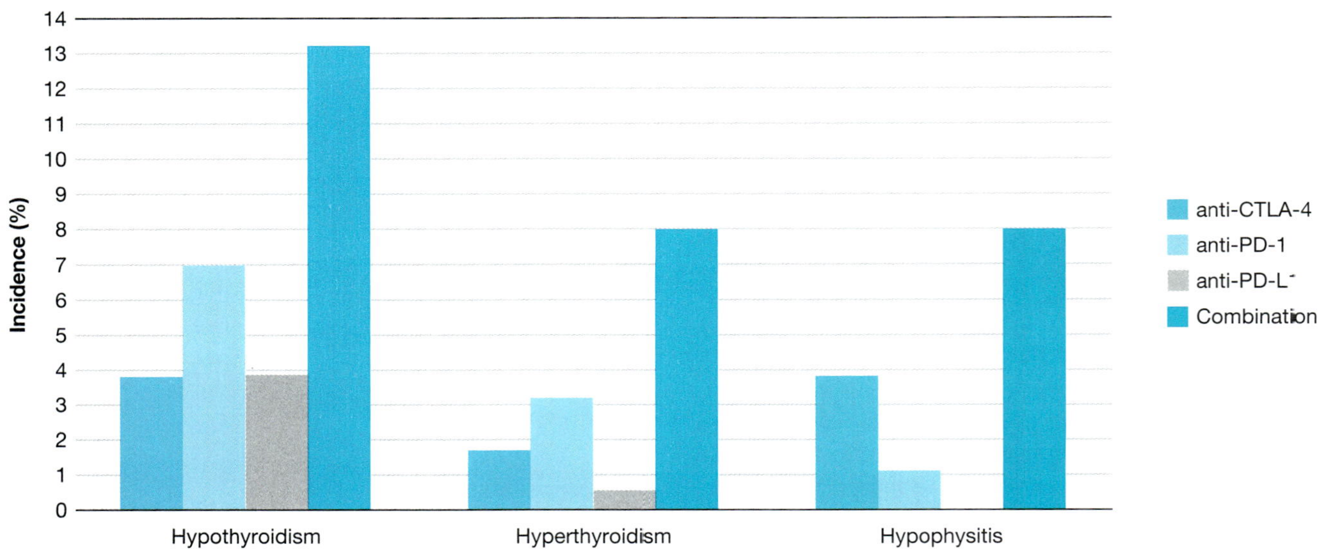

FIGURE 5.4. Incidence of hypothyroidism, hyperthyroidism and hypophysitis after the use of different immune check point inhibitors. (From Barroso-Sousa R, Ott PA, Hodi FS, Kaiser UB, Tolaney SM, Min L. Endocrine dysfunction induced by immune checkpoint inhibitors: practical recommendations for diagnosis and clinical management. *Cancer.* 2018;124(6):1111–21. doi:10.1002/cncr.31200.)

Bone Loss

Bone loss is a silent and gradual process that leads to osteopenia and eventually to **osteoporosis**. At least 40% of postmenopausal women without cancer and 15% to 30% of men without cancer will experience a fracture associated with fragility (54). Peak bone mass in a human body is attained by 30 years of age and then begins a gradual decline with age, menopause, and exposure to bone wasting substances caused by smoking, excessive alcohol consumption, and some cancer treatments (Box 5.4).

Osteoporosis is severe bone loss and increases the risk for fracture and can occur in men and women (55-58). Bone loss is measured by dual-energy x-ray absorptiometry (DEXA scan) that measures the mineral content of bone. Fracture risk increases as the bone mineral density (BMD) decreases and the bone becomes more porous. Bone loss is categorized by T-scores. The lower the score, the more porous or fragile the bone is, meaning that the person is at increased risk for fracture. A T-score of −1 to −2.5 is classified as osteopenia and a T-score of −2.5 and lower is classified as osteoporosis (Figure 5.5).

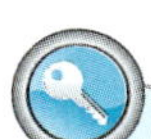

Osteoporosis. A silent bone disease with no symptoms. It causes the bone mass and bone density to decrease and compromises the strength and structure of the bones. It increases the risk of bone fracture.

People with osteoporosis have a 4-fold increased risk of fracture compared with an individual with normal BMD (Figure 5.6). Women with osteopenia have 1.8-fold higher risk of fracture than men. Osteoporosis is associated with a significantly higher number of fractures than osteopenia. However, fracture risk is still significant in people with osteopenia.

Bone loss is accelerated by many chemotherapy drugs (eg, doxorubicin), steroids (eg, dexamethasone), and hormonal

Box 5.4 Risk Factors for Bone Loss

The following are risk factors for bone loss:

- Female
- Advanced age female or male
- Low body weight
- Early menopause
- Surgical menopause
- Hypogonadism
- Menopause
- Cigarette smoking
- Excess alcohol consumption
- Sedentary lifestyle
- Chronic corticosteroid use

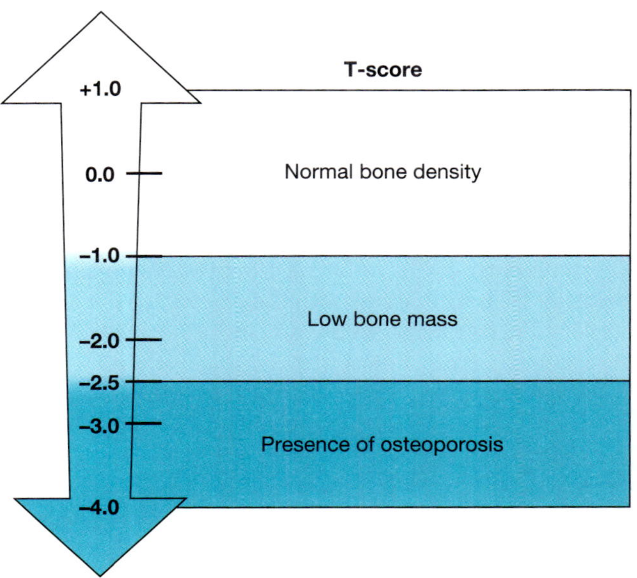

FIGURE 5.5. Bone density T-score from the normal range (white) to osteopenia (light blue) and osteoporosis (dark blue).

treatments (eg, androgen ablation and estrogen suppression). Activities that stress the bones help to promote bone growth. During treatment exercise has a bone-preserving effect and posttreatment exercise helps to promote bone health (59).

Psychosocial Challenges

Psychosocial challenges including anxiety, depression, and fear of cancer recurrence are common among people living beyond cancer (60-62). Although anxiety and depression can be medically treated, fear of recurrence may be an ongoing concern that can have a negative effect on QoL. A systematic review observed that as many as 20% to 30% of people living beyond cancer reported problems related to their cancer treatment, including lower QoL, physical problems, psychological distress, sexual problems, problems with social relationships, and financial concerns (12). Moderate to high levels of fear of recurrence are reported by 30% to 70% of PLWBC (12). Cancer is a disease that has lifelong effects.

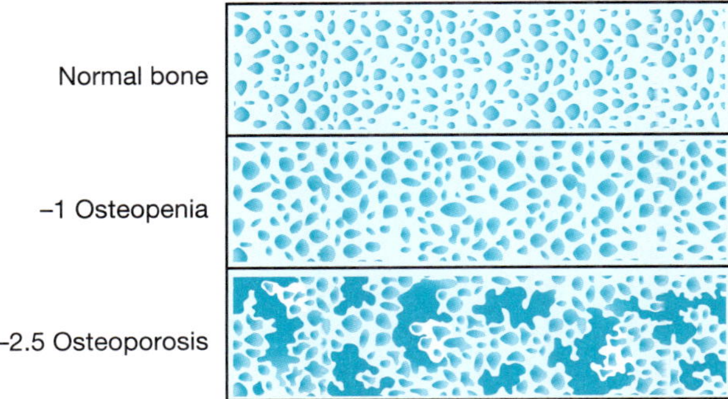

FIGURE 5.6. Bone density scores ranging from normal to osteoporosis. Normal bone is less porous (dark spots).

RECURRENCE

When cancer recurs after successful treatment, it is called a **recurrence**. It is a recurrence of the same tumor type. Recurrence develops because some cancer cells survived the first cancer treatment. When treatment was initially completed, these cells were too small to detect, but over time the cells developed into a detectable recurrence. Cancer can recur in different ways: local, regional, or distant. A local recurrence develops at the original site or very close to it. A regional recurrence means that the cancer cells have spread into surrounding tissue or lymph nodes that are close to the original site of disease. A distant recurrence, or metastatic disease, means that the disease has spread to distant parts of the body. The common patterns, or places, that cancer spreads to are lymph nodes, liver, lungs, bones, and brain. If people with breast or prostate cancer develop metastatic disease in their bones, they still have breast or prostate cancer. They do not have bone cancer.

Sometimes, PLWBC develop secondary cancers (37). This is called a secondary primary cancer because it is different than the first cancer, and it is not a recurrence of the primary cancer. Second primary cancers can occur years after treatment for a primary cancer as a result of exposure to chest radiation or certain chemotherapy treatments. For example, treatment with cyclophosphamide is associated with the development of leukemias; treatment for lymphoma often includes chest radiation (mantle field) that increases a person's risk for developing breast cancer.

Recurrence or development of a second cancer requires restaging to determine the extent of a recurrence. Laboratory tests, radiologic imaging, and sometimes biopsies are required to establish how far the disease has spread (**metastasized**). Once the staging is complete, the type(s) of treatment will be made in the same fashion as at the initial diagnosis. Often a local and regional recurrence can be treated with a cure in mind, but metastatic disease is generally treated with the intent of controlling disease and looking at cancer as a chronic disease.

Psychological Impacts

Recurrent cancer is a devastating emotional blow to anyone living beyond cancer. The disbelief, anger, sadness, and fear of the unknown symptoms and death descend upon the individual and their loved ones as they struggle with making treatment decisions, and family and work plans (60-62). Some people see a cancer recurrence as a wake-up call. But for almost all people,

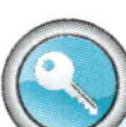

Recurrence. When the same type of cancer reoccurs or comes back. It is also called relapse. Cancer can come back in the original site (primary) or another place in the body.

Metastasis. Cancer that has spread from the primary site to a distant site. The most common sites of metastasis for solid tumors are the lungs, liver, bones, and brain.

a recurrence is a reminder to live a full and meaningful life and to focus on what is important to them. Everyone finds meaning in their life in a different way. It may be through prayer, walking in the woods, being with grandchildren or people you love, or pursing work or activities that are important. PLWBC will embrace the things that bring joy and comfort and help to allay the overwhelming anxiety and fear that fill the mind at night and in the quiet hours.

Treatment

Treatment for recurrent disease is different than at initial diagnosis (63). If the recurrence is local or regional, it may be focused on achieving a complete remission, but different treatment approaches are commonly used, and the treatments are often more aggressive and difficult to tolerate; side effects may be harder to manage or have a great impact on the person. Figure 5.7 shows the rate of recurrence for **locoregional recurrence** by type of cancer (64). If the treatment is for metastatic disease, then the goal is to control the disease and treat the cancer more like a chronic disease. The intent of treatment is to provide the person living with cancer a treatment that has fewer or less intense side effects so that they may enjoy as many years of QoL as possible. Depending on the specific type, site, and extent of recurrent cancer, there are many treatment options that may be considered, including surgery, radiation therapy, chemotherapy, biologic or immunotherapy, or blood and marrow transplant. The oncology team will discuss with the person living with cancer what the treatment options are, including the possibility of participating in a clinical trial.

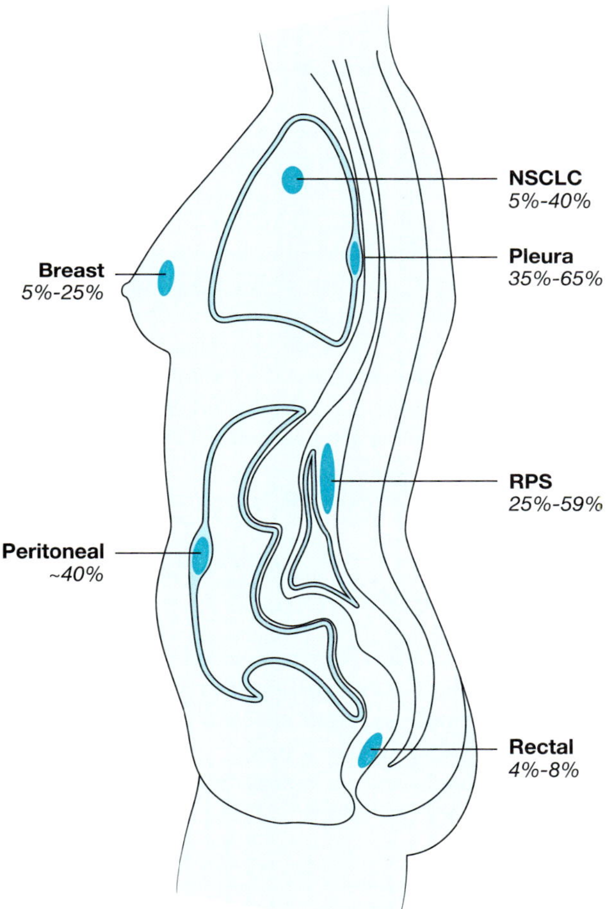

FIGURE 5.7. A summary of local recurrence rates for various common malignancies after surgery. Abbreviations: NSCLC, non-small cell lung cancer; RPS, retroperitoneal sarcoma. (From Mahvi DA, Liu R, Grinstaff MW, Colson YL, Raut CP. Local cancer recurrence: the realities, challenges, and opportunities for new therapies. *CA Cancer J Clin.* 2018;68(6):488–505. doi:10.3322/caac.21498.)

When metastatic cancer is treated as a chronic disease, the focus is on giving the person living with cancer the optimal QoL. Treatment is often given at a lower dose to keep the disease stable, limit growth, and minimize side effects. Managing side effects of treatment is foremost so that life can be enjoyed and lived fully. PLWC need to celebrate life, travel, and live. Treatments are carefully scheduled around family reunions, vacations, and other adventures or celebrations.

CLINICAL TRIALS

A **clinical trial** is a rigorously controlled research study to find better treatments for cancer. All clinical trials must undergo careful scientific oversight by an Institutional Review Board (IRB) that determines the safety, risks, benefits, and ethical value of the study. Clinical trials have specific enrollment or eligibility criteria that an individual must meet to be able to participate. Before a participant enrolls in a trial, they must be informed of all the potential risks and benefits of the study and all the study procedures and sign the Informed Consent form to participate.

There are different phases of clinical trials (Table 5.5). Phase 0 clinical trials are preclinical studies that examine the effects of a new drug or treatment in animals. Phase 1 clinical trial tests a promising drug to determine what dose is safe and how it should be given. Phase II trials study how cancer responds to the new drug or treatment to determine if it is effective. Phase III trials look at the best treatment available today (standard of care) and compare it to what science suggests may be an even better treatment. Phase IV trials are large studies examining the long-term benefits and side effects of a treatment that has Food and Drug Association (FDA) approval. These trials are conducted in by community-based physicians, or their research associates, taking responsibility for the data collected at their site and the transmission of the data to the leading principal investigators.

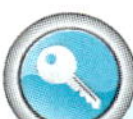

Locoregional recurrence. Recurrence of a tumor affecting lymph nodes or structures (eg, chest wall) adjacent to the original site of disease.

Clinical trial. A rigorously controlled research study to find better treatments for cancer.

Table 5.5 Phases of Clinical Trials

PHASE	PRIMARY GOAL	PRIMARY RESEARCHER	SUBJECT TYPE	COMMENTS
Preclinical	Nonhuman efficacy Toxicity PK	PhD, MD, PharmD, or any researcher	Cell lines (animal)	
0	Determining PK and PD	Clinical researcher	Human	Focuses on determining oral bioavailability and half-life Often combined with Phase 1
1	Evaluation of safety and adverse events	Clinical researcher	Human	May be expanded or combined with Phase 2
2	Examine efficacy and dose range	Clinical researcher	Human	May help in optimizing dose, schedule, and select disease types
3	Expanded study to substantiate efficacy and safety	Clinical researcher	Human (N = large range)	Generally includes multiple sites and investigators
4	Postmarketing surveillance	Primary physician	Human (N = all patients taking the drug)	Determines long-term effects

PD, pharmacodynamic; PK, pharmacokinetic.
From Mahipal A, Nguyen D. Risks and benefits of phase 1 clinical trial participation. *Cancer Control.* 2014;21(3):193–9. doi:10.1177/107327481402100303.

END OF LIFE

Living with Stage IV cancer may continue for decades, and death may not be because of cancer. Treatments for people living with metastatic breast cancer have improved so much, in part due to clinical trials, that many people live for years. The 5-year survival rate for women is 28% and for men is 22% (65). Table 5.6 shows the survival rate for breast cancer at different stages for women diagnosed with breast cancer between 2010 and 2016 (66). These data are collected by the Surveillance, Epidemiology, and End Results (SEER) Program of the NCI and the Division of Cancer Control and Population Sciences (DCCPS). SEER collects data on cancer statistics to report on the burden of cancer among the US population.

Table 5.6 Five-Year Survival Rates for Breast Cancer

SEER STAGE	FIVE-YEAR RELATIVE SURVIVAL RATE (%)
Localized	99
Regional (spread to lymph nodes)	86
Distant (Metastatic)	30
All SEER stages combined	91

From American Cancer Society. *Survival Rates for Breast Cancer* [Internet]. 2023. Available from https://www.cancer.org/cancer/breast-cancer/understanding-a-breast-cancer-diagnosis/breast-cancer-survival-rates.html.

People living with metastatic disease are often actively receiving treatment during this time, but the goal is to enable the control of disease spread while allowing the individual to engage and embrace a full and meaningful life. Sometimes people living with metastatic disease die from heart disease, which is the number 1 cause of death in the US (67). However, for most people living with metastatic disease, death is because of cancer. When cancer is no longer responsive to treatment, it is called the end-stage or terminal cancer. There still may be clinical trial options, but many people choose palliative care or hospice to help control their side effects and symptoms, and maximize the quality of their remaining life (68, 69). Clinical trials for people with end-stage diseases are in early phase trials (Phase I or II), examining the safety, efficacy, and optimal dosing of the study drug. People living with end-stage disease join these early clinical trials with the hopes that the new study drug may cure or slow their disease, or for the altruistic reason to help future PLWC by participating in the trial.

Palliative care is focused on symptom management. The purpose of palliative care is to control side effects to allow an

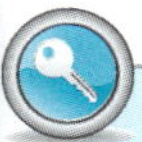

Palliative care. Specialized medical care focusing on managing symptoms to improve the QoL for people living with a serious illness.

individual to live the fullest life possible. Palliative care is not restricted to people at the end of life; it is for all, regardless of age, stage of disease, or prognosis (70-72). Procedures or medication are given to reduce pain or make the person feel more comfortable. If a mass is pressing on nerves or vital organs and causing pain, surgery may be performed to remove the mass and alleviate the pain. Radiation therapy may also be used in a focused area to reduce pain. For example, a person with pain from bone metastasis that limits walking and sitting comfortably could have radiation to the bone lesion that is causing pain. Chemotherapy may be given to reduce the size or try to slow the growth of a tumor. This topic is covered in greater detail in Chapter 16.

Hospice is the final transition in cancer care. At this stage, the person living with cancer is no longer receiving any type of cancer care. Hospice care is focused on relieving symptoms and providing support at the end of life, not extending life. Hospice is not focused on dying. Rather, it is focused on living a good quality life and living each day as comfortably as possible by controlling pain and other symptoms. Hospice does not hasten death, and it does not mean the person living with cancer has given up. Every person living with cancer, especially at the end of life, has a choice as to how they would like to live and with whom they would like to spend their time. At the end of life, spending time with loved ones and friends becomes even more meaningful and important.

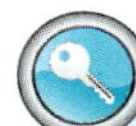

Hospice. Provided to people with a terminal disease, who are no longer receiving treatment to cure or control their disease. A health care provider must determine that the individual has 6 months or less to live.

People can be admitted to hospice when certified by a health care provider who determines that the person has a life expectancy of 6 months or less. If a person is able, they must sign consent for hospice care. If the person lives beyond the expected 6 months, they can be re-enrolled on hospice as long as the need for hospice care is demonstrated by the hospice providers and the person consents to continuing on hospice. The person on hospice can, at any time, decide that s/he no longer wants to be on hospice. Reasons for this may include wanting to resume cancer treatment, joining a clinical trial, or an unexpected improvement in a physical condition.

Hospice can be provided in different places: a person's home, a hospital, or a nursing home. Often families feel that it would be impossible to keep a loved one at home because they do not have the equipment or supplies or support, but hospice services are extensive. They include medical, nursing, physical, occupational and speech therapy services, medical supplies and equipment, medications for pain and symptom management, volunteers to give caregivers respite, counseling and spiritual care, and grief counseling for loved ones. Hospice workers and volunteers are especially trained to provide support for both the person at the end of life and their loved ones.

SUMMARY

Cancer treatments can cause side effects that linger many years after treatment ends, side effects that never go away, and side effects that insidiously develop years after treatment ends. PLWBC need to learn to live with and manage these side effects. Exercise trainers must be aware of the potential for these effects and be creative in determining ways for people to engage in exercise and physical activities despite their limitations. Cancer recurrence and end of life pose 2 very different aspects of exercise programing that are important to the person living with cancer who deeply aspires to remain as independent as possible. The third section of this book will focus on prescribing exercise for PLWBC at all stages along the cancer journey.

Case Study #1

Jim was a 48-year-old helicopter pilot who noticed a dark irregular mole on the bottom of his foot, which was diagnosed as malignant melanoma. The lesion was surgically excised, and after about 6 weeks of recovery, he was treated with immunotherapy (interferon-alpha) for almost 12 months. It has been now 3 years since his treatment, and he has resumed his job flying a rescue helicopter at the Grand Canyon. He states that he feels too tired to exercise. He complains that he gets fatigued easily, notices his muscles have atrophied (wasting away or decreased muscle mass from disuse), and he is much weaker than he used to be.

Questions

1. Why is Jim become weaker?
2. Why would Jim have sarcopenia?
3. Why Jim feels fatigued 3 years after treatment ended?

Case Study #2

Sarah was a 62-year-old woman with an 8-year history of breast cancer. She was initially treated surgically with a mastectomy; chemotherapy that included doxorubicin, cyclophosphamide, and paclitaxel; followed by radiation therapy and 5 years of antiestrogen therapy. She lived a full life with 3 daughters who had graduated from college. She loved to travel and was physically active and focused on living and eating well. Three years after completing all treatments, she developed bone metastasis in her left femur. She was started on denosumab, a bisphosphonate used to treat bone metastasis and paclitaxel, which caused CIPN, low platelet counts, and anemia. Sarah was distraught and depressed by her diagnosis and knew that she had limited time to live, and hence she wanted to be with her family and live life fully. She made the most of her time by traveling to Tahiti to snorkel and scuba dive on remote islands and trained to be fit enough to complete a 32-mile backpack trip in 3 days, carrying her own gear and pack. She negotiated travel, backpacking, and family trips with her oncology team who planned her treatments and boosted her with transfusions, as needed, so that she would feel well when she went off on her adventures.

Questions

1. What is/are the risk(s) of a low platelet count?
2. What is/are the risk(s) of hiking with chemotherapy-induced peripheral neuropathy?
3. How did Sarah carry a backpack with bone metastasis to her femur?

Meet the Expert

FEATURED PROFESSIONAL

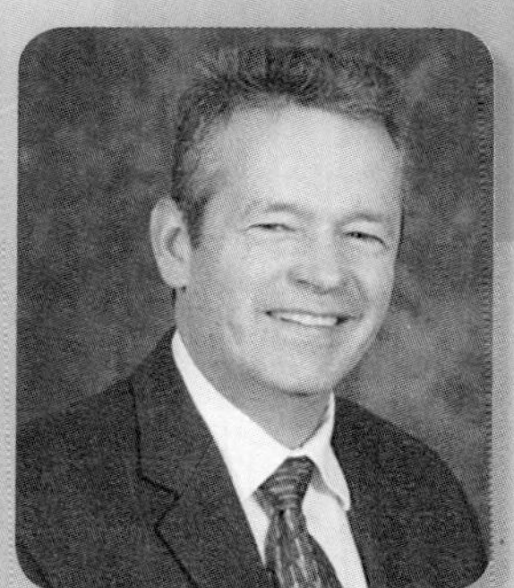

Kerry S. Courneya, PhD

Professor and Canada Research Chair in Physical Activity and Cancer
Director, Behavior Medicine Laboratory and Fitness Center
Faculty of Kinesiology, Sport and Recreation
University of Alberta

Q: "Where did you grow up?"

London, Ontario Canada

Q: "Where did you train? What is your training?"

I attended Western University and received my BA (1987) and MA (1989) in Kinesiology. I then attended the University of Illinois at Urbana-Champaign where I completed my PhD in Kinesiology (1992).

Q: "What are you best known for?"

My initial research interests in exercise oncology focused on motivation, quality of life, and symptom management. I published many studies on these topics in different cancer patient groups. More recently, my research interests have expanded to include cancer outcomes, such as tumor response, recurrence, progression, and survival. I have also mentored many trainees who are now contributing to the field.

Q: "What are you currently working on?"

I am currently part of the Colon Health and Life-Long Exercise Change (CHALLENGE) trial that is the first large-scale trial examining the effects of exercise on disease-free survival in 962 colon cancer survivors.

Q: "Anything else you want to include?"

Exercise oncology is an exciting field that is improving the lives of cancer patients and their families. Even after 30 years, I am still passionate about studying exercise oncology!

Favorite Quote:

"You cannot fix by analysis that which is bungled by design. By Design: Planning Research on Higher Education."
—*Richard J. Light (Author), Judith D. Singer (Author), John B. Willett (Author)*

STUDY QUESTIONS

1. What are 2 organizations that set standards for care in oncology?
2. What is the most common side effect after treatment has ended?
3. What causes muscle weakness?
4. Which treatment is better to improve muscle strength for people living beyond cancer?
   a. Aerobic exercise
   b. Flexibility exercise
   c. Resistance exercise
   d. Yoga exercise
5. List 3 signs of chemotherapy-induced neuropathy.
6. What is the difference between osteopenia and osteoporosis?
7. True or false. Only women get osteoporosis.
8. What is the intent of treatment for metastatic disease?
9. What is the focus of palliative care?
10. What is the purpose of hospice care?

REFERENCES

1. Denlinger CS, Sanft T, Moslehi JJ, et al. NCCN guidelines insights: survivorship, version 2.2020: featured updates to the NCCN guidelines. *J Natl Compr Canc Netw*. 2020;18(8):1016–23. doi: 10.6004/jnccn.2020.0037
2. Commission on Cancer. Chicago (IL): American College of Surgeons. [Internet]. 2021. Available from https://www.facs.org/quality-programs/cancer/coc
3. Demark-Wahnefried W, Aziz NM, Rowland JH, Pinto BM. Riding the crest of the teachable moment: promoting long-term health after the diagnosis of cancer. *J Clin Oncol*. 2005;23(24):5814–30. doi:10.1200/JCO.2005.01.230
4. Fisher MI, Cohn JC, Harrington SE, Lee JQ, Malone D. Screening and assessment of cancer-related fatigue: a clinical practice guideline for health care providers. *Phys Ther*. 2022;102(9):pzac120. doi:10.1093/ptj/pzac120
5. Boelhouwer IG, Vermeer W, van Vuuren T. Late effects of cancer (treatment) and work ability: guidance by managers and professionals. *BMC Public Health*. 2021;21(1):1255. doi:10.1186/s12889-021-11261-2
6. Jankowski C, Carpenter KM, Aranha O, et al. NCCN clinical practice guidelines in oncology: cancer related fatigue. Version 2.2024-October 2023 MS-1-23. https://www.nccn.org/professionals/physician_gls/pdf/fatigue.pdf
7. Todd KH. A review of current and emerging approaches to pain management in the emergency department. *Pain Ther*. 2017;6(2):193–202. doi:10.1007/s40122-017-0090-5
8. van den Beuken-van Everdingen MHJ, Hochstenbach LMJ, Joosten EAJ, Tjan-Heijnen VCG, Janssen DJA. Update on prevalence of pain in patients with cancer: systematic review and meta-analysis. *J Pain Symptom Manage*. 2016;51(6):1070–90.e9. doi:10.1016/j.jpainsymman.2015.12.340
9. Gallaway MS, Townsend JS, Shelby D, Puckett MC. Pain among cancer survivors. *Prev Chronic Dis*. 2020;17:E54. doi:10.5888/pcd17.190367
10. Simon S. *One in 3 cancer survivors has chronic pain*. [Internet]. 2019. Available from https://www.cancer.org/latest-news/one-in-3-cancer-survivors-has-chronic-pain.html
11. Caruso R, Breitbart W. Mental health care in oncology: contemporary perspective on the psychosocial burden of cancer and evidence-based interventions. *Epidemiol Psychiatr Sci*. 2020;29:e86. doi:10.1017/S2045796019000866
12. Hall DL, Luberto CM, Philpotts LL, Song R, Park ER, Yeh GY. Mind-body interventions for fear of cancer recurrence: a systematic review and meta-analysis. *Psychooncology*. 2018;27(11):2546–58. doi:10.1002/pon.4757
13. Seretny M, Currie GL, Sena ES, et al. Incidence, prevalence, and predictors of chemotherapy-induced peripheral neuropathy: a systematic review and meta-analysis. *PAIN®*. 2014;155(12):2461–70. doi:10.1016/j.pain.2014.09.020
14. Selvy M, Kerckhove N, Pereira B, et al. Prevalence of chemotherapy-induced peripheral neuropathy in multiple myeloma patients and its impact on quality of life: a single center cross-sectional study. *Front Pharmacol*. 2021;12:637593. doi:10.3389/fphar.2021.637593
15. Selvy M, Pereira B, Kerckhove N, et al. Long-term prevalence of sensory chemotherapy-induced peripheral neuropathy for 5 years after adjuvant FOLFOX chemotherapy to treat colorectal cancer: a multicenter cross-sectional study. *J Clin Med*. 2020;9(8):2400. doi:10.3390/jcm9082400
16. Clark RA, Marin TS, McCarthy AL, et al. Cardiotoxicity after cancer treatment: a process map of the patient treatment journey. *CardioOncology*. 2019;5(1):14. doi:10.1186/s40959-019-0046-5
17. Feijen EAM, Font-Gonzalez A, Van der Pal HJH, et al. Risk and temporal changes of heart failure among 5-year childhood cancer survivors: a DCOG-LATER study. *J Am Heart Assoc*. 2019;8(1):e009122. doi:10.1161/JAHA.118.009122
18. Huang T-T, Hudson MM, Stokes DC, Krasin MJ, Spunt SL, Ness KK. Pulmonary outcomes in survivors of childhood cancer: a systematic review. *Chest*. 2011;140(4):881–901. doi:10.1378/chest.10-2133
19. Ng AK, van Leeuwen FE. Hodgkin lymphoma: late effects of treatment and guidelines for surveillance. *Semin Hematol*. 2016;53(3):209–15. doi:10.1053/j.seminhematol.2016.05.008
20. Fidler MM, Reulen R, Bright CJ, et al. Respiratory mortality of childhood, adolescent and young adult cancer survivors. *Thorax*. 2018;73(10):959–68. doi:10.1136/thoraxjnl-2017-210683
21. Cella D, Lai J-S, Chang C-H, Peterman A, Slavin M. Fatigue in cancer patients compared with fatigue in the general United States population. *Cancer*. 2002;94(2):528–38. doi:10.1002/cncr.10245
22. Hammermüller C, Hinz A, Dietz A, et al. Depression, anxiety, fatigue, and quality of life in a large sample of patients suffering from head and neck cancer in comparison with the general population. *BMC Cancer*. 2021;21(1):94. doi:10.1186/s12885-020-07773-6
23. Du S, Hu L, Dong J, et al. Patient education programs for cancer-related fatigue: a systematic review. *Patient Educ Couns*. 2015;98(11):1308–19. doi:10.1016/j.pec.2015.05.003
24. Halle JL, Counts BR, Carson JA. Exercise as a therapy for cancer-induced muscle wasting. *Sports Med Health Sci*. 2020;2(18):186–94. doi:10.1016/j.smhs.2020.11.004
25. Swartz MC, Lewis ZH, Lyons EJ, et al. Effect of home- and community-based physical activity interventions on physical function among cancer survivors: a systematic review and meta-analysis. *Arch Phys Med Rehabil*. 2017;98(8):1652–65. doi:10.1016/j.apmr.2017.03.017
26. Winters-Stone KM, Dobek JC, Bennett JA, et al. Resistance training reduces disability in prostate cancer survivors on androgen deprivation therapy: evidence from a randomized controlled trial. *Arch Phys Med Rehabil*. 2015;96(1):7–14. doi:10.1016/j.apmr.2014.08.010

27. Irwin ML, Cartmel B, Gross CP, et al. Randomized exercise trial of aromatase inhibitor-induced arthralgia in breast cancer survivors. *J Clin Oncol.* 2015;33(10):1104–11. doi:10.1200/JCO.2014.57.1547
28. McNeely ML, Parliament MB, Seikaly H, et al. Effect of exercise on upper extremity pain and dysfunction in head and neck cancer survivors. *Cancer.* 2008;113(1):214–22. doi:10.1002/cncr.23536
29. Ciaramella A, Poli P. Assessment of depression among cancer patients: the role of pain, cancer type and treatment. *Psychooncology.* 2001;10(2):156–65. doi:10.1002/pon.505
30. Andersen BL, DeRubeis RJ, Berman BS, et al. Screening, assessment, and care of anxiety and depressive symptoms in adults with cancer: an American Society of Clinical Oncology guideline adaptation. *J Clin Oncol.* 2014;32(15):1605–19.
31. Capuron L, Ravaud A, Neveu PJ, Miller AH, Maes M Dantzer R. Association between decreased serum tryptophan concentrations and depressive symptoms in cancer patients undergoing cytokine therapy. *Mol Psychiatry.* 2002;7(5):468–73. doi:10.1038/sj.mp.4000995
32. Corbett T, Groarke A, Walsh JC, McGuire BE. Cancer-related fatigue in post-treatment cancer survivors: application of the common sense model of illness representations. *BMC Cancer.* 2016;16(1):919. doi:10.1186/s12885-016-2907-8
33. Teng C, Cohen J, Egger S, Blinman PL, Vardy JL. Systematic review of long-term chemotherapy-induced peripheral neuropathy (CIPN) following adjuvant oxaliplatin for colorectal cancer. *Support Care Cancer.* 2022;30(1):33–47. doi:10.1007/s00520-021-06502-4
34. Ogle T, Alexander K, Yates P, et al. Occurrence and perceived effectiveness of activities used to decrease chemotherapy-induced peripheral neuropathy symptoms in the feet. *Eur J Oncol Nurs.* 2021;54:102025. doi:10.1016/j.ejon.2021.102025
35. Varga I, Mravec B. Nerve fiber types. In: Tubbs RS, Rizk E, Shoja MM, Loukas M, Barbaro N, Spinner RJ, editors. *Nerves and Nerve Injuries.* San Diego (CA): Academic Press; 2015. Chapter 8, pp. 107–13. Available from https://www.sciencedirect.com/science/article/pii/B9780124103900000081
36. Helgers RJA, Winkens B, Slangen BFM, Werner HMJ. Lymphedema and post-operative complications after sentinel lymph node biopsy versus lymphadenectomy in endometrial carcinomas: a systematic review and meta-analysis. *J Clin Med.* 2021;10(1):120. doi:10.3390/jcm10010120
37. Allam O, Park KE, Chandler L, et al. The impact of radiation on lymphedema: a review of the literature. *Gland Surg.* 2020;9(2):596–602. doi:10.21037/gs.2020.03.20
38. Schmitz KH, Ahmed RL, Troxel A, et al. Weight lifting in women with breast-cancer-related lymphedema. *N Engl J Med.* 2009;361(7):664–73. doi:10.1056/NEJMoa0810118
39. Schmitz KH, Ahmed RL, Troxel AB, et al. Weight lifting for women at risk for breast cancer–related lymphedema: a randomized trial. *JAMA.* 2010;304(24):2699–705. doi:10.1001/jama.2010.1837
40. Stone JR, Kanneganti R, Abbasi M, Akhtari M. Monitoring for chemotherapy-related cardiotoxicity in the form of left ventricular systolic dysfunction: a review of current recommendations. *JCO Oncol Pract.* 2021;17(5):228–36. doi:10.1200/op.20.00924
41. Maltser S, Cristian A, Silver JK, Morris GS, Stout NL. A focused review of safety considerations in cancer rehabilitation. *PM&R.* 2017;9(suppl 2):S415–28. doi:10.1016/j.pmrj.2017.08.403
42. Dent SF, Kikuchi R, Kondapalli L, et al. Optimizing cardiovascular health in patients with cancer: a practical review of risk assessment, monitoring, and prevention of cancer treatment–related cardiovascular toxicity. *Am Soc Clin Oncol Educ Book.* 2020(40):501–15. doi:10.1200/edbk_286019
43. Leerink JM, de Baat EC, Feijen EAM, et al. Cardiac disease in childhood cancer survivors: risk prediction, prevention, and surveillance. *JACC: CardioOncology.* 2020;2(3):363–78. doi:10.1016/j.jaccao.2020.08.006
44. Smith WA, Li C, Nottage KA, et al. Lifestyle and metabolic syndrome in adult survivors of childhood cancer: a report from the St. Jude Lifetime Cohort Study. *Cancer.* 2014;120(17):2742–50. doi:10.1002/cncr.28670
45. Armstrong GT, Oeffinger KC, Chen Y, et al. Modifiable risk factors and major cardiac events among adult survivors of childhood cancer. *J Clin Oncol.* 2013;31(29):3673–80. doi:10.1200/JCO.2013.49.3205
46. Anazodo AC, Choi S, Signorelli C, et al. Reproductive care of childhood and adolescent cancer survivors: a 12-year evaluation. *J Adolesc Young Adul Oncol.* 2021;10(2):131–41. doi:10.1089/jayao.2020.0157
47. Nguyen PL, Alibhai SM, Basaria S, et al. Adverse effects of androgen deprivation therapy and strategies to mitigate them. *Eur Urol.* 2015;67(5):825–36. doi:10.1016/j.eururo.2014.07.010
48. Pyrgidis N, Vakalopoulos I, Sountoulides P. Endocrine consequences of treatment with the new androgen receptor axis-targeted agents for advanced prostate cancer. *Hormones (Athens).* 2021;20(1):73–84. doi:10.1007/s42000-020-00251-5
49. Rønjom MF. Radiation-induced hypothyroidism after treatment of head and neck cancer. *Dan Med J.* 2016;63(3):B5213.
50. Macklin-Doherty A, Jones M, Coulson P, et al. Risk of thyroid disorders in adult and childhood Hodgkin lymphoma survivors 40 years after treatment. *Leukemia & Lymphoma.* 2022;63(3):562–72. doi:10.1080/10428194.2021.1999445
51. Barroso-Sousa R, Ott PA, Hodi FS, Kaiser UB, Tolaney SM, Min L. Endocrine dysfunction induced by immune checkpoint inhibitors: practical recommendations for diagnosis and clinical management. *Cancer.* 2018;124(6):1111–21. doi:10.1002/cncr.31200
52. Osorio JC, Ni A, Chaft JE, et al. Antibody-mediated thyroid dysfunction during T-cell checkpoint blockade in patients with non-small-cell lung cancer. *Ann Oncol.* 2017;28(3):583–9. doi:10.1093/annonc/mdw640
53. Moeller LC, Führer D. Thyroid hormone, thyroid hormone receptors, and cancer: a clinical perspective. *Endocr Relat Cancer.* 2013;20(2):R19–29. doi:10.1530/erc-12-0219
54. International Osteoporosis Foundation. *Osteoporosis Epidemiology.* [Internet]. 2021. Available from https://www.osteoporosis.foundation/health-professionals/about-osteoporosis/epidemiology
55. Winters-Stone KM, Leo MC, Schwartz A. Exercise effects on hip bone mineral density in older, post-menopausal breast cancer survivors are age dependent. *Arch Osteoporos.* 2012;7(1):301–6. doi:10.1007/s11657-012-0071-6
56. Winters-Stone KM, Schwartz AL, Hayes SC, Fabian CJ, Campbell KL. A prospective model of care for breast cancer rehabilitation: bone health and arthralgias. *Cancer.* 2012;118(S8):2288–99. doi:10.1002/cncr.27465
57. Leslie WD, Edwards B, Al-Azazi S, et al. Cancer patients with fractures are rarely assessed or treated for osteoporosis: a population-based study. *Osteoporos Int.* 2021;32(2):333–41. doi:10.1007/s00198-020-05596-6
58. Johns Hopkins Medicine. *Bone Densitometry.* [Internet]. 2021. Available from https://www.hopkinsmedicine.org/health/treatment-tests-and-therapies/bone-densitometry
59. Schwartz AL. Health maintenance for the long run. In: Curtiss C, Haylock P, editors. *Cancer Survivorship: Interprofessional, Patient-Centered Approaches to the Seasons of Survival.* Pittsburgh (PA): Oncology Nursing Society; 2019.
60. Niedzwiedz CL, Knifton L, Robb KA, Katikireddi SV, Smith DJ. Depression and anxiety among people living with and beyond cancer: a growing clinical and research priority. *BMC Cancer.* 2019;19(1):943. doi:10.1186/s12885-019-6181-4
61. Séguin Leclair C, Lebel S, Westmaas JL. Can physical activity and healthy diet help long-term cancer survivors manage their fear of recurrence? *Front Psychol.* 2021;12(2210). doi:10.3389/fpsyg.2021.647432
62. Wang X, Wang N, Zhong L, et al. Prognostic value of depression and anxiety on breast cancer recurrence and mortality: a systematic review and meta-analysis of 282,203 patients. *Mol Psychiatry.* 2020;25(12):3186–97. doi:10.1038/s41380-020-00865-6
63. Waks AG, Winer EP. Breast cancer treatment: a review. *JAMA.* 2019;321(3):288–300. doi:10.1001/jama.2018.19323
64. Mahvi DA, Liu R, Grinstaff MW, Colson YL, Raut CP. Local cancer recurrence: the realities, challenges, and opportunities for new

therapies. *CA Cancer J Clin.* 2018;68(6):488–505. doi:10.3322/caac.21498

65. Siegel RL, Miller KD, Jemal A. Cancer statistics, 2020. *CA Cancer J Clin.* 2020;70(1):7–30. doi:10.3322/caac.21590
66. American Cancer Society. *Survival Rates for Breast Cancer* [Internet]. 2021. Available from https://www.cancer.org/cancer/breast-cancer/understanding-a-breast-cancer-diagnosis/breast-cancer-survival-rates.html
67. Ahmad FB, Anderson RN. The leading causes of death in the US for 2020. *JAMA.* 2021;325(18):1829–30. doi:10.1001/jama.2021.5469
68. Balogun JA. Emerging trends and best practices in hospice and palliative care. In: Okonofua F, Balogun JA, Odunsi K, Chilaka VN, editors. *Contemporary Obstetrics and Gynecology for Developing Countries.* Cham: Springer International Publishing; 2021, pp. 663–86.
69. Dans M, Kutner JS, Agarwal R, et al. NCCN Guidelines® insights: palliative care, version 2.2021: featured updates to the NCCN Guidelines. *J Natl Compr Canc Netw.* 2021;19(7):780–8. doi:10.6004/jnccn.2021.0033
70. Radbruch L, De Lima L, Knaul F, et al. Redefining palliative care: a new consensus-based definition. *J Pain Symptom Manage.* 2020;60(4):754–64. doi:10.1016/j.jpainsymman.2020.04.027
71. World Health Organization. *Ensuring Balance in National Policies on Controlled Substances: Guidance for Availability and Accessibility of Controlled Medicines.* Geneva: World Health Organization; 2011. Available from https://apps.who.int/iris/handle/10665/44519
72. National Cancer Institute. *Palliative Care in Cancer.* [Internet]. 2022. Available from https://www.cancer.gov/about-cancer/advanced-cancer/care-choices/palliative-care-fact-sheet

SECTION

2

Mechanisms Linking Exercise and Cancer Outcomes

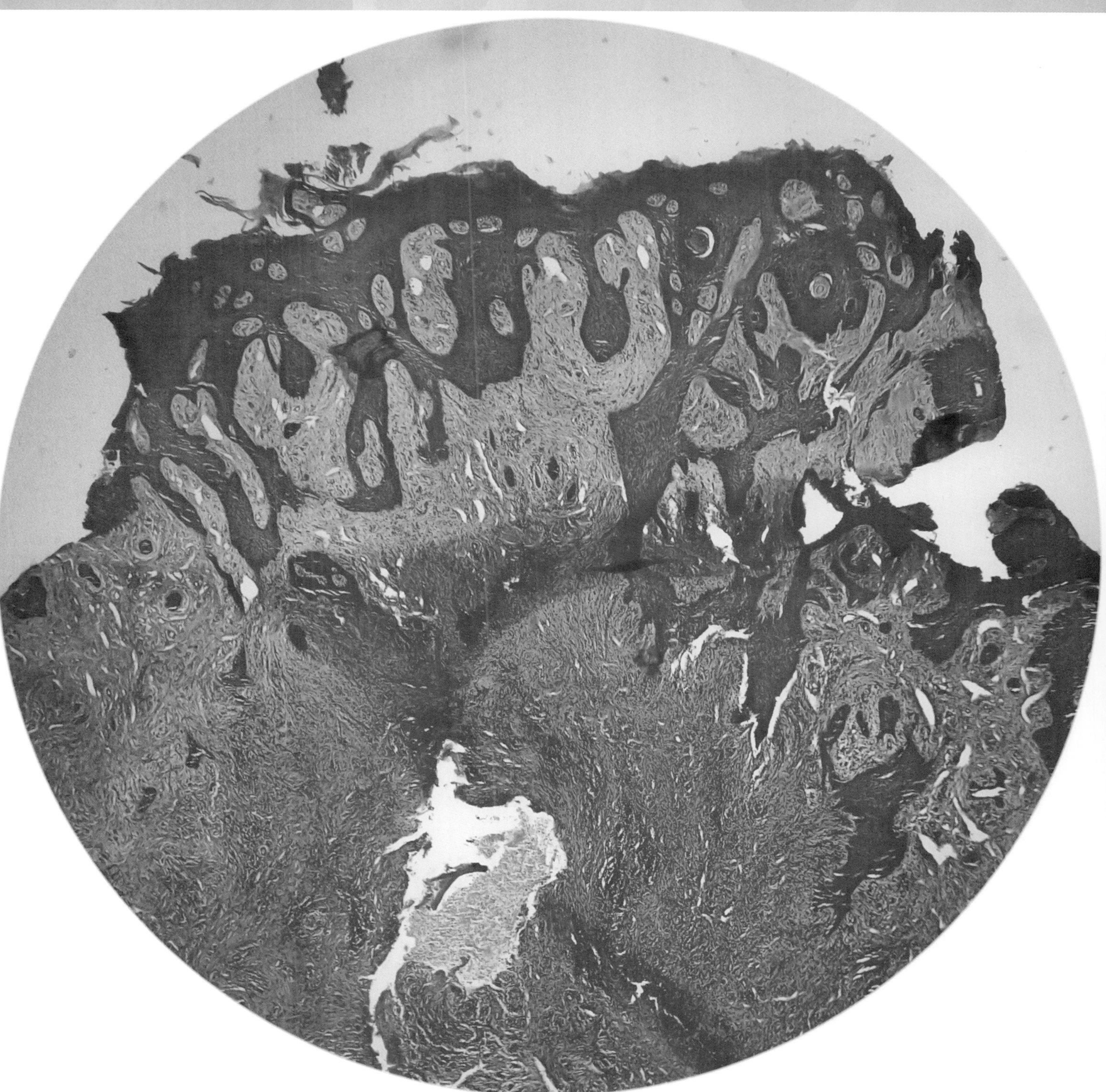

CHAPTER

6

Mechanisms Linking Exercise and Obesity to Cancer Outcomes: An Overview

OUTLINE

1. Introduction
2. Epidemiology of Exercise, Obesity, and Cancer
   a. Exercise, Obesity, and Cancer Incidence
   b. Exercise, Obesity, and Cancer Recurrence
   c. Exercise, Obesity, and Cancer Mortality
3. Mechanisms for the Link Between Exercise, Obesity, and Cancer
   a. Insulin
   b. Cellular Growth Factors (IGF and Binding Proteins)
   c. Estrogens and Androgens
   d. Inflammation
   e. Oxidative Stress
   f. Immune Function
   g. Adipokines
   h. Synergy: All Factors Acting Together
   i. Chemotherapy Completion Rate: Relative Dose Intensity
4. Weight Loss: Bariatric Surgery Offering Clues
5. Effects of Exercise Training on Obesity and Body Composition
   a. Effects of Exercise on Weight Loss and Weight Gain Prevention
   b. Exercise Intended to Promote Fat Loss
   c. Exercise Intended to Promote Muscle Gain
6. Summary
7. Case Study
8. Meet the Expert
9. Study Questions
10. References

OBJECTIVES

After completing review of this chapter, students will be able to:

1. Distinguish the association of exercise, obesity, and cancer incidence, recurrence, and mortality.
2. Comprehend the mechanisms for the hypothesized link between exercise, obesity, and cancer.
3. Apply the effects of exercise training on obesity and body composition relevant to cancer.

INTRODUCTION

Achieving and maintaining a healthy body weight is among the most important cancer risk reduction recommendations, for 3 reasons. First, the majority of Americans are overweight or obese (1), so the majority of the population is exposed to this cancer risk factor. Second, obesity is associated with a higher incidence of 13 common types of cancer (2). Third, these 13 types of cancer account for 40% of all cancer diagnoses in the US each year. Achieving and maintaining a healthy body weight is second only to avoiding tobacco in terms of steps that can be taken to reduce cancer risk (3). Exercise is relevant to the goal of achieving and maintaining a healthy body weight, and part (but not all) of the association between exercise and cancer risk reduction is through effects on body weight and obesity (4).

Within this chapter we discuss exercise, obesity, and cancer in 4 sections: epidemiology, mechanisms, weight loss, and the role of exercise. But first, let us define some terms important to our discussion.

Overweight and *obesity* are defined as a body weight that is higher than what is considered healthy for a given height. The metric most often used to discern whether someone is overweight or obese is **body mass index (BMI)**, which is weight in kilograms divided by height in meters squared (kg/m^2). In Table 6.1, we present a chart of BMI values for specific weights

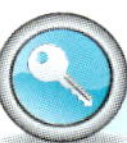

Body Mass Index (BMI). The most commonly used measure to define overweight or obesity. It is calculated as weight in kilograms divided by height in meters squared (kg/m^2). A healthy BMI is <25 kg/m^2.

Table 6.1 Adult Body Mass Index Chart[a]

BMI	19	20	21	22	23	24	25	26	27	28	29	30	31	32	33	34	35
HEIGHT	WEIGHT IN POUNDS																
4′10″	91	96	100	105	110	115	119	124	129	134	138	143	148	153	158	162	167
4′11″	94	99	104	109	114	119	124	128	133	138	143	148	153	158	163	168	173
5′	97	102	107	112	118	123	128	133	138	143	148	153	158	163	168	174	197
5′1″	100	106	111	116	122	127	132	137	143	148	153	158	164	169	174	180	185
5′2″	104	109	115	120	126	131	136	142	147	153	158	164	169	175	180	186	191
5′3″	107	113	118	124	130	135	141	146	152	158	163	169	174	180	186	191	197
5′4″	110	116	122	128	134	140	145	151	157	163	169	174	180	186	192	197	204
5′5″	114	120	126	132	138	144	150	156	162	168	174	180	186	192	198	204	210
5′6″	118	124	130	136	142	148	155	161	167	173	179	186	192	198	204	210	216
5′7″	121	127	134	140	146	153	159	166	172	178	185	191	198	204	211	217	223
5′8″	125	131	138	144	151	158	164	171	177	184	190	197	203	210	216	223	230
5′9″	128	135	142	149	155	162	169	176	182	189	196	203	209	216	223	230	236
5′10″	132	139	146	153	160	167	174	181	188	195	202	209	216	222	229	236	243
5′11″	136	143	150	157	165	172	179	186	193	200	208	215	222	229	236	243	250
6′	140	147	154	162	169	177	184	191	199	206	213	221	228	235	242	250	258
6′1″	144	151	159	166	174	182	189	197	204	212	219	227	235	242	250	257	265
6′2″	148	155	163	171	179	186	194	202	210	218	225	233	241	249	256	264	272
6′3″	152	160	168	176	184	192	200	208	216	224	232	240	248	256	264	272	279
	Healthy weight						Overweight					Obese					

[a]Search first for the current height, scan across to find the current weight, and look up to the top of the column to determine BMI. BMI categories are provided at the bottom row. This figure does not include class II (BMI 35-39.9) or class III (BMI 40 or greater) obesity.
From U.S. Department of Health and Human Services, National Institutes of Health, National Health, Lung, and Blood Institute. *The Clinical Guidelines on the Identification, Evaluation, and Treatment of Overweight and Obesity in Adults: Evidence Report.* September 1998 [NIH pub. NO. 98-4083].

and heights, starting with feet and inches for height and pounds for weight (US measurements). BMI is classified by the World Health Organization as follows: underweight (BMI > 18 kg/m^2), normal weight (BMI of 18-24.99 kg/m^2), overweight (BMI of 25-29.99 kg/m^2); class I obesity (BMI of 30-34.99 kg/m^2); class II obesity (BMI of 35-39.99 kg/m^2); and class III obesity (BMI of 40 kg/m^2 or greater).

Although BMI is exceptionally useful for public health purposes, there are aspects of body composition not well captured with a crude measure of weight over height. The majority of adults are relatively sedentary and, as a result, there is usually an increase in fat, leading to an increase in their body weight. The BMI categories assume that to be the case. But if someone starts to do progressive resistance training and increases muscle mass by 10 pounds, increasing BMI by 1 to 2 points, they are not at a greater risk for chronic diseases such as cancer. A heavily muscled, healthy athlete might well have a BMI in the unhealthy range, as depicted in Figure 6.1. This is the limitation of BMI as a measurement for tracking health.

Further, there are specific aspects of body composition that are relevant to cancer incidence, recurrence, and mortality. These include muscle mass and fat mass. These two aspects of body composition may be measured in a variety of ways in research studies, including **CT scans**, dual energy x-ray absorptiometry (DXA), D_3-creatine dilution, and bioelectrical impedance analysis. CT scans are typically obtained clinically for a section of the torso and cross-sectional slices of CT images, often at the level of the third lumbar vertebrae, and can be analyzed for the amount and quality of both muscle and fat, including the fat close to the center of the belly (called visceral fat). **DXA scans** use an x-ray technique to look at the density of the body to estimate the amount of lean muscle and fat tissue. One measure of particular interest from DXA scans is appendicular skeletal muscle mass. This refers to a measure of body muscle content in the 4 limbs. **D_3-creatine dilution** is a measure of muscle mass. It works by providing a direct measurement of creatine pool size. The participant swallows a pill with 30 mg of an oral tracer dose of D_3-creatine. They fast (water allowed, no caloric intake) prior to collecting urine after a specific number of days. A constant fraction of creatine is converted to creatinine (a waste product that forms when creatine breaks down), which is rapidly excreted in urine. The urine is tested for the amount of creatinine. The creatine pool size, and thus muscle mass, is determined from urine D_3-creatine enrichments in special laboratory tests (2). Finally, **bioelectrical impedance analysis** is a noninvasive test that involves the placement of 2 electrodes on the right hand and the foot. A low-level electrical current is sent through the body to detect the amount of water in the body. Tissues with higher water content (blood and muscle tissues) have high electrical conductivity. Tissues

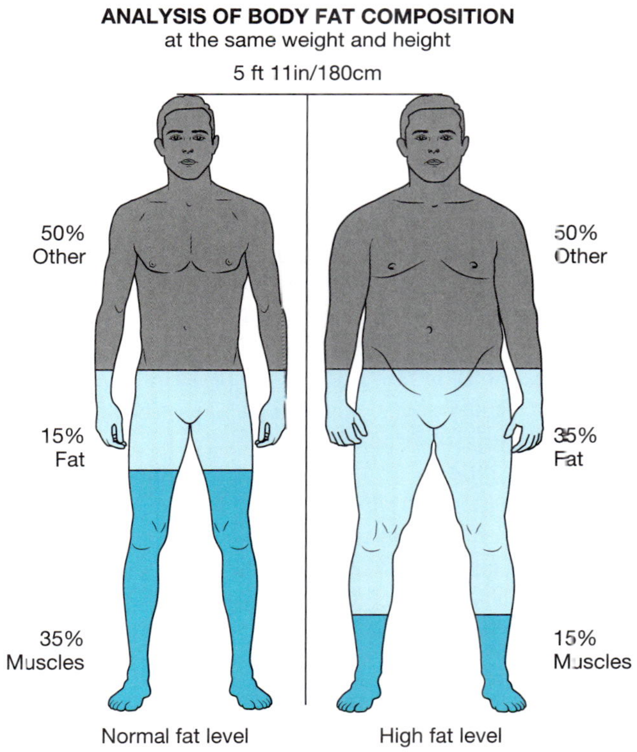

ANALYSIS OF BODY FAT COMPOSITION
at the same weight and height
5 ft 11in/180cm
50% Other
15% Fat
35% Muscles
Normal fat level
50% Other
35% Fat
15% Muscles
High fat level

FIGURE 6.1. Body mass index (BMI) versus body composition. BMI is a crude measure of weight for height but does not account for differences in body composition. This can result in inaccurately labeling a well-muscled athlete as "obese."

Computed tomography (CT) scan. Takes a series of x-ray images from different angles around the body and uses computer processing to create cross-sectional images (slices) of the bones, blood vessels, and soft tissues in the body. CT scans can be analyzed with the help of a computer to discern the amount of muscle and fat in a given slice. This is commonly done at the level of the abdomen when scientists or clinicians are interested in body composition measurements.

Dual energy x-ray absorptiometry (DXA) scan. This test uses very low levels of radiation to measure body tissues, including bone, fat, and lean tissues. The test can be used to discern bone density, body composition, visceral fat, and appendicular skeletal muscle mass.

D_3-creatine dilution. Measurement of total body creatine pool size provides and the assessment of muscle mass, given that 98% of creatine in the body is found in muscle cells. To complete this assessment, the participant swallows a dose of radiolabeled creatine (D_3Cr). Approximately 3 days later, a urine sample is provided. The amount of D_3-creatinine in the urine is used to determine the total body creatine pool size and, in turn, the total body muscle mass.

Bioelectrical impedance analysis. Measures body composition based on the rate at which an electrical current travels through the body, given the observation that electricity is conducted at a different rate through water than fat.

Table 6.2 Commonly Used Body Composition Methods

METHOD	BASIS	ASSUMPTIONS	BODY COMPOSITION MEASURED
Computed tomography of torso	Clear anatomic boundaries can be visualized between subcutaneous and visceral adipose tissue, skeletal muscle, visceral organs, and skeleton	The results seen in the slice reviewed reflect the whole body	Visceral fat, subcutaneous fat, skeletal muscle, amounts and density
Dual energy x-ray absorptiometry scan	Absorption of 2 different energy x-rays	X-ray absorption is directly related to bone, fat, and lean mass	Direct measure of bone density, fat, and lean mass overall (not a direct measure of muscle mass)
D_3-creatine dilution	Enrichment of D_3-creatinine in single urine sample	Urine D_3-creatinine represents muscle D_3-creatine enrichment; creatine pool size is a measurement of muscle mass	Total body creatine pool size, skeletal muscle mass
Bioelectrical impedance analysis	Electrical conductivity of tissues with more versus less water content	Hydration is the same between people and within person over time	Body fat % and (by subtraction) lean mass

with lower water content (fat and bone tissues) have lower electrical conductivity. Bioelectrical impedance analysis determines resistance to the flow of the electrical current as it passes through the body to determine body fat. It is highly responsive to hydration levels, and as such not considered to be as useful in research settings. Table 6.2 reviews methods, basis, assumptions, and elements of body composition measured for each of the reviewed methods.

EPIDEMIOLOGY OF EXERCISE, OBESITY, AND CANCER

Exercise, Obesity, and Cancer Incidence

Exercise has been shown to be associated with the prevention of 7 to 8 types of cancer, including breast, colon, endometrial, kidney, bladder, esophageal, and stomach (5). The magnitude of risk reduction is between 10% and 20%, depending on the cancer site. A consortium of researchers, led by Dr. Steven Moore, pooled results from many cohort studies across North America and Europe to examine the effects of exercise on cancer prevention. In their analysis, they showed the effects of regular physical activity before and after accounting for the effects on obesity. The only cancer for which there was no longer any effect of physical activity after accounting for obesity was endometrial cancer (6). This means that there are likely independent effects of physical activity on cancer incidence risk, beyond the effects on obesity (excepting for endometrial cancer). That said, the mechanisms through which obesity and physical activity influence cancer risk are similar, as will be reviewed in this chapter.

As noted in the section "Introduction," obesity is associated with increased risk for 13 types of cancer: breast, colorectal, endometrial, esophageal, gallbladder, kidney, liver, oral, ovarian, pancreatic, prostate, certain types of brain cancers, and stomach cancers. The scientific research that has detected these associations is largely observational. Cohort studies that gather data from a large group of people and follow them for the long term are crucial to our understanding of long-term health consequences of lifestyle factors, including obesity. Two such studies are the Nurses' Health Study and the Health Professionals Follow-Up Study, both of which are conducted at Harvard University. In an analysis of data from these 2 cohorts that assessed the trajectory of body shape (eg, BMI) from age 5 to 60, including 73,581 women and 32,632 men, researchers observed relationships between a more consistent obese body shape since early age and a higher risk of colorectal, esophagus, pancreas, kidney, endometrial, and breast cancers (7). These findings support the need to avoid obesity early in life, as early exposure is associated with risk for many types of cancer.

There is little to no research on the potential role of body composition and risk of cancer incidence. This may be because the measurements needed to accurately assess muscle mass and fat mass are relatively expensive, and the size of the studies needed to detect effects is quite large (see the sample size from the cohort studies in the previous paragraph).

Exercise, Obesity, and Cancer Recurrence

There are scant data on the topic of exercise training and cancer recurrence. In a recent meta-analysis (8), there were 3 RCTs that could be included in an analysis of this topic. All of the studies were performed with breast cancer survivors. The analysis suggests that there is a substantive (48%) reduction of recurrence risk for breast cancer survivors who are physically active as compared with the control groups in these studies. However, there are methodologic concerns and the number of studies is small. More research is needed on this topic to draw firm conclusions (8).

Although obesity is an established risk factor for the incidence of several cancers, the impact of obesity on cancer survival is not well understood. It is unknown whether the greatest risk associated with obesity occurs before diagnosis (reflecting the role of obesity as a risk factor for incident disease) or weight gain or loss during or after treatment has a greater influence on prognosis. Clearly, each could be relevant. Understanding the difference is important to developing appropriate interventions to reduce the burden of cancer (9).

There has been far less research on the role of obesity on cancer recurrence than cancer incidence. In one cohort study of patients with prostate cancer, postdiagnosis weight gain was associated with a 2-fold increased risk of prostate cancer recurrence (10). In a group of 4,381 patients with colon cancer participating in adjuvant therapy trials, patients who were obese postdiagnosis had a higher risk of death than those who were not obese (11). More specifically, men with a BMI of 35 or higher had a 35% increased risk of death than men of normal weight. Among women, those with a BMI over 30 had a 24% increased risk of death as compared with women of normal weight. Obesity is also associated with poorer **disease-free survival** in breast cancer patients (12).

As with risk for cancer incidence, there is little to no published data on the topic of whether specific aspects of body composition (muscle or fat mass) influence cancer recurrence.

Exercise, Obesity, and Cancer Mortality

Epidemiological evidence suggests that there are 3 cancers for which exercise may reduce risk of cancer-specific and all-cause mortality: breast, prostate, and colon (5). The magnitude of the effects is between 30% and 50%, making exercise a potent risk reduction strategy for cancer mortality for these cancer sites.

In 2003, Dr. Eugenie Calle published a landmark paper (2) on the relationship between obesity and cancer mortality based on data from a very large cohort study conducted by the ACS. Figures from that paper are presented in Figure 6.2. The risk of death from cancer was compared between those with an elevated BMI (of 30, 35, or 40, shown in the left-most column of the figure) with those with a BMI of less than 25. The numbers in the graph depict the percentage increase in cancer mortality for the obese compared with the nonobese cohort members. For example, for prostate cancer, the value 1.34 in the figure for men refers to a 34% increased risk of cancer mortality among men with a BMI of 35 or greater as compared with men with a BMI less than 25. Notably, the elevated risk of cancer mortality from obesity varied by cancer type, from a 34% increase in prostate cancer to a 452% increase in liver cancer mortality in men who are obese. For women, the lowest increased risk for cancer mortality with obesity was multiple myeloma with a 44% increase, and the highest was for uterine (endometrial) cancer (625% increased risk of mortality among women who are obese as compared with women who are not obese). The paper by Dr. Calle, published in the prestigious *New England Journal of Medicine*, has had a strong influence on research about obesity and cancer outcomes. At the time of publication, there were few studies on the mechanisms through which these relationships might occur. As will be seen in the following section, research on mechanisms explaining the obesity cancer link has since flourished.

There is a paradox regarding obesity and cancer outcomes that deserves attention. It is observed that obesity is associated with cancer incidence in a linear manner. On the contrary, overweight and class I obesity (BMI 25-35) in survivors is commonly associated with improved survival as compared with patients who are not obese. The excess risk of cancer mortality associated with obesity is noted only in the most obese (class III, BMI over 35). The explanation for this is likely to be about body composition. As noted above, BMI is a poor proxy for adiposity and does not distinguish muscle from fat, nor does it describe the distribution of fat (visceral vs subcutaneous). Low muscle mass is associated with a higher risk of recurrence, overall, and cancer-specific mortality (as well as treatment toxicities) (13). Patients who are overweight carry more muscle mass; therefore, perhaps a small amount of obesity, accompanied by added muscle mass, is protective in the setting of cancer mortality risk. This hypothesis is an active area of research.

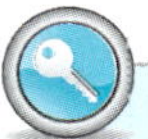

Disease-free survival. Length of time after primary treatment for a cancer ends that a patient survives without any signs or symptoms of that cancer.

MECHANISMS FOR THE LINK BETWEEN EXERCISE, OBESITY, AND CANCER

The mechanisms to explain the associations of exercise and obesity with the risks of cancer incidence, recurrence, or mortality need to be associated with 1. exercise or 2. obesity or body composition and cancer incidence, recurrence, or mortality. Ideally, randomized trials in humans would be conducted to show that exercise interventions alone (regardless of obesity or body composition changes), or interventions leading to changes in obesity or body composition, result in changes in the mechanism and cancer incidence. However, the follow-up would need to be a decade or longer to observe

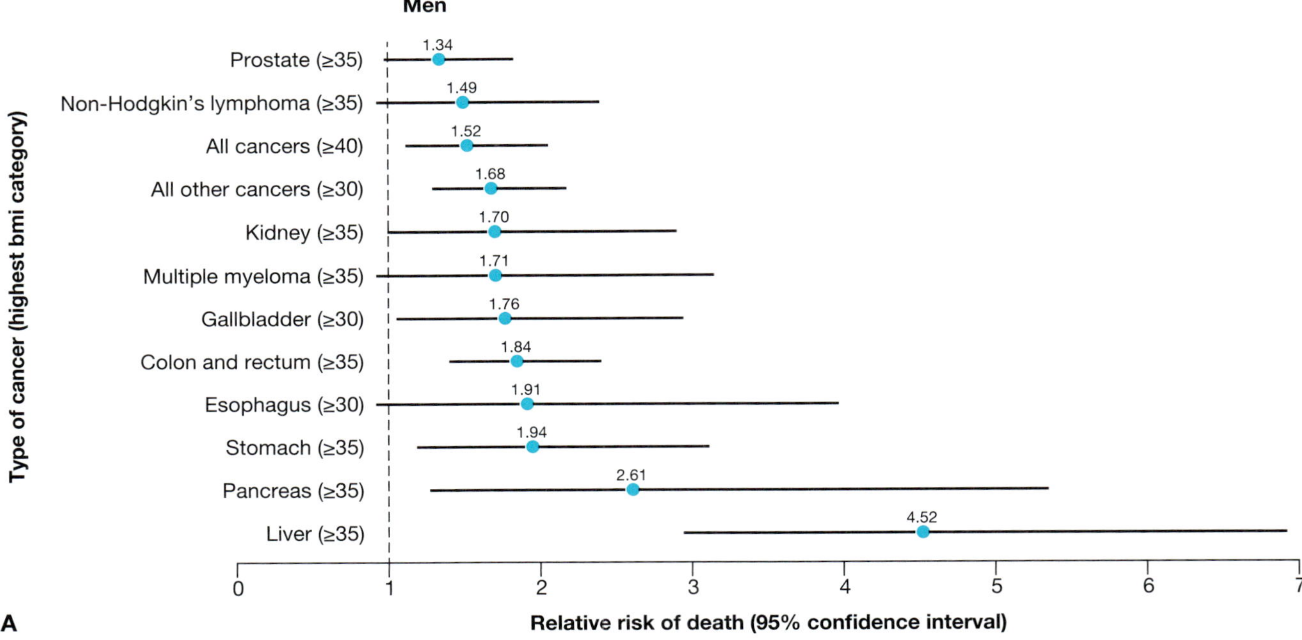

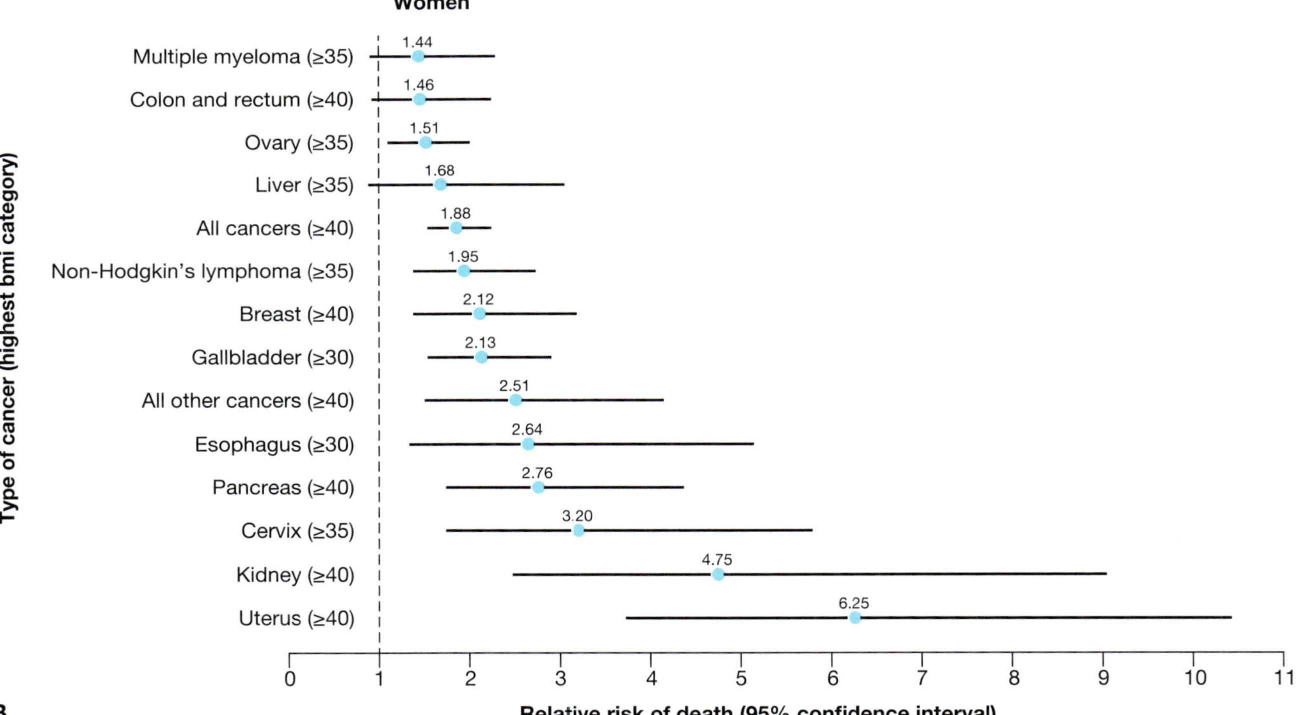

FIGURE 6.2. Relative risks of death from various types of cancer according to BMI for US men (A) and US women (B). The relative risks are the numbers above each line and can be interpreted as a percent increase in risk over normal-weight individuals. For example, women with a BMI ≥ 40 have a 625% increase in risk of death from uterine cancer as compared with women with a BMI of 18-24.99. By contrast, women with a BMI ≥ 35 have a 44% increased risk of death from multiple myeloma as compared to women with a BMI of 18-24.99. (Redrawn from figures 1 and 2 in Calle EE, Rodriguez C, Walker-Thurmond K, Thun MJ. Overweight, obesity, and mortality from cancer in a prospectively studied cohort of U.S. adults. *N Engl J Med.* 2003;348(17):1625–38. doi:10.1056/NEJMoa021423.)

effects on cancer incidence. Therefore, it is challenging to directly observe effects of exercise on obesity on cancer incidence. Instead, we rely on observational evidence from large epidemiological studies to assist in making connections between exercise, obesity, mechanisms, and cancer outcomes. In the sections that follow, we present both the mechanistic and epidemiological evidence associated with the mechanism.

Insulin

Regular physical activity is associated with a reduced likelihood of hyperinsulinemia and normalization of blood glucose. Regular physical activity also reduces the incidence of type II diabetes. Although this effect is observed across all BMI categories (normal weight, overweight, and obese), there is a mechanistic overlap of the roles of obesity and physical activity with regard to insulin-related outcomes (14). In addition to physical inactivity, obesity leads to hyperinsulinemia and **insulin** resistance, and eventually type II diabetes (which is also associated with cancer incidence) (15). How does this happen?

When you take in more calories than you use (or exercise less than you eat), the excess energy is stored as fat. While fat tissue can be burned for energy, it also releases fatty acids, hormones, and pro-inflammatory cytokines (inflammation causing small signaling molecules). The release of pro-inflammatory cytokines can lead to chronic low-grade inflammation, lasting weeks, months, or even years. Chronic low-grade inflammation blocks normal insulin signaling pathways, making it more difficult for insulin to do its primary job of getting glucose into cells. This leads to increased glucose in the blood and an increase in insulin production from the liver to make up for the blocked pathways (leading to hyperinsulinemia). But eventually, resistance to insulin reaches a point where no amount of extra insulin can help in getting the excess glucose into the cells.

Lean mass also plays a role in insulin. Increased lean mass increases skeletal muscle glucose uptake and improves insulin sensitivity (16). This can occur even in participants with obesity.

The excess glucose and insulin resistance caused by obesity lead to type II diabetes. The epidemiological observational studies relevant to this section focus on the association of type II diabetes with cancer incidence and mortality. Type II diabetes is diagnosed when blood glucose is elevated (126 mg/dL or higher) and/or hemoglobin A1C (a measure of average blood glucose levels over the past 3 months) is 6.5% or higher. It is notable that in large epidemiological studies, insulin resistance (type II diabetes) is observed to be associated with many of the same cancers associated with inactivity and obesity, including esophageal, colorectal, pancreatic, liver, kidney, breast, endometrial, and bladder (17).

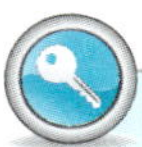

Insulin. A hormone produced by the pancreas that regulates the amount of glucose in the blood.

Cellular Growth Factors (IGF and Binding Proteins)

Insulin-like growth factor (IGF) is a polypeptide hormone structurally similar to insulin that binds to a tyrosine kinase receptor (IGF1-R) in order to function as a major mediator of growth-hormone-stimulated somatic growth, as well as a mediator of growth-hormone-independent growth responses in many cells. IGFs directly regulate protein, carbohydrate, and fat metabolism. The IGFs and their binding proteins play a central role in growth, metabolism, and reproduction. There are 2 types of IGFs (IGF-1 and IGF-2), but the one most relevant for cancer is IGF-1. There are several binding proteins for IGF-1 that mediate its action. Obesity results in altered IGF-1 responsiveness to growth hormone and suppressed binding protein levels, resulting in greater IGF-1 activity than the nonobese state (18).

The effects of changing muscle mass on IGF-1 activity vary by study. In general, it would be expected that circulating IGF-1 would be positively associated with muscle mass, but results from research on this topic are inconsistent. Further, the effects of higher IGF-1 in patients with more muscle might differ from the effects of elevated IGF-1 in patients with more fat mass, particularly with regard to the development of cancer. Exercise training studies are not consistently observed to alter IGF-1 or its binding proteins (19).

The binding of IGF-1 to IGF-1R initiates a cascade of downstream signal transduction pathways known to be involved in cell growth, proliferation, and cancer, including RAS/RAF and P13K/Akt/MTOR (see Chapter 2 for more on these pathways). Not surprisingly then, IGF-1 has been found to be associated with increased risk of developing a number of common cancers, including lung, breast, colorectal, and prostate. It is hypothesized that IGF-1 has a particular role in the progression of cancer cells to clinical cancer diagnoses, by increasing the activity in cancer cells, leading to increased cell proliferation, and blocking apoptosis, as shown in Figure 6.3 (20).

Estrogens and Androgens

Estrogens

Estrogens are involved in a broad spectrum of physiologic functions, from the regulation of the menstrual cycle and

Insulin-like growth factor (IGF). A protein made by the body that stimulates the growth of many types of cells.
Estrogens. A group of steroid hormones that promote the development and maintenance of female characteristics in the body.

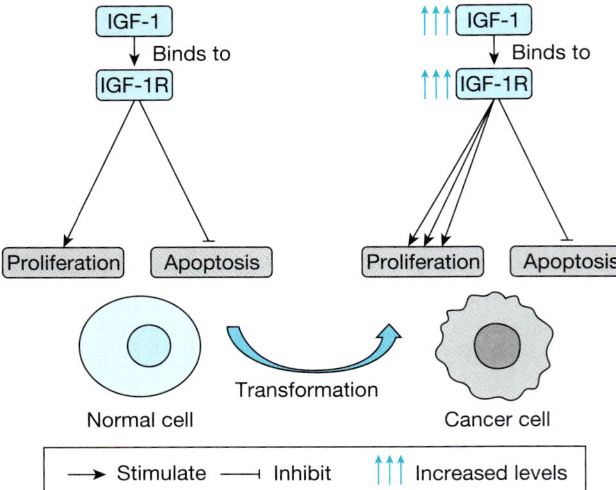

FIGURE 6.3. Effects of insulin-like growth factor 1 on cell proliferation and apoptosis in the setting of normal and cancer cells. (Redrawn from Shanmugalingam T, Bosco C, Ridley AJ, Van Hemelrijck M. Is there a role for IGF-1 in the development of second primary cancers? *Cancer Med.* 2016;5(11):3353–67, Figure 1. https://doi.org/10.1002%2Fcam4.871; https://onlinelibrary.wiley.com/doi/abs/10.1002/cam4.871.)

reproduction to the modulation of bone density, brain function, and cholesterol mobilization. The effects of exercise alone on estrogens are small when compared with interventions that combine exercise with caloric restriction (21). In a meta-analysis of 6 RCTs with 1,588 postmenopausal women, combined interventions that included both caloric restriction and exercise resulted in reduced total estradiol by 18%.

The role of obesity in estrogens depends on menopausal status. Among women who are premenopausal, obesity generally reduces estrogen levels. But after menopause, higher body weight is associated with elevated estrogen levels (22). This is depicted in Figure 6.4 from the Penn Ovarian Aging Study that included 436 women from premenopausal status to postmenopausal status and measured hormones and BMI over 12 years of follow-up. As shown, the women with a BMI of 30 or greater had the lowest estrogen (estradiol) levels in the premenopausal stages of follow-up, but the highest levels at the point of having reached postmenopause. In the very same study, an analysis of women who were at the latter part of the menopausal transition demonstrated that estrogen levels were lower in those who were more active. This was not observed in any other age group (23).

As to muscle mass, the relationship is somewhat in reverse. There is evidence that higher estrogen levels are beneficial to the intrinsic quality of skeletal muscle, if not muscle size (24). It is unclear whether this has relevance to cancer risk.

The cancers associated with higher levels of estrogen include breast, ovarian, endometrial, prostate, lung, and colon (25). More specifically, for postmenopausal women, elevated estrogens are associated with increased cancer risk. The primary source of estrogens in postmenopausal women is adipose tissue. Further, extended exposure to exogenous estrogens (eg, hormone replacement therapy) is also associated with elevated breast cancer risk, likely because of the

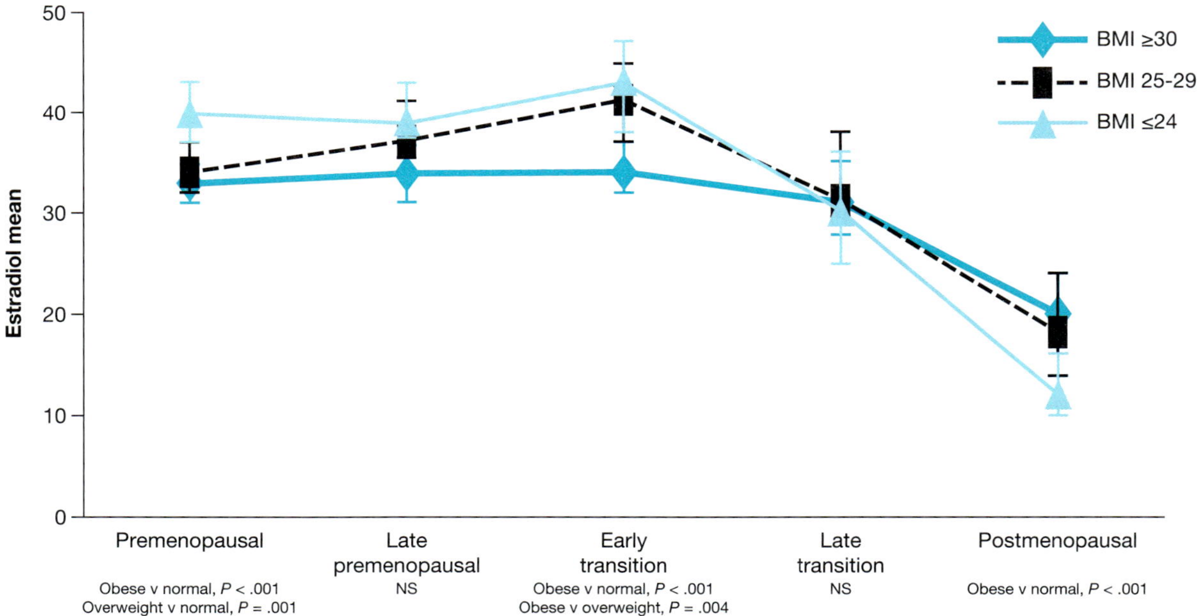

FIGURE 6.4. Relationship between BMI and estradiol levels throughout the menopausal transition. At premenopause, higher BMI is associated with lower estradiol levels. By postmenopause, this is reversed: higher BMI is associated with higher estradiol levels. (Redrawn from Schmitz KH, Lin H, Sammel MD, et al. Association of physical activity with reproductive hormones: the Penn Ovarian Aging Study. *Cancer Epidemiol Biomarkers Prev.* 2007;16(10): 2042–7.)

marked proliferative effect on breast epithelial tissue (26). Most of what we know about the role of estrogen and cancer risk comes from studies of breast and endometrial cancer. For example, in an analysis of 9 prospective cohort studies, the risk for breast cancer increased with increased circulating concentrations of estrogens. There was a 2-fold risk of breast cancer, when comparing women with the lowest to the highest quintile of estrogens (27). This is one of few mechanisms for which there are clinical trial data. Clinical trials document that reducing estrogen exposure through drug therapies (tamoxifen or aromatase inhibitors) reduces the incidence of breast cancer among women at elevated risk (25).

Androgens

Testosterone is the most common **androgens** in the body and occurs in both men and women. Similar to estrogens, exercise interventions alone, in the absence of caloric restriction, do not have a meaningful impact on testosterone in postmenopausal women (21). In the same meta-analysis mentioned in the estrogen section above, interventions that combine caloric restriction with exercise reduced free testosterone by 14% (22). Among insufficiently active men, exercise has no effect on resting testosterone levels.

Among men, obesity is associated with a reduction of testosterone (28). Whether this alters risk for prostate cancer is unclear (29). However, obesity is associated with increased risk for prostate cancer through other mechanisms discussed in this chapter (eg, insulin, growth factors, and inflammation) (30).

Among women, obesity is consistently associated with elevated androgens (31). This is problematic because androgens (principally testosterone) are also associated with elevated risk for breast and endometrial cancers among women (31). The primary hypothesized mechanism through which excess androgen contributes to breast and endometrial cancer risk is through conversion of testosterone to estradiol (through aromatization), leading to a marked proliferation of epithelial tissues. That said, testosterone itself has antiproliferative effects on the breast and, when given in combination with an aromatase inhibitor (to prevent conversion to estradiol), prevents breast cancer from occurring.

Inflammation

Physical inactivity is associated with a state of excess **inflammation** in the body, at least in part due to excess adipose tissue (32). There is evidence of an independent effect of physical inactivity on inflammation beyond obesity (33), but both are so inextricably linked that it makes sense to talk about them together.

Both physical inactivity and obesity are states of taking in more calories than are used and, as a result, having an increase in fat tissue (adipose tissue). The excess of fat in the adipose tissue results in an increased secretion of pro-inflammatory cytokines, as discussed in the earlier section about insulin. In particular, 1 study showed that in obese subjects, inflammatory

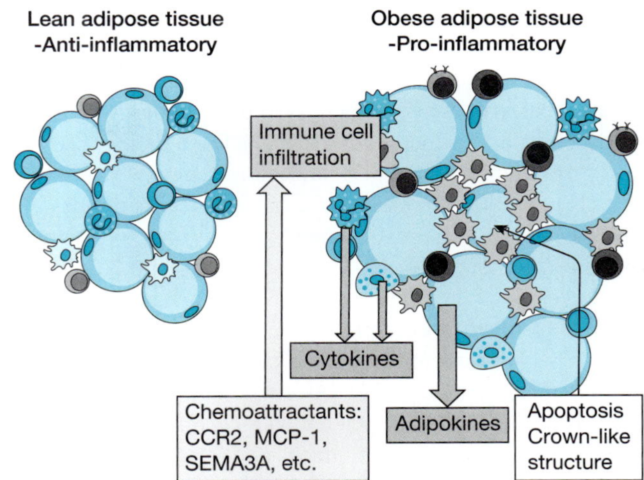

FIGURE 6.5. Lean versus obese adipose tissue. Differences in immune cells inflammation, apoptosis, and crown-like structures. (Modified and redrawn from Kawai T, Autieri MV, Scalia R. Adipose tissue inflammation and metabolic dysfunction in obesity. *Am J Physiol Cell Physiol.* 2021;320(3):C375–91, Figure 1.)

changes and enhanced secretion of pro-inflammatory cytokines were able to induce insulin resistance by inactivating the insulin receptor (34). Low-grade chronic inflammation is consistently associated with excess body fat and characterized by more activity from immune cells that produce additional pro-inflammatory cytokines. The mechanisms by which insulin and inflammation explain the obesity and cancer link are highly connected. A hallmark of the inflammatory process in adipose tissue is the presence of crown-like structures, which are microscopic examples of dying adipose cells surrounded by immune cells called **macrophages**. In Figure 6.5, we depict a cartoon of anti-inflammatory lean adipose tissue as compared with pro-inflammatory obese adipose tissue.

As with other mechanisms, there is an inverse association between muscle and inflammation. Whether it is relevant to cancer is unclear. Increased muscle activity is related to the release of anti-inflammatory cytokines, including IL-6, which

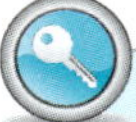

Androgens. A group of steroid hormones typically associated with the development and maintenance of male characteristics in the body. Androgens are hormones that contribute to growth and reproduction in both men and women.

Inflammation. At a local level, inflammation is a physical condition in which part of the body becomes reddened, swollen, hot, and often painful, especially as a reaction to injury or infection. Chronic inflammation is distinct from this phenomenon and is defined as a slow, long-term inability to clear the elevated signs of inflammation. There is a strong relationship between chronic inflammation and immune system function.

Macrophage. Type of white blood cell that surrounds and kills microorganisms, removes dead cells, and stimulates the action of other immune system cells.

may act to temper the pro-inflammatory cytokine activity arising from adipose cells. In addition, low-grade inflammation has been observed to reduce muscle mass, strength, and physical performance, particularly in older patients (35).

Chronic inflammation can damage DNA or alter the way cells grow and divide, which can lead to cancer. The concept that chronic inflammation could cause cancer is not new. In 1865, a German scientist named Rudolf Virchow proposed that the origin of cancer was chronic inflammation (36). This was based on the observation that the application of some irritants resulted in inflammation and greater cell proliferation. What we now understand is that inflammation is part of a larger story, including DNA changes, growth factors, and the TME. The cancers associated with chronic inflammation include colorectal, liver, stomach, and breast cancers (36). It could be hypothesized that chronic inflammation has the potential to contribute to all types of cancer, given effects on DNA and cell proliferation.

Oxidative Stress

The body seeks a balance between the normal production of highly reactive molecules called ROS or "free radicals" and antioxidants in the body. The term "oxidative stress" refers to the condition of excess free radicals as compared to antioxidants in the body. This can occur in several ways, including through environmental stressors, cigarette smoking, alcohol consumption, inactivity, or obesity. Muscle activity has a net zero effect on oxidative stress, because muscle increases both free radicals and antioxidants. The effects of **oxidative stress** on the body include damage to cell membranes, modifications that could altered the activity of proteins, and DNA damage. There may also be epigenetic changes because of oxidative stress. If not controlled, oxidative stress can be responsible for the development of multiple disease states, including cancer. Adipose tissue has properties that contribute to endocrine functions in the body, secreting hormones and cytokines. In certain pathological conditions, including obesity, adipose tissue contributes to the production of free radicals. The process by which this occurs is strongly related to the pro-inflammatory processes described earlier. In a vicious cycle in the setting of obesity, immune cells generate free radicals, and the free radicals promote inflammation (37).

Oxidative stress, like inflammation, is likely associated with the development of all cancer types. A key activity of ROS is to damage DNA, a hallmark activity for cancer initiation, promotion, and progression. In addition, free radicals play a key role in growth factor receptor signaling, another pathway through which oxidative stress contributes to carcinogenesis.

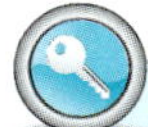

Oxidative stress. An imbalance of the production of reactive oxygen species (free radicals) and antioxidants in the body intended to clear the body of free radicals.

Immune Function

Exercise has well documented positive effects on immune function. The relationship is described as having an upside-down J shape, in that the benefits to immune function continue to accrue until a threshold of exercise volume is reached, above which immunity is inversely effected.

One of the ways that physical inactivity and obesity effects the immune system is through chronic inflammation. The state of chronic inflammation leads to a series of steps culminating in the infiltration of immune cells called macrophages in the adipose tissue, leading to the crown-like structures described in the section on inflammation. Macrophages encircle the adipose tissue cells after the inflammatory stresses lead to cell death. This is important in the setting of cancer because these crown-like structures have been found in half of the patients with breast cancer, and their presence is associated with excess adiposity. The inflammation associated with obesity also decreases the level of regulatory T-cells (a type of immune cell). There have also been observations of increased proportions of multiple types of immune cells in inflamed adipose tissue. In addition, obesity-related changes in the function of adipose cells result in the alteration and production of immune cells in the bone marrow. Finally, obesity is linked to the reduction of the diversity of T-cell receptors, altering the capacity of T-cells to function normally (38).

There is a potential mechanism for muscle mass to play a role in immune system activity relevant to cancer. Muscle activity leads to the increased production of glutamine that is fuel for the immune system. This, in turn, could contribute to the body's natural defense systems against cancer. Little research has explored whether muscle mass alters the immune system function in a manner relevant to cancer. This is an area of active scientific enquiry.

It is likely that the effects of obesity on the immune system affect the development of many cancers. One recent study can be used to illustrate the mechanisms by which this may occur. Mice were given a high fat diet, which impaired immune cell function in the TME (altering a particular type of immune cell: $CD8^{+}$ T cells), which accelerated tumor cell growth. This was tested using mouse models of colorectal, breast, melanoma, and lung cancers (39). The effect of a high fat diet of impairing immune cell function and accelerating cell growth was the same in all cancer types.

Adipokines

Adipokines are factors produced by adipose tissue that influence metabolic homeostasis, the feeling of fullness (called satiety), and

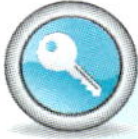

Adipokines. Molecules made by fat cells in the body. They circulate in the blood and help control many important functions such as appetite, fat storage, glucose and fat metabolism, blood pressure, inflammation, and immune response.

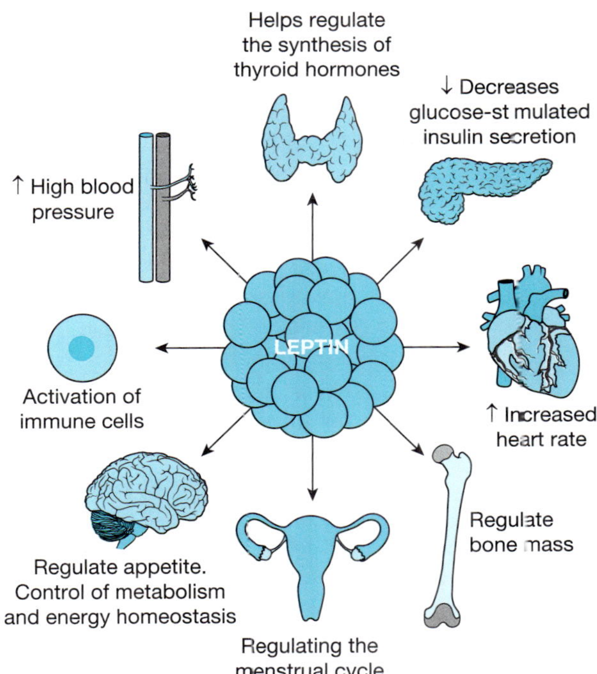

FIGURE 6.6. Leptin is a hormone made by adipose cells that helps regulate appetite, control of metabolism, energy homeostasis, activation of immune cells, and other functions. (From iStock, Getty Images, credit ttsz.)

reproduction, among other roles. The most commonly studied adipokines that play a role in cancer are leptin and adiponectin. Leptin decreases appetite by telling the brain that the fat cells are full. Some people can become leptin resistant, meaning that the signal to tell the brain that the fat cells are full does not work. Leptin plays an important role at the intersection of metabolism and inflammation because leptin production by fat cells leads to the secretion of pro-inflammatory cytokines. Other roles of leptin include the regulation of blood pressure, thyroid function, insulin secretion, heart rate regulation, regulation of bone mass, and regulation of the menstrual cycle, as shown in Figure 6.6. Adiponectin has multiple physiologic effects, including the reduction of inflammation and enhancing the response of cells to insulin (40). The anti-inflammatory properties of adiponectin may help explain observations that it is beneficial for both insulin resistance and cancer risk. Figure 6.7 shows the activities of adiponectin, including the activities suppressed (shown in white) and the activities promoted (shown in blue).

According to a recent meta-analysis that focuses on overweight and obese persons, exercise training decreases leptin and increases adiponectin (41). In another review of studies in breast cancer survivors, exercise reduced leptin but did not alter adiponectin (42). It is unclear why results differed.

Metabolism within muscle cells is regulated, in part, by leptin and adiponectin. The role of adiponectin signaling in skeletal muscle also includes several aspects of skeletal muscle function and maintenance critical to muscle health. If there is a role of muscle in regulating adipokines that is relevant to cancer risk, it has not been studied yet.

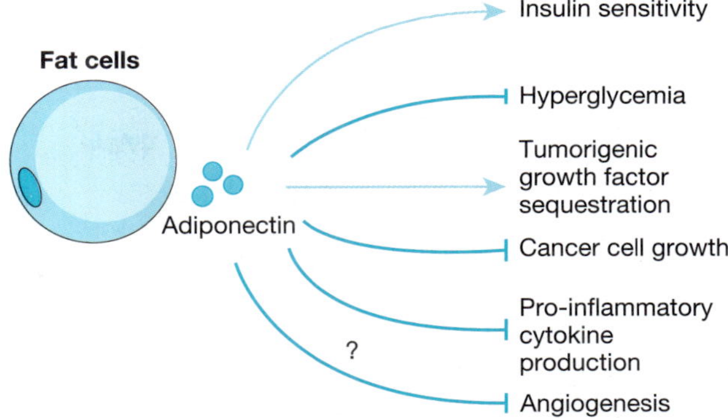

FIGURE 6.7. Physiologic effects of the release of adiponectin. The dark blue lines depict things stopped by adiponectin, and the light blue lines depict things promoted by adiponectin release from adipose cells. (Redrawn from Saxena NK, Sharma D. Metastasis suppression by adiponectin. *Cell Adh Migr.* 2010;4(3):358–62. doi:10.4161/cam.4.3.11541.)

Evidence that adipokines are associated with cancer risk arises from the epidemiologic literature (43-46). Higher circulating adiponectin has been associated with *lower* risk for colorectal cancer, postmenopausal breast cancer, kidney cancer, and liver cancer. Higher circulating levels of leptin have been found to be associated with *higher* risk of colorectal cancer. Studies of the association of leptin levels with risk for breast, endometrial, and pancreatic cancers were inconclusive. There are other types of evidence that leptin plays a role in the development of cancer, including the finding that leptin receptors are found in preserved human colon and breast cells (47).

Synergy: All Factors Acting Together

As we have seen, increases in adipose tissue lead to a cascade of physiologic changes that all contribute to the development of cancer. Further, the role of muscle mass in cancer risk is much less studied. Herein we discuss the synergy of the mechanisms by which exercise and obesity contribute to the development of cancer. Figure 6.8 provides a unifying overview of all the mechanisms reviewed in this chapter (47). Starting from the top dark blue oval: inactivity leads to increased adipose tissue, increased amounts of leptin, and decreased adiponectin, and contributes to increases in sex-steroid hormones, including estrogens. These activities contribute directly and indirectly to changes in cells that may be primed to become cancer cells or that are already cancer cells (in light blue), contributing to reduced apoptosis, increased cell proliferation, and increased angiogenesis. The intermediate factors along the way between the dark and light blue ovals are insulin resistance, insulin, IGF and its binding proteins, and inflammation and oxidative stress. As shown in Figure 6.8, these mechanisms explain the observed increased risk for colorectal, pancreatic, prostate, postmenopausal breast, and endometrial cancer.

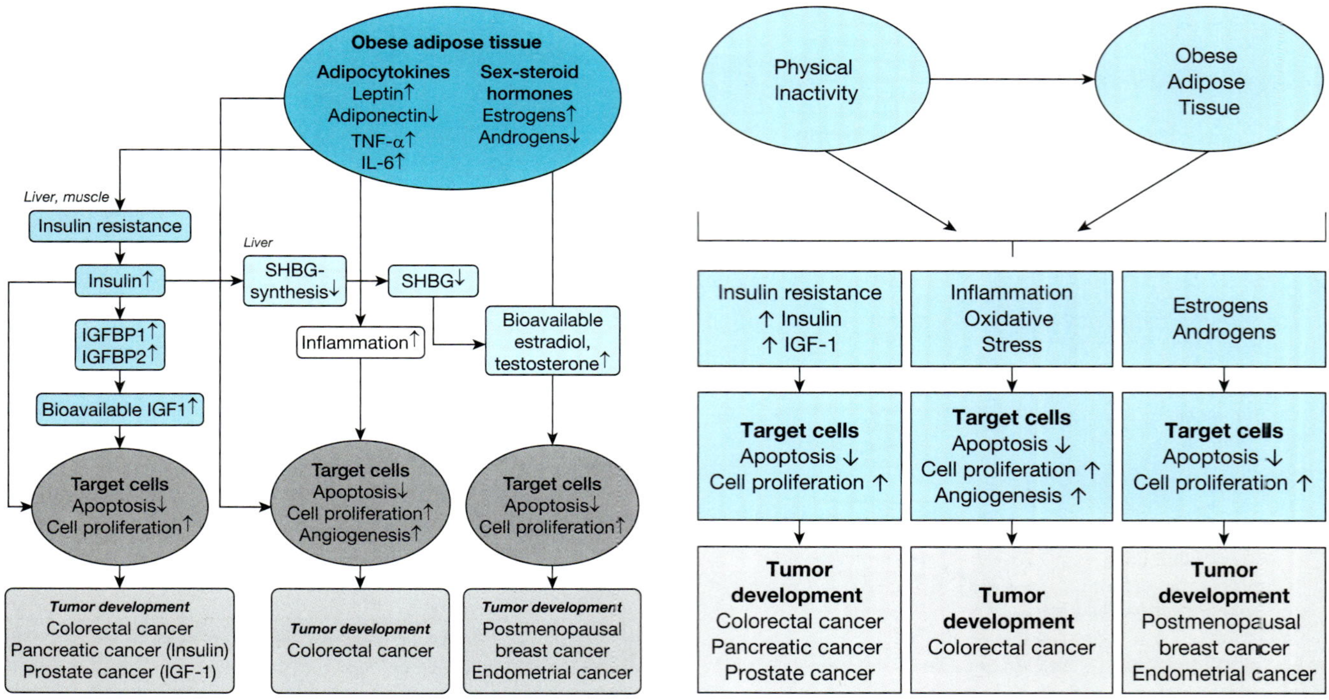

FIGURE 6.8. Synergistic effects of adipokines, sex steroid hormones, inflammation, insulin, and IGF-1 on cancer.

Chemotherapy Completion Rate: Relative Dose Intensity

When patients with cancer are prescribed chemotherapy, there is a specific dose of each of the chemotherapy drugs that is prescribed, generally in relation to the body surface area. It is not uncommon for oncologists to need to reduce the dose from what was originally prescribed because the patient experiences toxic responses to the drugs, such as excessive nausea and vomiting, fevers and infections, loss of sensation in hands and feet, or drastic changes in blood cell counts. It has been observed that receiving at least 85% of the originally prescribed chemotherapy dose is associated with improved long-term cancer survival (48). The percentage of originally prescribed chemotherapy received is often referred to as **relative dose intensity (RDI)**. Approximately 40% of obese patients receive a reduced chemotherapy dose, as compared to 6% among patients with a body weight in the normal range. This may contribute to the observation that inactive and obese cancer patients may have worse overall survival (29).

The hypothesized mechanisms for this include the possible shift in the way chemotherapy drugs are cleared from the body in obese compared with lean patients, which may contribute to the worse chemotherapy toxicity profile in obese patients. There is also ongoing research interest in the potential role of muscle mass in chemotherapy tolerance (49, 50).

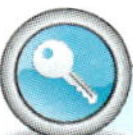

Relative dose intensity (RDI). Ratio of the chemotherapy dose intensity delivered to the reference standard dose intensity.

WEIGHT LOSS: BARIATRIC SURGERY OFFERING CLUES

We have presented compelling evidence that both exercise and obesity are associated with cancer risk. One ongoing question, based on the data shared so far in this chapter, is whether weight loss would reduce risk for cancer. Studies of weight loss and cancer incidence are challenging, given the long follow-up time required and the difficulty in obtaining meaningful weight loss that can be sustained. There has been some provocative research on a cohort of patients who have received bariatric surgery (weight loss surgery) that is relevant to this question.

The Swedish Obese Subjects study (51) examined long-term outcomes after bariatric surgery as compared with the more typical approaches to weight loss (eg, behavioral weight loss and meal replacement systems). The study started with 701 obese patients. Of these, 393 underwent bariatric surgery. The rest received more conventional behaviorally based weight loss intervention (behavioral counseling, advice to exercise, and meal replacements). These patients have been followed for 21 years on average. The patients who underwent bariatric surgery maintained

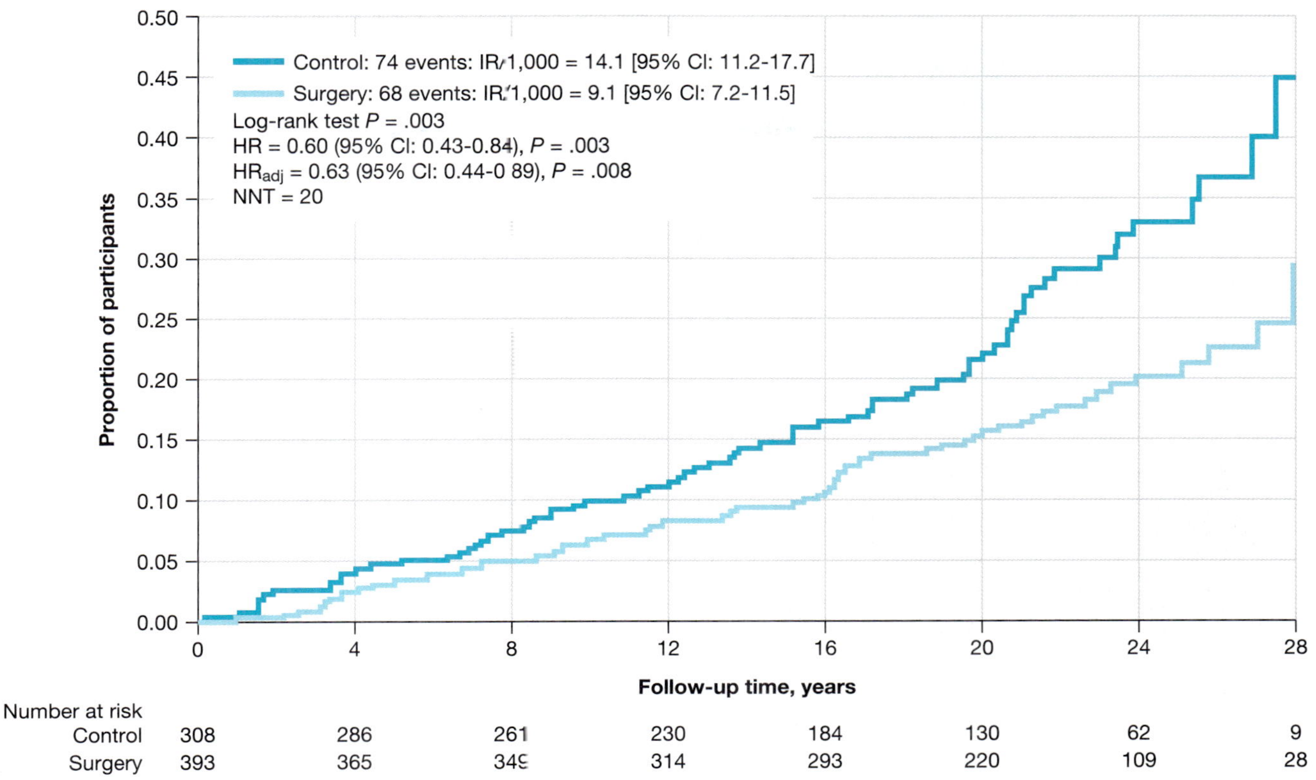

FIGURE 6.9. Long-term follow-up of obese patients who received weight loss surgery (light blue) versus usual weight loss approaches (dark blue). The outcome is cancer incidence. The lower light blue line depicts a lower incidence of cancer among obese patients who underwent weight loss surgery. (Modified from Sjoholm K, Carlsson LMS, Svensson PA, et al. Association of bariatric surgery with cancer incidence in patients with obesity and diabetes: long term results from the Swedish Obese Subjects study. *Diabetes Care*. 2021;45(2): 444–50. doi:10.2337/dc21-1335. https://diabetesjournals.org/care/article/45/2/444/138993/Association-of-Bariatric-Surgery-With-Cancer.)

weight losses of 22.5 kg over 10 years. The patients who underwent more conventional weight loss intervention lost 4.8 kg over 10 years. The incidence of any type of cancer was 9.1 per 1,000 in the bariatric surgery patients compared with 14.1 per 1,000 in the usual weight loss group. This is a 37% reduction in risk of cancer. Figure 6.9 documents the incidence of cancer in the 2 groups over the full length of follow-up. The dark blue line represents the usual weight loss group, that is, the control group, and the light blue line depicts the incidence of cancer over time in the bariatric surgery group.

EFFECTS OF EXERCISE TRAINING ON OBESITY AND BODY COMPOSITION

In addition to weight loss strategies, exercise training may play an important role in addressing the obesity-related mechanisms for cancer risk. These effects may be specific to activities to promote weight loss (aerobic or resistance exercise) and reduce fat mass (aerobic exercise) versus activities to increase muscle mass (resistance exercise).

Effects of Exercise on Weight Loss and Weight Gain Prevention

The ACSM® has published a position stand on the Appropriate Physical Activity Intervention Strategies for Weight Loss and Prevention of Weight Regain in Adults. The summary of the evidence is shown in Table 6.3 (52). The evidence categories referred to are A (RCTs, extensive body of data) and B (RCTs, limited body of data). To summarize the table, exercise alone, with no dietary component, is insufficient to cause meaningful weight loss, but it is useful in the setting of weight maintenance and preventing weight regain.

Exercise Intended to Promote Fat Loss

The amount of exercise recommended for cancer prevention and general health is often quoted to be 150 minutes per week of aerobic exercise and twice weekly strength training. However, the amount of exercise needed for substantive changes in fat mass may be more. For example, a study of 52 overweight and obese adults randomly assigned

Table 6.3 Level of Evidence From American College of Sports Medicine® on Physical Activity and Weight Loss and Weight Control

EVIDENCE STATEMENT	EVIDENCE CATEGORY
Physical activity (PA) to prevent weight gain. PA of 150 to 250 minutes per week with an energy equivalent of 1,200 to 2,000 minutes per week will prevent weight gain greater than 3% in most adults.	A
PA for weight loss. PA < 150 minutes per week promotes minimal weight loss, PA > 150 minutes week results in modest weight loss of ~2-3 kg, PA > 225-420 minutes per week results in 5- to 7.5-kg weight loss, and a dose-response exists.	B
PA for weight maintenance after weight loss. Some studies support the value of ~200 to 300 minutes per week PA during weight maintenance to reduce weight regain after weight loss, and it seems that "more is better." However, there are no correctly designed, adequately powered, energy balance studies to provide evidence for the amount of PA to prevent weight regain after weight loss.	B
Lifestyle PA is an ambiguous term and must be carefully defined to evaluate the literature. Given this limitation, it seems lifestyle PA may be useful to counter the small energy imbalance responsible for obesity in most adults.	B
PA and diet restriction. PA will increase weight loss if diet restriction is modest but not if diet restriction is severe (ie, <kcal per week needed to meet RMR).	A
Resistance training (RT) for weight loss. Research evidence does not support RT as effective for weight loss with or without diet restriction. There is limited evidence that RT promotes gain or maintenance of lean mass and loss of body fat during energy restriction and there is some evidence RT improves chronic disease risk factors (ie, HDL-C, LDL-C, insulin, blood pressure).	B

From Donnelly JE, Blair SN, Jakicic JM, Manore MM, Rankin JW, Smith BK. Appropriate physical activity intervention strategies for weight loss and prevention of weight regain for adults. *Med Sci Sports Exerc.* 2009;41(2):459–71. doi:10.1249/MSS.0b013e3181949333.

participants to 6, 2, or no exercise sessions per week over a 12-week intervention period (53). The participants in the twice weekly group were asked to do 90 to 120 minutes of self-selected intensity with a minimal heart rate goal (total of 180-240 minutes per week). The participants in the 6 times a week group were asked to do 40 to 60 minutes of exercise with the same intensity goal (total of 240-360 minutes per week). The percentage fat loss in the 6 times per week group was 7.7 as compared with 1.45 and 0.38 of losses in the 2 and 0 times per week groups respectively. These differences were statistically significant. This study is 1 example of multiple studies that show for substantive fat loss, the dose of exercise will need to be at or around 300 minutes per week. Notably, the percentage weight losses in the 3 groups were 1.48, 0.84, and 1.09 in the 6, 2, and 0 times per week groups respectively, clearly denoting the importance of measuring body composition rather than just weight loss.

The potential for such programs and fat loss to have meaningful effects on cancer risk reduction seems quite promising, given the mechanisms reviewed earlier. Notably, exercise interventions have been shown to improve many of the mechanisms reviewed earlier, including reduced insulin, improved insulin sensitivity, reduced leptin, increased adiponectin, improved immune function, reduced chronic inflammation, and reduced estrogens (19). The effects of exercise training on IGF pathway is less clear (54).

Exercise Intended to Promote Muscle Gain

Progressive resistance exercise reliably increases muscle mass. The potential for increased muscle mass to result in improved cancer risk may lie in the well-established effects of resistance exercise to improve insulin sensitivity and to reduce chronic inflammation (55).

SUMMARY

There is strong observational epidemiological evidence that obesity is associated with increased risk for 13 different cancers. Physical inactivity is associated with increased risk for 7 cancers. The mechanisms thought to link exercise, obesity, and cancer risk include elevated insulin, insulin resistance, growth factors (IGF-1), estrogen, inflammation, oxidative stress, immune function, increased leptin, and decreased adiponectin. A large study of patients who underwent surgical weight loss supports the notion that weight loss does reduce risk for cancer. Further, there is evidence that exercise training can improve many of the mechanisms reviewed in this chapter without substantive weight loss.

Areas that require further research include:

- role of exercise in the prevention of less common cancers,
- role of body composition (muscle and fat mass in particular) in cancer incidence and recurrence,
- effect of exercise training on cancer recurrence,
- impact of obesity on cancer survival, and
- further explanation of the obesity paradox through rigorous research involving measurement of body composition.

All of the mechanisms reviewed herein included a statement about the hypothesized reason for the effects, underscoring the need for future rigorous science to explicate the mechanisms connecting exercise, obesity, and cancer.

Case Study

Darnell is 49 years old, a father of 2, and has a BMI of 33. He reports having performed no exercise in the past 2 years since his twins were born. His father died of colon cancer, and he is worried about whether he is also at risk for colon cancer. He wants to see his twins grow up and has come for advice on how best to reduce his risk for colon cancer through lifestyle changes.

Questions

1. What would be the first recommendation for Darnell: exercise, weight loss, or some combination? Why?
2. How would you get Darnell started with an exercise program?
3. Should Darnell do resistance exercise?

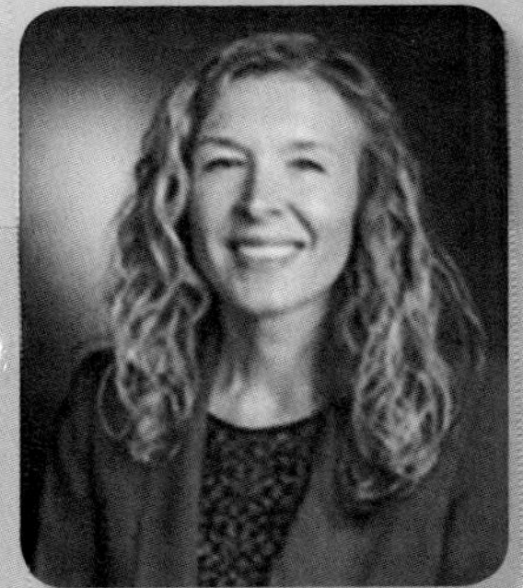

Meet the Expert

FEATURED PROFESSIONAL

Jennifer Ligibel, MD, FASCO

Director, Leonard P. Zakim Center for Integrative Therapies and Healthy Living
Director, Center for Faculty Well-Being
Associate Professor of Medicine, Harvard Medical School
Dana-Farber Cancer Institute
Medical Oncologist

Q: "Where did you grow up?"

Toledo, OH.

Q: "Where did you train? What is your training?"

I received an undergraduate degree in Zoology from Duke University and went to medical school at Washington University in St. Louis, MO. I moved to Boston to train in internal medicine at Massachusetts General Hospital and completed a fellowship in medical oncology at the Dana-Farber Cancer Institute.

Q: "What are you best known for?"

I am the Principal Investigator of the Breast Cancer Weight Loss (BWEL) study (A011401) and was the chair of the American Society of Clinical Oncology Obesity and Energy Balance Sub-Committee.

Q: "What are you currently working on?"

I am currently working to complete the BWEL trial and am working with Drs. Katie Schmitz and Nate Berger on the THRIVE-65 Study, part of the NCI ENICTO Consortium.

Favorite Quote:

Not a quote but a question. My work is dedicated to the countless women who have asked me over the years: "Dr. Ligibel, what can *I* do to beat breast cancer?"

—*Jennifer Ligibel*

STUDY QUESTIONS

1. What are 4 cancers associated with obesity?
2. The methods of assessing body composition commonly used in research on exercise, obesity, and cancer are:
   a. DXA, total body water, and BMI
   b. DXA, CT scan, and D_3-creatine dilution
   c. DXA, BMI, and bioimpedance
   d. All of the above
3. True or false. There is less knowledge about body composition and cancer incidence than obesity and cancer incidence.
4. As insulin goes up, cancer risk goes:
   a. Up
   b. Down
   c. Stays the same
   d. Depends on other factors
5. Estrogen is ________________ in postmenopausal women who are obese, as compared with postmenopausal women who are not obese.
   a. The same
   b. Lower
   c. Higher
   d. Depends on other factors
6. What is a crown-like structure?
   a. A ring of IGF-1 around muscle cells denoting buffness
   b. A ring of macrophages surrounding tumor cells that kill the tumor cells
   c. A ring of pro-inflammatory cytokines surrounding a dead fat cell
   d. A ring of macrophages surrounding a dead fat cell
7. Name 3 functions of leptin.
8. In the Swedish Obese Study, they followed patients that received weight loss surgery and patients that did more conventional (dietary) weight loss. The result with regard to cancer risk was that over 21 years the likelihood of cancer was ___% lower among those who had the weight loss surgery.
   a. 10
   b. 90
   c. 5
   d. 37
9. True or false. Exercise alone often leads to weight loss.
10. True or false. Exercise training can improve many of the factors on the mechanistic pathway between obesity and cancer risk, regardless of not producing weight loss.

REFERENCES

1. Hales CM, Carroll MD, Fryar CD, Ogden CL. Prevalence of obesity and severe obesity among adults: United States, 2017–2018. *NCHS Data Brief.* 2020(360):1–8.
2. Calle EE, Rodriguez C, Walker-Thurmond K, Thun MJ. Overweight, obesity, and mortality from cancer in a prospectively studied cohort of U.S. adults. *N Engl J Med.* 2003;348(17):1625–38. doi:10.1056/NEJMoa021423
3. Rock CL, Thomson C, Gansler T, et al. American Cancer Society guideline for diet and physical activity for cancer prevention. *CA Cancer J Clin.* 2020;70(4):245–71. doi:10.3322/caac.21591
4. Patel AV, Friedenreich CM, Moore SC, et al. American College of Sports Medicine® roundtable report on physical activity, sedentary behavior, and cancer prevention and control. *Med Sci Sports Exerc.* 2019;51(11):2391–402. doi:10.1249/MSS.0000000000002117
5. McTiernan A, Friedenreich CM, Katzmarzyk PT, et al. Physical activity in cancer prevention and survival: a systematic review. *Med Sci Sports Exerc.* 2019;51(6):1252–61. doi:10.1249/MSS.0000000000001937
6. Moore SC, Lee IM, Weiderpass E, et al. Association of leisure-time physical activity with risk of 26 types of cancer in 1.44 million adults. *JAMA Intern Med.* 2016;176(6):816–25. doi:10.1001/jamainternmed.2016.1548
7. Song M, Willett WC, Hu FB, et al. Trajectory of body shape across the lifespan and cancer risk. *Int J Cancer.* 2016;138(10):2383–95. doi:10.1002/ijc.29981
8. Morishita S, Hamaue Y, Fukushima T, Tanaka T, Fu JB, Nakano J. Effect of exercise on mortality and recurrence in patients with cancer: a systematic review and meta-analysis. *Integr Cancer Ther.* 2020;19:1534735420917462. doi:10.1177/1534735420917462
9. Schmitz KH, Neuhouser ML, Agurs-Collins T, et al. Impact of obesity on cancer survivorship and the potential relevance of race and ethnicity. *J Natl Cancer Inst.* 2013;105(18):1344–54. doi: 10.1093/jnci/djt223
10. Joshu CE, Mondul AM, Menke A, et al. Weight gain is associated with an increased risk of prostate cancer recurrence after prostatectomy in the PSA era. *Cancer Prev Res (Phila).* 2011;4(4):544–51. doi:0.1158/1940-6207
11. Sinicrope FA, Foster NR, Sargent DJ, O'Connell MJ, Rankin C. Obesity is an independent prognostic variable in colon cancer survivors. *Clin Cancer Res.* 2010;16(6):1884–93. doi:10.1158/1078-0432.CCR-09-2636
12. Protani M, Coory M, Martin JH. Effect of obesity on survival of women with breast cancer: systematic review and meta-analysis. *Breast Cancer Res Treat.* 2010;123(3):627–35. doi:10.1007/s10549-010-0990-0
13. Caan BJ, Cespedes Feliciano EM, Kroenke CH. The importance of body composition in explaining the overweight paradox in cancer-counterpoint. *Cancer Res.* 2018;78(8):1906–12. doi:10.1158/0008-5472.CAN-17-3287

14. U.S. Department of Health and Human Services. *2018 Physical Activity Guidelines Advisory Committee Scientific Report.* [Internet]. Washington, DC, 2018. Available from https://health.gov/sites/default/files/2019-09/PAG_Advisory_Committee_Report.pdf
15. Ballotari P, Vicentini M, Manicardi V, et al. Diabetes and risk of cancer incidence: results from a population-based cohort study in northern Italy. *BMC Cancer.* 2017;17(1):703. doi:10.1186/s12885-017-3696-4
16. Shou J, Chen PJ, Xiao WH. Mechanism of increase risk of insulin resistance in aging skeletal muscle. *Diabetol Metab Syndr.* 2020;12(14):1–10. doi:10.1186/s13098-020-0523-x
17. Orgel E, Mittelman SD. The links between insulin resistance, diabetes, and cancer. *Curr Diab Rep.* 2013;13(2):213–22. doi:10.1007/s11892-012-0356-6
18. Lewitt MS, Dent MS, Hall K. The insulin-like growth factor system in obesity, insulin resistance and type 2 diabetes mellitus. *J Clin Med.* 2014;3(4):1561–74. doi:10.3390/jcm3041561
19. Kang DW, Lee J, Suh SH, Ligibel J, Courneya KS, Jeon JY. Effects of exercise on insulin, IGF axis, adipocytokines, and inflammatory markers in breast cancer survivors: a systematic review and meta-analysis. *Cancer Epidemiol Biomarkers Prev.* 2017;26(3):355–65. doi:10.1158/1055-9965.EPI-16-0602
20. Shanmugalingam T, Bosco C, Ridley AJ, Van Hemelrijck M. Is there a role for IGF-1 in the development of second primary cancers? *Cancer Med.* 2016;5(11):3353–67. doi:10.1002/cam4.871
21. de Roon M, May AM, McTiernan A, et al. Effect of exercise and/or reduced calorie dietary interventions on breast cancer-related endogenous sex hormones in healthy postmenopausal women. *Breast Cancer Res.* 2018;20(1):81. doi:10.1186/s13058-018-1009-8
22. Freeman EW, Sammel MD, Lin H, Gracia CR. Obesity and reproductive hormone levels in the transition to menopause. *Menopause.* 2010;17(4):718–26. doi:10.1097/gme.0b013e3181cec85d
23. Schmitz KH, Lin H, Sammel MD, et al. Association of physical activity with reproductive hormones: the Penn Ovarian Aging Study. *Cancer Epidemiol Biomarkers Prev.* 2007;16(10):2042–7. doi:10.1158/1055-9965.EPI-07-0061
24. Lowe DA, Baltgalvis KA, Greising SM. Mechanisms behind estrogen's beneficial effect on muscle strength in females. *Exerc Sport Sci Rev.* 2010;38(2):61–7. doi:10.1097/JES.0b013e3181d496bc
25. Liang J, Shang, Y. Estrogen and cancer. *Annu Rev Physiol.* 2013;75:225–40.
26. Travis RC, Key TJ. Oestrogen exposure and breast cancer risk. *Breast Cancer Res.* 2003;5(5):239–47. doi:10.1186/bcr628
27. Newell SA, Sanson-Fisher RW, Savolainen NJ. Systematic review of psychological therapies for cancer patients: overview and recommendations for future research. *J Natl Cancer Inst.* 2002;94(8):558–84. doi:10.1093/jnci/94.8.558
28. Fui MN, Dupuis P, Grossmann M. Lowered testosterone in male obesity: mechanisms, morbidity and management. *Asian J Androl.* 2014;16(2):223–31. doi:10.4103/1008-682X.122365
29. Loughlin KR. The testosterone conundrum: the putative relationship between testosterone levels and prostate cancer. *Urol Oncol.* 2016;34(11):482 e1–e4. doi:10.1016/j.urolonc.2016.05.023
30. Freedland SJ, Aronson WJ. Examining the relationship between obesity and prostate cancer. *Rev Urol.* 2004;6(2):73–81.
31. Kaaks R, Lukanova A, Kurzer MS. Obesity, endogenous hormones, and endometrial cancer risk: a synthetic review. *Cancer Epidemiol Biomarkers Prev.* 2002;11(12):1531–43.
32. Burini RC, Anderson E, Durstine JL, Carson JA. Inflammation, physical activity, and chronic disease: an evolutionary perspective. *Sports Med Health Sci.* 2020;2(1):1–6. doi:10.1016/j.smhs.2020.03.004
33. Fischer CP, Berntsen A, Perstrup LB, Eskildsen P, Pedersen BK. Plasma levels of interleukin-6 and C-reactive protein are associated with physical inactivity independent of obesity. *Scand J Med Sci Sports.* 2007;17(5):580–7. doi:10.1111/j.1600-0838.2006.00602.x
34. Zatterale F, Longo M, Naderi J, et al. Chronic adipose tissue inflammation linking obesity to insulin resistance and type 2 diabetes. *Front Physiol.* 2019;10:1607. doi:10.3389/fphys.2019.01607
35. Rahbek CB, Kamper RS, Haddock B, Andersen H, Jorgensen N, Suetta, C. The relationship between low-grade inflammation and muscle mass, strength, and physical performance in a geriatric outpatient population. *J Geriatr Med Gerentol.* 2021;7(3):1–8. doi:10.23937/2469-5858/1510119.
36. Libby P, Ridker PM, Maseri A. Inflammation and atherosclerosis. *Circulation.* 2002;105(9):1135–43. doi:10.1161/hc0902.104353
37. Marseglia L, Manti S, D'Angelo G, et al. Oxidative stress in obesity: a critical component in human diseases. *Int J Mol Sci.* 2015;16:378–400. doi:10.3390/ijms16010378.
38. Woodall MJ, Neumann S, Campbell K, Pattison ST, Young SL. The effects of obesity on anti-cancer immunity and cancer immunotherapy. *Cancers (Basel).* 2020;12(5). doi:10.3390/cancers12051230
39. Ringel AE, Drijvers JM, Baker GJ, et al. Obesity shapes metabolism in the tumor microenvironment to suppress anti-tumor immunity. *Cell.* 2020;183(7):1848–66 e26. doi:10.1016/j.cell.2020.11.009
40. Saxena NK, Sharma D. Metastasis suppression by adiponectin: LKB1 rises up to the challenge. *Cell Adh Migr.* 2010;4(3):358–62. doi:10.4161/cam.4.3.11541
41. Yu N, Ruan Y, Gao X, Sun J. Systematic review and meta-analysis of randomized, controlled trials on the effect of exercise on serum leptin and adiponectin in overweight and obese individuals. *Horm Metab Res.* 2017;49(3):164–73. doi:10.1055/s-0042-121605
42. Bruinsma TJ, Dyer AM, Rogers CJ, Schmitz KH, Sturgeon KM. Effects of diet and exercise-induced weight loss on biomarkers of inflammation in breast cancer survivors: a systematic review and meta-analysis. *Cancer Epidemiol Biomarkers Prev.* 2021;30(6):1048–62. doi:10.1158/1055-9965.EPI-20-1029
43. Tessitore L, Vizio B, Jenkins O, et al. Leptin expression in colorectal and breast cancer patients. *Int J Mol Med.* 2000;5(4):421–6. doi:10.3892/ijmm.5.4.421
44. Ho GY, Wang T, Gunter MJ, et al. Adipokines linking obesity with colorectal cancer risk in postmenopausal women. *Cancer Res.* 2012;72(12):3029–37. doi:10.1158/0008-5472.CAN-11-2771
45. Aleksandrova K, Boeing H, Jenab M, et al. Leptin and soluble leptin receptor in risk of colorectal cancer in the European Prospective Investigation into Cancer and Nutrition cohort. *Cancer Res.* 2012;72(20):5328–37. doi:10.1158/0008-5472.CAN-12-0465
46. Yamauchi N, Takazawa Y, Maeda D, et al. Expression levels of adiponectin receptors are decreased in human endometrial adenocarcinoma tissues. *Int J Gynecol Pathol.* 2012;31(4):352–7. doi:10.1097/PGP.0b013e3182469583
47. Nimptsch K, Pischon, T. Obesity biomarkers, metabolism, and risk of cancer: an epidemiological perspective. *Recent Results Cancer Res.* 2016;208:199–217. doi:10.1007/978-3-319-42542-9_11
48. McMeekin S, Dizon D, Barter J, et al. Phase III randomized trial of second-line ixabepilone versus paclitaxel or doxorubicin in women with advanced endometrial cancer. *Gynecol Oncol.* 2015;138(1):18–23. doi:10.1016/j.ygyno.2015.04.026
49. Cheng E, Caan BJ, Cawthon PM, et al. Body composition, relative dose intensity, and adverse events among patients with colon cancer. *Cancer Epidemiol Biomarkers Prev.* 2023. doi:10.1158/1055-9965.EPI-23-0227
50. Cespedes Feliciano EM, Chen WY, Lee V, et al. Body composition, adherence to anthracycline and taxane-based chemotherapy, and survival after nonmetastatic breast cancer. *JAMA Oncol.* 2020;6(2):264–70. doi:10.1001/jamaoncol.2019.4668
51. Sjoholm K, Carlsson LMS, Svensson PA, et al. Association of bariatric surgery with cancer incidence in patients with obesity and diabetes: long-term results from the Swedish obese subjects study. *Diabetes Care.* 2022;45(2):444–50. doi:10.2337/dc21-1335

52. Donnelly JE, Blair SN, Jakicic JM, et al. American College of Sports Medicine® position stand: appropriate physical activity intervention strategies for weight loss and prevention of weight regain for adults. *Med Sci Sports Exerc.* 2009;41(2):459–71. doi:10.1249/MSS.0b013e3181949333
53. Flack KD, Hays HM, Moreland J, Long DE. Exercise for weight loss: further evaluating energy compensation with exercise. *Med Sci Sports Exerc.* 2020;52(11):2466–75. doi:10.1249/MSS.0000000000002376
54. Devin JL, Bolam KA, Jenkins DG, Skinner TL. The influence of exercise on the insulin-like growth factor axis in oncology: physiological basis, current, and future perspectives. *Cancer Epidemiol Biomarkers Prev.* 2016;25(2):239–49. doi:10.1158/1055-9965.EPI-15-0406
55. Hardee JP, Porter RR, Sui X, et al. The effect of resistance exercise on all-cause mortality in cancer survivors. *Mayo Clin Proc.* 2014;89(8):1108–15. doi:10.1016/j.mayocp.2014.03.018

CHAPTER

7

Inflammation and the Immune System

OUTLINE

1. Introduction
2. What Is Inflammation?
   a. Acute Inflammatory Response
   b. Chronic Inflammatory Response
3. The Immune System
   a. Innate and Acquired Immunity
4. Chronic Inflammation and Cancer
   a. Induction of Cancer-Associated Inflammation
5. Inflammatory Markers and Cancer Prognosis
6. The Immune System and Cancer
7. Normal Inflammatory and Immune Responses to Exercise
   a. Inflammatory Response to Acute Bout of Exercise
   b. Inflammatory Response to a Prolonged Period of Exercise Training
   c. Cellular Immune Response to Exercise
8. Impact of Exercise on the Inflammatory and Immune Responses in Cancer Survivors
9. Effect of Cancer Treatments on the Immune System
   a. Effect of Cancer Treatments on Innate Immunity
   b. Effect of Chemotherapy on the Immune System
   c. Effect of Radiation Therapy on the Immune System
   d. Effect of High-Dose Steroids on the Immune System
10. Immunotherapy/Targeted Treatments
   a. Monoclonal Antibodies
   b. Adoptive Cell Transfer
   c. Vaccines
   d. Cytokines
11. Exercise Precautions With Patients Who Have Cancer and a Compromised Immune System Because of Treatment
12. Summary
13. Case Study
14. Meet the Expert
15. Study Questions
16. References

OBJECTIVES

After completing review of this chapter, students will be able to:

1. Understand the concept of inflammation and the cells and mediators involved in an inflammatory/immune response.
2. Recognize the roles and responses of the inflammatory and immune system to cancer.
3. Evaluate the role that exercise plays in the inflammatory and immune responses in a cancer setting.
4. Be aware of the contraindications and safety requirements when exercising a cancer survivor with a compromised immune system.

INTRODUCTION

Inflammation and the immune system are important to the field of exercise oncology. Inflammation is commonly considered as an immediate (acute) response to a tissue injury or a bacterial infection, but it is much more complex. The response to an infection or tissue damage involves the local production of small polypeptides called **cytokines** that facilitate an influx of various immune cells. This is accompanied by a **systemic** response that is elicited within a few hours after the initial insult and usually subsides over a period of 24 to 72 hours when the body returns to homeostasis (normal function) and the infection is killed or the trauma healed. This inflammatory response is also the first line of defense against carcinogens that stimulate abnormal cell growth and proliferation.

Conversely, if the inflammation develops into a low-grade continuous (chronic) response, this may contribute to changes in the **tumor stroma** and tumor growth at the stages of tumor initiation, proliferation, or progression. Over the past 20 years, efforts have been made to elucidate the effect of exercise on inflammation and the immune system in cancer survivors. This chapter will demonstrate that staying active after a cancer diagnosis has mostly a positive influence on the inflammatory process and the immune system. From an exercise prescription perspective, the importance of being aware of the immune/inflammatory status of a cancer survivor and ensuring that the prescribed activities do not compromise or exacerbate a treatment-related inflammatory or immune response will be considered.

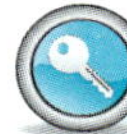

Cytokine. A small polypeptide that is made by certain immune and nonimmune cells and has an immunoregulatory role.

Systemic. Having an effect on the whole body.

Tumor stroma. The noncancer cell and nonimmune cell structural components of tumors that hold the tumor tissues together.

WHAT IS INFLAMMATION?

Inflammation is a highly conserved process that has evolved as a protective reaction to injury, disease, or irritation of the tissues and involves activation, recruitment, and engagement of immune cells and their mediators.

Inflammation was originally described in ancient Rome (30-38 BC) as being present when 5 specific symptoms were observed: redness (*rubor*), swelling (*tumor*), heat (*calor*), pain (*dolor*), and loss of function (*functio laesa*) (1). The sensation of heat is caused by an increased volume of blood moving through dilated, permeable blood vessels into the area of injury, which results in the redness because of the increased number of localized erythrocytes (red blood cells, ie, RBCs). The migration of fluid into the surrounding tissues from the permeable blood vessels then causes swelling (described as **edema**). Pain is caused by the direct effects of the initial damage or is a result of the inflammatory response itself. Finally, the loss of function is either because of the loss of mobility in a joint (owing to swelling or pain) or because of the replacement of functional cells with scar tissue (Figure 7.1).

It is now recognized that inflammation is more complex and diverse than the simple description provided above. Inflammation can be categorized several ways: the stage in

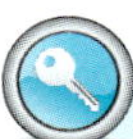

Edema. A swelling of tissues caused by the capillary blood vessels pushing fluid, mostly water, into the intercellular spaces of the body.

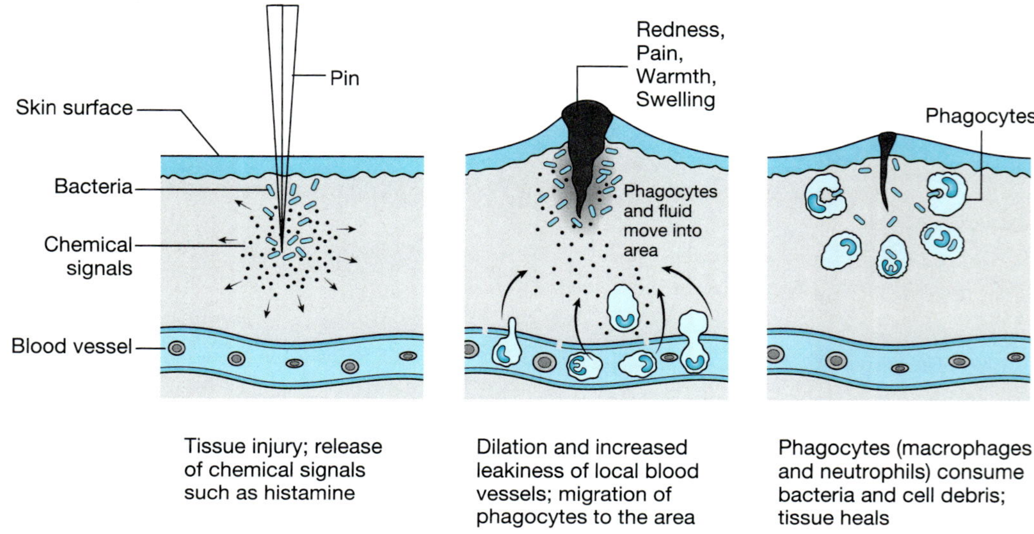

FIGURE 7.1. Entitled symptoms of inflammation.

Table 7.1 Main Differences Between Acute and Chronic Inflammation

	ACUTE	CHRONIC
Causative agent	Pathogens, irritants, cellular stress, trauma	Persistent acute infection, persistent foreign bodies, autoimmune reaction, tissue damage, metabolic dysfunction
Onset	Immediate	Delayed
Duration	Short term (a few days)	Persistent nonresolving (months or years)
Magnitude	High grade	Low grade
Outcomes	Resolution, irritant removal, tissue repair, chronic inflammation	Tissue destruction, fibrosis, collateral damage
Major cells	Neutrophils, monocytes, macrophages	Monocytes, macrophages, lymphocytes, plasma cells, fibroblasts
Biomarkers	IL-6, TNF-α, IL-1 beta, CRP	No recognized standard biomarkers

the process of inflammation; the type of pathogen, chemical, autoimmune, or physical injury that initiated the inflammation; the tissue or organ involved; and whether the inflammation is an acute, resolving form or a chronic, nonresolving, long-lasting response (Table 7.1).

Acute Inflammatory Response

The initial acute response to an infection, trauma, autoimmune disease, and some tumors involves the local production of cytokines that induce an influx of lymphocytes, neutrophils, monocytes, and other cells into the affected area. This is accompanied by a systemic response (known as the acute-phase response) in which the serum concentrations of cytokines and cytokine inhibitors increase or decrease by at least 25% during the inflammatory phase (2). This general (innate) inflammatory response is the first line of defense against carcinogens that stimulate abnormal cell proliferation. Nonspecific immune cells such as NK cells sense cellular changes associated with tumor development, including modifications in cell metabolism, tissue metabolism (such as hypoxia), or tissue anatomy (such as organ lesions). This response can be harnessed as a cancer treatment; for example, an induced acute inflammation is used in the treatment of bladder cancer. Patients receive an antituberculosis vaccine containing attenuated *Mycobacterium bovis* bacillus directly into the urinary bladder, which induces an acute inflammatory response against the squamous cancer bladder cells (3).

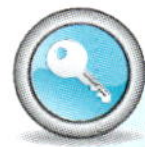

Pathogen. Any organism that can produce disease.
Acute inflammation. An immediate adaptive response to a noxious stimulus that lasts only a few days.

Chronic Inflammatory Response

If the acute inflammatory response is not resolved, it can result in a state of low-grade, systemic chronic inflammation with neutrophils being replaced in the tissue site by an infiltration of macrophages, lymphocytes, and plasma cells, which produce inflammatory cytokines, growth factors, and enzymes, contributing to increased tissue damage. A chronic inflammatory response increases the risk for various noncommunicable diseases (Figure 7.2) (4). Worldwide, 3 out of 5 people die of chronic inflammatory diseases, such as cardiovascular disorders, chronic respiratory diseases, cancer, obesity, and diabetes.

Chronic inflammation can regulate carcinogenesis on the levels of tumor initiation, proliferation, and progression by several mechanisms, including accelerated cell proliferation, evasion from apoptosis, enhanced angiogenesis, and metastasis (5). For example, a low-grade chronic inflammatory response can promote cytokine-induced DNA damage and increased genetic instability, leading to the accumulation of random genetic alterations in cancer cells (6). Chronic inflammation can also lead to uncontrolled T-cell stimulation, resulting in poor T-cell antigen response to avoid autoimmunity, and T cells ultimately entering a quiescence state also known as T-cell exhaustion. See Table 7.1 for a comparison of acute and chronic inflammation.

Chronic inflammation. Slow, long-term inflammation lasting for prolonged periods of several months to years.
Antigen. A molecule or structure that can bind to a specific antibody or T-cell receptor and then trigger an immune response.

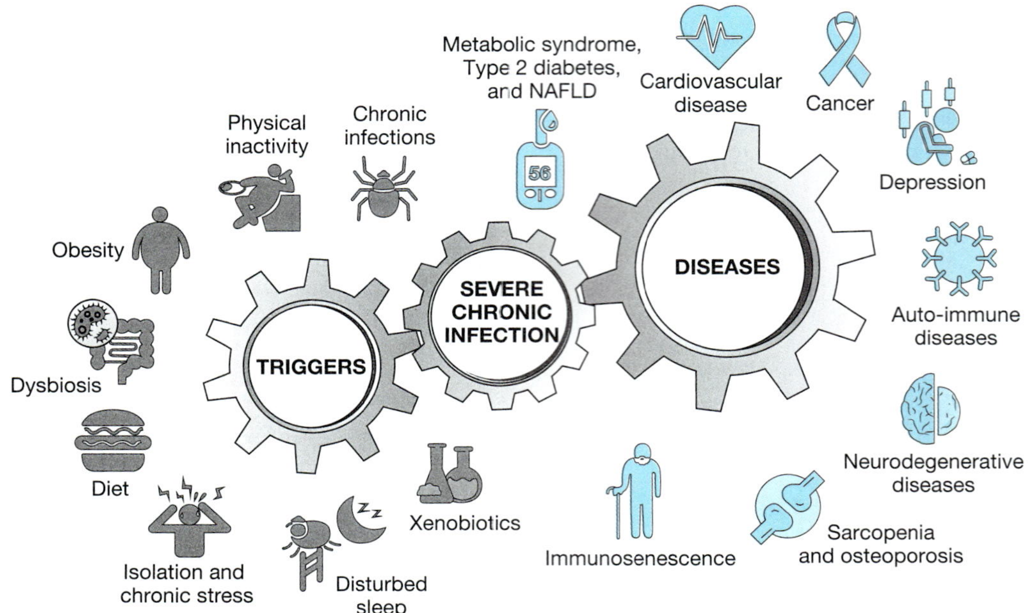

FIGURE 7.2. Causes and consequences of low-grade SCI. Several causes of low-grade SCI and their consequences have been identified. As shown on the left, the most common triggers of SCI (in the counter-clockwise direction) include chronic infections, physical inactivity, visceral obesity, intestinal dysbiosis, diet, social isolation, psychological stress, disturbed sleep and disrupted circadian rhythm, and exposure to xenobiotic, such as air pollutants, hazardous waste products, industrial chemicals, and tobacco smoking. As shown on the right, the consequences of SCI (in the clockwise direction) include metabolic syndrome, type II diabetes, nonalcoholic fatty liver disease, cardiovascular disease, cancer, depression, autoimmune diseases, neurodegenerative diseases, sarcopenia, osteoporosis, and immunosenescence. Abbreviations: SCI, systemic chronic inflammation; NAFLD, nonalcoholic fatty liver disease. (Redrawn from Furman D, Campisi J, Verdin E, et al. Chronic inflammation in the etiology of disease across the life span. *Nat Med.* 2019;25(12):1822–32, Figure 1.)

THE IMMUNE SYSTEM

The immune system is comprised of cellular and soluble proteins: white blood cells that originate from the bone marrow from common stem cells (Figure 7.3) and soluble factors that activate the white blood cells or neutralize foreign agents or regulate the immune response.

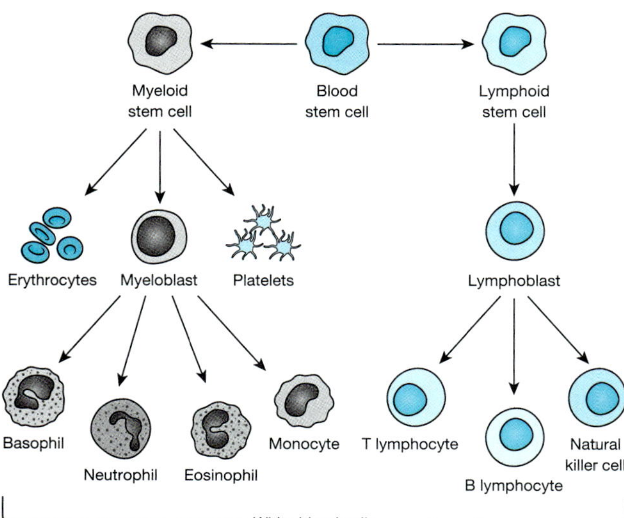

FIGURE 7.3. Origins of and links among white blood cells.

Innate and Acquired Immunity

The immune system can be divided into 2 groups: innate (natural or nonspecific) and adaptive (required or specific); each consists of specific cellular and soluble components (Table 7.2) (7).

When the body is under attack, the *innate* system is typically activated first, and **phagocytes** and NK cells are the first responders. NK cells are lymphocytes that are found in the bone marrow, lymph nodes, spleen, and peripheral blood. Upon activation, NK cells release their granule contents that cause the formation of pores on the cell membrane of the infected or transformed (malignant) cell, then causing it to disintegrate and die. If the innate response fails to eliminate the object/organism/rogue cell, the adaptive immune system responds. The essence of **adaptive immunity** is the

Phagocytes. Macrophages, neutrophils, monocytes, dendritic cells, and osteoclasts are professional phagocytes that are responsible for removing microorganisms and presenting antigens to lymphocytes in order to activate an adaptive immune response.

Adaptive immunity. A subsystem of the immune system that is composed of specialized, systemic cells and processes that eliminate pathogens or prevent their growth.

Table 7.2 Main Cellular and Soluble Components of the Immune System

INNATE CELLULAR COMPONENTS	ADAPTIVE CELLULAR COMPONENTS
Natural killer cells (CD16$^+$, CD56$^+$)	T cells (CD3$^+$, CD4$^+$, CD8$^+$)
Phagocytes (neutrophils, eosinophils, basophils, monocytes, macrophages)	B cells (CD19$^+$, CD20$^+$, CD22$^+$)
INNATE SOLUBLE COMPONENTS	**ADAPTIVE SOLUBLE COMPONENTS**
Acute-phase proteins, eg, CRP	IgM
Cytokines, eg, IL-6	IgG
Complement, eg, C3 convertase	IgA
Growth factors eg, EGF	IgD
Lymphokines, eg, GM-CSF	
Chemokines, eg, IL08	

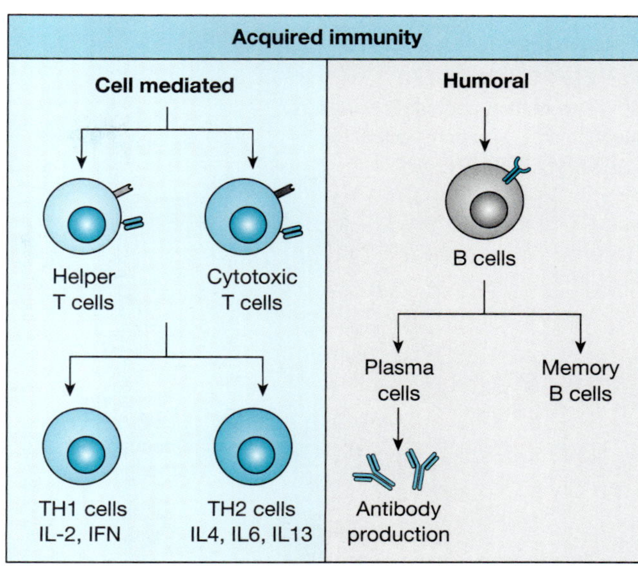

FIGURE 7.4. Major components of adaptive immunity.

body's ability to distinguish between *self* and potential **immunogenic** pathogens or more accurately to discriminate between molecular entities signaling as potential danger and those that do not (8). An adaptive immune response will result in the proliferation of T cells either to attack the invader directly or produce specific mediator proteins and antigen activation of specific B cells, which then differentiate into plasma calls to produce antigen-specific antibodies (a **humoral response**). These extracellular responses are matched by equally complex intracellular signaling control mechanisms, with the ability of cells to assemble and disassemble a range of signaling pathways as they move from inactive to dedicated roles within the immune response site.

Adaptive immune response is based on antigen-specific responses by antibodies and **cell-mediated responses/reactions** (Figure 7.4). It is important to note that chronic inflammation and an impaired immune response increase one's risk of developing cancer. The incidence of a majority of cancers is linked to external factors triggering some form of chronic inflammation. Up to 20% of cancers are linked to chronic infections, 30% can be attributed to tobacco smoking and inhaled pollutants (such as asbestos), 35% to dietary factors, and 20% of cancer burden is linked to obesity (9).

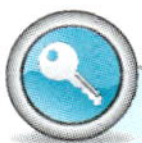

Immunogenicity. The ability of a foreign or abnormal structure to provoke an immune response in the body of a human.

Humoral response. The immune response involving the transformation of B cells into plasma cells that produce and secrete antibodies to a specific antigen.

Cell-mediated response. Response to an antigen that involves the activation of various immune cells, including phagocytes, antigen-specific cytotoxic T lymphocytes, and also the release of various cytokines.

CHRONIC INFLAMMATION AND CANCER

In order to deconstruct the roles and the mechanisms of action of inflammation in cancer, it is important to understand how inflammation is induced and maintained in the first place, both in terms of time and stimulus.

Induction of Cancer-Associated Inflammation

Cancer-associated inflammation can be generated at different time points of tumor development:

- It may precede carcinogenesis and is a result of an infection or autoimmune process.
- It can be induced by the tumor microenvironment (TME).
- It can be triggered by cancer treatments.

Chronic Inflammation Preceding Tumor Formation

Around 15% to 20% of all cancer cases are preceded by chronic inflammation at the tissue or organ site of the cancer. Examples include inflammatory bowel disease (IBD), chronic hepatitis, and *Helicobacter pylori*-induced gastritis, all of which increase the risk of developing colorectal cancer, liver cancer, and stomach cancer, respectively (10). In these cases, the inflammation exists long before the tumor

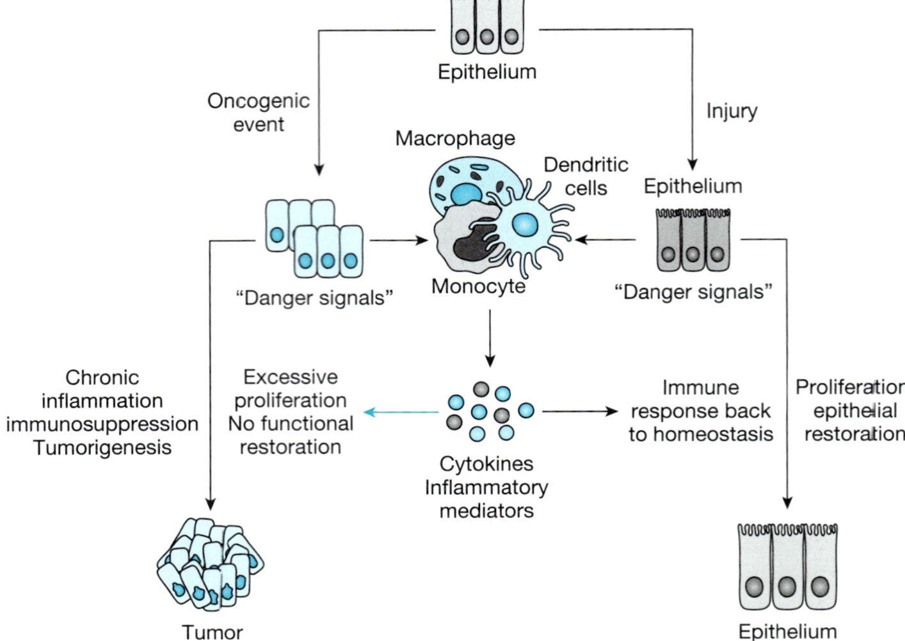

FIGURE 7.5. Normal inflammation compared with inflammation in cancer. (Redrawn from Greten FR, Grivennikov SI. Inflammation and cancer: triggers, mechanisms, and consequences. *Cell Press.* 2019;51(1):27–41.)

formation. Various environmental carcinogens also partly or completely cause cancer by the induction of chronic inflammation. For example, inhalation of tobacco smoke and asbestos particles cause significant lung and airway inflammation and significantly increase the risk of developing lung cancer and mesothelioma respectively. Systemic low-grade chronic inflammation induced by obesity, hyperglycemia, and excessive lipid accumulation can also promote or increase the risk of many different cancers, including liver, pancreatic, colon, and breast (9). Local white adipose tissue in people who are obese is infiltrated by immune cells, including macrophages, lymphocytes, and pro-inflammatory mediators, potentially promoting tumor growth. Obesity-associated chronic inflammation in mammary adipose tissue has been shown to drive the correlation between obesity and breast cancer risk (11).

Tumor Microenvironment-Induced Inflammation

TME closely resembles a healing wound, but instead of restoring normal epithelial homeostasis, this chronic inflammation and cytokine-driven proliferation facilitate further tumor growth (Figure 7.5).

Within the tumor there is a network of proliferating tumor cells, stromal cells comprised of fibroblasts and mesenchymal stroma cells, extracellular matrix, blood vessels, and inflammatory immune cells that form the TME. Chronic inflammation influences the composition of the TME, and in particular, the plasticity of both tumor and stromal cells. Plasticity refers to the ability of cancer cells to modify their physiological characteristics, permitting them to survive hostile microenvironments and resist therapy. The pro-tumorigenic inflammatory response causes an increase in the numbers of macrophages and fibroblasts migrating into the affected tissue site and in the recruitment and release of specific inflammatory mediators and cytokines (12). This has a direct effect on cancer cells by increasing their proliferation and resistance to apoptosis; this has led to the term tumor-elicited inflammation (TEI) (Figure 7.6).

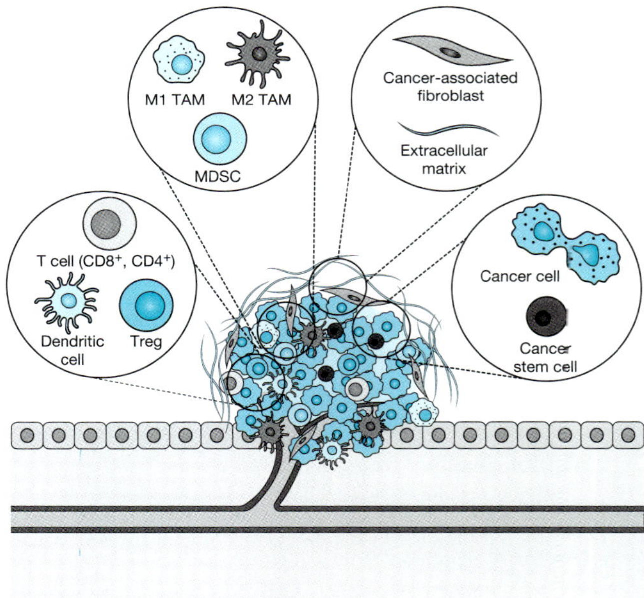

FIGURE 7.6. The tumor microenvironment. Abbreviations: MDSC, myeloid derived suppressor cells; TAM, tumor-associated macrophages. (Redrawn from Benavente S, Sanchez-Garcia A, Naches S, LLeonart ME, Lorente J. Therapy-induced modulation of the tumor microenvironment: new opportunities for cancer therapies. *Front Oncol.* 2020;10:582884.)

Pro-inflammatory signals stimulate the TME to induce immunosuppression and enhance the recruitment, proliferation, and functions of other pro-tumorigenic auxiliary cells within the TME (such as fibroblasts, myeloid cells, regulatory T cells (Tregs), and the endothelium of new blood vessels). Adipocytes are a primary component in the breast cancer TME, driving enhanced tumor growth and progression through dynamic communication between tumor cells and adipocytes.

Cancer Treatment-Induced Inflammation

Cancer treatment-induced inflammation often develops in response to cancer treatments such as chemotherapy, radiotherapy, targeted biological therapies, and immunotherapies (see the section "Immunotherapy/Targeted Treatments"). Partial destruction of the tumor by these treatments results in the release of dead cell material that stimulates an inflammatory response, resembling normal tissue injury with subsequent wound healing and tissue repair. However, the recognition of the dying tumor cells also stimulates the production of cytokines and growth factors (such as tumor necrosis factor [TNF], epidermal growth factor [EGF], and interleukin-6 [IL-6]) by the cells of the TME. These growth factors then paradoxically serve as anti-cell death signals, which then decrease the effectiveness of the anticancer treatment (13). This has implications for the impact of treatment-related inflammation on exercise prescription, discussed in the section "Immunotherapy/Targeted Treatments."

INFLAMMATORY MARKERS AND CANCER PROGNOSIS

The definition of prognosis is "an expert prediction of the outcome based on an accurate diagnosis, knowledge of the natural history of the disease, the disease's response to treatment, and the progression of the disease in the patient in question" (14). Often predicting a cancer patient's outcome by investigating tumor size, histological grade, histological subtype, etc fails to accurately stratify low- and high-risk patients. Thus, the systemic inflammatory response in cancer has been well established in observational studies and systematic reviews as a prognosis tool. Over the past 30 years, markers such as C-reactive protein (CRP), albumin, neutrophil count, and lymphocyte count are measured as a means of predicting disease-free and overall survival rates in patients with cancer at all stages of disease (15).

THE IMMUNE SYSTEM AND CANCER

One phenomenon that has puzzled immunologists for a long time is how and why abnormal cancer cells manage to avoid destruction by the host's immune system. Theoretically, cancer cell proliferation and tumor development should be prevented by the body's innate and adaptive immune cells. Indeed, NK cells and macrophages, as part of **innate immunity**, are the first line of defense against malignant cells. These cells and adaptive immunity cells comprise the cancer immunosurveillance network that interacts with the highly immunogenic tumor cells present at the beginning of the carcinogenic process to eradicate the growing tumor and protect the host from tumor formation (16). The cancer immunoediting process is where the immune system either protects against cancer development or promotes growth of cancers capable of escaping immune control (elimination, equilibrium, escape). Although not completely understood, immune escape strategies include 1. sneaking through, 2. modulating tumor antigens, 3. masking tumor antigens, 4. inducing tolerance, 5. producing blocking antibodies, and 6. producing or expressing immunosuppressants (7). As the tumor develops, cancer cells evolve ways to mimic peripheral **immune tolerance** (the normal process that ensures that self-reactive T and B cells do not cause autoimmune diseases) and thus avoid being recognized and attacked. Checkpoint receptors on T cells such as programmed death-1 (PD-1) bind to the partner protein on the cancer cell, for example, programmed death ligand-1 (PD-L1) sends a switch-off signal to the T cells, thus preventing the immune system from destroying the cancer (Figure 7.7).

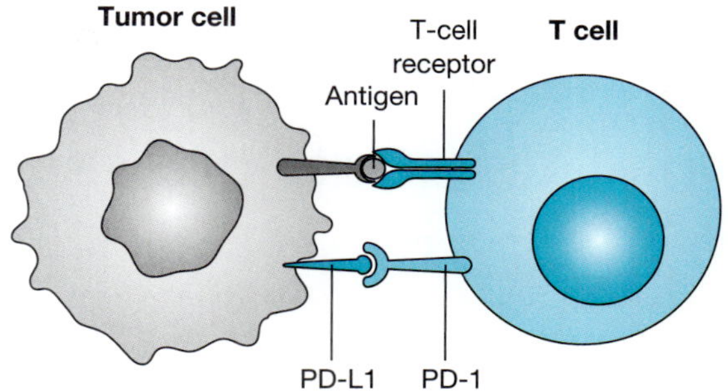

FIGURE 7.7. Immune checkpoint inhibitor (PD-1). Abbreviations: PD-1, programmed cell death-1; PD-L1, programmed death ligand-1.

In addition, the innate and adaptive immune response may increase tumor development by enabling the more aggressive tumor clones to survive and multiply. During the early stages of tumor development, cytotoxic immune cells, such as NK and $CD8^+$ T cells, recognize and eliminate more immunogenic cancer cells. This elimination ultimately results in the survival and proliferation of the less immunogenic cancer cell variants that are therefore less visible to immune detection. Recent cancer treatments, such as CAR

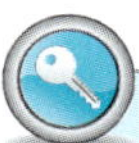

Innate immunity. Nonspecific general immune response that quickly forms the first line of defense in the immune response.

Immune tolerance. A state of unresponsiveness of the immune system to substances or tissue that have the capacity to elicit an immune response.

T-cell therapy and immunotherapy, have found ways to enable the immune system to re-recognize and destroy the tumor cells (see the section "Effect of Cancer Treatments on the Immune System").

NORMAL INFLAMMATORY AND IMMUNE RESPONSES TO EXERCISE

Before examining the effect of exercise on the immune and inflammatory responses in a cancer setting, it is important to briefly review the normal responses to exercise in healthy individuals.

Inflammatory Response to Acute Bout of Exercise

All structured physical activities that involve the contraction of skeletal muscles promote the synthesis and secretion of anti-inflammatory cytokines and peptides from fused myoblasts (myotubes)—mediators commonly termed *myokines.* A single bout of moderate-to-vigorous intensity aerobic exercise lasting 30 to 60 minutes in duration stimulates elevated plasma concentrations of muscle-derived IL-6, which subsequently initiates the secretion of the IL-1 receptor agonist and IL-10 from monocytes and lymphocytes respectively. This promotes a range of benefits in vascular reactivity, lipid and glucose metabolism, and the suppression of pro-inflammatory cytokines (17) (Box 7.1 and Figure 7.8).

The magnitude of change in these mediators of inflammation depends on the overall exercise workload. During a single bout of exercise as the IL-6 levels increase, the levels of the pro-inflammatory mediators IL-1b and TNF-α remain suppressed. Furthermore, there is a decrease in the pro-inflammatory subtype 1 (M1) macrophages resident in the muscle and an increase in the anti-inflammatory subtype 2 (M2) macrophages in response to the exercise. Overall, these observations suggest that exercise acutely promotes an anti-inflammatory environment within the body.

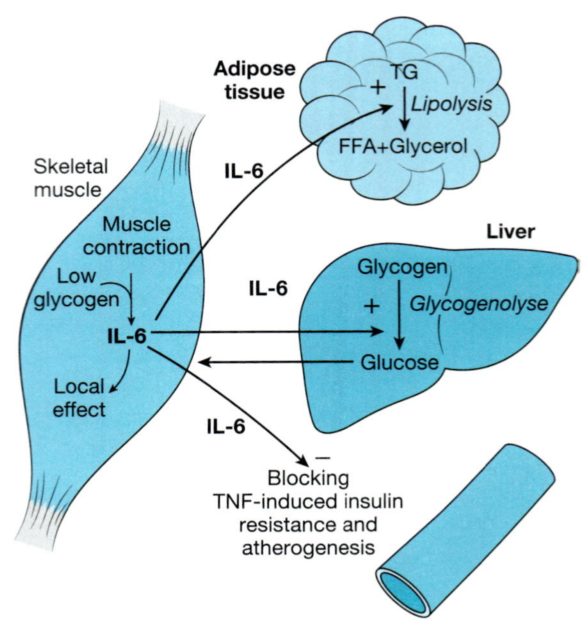

FIGURE 7.8. Schematic presentation of the possible biological effects of muscle-derived IL-6. Abbreviations: TG, triglyceride; FFA, free fatty acid. (Redrawn from Pedersen BK, Steensberg A, Schjerling P. Muscle-derived interleukin-6: possible biological effects. *J Physiol.* 2001;536(2):329–37. Available from https://physoc.onlinelibrary.wiley.com/doi/full/10.1111/j.1469-7793.2001.0329c.xd?sid=nlm%3Apubmed.)

Box 7.1 Results of Acute Exercise Bout and Release of IL-6

- increased intramuscular glucose uptake and the translocation of GLUT4 to the sarcolemma (38);
- activation of AMPK (50 AMP-activated protein kinase) signaling and downstream alterations in cellular metabolism (39);
- increased hepatic glucose production and output (40);
- induction of lipolysis and fatty acid oxidation in adipose tissue (41);
- initiates the secretion of cytokines IL-8, IL-10, IL-18, IL-1 receptor antagonist (IL-1ra), G-CSF, and monocyte chemoattractant protein 1 from monocytes and lymphocytes.

Data from Petersen AM, Pedersen BK. The anti-inflammatory effect of exercise. *J Appl Physiol (1985).* 2005;98(4):1154–62.

Inflammatory Response to a Prolonged Period of Exercise Training

Evidence from epidemiological observational studies suggests that regular exercise has an overall anti-inflammatory effect mediated through various pathways, such as the improved control of pro-inflammatory signaling pathways, release of muscle myokines that stimulate the production of IL-1ra and IL-10, a decrease in dysfunctional adipose tissue and pro-inflammatory adipokine secretion, and an enhanced innate immune function (18). High levels of physical activity are associated with 20% to 60% reduced levels of peripheral inflammatory mediators compared with a sedentary lifestyle. This effect is independent of age, sex, and obesity as measured by BMI or blood glucose (19). Systematic reviews, for example, in postmenopausal women (20) or older adults (21) demonstrate that regular exercise lowers the circulating levels of the inflammatory mediators CRP, IL-6, and TNF-α.

Box 7.2 The Alpha Study: Effect of Exercise on Inflammatory Markers in Postmenopausal Women at a Higher Risk of Breast Cancer

The Alberta Physical Activity and Breast Cancer Prevention Trial (ALPHA trial) randomized 320 inactive postmenopausal women to either 1 year of moderate-to-vigorous aerobic exercise or usual inactivity. Baseline, 6-month, and 12-month serum was analyzed for CRP, IL-6, and TNF-α. Statistically significant differences in CRP levels were observed over 12 months for exercisers versus controls but not in IL-6 or TNF-α. A statistically significant trend of decreasing CRP with increasing exercise adherence and stronger intervention effects on CRP in women with higher baseline physical fitness were found. The intervention effect on CRP seemed to be mediated by fat loss. Subanalysis suggested that IL-6 decreases were greater in women with higher baseline BMI, which in turn correlated significantly with body fat changes during the trial.

This group followed the ALPHA trial with the BETA trial which examined whether high volume of exercise decreased inflammatory biomarkers, associated with postmenopausal breast cancer risk, more than a moderate volume of exercise. It was 2-armed randomized trial in 400 inactive, healthy, postmenopausal women, aged 50 to 74 years, with a BMI of 22 to 40 kg/m^2. Participants were randomized to high (300 minutes per week) or moderate (150 minutes per week) volumes of aerobic exercise while maintaining usual diet. Fasting blood concentrations of CRP, IL6, and TNF-α were measured at baseline 6 and 12 months. Analyses of 386 (97%) participants showed prescribing 300 minutes per week of moderate-to-vigorous aerobic exercise did *not* improve inflammatory markers compared with 150 minutes per week in postmenopausal women. In further analysis, it was observed that CRP decreased by 22.45% for those participants who exercised >246 minutes per week (highest quintile) and increased by 0.07% for those who exercised <110 minutes per week.

Data from Friedenreich CM, Neilson HK, Woolcott CG, et al. Inflammatory marker changes in a yearlong randomized exercise intervention trial among postmenopausal women. *Cancer Prev Res (Phila).* 2012;5(1):98–108; Friedenreich CM, Neilson HK, O'Reilly R, et al. Effects of a high vs moderate volume of aerobic exercise on adiposity outcomes in postmenopausal women: a randomized clinical trial. *JAMA Oncol.* 2015;1(6):766–76.

An example of 2 related relevant RCTs that examined the effect of a year-long intervention on inflammatory markers on postmenopausal women at a high risk of breast cancer is outlined in Box 7.2.

Cellular Immune Response to Exercise

Acute moderate-intensity exercise results in a 10-fold mobilization of NK cells and a 2.5-fold increase in CD8$^+$ T lymphocytes. Exercise-induced mobilization of NK cells is a very rapid phenomenon and occurs within minutes of undertaking moderate-to-vigorous intensity activity. The maximum level of circulating NK cells is reached within 30 minutes of endurance exercise, and then no further increases in NK cells numbers are observed (22). A single session of exercise of climbing 10 flights of stairs in a young healthy cohort showed an increased cytotoxic activity of T cells toward the tumor antigens (22). In a study comparing older adults (aged 55-79 years), who were either sedentary or master athletes (men with the ability to cycle 100 km in 6.5 hours or women with the ability to cycle 60 km in 5.5 hours), the master athletes had higher numbers of naive CD4$^+$ T cells compared to the sedentary older adult suggestive of improved T-cell functions. Also, the immune composition of T cells for master athletes was similar to those of young (aged 20–36 years) healthy adults (23). These findings suggest that both single exercise sessions and prolonged exercise training could improve clinically relevant NK- and T-cell functions and promote treatments such as T-cell adoptive therapy described in Section 10.

Within approximately 15 minutes after the exercise, there is a dramatic decrease in the frequency of NK- and CD8$^+$ T cells in the bloodstream and they return to resting levels. This is caused by the redistribution of the NK cells from the bloodstream into the peripheral tissue to conduct **immune surveillance**, that is, to identify and eradicate infected cells or cells that have become damaged or malignant. This process is termed the acute stress/exercise immune-enhancement hypothesis. An important study by Kruger and colleagues (24) using fluorescent cell tracking in rodents found that following a single bout of exercise, T cells are indeed redeployed in large numbers to peripheral tissues, including the gut, lungs, and bone marrow.

In healthy humans, an exercise session on a treadmill at 80% of VO_2 max until exhaustion results in a rapid redistribution of NK cells and killer T cells presumably among various organs. Each bout of moderate-intensity exercise promotes a transient immunosurveillance response that, when repeated on a regular basis, dampens systemic inflammation (Figure 7.9).

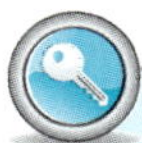

Immune Surveillance. The monitoring process by which cells of the immune system detect and destroy premalignant or malignant cells in the body.

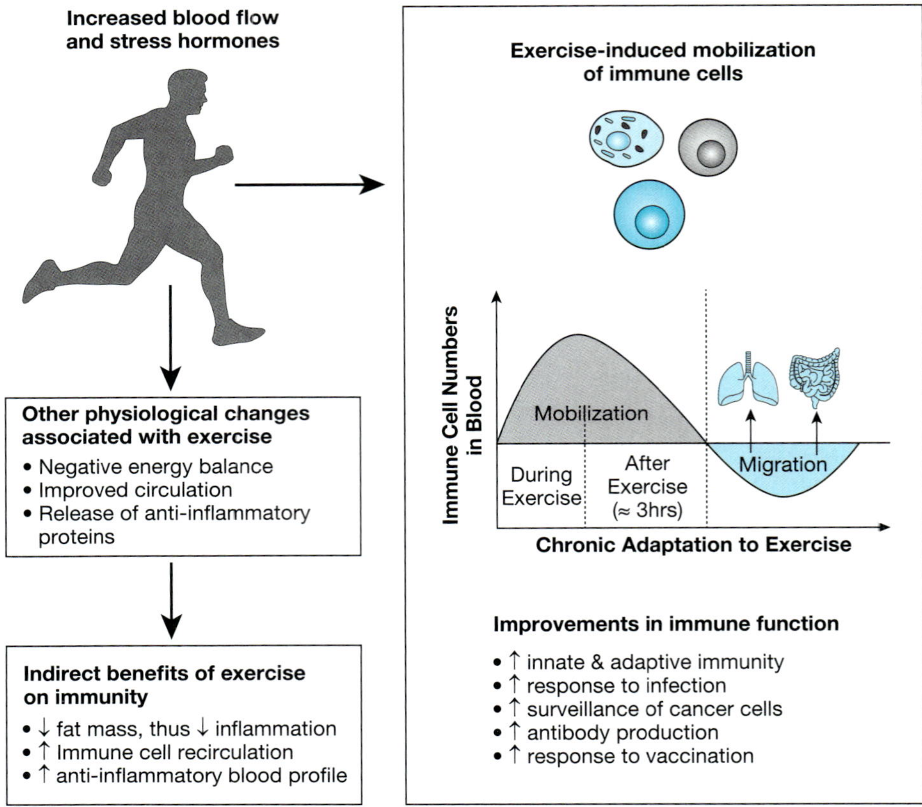

FIGURE 7.9. Mobilization and migration of immune cells with exercise.

IMPACT OF EXERCISE ON THE INFLAMMATORY AND IMMUNE RESPONSES IN CANCER SURVIVORS

In sections 4, 5 and 6 described how cancer cells and the TME influence immune and inflammatory responses and vice versa. In addition, the section "Normal Inflammatory and Immune Responses to Exercise" has explored the positive effect exercise has on the immune system and inflammation in healthy individuals. This section will now examine the evidence on the effect of exercise on the inflammatory and immune functions in the cancer setting.

To date, most of the research in this area has been preclinical studies conducted in mice and rats bearing tumor grafts or in genetically engineered mouse models of breast and prostate cancers. In these studies, it has been shown that a bout of exercise does provides beneficial antitumor immune responses, such as the infiltration of NK cells and T lymphocytes into the TME. Exercise also induces a favorable switch in the tumors of the exercising mice to include macrophages that respond and kill tumor cells (M1) rather than to the usual M2 phenotype of macrophages that are immune suppressive and support tumor progression. Similarly, habitual exercise results in an increased tumor density of NK cells and the increased infiltration and activation of CD8$^+$ T cells, which also contributes to tumor suppression (25) (Figure 7.10).

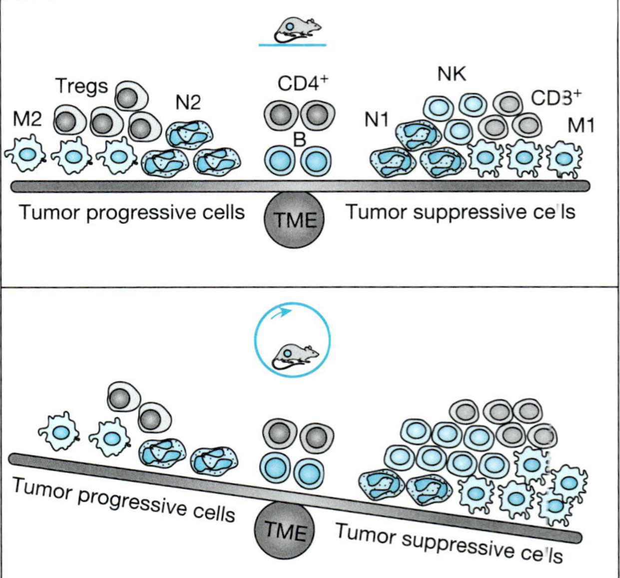

FIGURE 7.10. Exercise is shown to enhance infiltration of tumor-suppressive immune cells and to reduce infiltration of tumor-progressive immune cells, preventing tumor growth. Abbreviations: TME tumor microenvironment; M2, macrophages type 2; Tregs, regulatory T lymphocytes; N2, neutrophils type 2; CD4$^+$, T helper lymphocytes; B, B lymphocytes; N1, neutrophils type 1; NK, natural killer cells; CD8$^+$, cytotoxic T lymphocytes; M1, macrophages type 1. (From Spiliopoulou P, Gavriatopoulou M, Kastritis E, Dimopoulos MA, Terzis G. Exercise-induced changes in tumor growth via tumor immunity. *Sports.* 2021;9(4):46. https://doi.org/10.3390/sports9040046.)

Recent studies are now showing similar positive effects of exercise on the inflammation and the immune system observed in humans. A recent review and meta-analysis of 27 studies concluded that exercise training decreases circulating pro-inflammatory markers, notably CRP and TNF in cancer survivors (26). Prostate and breast cancer survivors experienced the greater training-induced reductions in pro-inflammatory markers than the other cancer types analyzed. Combined aerobic and resistance exercise was the most widely studied training modality and was associated with the largest reductions in the concentration levels of the pro-inflammatory marker. Exercise training did not statistically change circulating anti-inflammatory cytokines or immune cell markers, although overall trends were positive for both groups of markers. Regular participation in a combination of resistance training and aerobic training in prostate and breast cancer survivors, therefore, appears to be associated with a decrease in low-grade inflammation with the implications for anti-inflammatory function still being unclear.

A specific review by Schauer and colleagues (27) on the role of exercise in the management of neutropenia during chemotherapy concluded that the evidence is weak. Some initial findings suggest a clinical improvement in the incidence or duration of neutropenia for participants randomized to the exercise intervention during chemotherapy, but none of the studies were designed to directly address this question. Some of the data from the larger trials in the review indicated that this prevention of neutropenia could potentially result in an increase of the tolerability and adherence to chemotherapy. However, a recent systematic review of 8 exercise trials including 1,044 individuals with cancer found that exercise was associated with a higher chemotherapy completion rate in only 2 studies with no differences observed in the remaining 6 trials (28). See Figures 7.11 and 7.12.

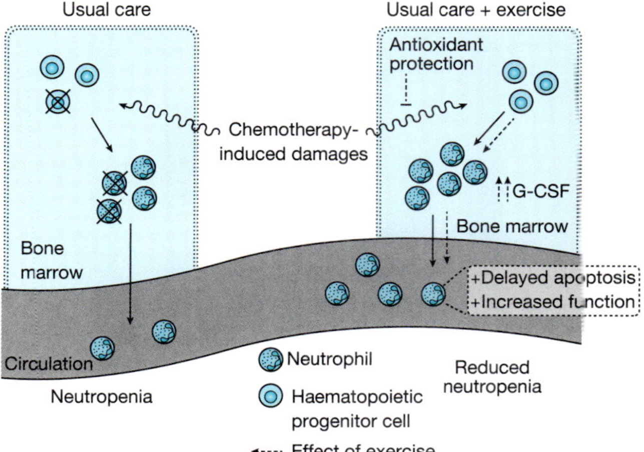

FIGURE 7.11. Proposed mechanisms of exercise modulating chemotherapy induced neutropenia. Abbreviation: G-CSF, granulocyte colony-stimulating factor. (Redrawn from Schauer T, Hojman P, Gehl J, Christensen JF. Exercise training as prophylactic strategy in the management of neutropenia during chemotherapy. *Br J Pharmacol.* 2022;179(12):2925–37. doi:10.1111/bph.15141, Figure 3.)

These recent promising studies suggest that exercise has the potential to boost the immune system and inflammatory reactions and assist in positive antitumor responses during and after cancer treatments.

EFFECT OF CANCER TREATMENTS ON THE IMMUNE SYSTEM

Cancers such as leukemia and lymphoma directly result in a weakened immune system as the tumor cells are derived from the immune cells of bone marrow and the lymphatic system.

Effect of Cancer Treatments on Innate Immunity

Cancer treatments may overcome and damage a cancer patient's innate immunity (29) as follows:

- Chemotherapy given intravenously in the arm or a wound from surgery may break the skin barrier, resulting in an infection.
- A catheter into the bladder can become a route for bacteria to get inside the bladder and cause infection.
- Antacids for heartburn may neutralize the stomach acid that kills bacteria.
- Chemotherapy can reduce the protective hair and immune cells around the nasal and mucosal cavities, making it harder to fight infections.
- Radiotherapy to the lung can damage the hairs and mucus producing cells in the lung that help to remove bacteria, resulting in conditions like pneumonia.

Effect of Chemotherapy on the Immune System

Chemotherapy treatments have a profound impact on the immune system. Some chemotherapeutic drugs (eg, anthracyclines) break the immunosuppressive barrier and direct the immune system toward tumor-cell death. On the other hand, most chemotherapeutic drugs target fast proliferating cells and therefore affect healthy as well as cancerous cells, which results in substantially depleted immune cell numbers that leave the immune system in a weak state. Neutrophils have a short half-life and a high turnover rate; therefore, they are very susceptible to bone marrow suppression by a wide range of chemotherapy regimens; *neutropenia* is one of the most common side effects. Chemotherapy reduces the production of neutrophils and RBCs by the bone marrow, and patients are particularly at risk of getting an infection 7 to 14 days after receiving chemotherapy, when the levels of neutrophils and RBCs are at their lowest. This time is called

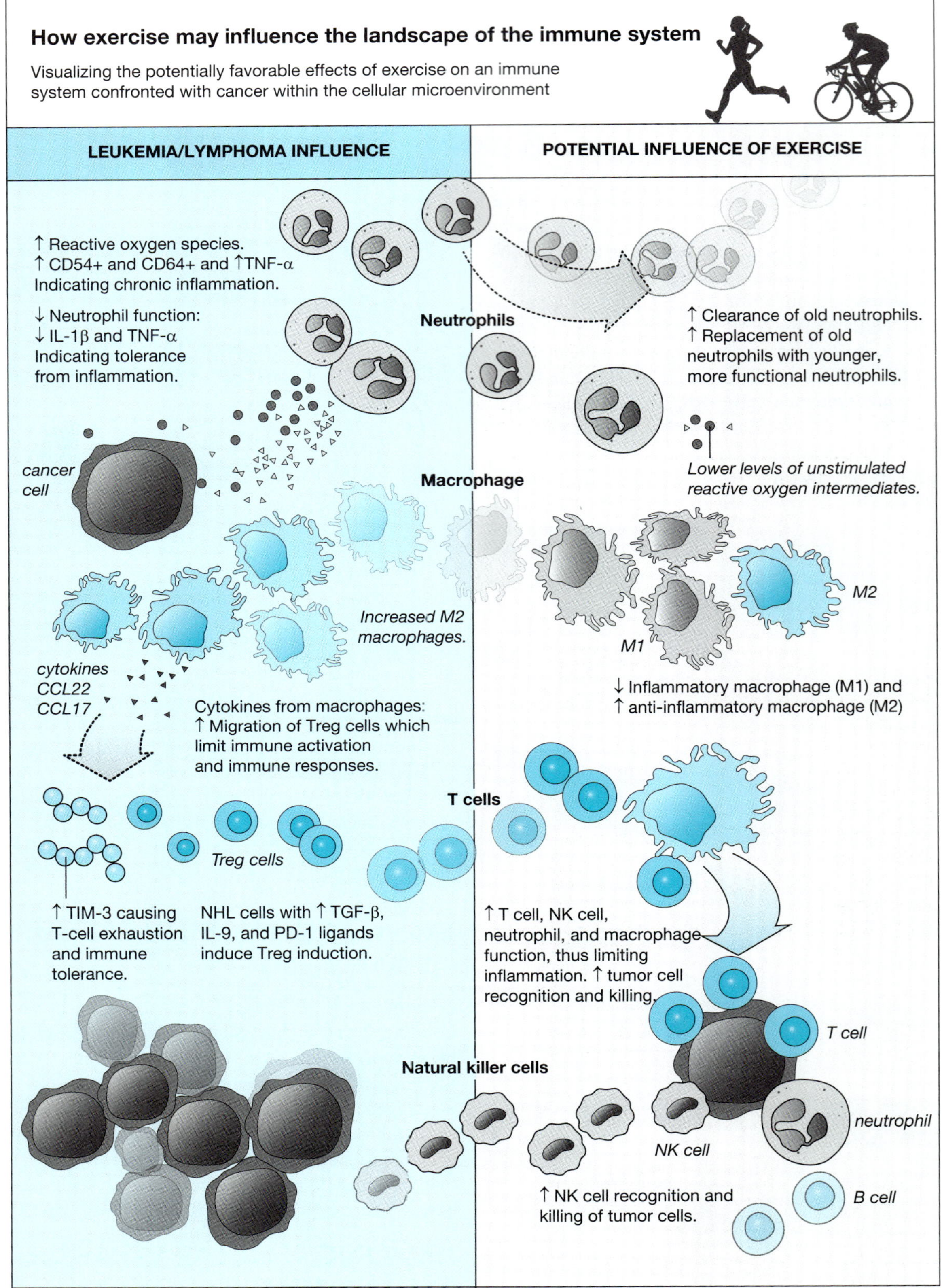

FIGURE 7.12. Potential positive effects of exercise within the cellular environment of an immune system challenged with cancer. Denotations and abbreviations: ↑, increased; ↓, decreased; PD-1, programmed cell death protein 1; TGF-β, transforming growth factor-β; TNF, tumor necrosis factor. (Redrawn from Sitlinger A, Brander DM, Bartlett DB. Impact of exercise on the immune system and outcomes in hematologic malignancies. *Blood Adv.* 2020;4(8):1801–11. https://doi.org/10.1182/bloodadvances.2019001317.)

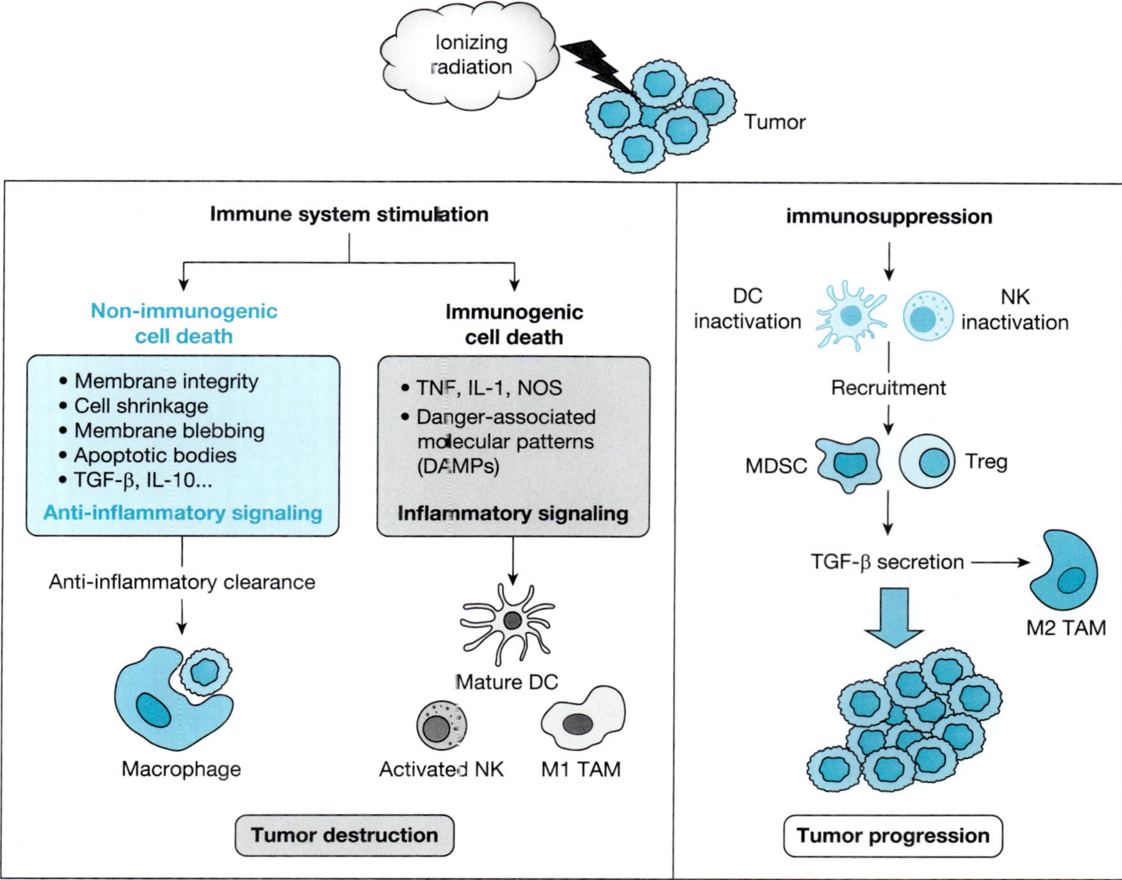

FIGURE 7.13. The effects of ionizing radiation on the immune system. Either stimulation or suppression of the immune system occurs. Stressed cells may simply undergo anti-inflammatory clearance, resulting in nonimmunogenic cell death or trigger inflammatory signaling that will release (DAMPs) with the activation of dendritic cells that initiate cytotoxic T-cell responses against tumor cells. On the other hand, the inactivation of these cells (DCs and cytotoxic T cells) with the recruitment of MDSCs and T-regulator lymphocytes and the secretion of TGF-β leads to the modification of the macrophage phenotype from a pro-inflammatory type M1 to an immunosuppressive type M2 that may allow tumor growth and progression. Abbreviations: TGF-β, tumor growth factor-β; IL, interleukin; RT, radiotherapy; HSP, heat shock proteins; HMGB1, high mobility group box 1 molecules; ATP, adenosine-5-triphosphate; TNF, tumor necrosis factor; NOS, nitrogen reactive species; DC, dendritic cells; NK, natural killer; MDSC, myeloid derived suppressor cells; Treg, T regulator lymphocyte; TAM, tumor-associated macrophages. (From Carvalho HA, Villar RC. Radiotherapy and immune response: the systemic effects of a local treatment. *Clinics (Sao Paulo).* 2018;73(suppl 1):e557s. doi:10.6061/clinics/2018/e557s. Copyright © 2018 CLINICS.)

the *nadir*, when it is important to take special care to avoid infections (30).

Effect of Radiation Therapy on the Immune System

Radiation therapy can negatively affect the immune system if the bone marrow is being directly irradiated. Radiation at other sites results in either stimulation or suppression of the immune system. Radiated tumor cells may undergo anti-inflammatory clearance, resulting in tumor-cell death, or radiation results in the inactivation of cytotoxic T cells and the modification of the macrophage phenotype from a pro-inflammatory type M1 to an immunosuppressive type M2 that ultimately enables the tumor growth and progression (31). See Figure 7.13.

Effect of High-Dose Steroids on the Immune System

Steroids dampen the inflammatory response and are immunosuppressive, causing the impairment of killer T-cell activation and the promotion of M2 macrophages. This can result in an increased risk of infections (32).

IMMUNOTHERAPY/TARGETED TREATMENTS

There are several cancer treatments that fall into the category of immunotherapy or targeted therapies and use the immune system to find and kill cancer cells.

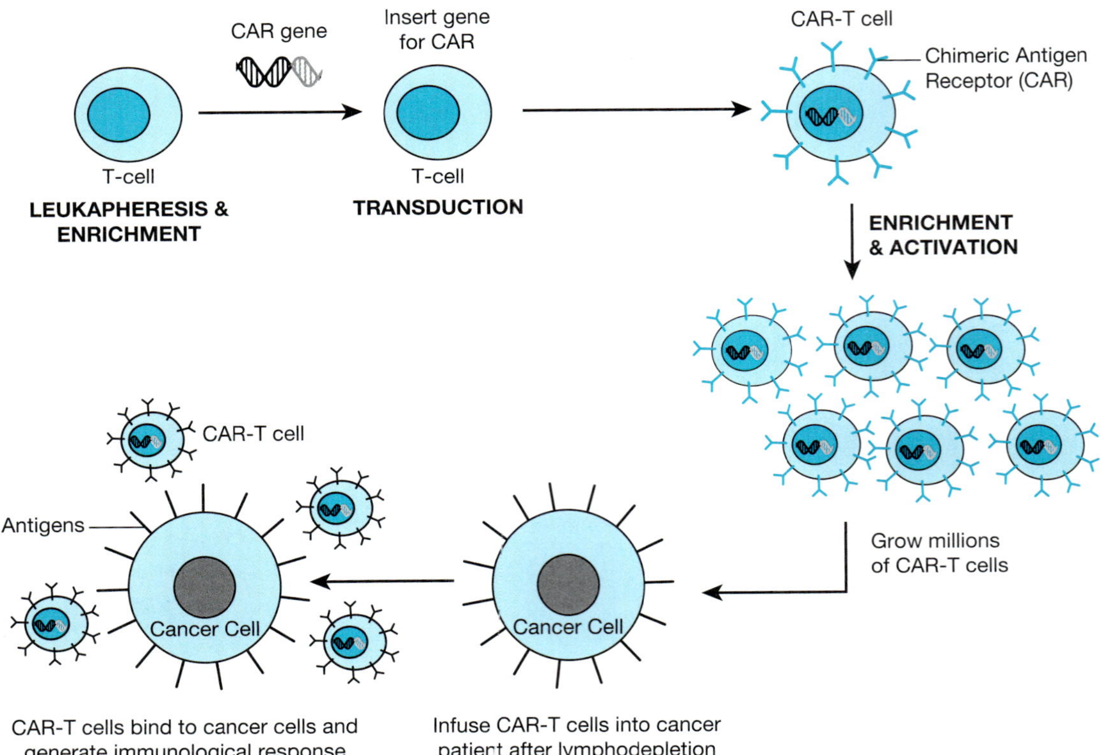

FIGURE 7.14. CAR-T cells-based immunotherapy against cancer cells. Abbreviation: CAR-T cells, chimeric antigen receptor T-cells.

Monoclonal Antibodies

MABs recognize and attack-specific protein receptors on the cancer cell surface. Some MABs work by antibody-dependent cell-mediated cytotoxicity, whereas others have drugs or radioactive substances attached to them.

Other MABs target proteins on cells of the immune system. This type of immunotherapy is called checkpoint inhibitors. Checkpoint inhibitors block the proteins on the cancer cells that have been stopping the immune system from attacking cancer cells. Checkpoint inhibitors block different proteins including:

- CTLA-4 (cytotoxic T-lymphocyte associated protein 4)
- PD-1 (programmed cell death protein-1)
- PD-L1 (programmed death ligand-1)

Some MABs stop growth factor receptors on cancer cells from working properly, either by directly blocking the receptor or binding to the signal protein. Some MABs block vascular endothelial growth factor from attaching to the receptors on the cells that line the blood vessels. These MABs are called antiangiogenic drugs (33).

Adoptive Cell Transfer

CARs are engineered synthetic receptors that function to redirect T-cell lymphocytes to recognize and eliminate cells expressing a specific target antigen (34). T cells are extracted from the patient's blood by apheresis. These T cells are then genetically engineered to produce a CAR on the T-cell surface that can recognize and target a specific protein on the cancer cells. The T cell is now a CAR-T cell that is infused back into the patient's bloodstream. The CAR binds to the target antigens expressed on the cell surface, resulting in vigorous T-cell activation and powerful antitumor responses. CAR T-cell therapy is currently mostly available for leukemia and lymphoma cancer patients. The success of anti-CD19 CAR T-cell therapy against B-cell malignancies resulted in its approval by the U.S. FDA in 2017. See Figure 7.14. The next potential generation of cellular immunotherapy is CAR-NK cells - incorporating chimeric antigen receptors into natural killer cells and harness their innate cytotoxic potential towards malignancies.

Vaccines

There are vaccines that can prevent healthy people from getting certain cancers caused by viruses. The most common is the HPV vaccine first licensed by the FDA in 2006 and recommended for use in females between the ages of 9 and 26 years for the prevention of cervical cancer along with various other HPV-associated cancers (eg, vaginal cancers, vulvar cancers, anal cancers, and HPV-induced oral cancers). Another example of a preventive vaccine is the HBV vaccine that protects against chronic hepatitis B infection that significantly increases the risk of hepatocellular carcinoma (35). There are also therapeutic vaccines that treat existing cancer, as was described in section 2a, with bacillus Calmette-Guérin (BCG) to activate the immune system in early-stage bladder cancer. Cancer-specific therapeutic vacccines are also in various stages of development e.g some glioblastoma tumour vaccine designs and strategies holds promise as a complementary therapy to standard care.

Cytokines

Cytokines are not used very often now as there are more effective immunotherapy drugs, but sometimes interferon 1 and interleukin 2 are used for some cancer types including:

- kidney cancer (renal cell cancer)
- some types of leukemia
- skin (cutaneous) lymphoma (36)

EXERCISE PRECAUTIONS WITH PATIENTS WHO HAVE CANCER AND A COMPROMISED IMMUNE SYSTEM BECAUSE OF TREATMENT

As outlined in Chapter 4 and above, cancer treatments can negatively affect the immune system and mediators of inflammation. Often during chemotherapy and targeted therapy treatments and with hematological cancers, the patient's immune system is compromised. Therefore, it is important to ensure that there is no exposure to any potential viral or bacterial infections during these cancer treatments. This does not mean that the patient cannot exercise but that they need to ensure no further stress to the immune system by ensuring that activities are of a low-to-moderate intensity and undertaken in a clean environment. Patients should be especially vigilant about neutropenia, a condition characterized by an abnormally low level of neutrophils. Clinically, neutropenia is defined as an absolute neutrophil count (ANC) in the blood below 1.5×10^9 cells per liter, and sometimes this is manifested by the patient as severe fatigue (Box 7.3). During neutropenia, patients are at a higher risk of infections or febrile neutropenia (37). Febrile neutropenia is described as an ANC in the blood below 0.5×10^9 cells per liter (ANC 500) with an oral temperature >38.5 °C or 2 readings of >38 °C for 2 hours.

Box 7.3 Signs and Symptoms of Febrile Neutropenia[a]

- A fever with a temperature of 100.5 °F (38 °C) or higher
- Chills or sweating
- Sore throat, sores in the mouth, or a toothache
- Any redness, swelling, or pain (especially around a cut, wound, or catheter)
- A cough or shortness of breath
- Abdominal pain
- Pain near the anus
- Pain or burning when urinating, or urinating often
- Diarrhea or sores around the anus
- Unusual vaginal discharge or itching

[a]All symptoms are not necessary for the diagnosis of febrile neutropenia.
From Conquer Cancer® The ASCO Foundation © 2005–2023 American Society of Clinical Oncology (ASCO). All rights reserved worldwide. Available from https://www.cancer.net/coping-with-cancer/physical-emotional-and-social-effects-cancer/managing-physical-side-effects/neutropenia.

Febrile neutropenia occurs in almost one-third of cancer patients throughout the treatment trajectory. Infections in combination with a weakened immune system can cause prolonged hospitalization periods and an increased mortality risk. Neutropenia is also considered a key determining factor for deciding whether patients will experience chemotherapy dose delays and dose reductions. In some patients, neutropenia is also associated with low platelet and RBC counts, and there is an increased risk of bruising and fatigue. A fever may be the first sign of neutropenia and must be considered an emergency. Although the evidence suggests that exercise may reduce the risk of neutropenia, if a patient is neutropenic, there are no specific guidelines concerning how much exercise can be undertaken. However, because of the increased risk of infection, patients should follow strict infection control guidelines; this includes that patients and instructors should wear face masks, maintain regular hand hygiene and sanitization of equipment, and patients should be treated inside their home instead of in communal areas. Neutropenia is typically managed by chemotherapy dose modification, dose interval delays, and/or initiation of primary prophylaxis with G-CSF.

SUMMARY

The links between inflammation, immunity, and exercise as relate to cancer are explained. The 2 types of inflammation (acute and resolving or chronic and cancer-promoting) are described, and the role of the immune system's innate and adaptive components in eliminating threats is discussed. Inflammation and immune functions are shown to influence cancer initiation, progression, and treatment. Chronic inflammation precedes approximately 15% to 20% of cancers. The TME can also induce inflammation and suppresses immune function, which results in increased cancer growth. New immunotherapies, such as CAR T-cell therapy, have been developed to counter the ability of cancer cells to evade immunity. In cancer survivors, exercise has been shown to lower some inflammatory markers, but it is still unclear what effect exercise has on the immune system. Chemotherapy can affect the immune system by causing neutropenia, which increases infection risk. With treatment-compromised immunity, patients should avoid infection risks but can still exercise at low intensity. Overall, with respect to cancer, exercise has a positive effect on immunity and inflammation, but precautions are needed with a compromised immune system.

Case Study

Christine is a self-employed physiotherapist and had been active most of her life with her main activities in her spare time being running and cycling. When she was 56, Christine was diagnosed with a low-grade follicular non-Hodgkin's lymphoma and was told that she would probably need little or no treatment for months or possibly years. She continued with her running and cycling, but after 2 years of active surveillance of her lymphoma, Christine, now aged 58, complained of bone pain, muscle weakness, and profound fatigue, which not only affected her ability to exercise but also her ability to work. A PET scan and a bone marrow biopsy showed that the cancer had developed into DLBCL. As she now had a high-risk disease, over the next 18 months, she was treated with different chemoimmunotherapy regimes consisting of different chemotherapy drugs, a steroid, and a targeted immunotherapy drug called rituximab.

Rituximab is an MAB that targets a cell receptor protein called CD20 that is found on the surface of B cells. Rituximab locks on to the CD20 receptor on the malignant B cells, then it triggers the body's immune system to attack the cells and destroy them. Rituximab destroys both abnormal and normal B cells. Once treatment is over, the body can replace the normal B cells. Christine had 6 cycles of R-CHOP (rituximab, cyclophosphamide, doxorubicin hydrochloride, vincristine, and prednisolone), R-CODOX-M (rituximab, cyclophosphamide, vincristine, doxorubicin, and methotrexate), followed by R-IVAC (rituximab, ifosfamide, etoposide, and cytarabine). During this treatment phase, Christine experienced 2 episodes of grade 4 neutropenia (neutrophil count $<0.5 \times 10^9$ per liter), the first of which progressed to febrile neutropenia and resulted in Christine spending 14 days in the hospital. Also, she suffered from mucositis often during chemotherapy treatment, making it difficult to eat. Christine continued to work part-time and still remained active by walking for 10 to 20 minutes most days apart from the nadir phase of her treatment.

At the end of the treatment regime, tests showed that Christine still had progressive disease. Autologous stem cell transplant was not possible, so she was offered either allogeneic stem cell therapy or CAR T-cell therapy. Christine was apprehensive about going for the allogeneic transplant because of the potential toxicities, but more so because it would mean a full year without income. So, she decided to go for the CAR-T treatment. In patients with lymphoma like Christine, over 80% of patients respond to this therapy, with over 50% of patients achieving a complete response. At an average of 6-month follow-up, about one-third of patients remain in remission. CAR-T treatment does have some potentially serious side effects caused by cytokine release syndrome and neurotoxicity. These toxicities, however, are manageable and fully reversible in most patients and typically resolve within the first 2 weeks following CAR T-cell infusion.

Christine tolerated her CAR T-cell infusion remarkably well apart for a few days of fever. Within 4 weeks, her PET scan showed that she had achieved a complete response, and by 6 weeks, she was back at work in her clinic. She is now 1 year from her infusion, and her scans show an ongoing remission; she feels better than ever, and her family, friends, and clients are all thrilled to have her back. She is now back on her bike and running about 5 miles twice a week.

Questions

1. What are the potential benefits of exercising during treatment to Christine's immune system and to her inflammatory response?
2. Why was Christine given rituximab?
3. Christine had neutropenia: What is neutropenia?
4. What would be the signs or symptoms that Christine had febrile neutropenia?
5. Can Christine now get back to exercising as prediagnosis?

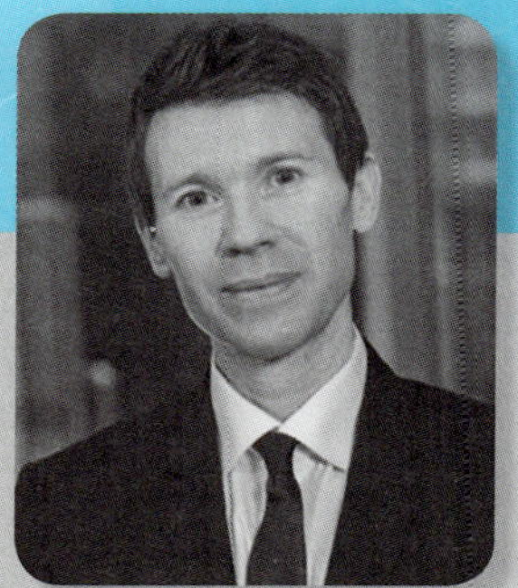

Meet the Expert

FEATURED PROFESSIONAL

Lee W. Jones, PhD

Member, Attending Physiologist
Division of Solid Tumor Oncology, Department of Medicine
Memorial Sloan Kettering Cancer Center
New York, NY

Q: "Where did you grow up?"

In the northwest of England in a city called Stoke-on-Trent (in between Birmingham and Manchester).

Q: "Where did you train? What is your training?"

I got my PhD in Physical Education (Exercise Psychology) from the University of Alberta (Canada) in the lab of Kerry Courneya. I also did a 2-year Postdoctoral Fellowship with Kerry.

Q: "What are you best known for?"

Not really sure, to be honest! My early work with Kerry was in the area of exercise promotion, specifically the role of the oncologist to promote exercise in cancer patients. I then started some work in the area of the physiological consequences of cancer therapy and the role of exercise to mitigate such effects. My recent work focuses on exercise to suppress cancer pathogenesis.

Q: "What are you currently working on?"

Trying to understand if exercise suppresses cancer growth and progression, and if so, what is the most appropriate dose, which patients/tumors response the best, and how it works mechanistically.

Q: "Anything else you want to include?"

Only that we've only started to scratch the surface on our understanding of how exercise might impact cancer and its treatment.

Favorite Quote:

"Inspiration exists, but it has to find you working."
—*Pablo Picasso*

STUDY QUESTIONS

1. Which one of the following is a characteristic of acute inflammation?
   a. Lasts for months or years
   b. Low-grade response
   c. Caused by trauma
   d. Mediated by macrophages, lymphocytes, and plasma cells
2. Which group below make up the innate immune system?
   a. T cells and B cells
   b. Macrophages and neutrophils
   c. Plasma cells and lymphocytes
   d. Natural killer cells and cytokines
3. What percentage of cancers can be linked to preceding chronic infections at the site of the cancer?
   a. 5 to 10
   b. 15 to 20
   c. 25 to 30
   d. 35 to 40
4. Which inflammatory marker is used to predict cancer prognosis?
   a. C-reactive protein
   b. IL-6
   c. Natural killer (NK) cells
   d. IgG
5. How do cancer cells avoid immune destruction?
   a. By immunosuppression
   b. Through inflammatory clearance
   c. Via peripheral tolerance
   d. By macrophage apoptosis
6. Studies with cancer survivors show that exercise training decreases with circulating cytokines?
   a. IL-6 and TNF-α
   b. CRP and TNF-α
   c. CRP and IL-6
   d. None of the above
7. How does chemotherapy affect the immune system?
   a. Stimulates neutrophil production
   b. Promotes NK cell cytotoxicity
   c. Causes bone marrow suppression
   d. Enhances B cell proliferation

8. CAR T-cell therapy involves:
   a. Radiation treatment
   b. Growth factor inhibitors
   c. Engineered T-cell receptors
   d. Antibody deletion
9. What is an example of a preventive anticancer vaccine?
   a. BCG
   b. Interferon
   c. HBV vaccine
   d. Rituximab
10. Exercise precautions in immunocompromised patients include:
   a. Avoiding infection exposures
   b. Including high-intensity activities
   c. Exercising only in communal areas
   d. No exercise restrictions

REFERENCES

1. Scott A, Khan KM, Cook JL, Duronio V. What is "inflammation"? Are we ready to move beyond Celsus? *Br J Sports Med.* 2004;38(3):248–9.
2. Kushner A. The phenomenon of the acute phase response. *Ann N Y Acad Sci.* 1982;389:39–48.
3. Korniluk A, Koper O, Kemona H, Dymicka-Piekarska V. From inflammation to cancer. *Ir J Med Sci.* 2017;186(1):57–62.
4. Furman D, Campisi J, Verdin E, et al. Chronic inflammation in the etiology of disease across the life span. *Nat Med.* 2019;25(12):1822–32.
5. Michels N, van Aart C, Morisse J, Mullee A, Huybrechts I. Chronic inflammation towards cancer incidence: a systematic review and meta-analysis of epidemiological studies. *Crit Rev Oncol Hematol.* 2021;157:103177.
6. Guven DC, Sahin TK, Erul E, Kilickap S, Gambichler T, Aksoy S. The association between the pan-immune-inflammation value and cancer prognosis: a systematic review and meta-analysis. *Cancers (Basel).* 2022;14(11):2675.
7. Adam JK, Odhav B, Bhoola KD. Immune responses in cancer. *Pharmacol Ther.* 2003;99(1):113–32.
8. Rich RR, Chaplin DD. The human immune response. *Clin Immunol.* 2019:3–17.e1.
9. Aggarwal BB, Vijayalekshmi RV, Sung B. Targeting inflammatory pathways for prevention and therapy of cancer: short-term friend, long-term foe. *Clin Cancer Res.* 2009;15(2):425–30.
10. Greten FR, Grivennikov SI. Inflammation and cancer: triggers, mechanisms, and consequences. *Immunity.* 2019;51(1):27–41.
11. Benavente S, Sanchez-Garcia A, Naches S, ME LL, Lorente J. Therapy-induced modulation of the tumor microenvironment: new opportunities for cancer therapies. *Front Oncol.* 2020;10:582884.
12. Iyengar NM, Gucalp A, Dannenberg AJ, Hudis CA. Obesity and cancer mechanisms: tumor microenvironment and inflammation. *J Clin Oncol.* 2016;34(35):4270–6.
13. Zhao H, Wu L, Yan G, et al. Inflammation and tumor progression: signaling pathways and targeted intervention. *Signal Transduct Target Ther.* 2021;6(1):263.
14. Mackillop WJ. The importance of prognosis in cancer medicine. *TNM Online.* [Wiley online]. New York (NY): John Wiley & Sons; 2006. https://onlinelibrary.wiley.com/doi/full/10.1002/0471463736.tnmp01.pub2
15. Dolan RD, Laird BJA, Horgan PG, McMillan DC. The prognostic value of the systemic inflammatory response in randomised clinical trials in cancer: a systematic review. *Crit Rev Oncol Hematol.* 2018;132:130–7.
16. Swann JB, Smyth MJ. Immune surveillance of tumors. *J Clin Invest.* 2007;117(5):1137–46.
17. Brown WM, Davison GW, McClean CM, Murphy MH. A systematic review of the acute effects of exercise on immune and inflammatory indices in untrained adults. *Sports Med Open.* 2015;1(1):35.
18. Gleeson M, Bishop NC, Stensel DJ, Lindley MR, Mastana SS, Nimmo MA. The anti-inflammatory effects of exercise: mechanisms and implications for the prevention and treatment of disease. *Nat Rev Immunol.* 2011;11(9):607–15.
19. Ertek S, Cicero A. Impact of physical activity on inflammation: effects on cardiovascular disease risk and other inflammatory conditions. *Arch Med Sci.* 2012;8(5):794–804.
20. Khalafi M, Malandish A, Rosenkranz SK. The impact of exercise training on inflammatory markers in postmenopausal women: a systemic review and meta-analysis. *Exp Gerontol.* 2021;150:111398.
21. Zheng G, Qiu P, Xia R, Lin H, Ye B, Tao J, et al. Effect of aerobic exercise on inflammatory markers in healthy middle-aged and older adults: a systematic review and meta-analysis of randomized controlled trials. *Front Aging Neurosci.* 2019;11:98.
22. Idorn M, Hojman P. Exercise-dependent regulation of NK cells in cancer protection. *Trends Mol Med.* 2016;22(7):565–77.
23. Duggal NA, Pollock RD, Lazarus NR, Harridge S, Lord JM. Major features of immunesenescence, including reduced thymic output, are ameliorated by high levels of physical activity in adulthood. *Aging Cell.* 2018;17(2):e12750.
24. Kruger K, Lechtermann A, Fobker M, Volker K, Mooren FC. Exercise-induced redistribution of T lymphocytes is regulated by adrenergic mechanisms. *Brain Behav Immun.* 2008;22(3):324–38.
25. Pedersen L, Christensen JF, Hojman P. Effects of exercise on tumor physiology and metabolism. *Cancer J.* 2015;21(2):111–16.
26. Khosravi N, Stoner L, Farajivafa V, Hanson ED. Exercise training, circulating cytokine levels and immune function in cancer survivors: a meta-analysis. *Brain Behav Immun.* 2019;81:92–104.
27. Schauer T, Hojman P, Gehl J, Christensen JF. Exercise training as prophylactic strategy in the management of neutropenia during chemotherapy. *Br J Pharmacol.* 2022;179(12):2925–37.
28. Bland KA, Zadravec K, Landry T, Weller S, Meyers L, Campbell KL. Impact of exercise on chemotherapy completion rate: a systematic review of the evidence and recommendations for future exercise oncology research. *Crit Rev Oncol Hematol.* 2019;136:79–85.
29. Deptula M, Zielinski J, Wardowska A, Pikula M. Wound healing complications in oncological patients: perspectives for cellular therapy. *Postepy Dermatol Alergol.* 2019;36(2):139–46.
30. Lyman C, Lyman G, Abgboola O. Risk models for predicting chemotherapy-induced neutropenia. *The Oncologist.* 2005;10:427–37.
31. Carvalho HA, Villar RC. Radiotherapy and immune response: the systemic effects of a local treatment. *Clinics (Sao Paulo).* 2018;73(suppl 1):e557s.
32. Della Corte CM, Morgillo F. Early use of steroids affects immune cells and impairs immunotherapy efficacy. *ESMO Open.* 2019;4(1):e000477.
33. Zahavi D, Weiner L. Monoclonal antibodies in cancer therapy. *Antibodies (Basel).* 2020;9(3):34.
34. Sterner RC, Sterner RM. CAR-T cell therapy: current limitations and potential strategies. *Blood Cancer J.* 2021;11(4):69.
35. Liu J. Anti-cancer vaccines: a one-hit wonder? *Yale J Biol Med.* 2014;87(4):481–9.

36. Bracarda S, Eggermont AM, Samuelsson J. Redefining the role of interferon in the treatment of malignant diseases. *Eur J Cancer*. 2010; 46(2):284–97.
37. Lustberg MB. Management of neutropenia in cancer patients. *Clin Adv Haematol Oncol*. 2012;10(12):825–6.
38. Knudsen JR, Steenberg DE, Hingst JR, et al. Prior exercise in humans redistributes intramuscular GLUT4 and enhances insulin-stimulated sarcolemmal and endosomal GLUT4 translocation. *Mol Metab*. 2020;39:100998.
39. Hardie DG. AMP-activated protein kinase: a key system mediating metabolic responses to exercise. *Med Sci Sports Exerc*. 2004;36(1): 28–34.
40. Trefts E, Williams AS, Wasserman DH. Exercise and the regulation of hepatic metabolism. *Prog Mol Biol Transl Sci*. 2015;135: 203–25.
41. Horowitz JF. Fatty acid mobilization from adipose tissue during exercise. *Trends Endocrinol Metab*. 2003;14(8):386–92.

CHAPTER

8

Mechanisms Underlying Noncancer Outcomes

OUTLINE

1. Introduction
2. Evaluating the Evidence
3. Strong Evidence
   a. Anxiety
   b. Depressive Symptoms
   c. Fatigue
   d. Health-Related Quality of Life
   e. Lymphedema
   f. Physical Function
4. Moderate Evidence
   a. Bone Health
   b. Sleep
5. Insufficient Evidence
   a. Cardiotoxicity
   b. Chemotherapy-Induced Peripheral Neuropathy
   c. Cognitive Function
   d. Falls
   e. Nausea
   f. Pain
   g. Sexual Function
   h. Treatment Tolerance
6. Summary
7. Case Study
8. Meet the Expert
9. Study Questions
10. References

OBJECTIVES

After completing review of this chapter, students will be able to:

1. Understand how levels of evidence are determined.
2. Know the 8 effects of exercise that have strong and moderate evidence.
3. Understand why 8 outcomes of exercise do not have sufficient evidence.
4. Explain how exercise reduces fatigue.
5. Describe how physical function effects anxiety, depression, fatigue, and QoL.

INTRODUCTION

This chapter will provide an overview of the **mechanisms** of noncancer **outcomes** that are affected by exercise. The science demonstrating the benefits of strong, moderate, and insufficient levels of evidence to determine the benefits of exercise for PLWBC will be described. The benefits of exercise during and following cancer treatment are well documented and form the basis for the *ACSM® Exercise Guidelines for Cancer Survivors* (1, 2). The speed with which exercise oncology research has progressed from the early research in the 1990s to today is remarkable and forms the underpinning for the evidence-based guidelines that have developed from the initial recommendations in 2010 to the more detailed guidelines in 2019. This chapter will focus on mechanisms, and Chapter 11 will detail the *ASCM Exercise Guidelines for Cancer Survivors* and exercise prescription during cancer treatment.

The focus here will be on the outcomes that are affected by cancer. Chapter 11 will delve into the actual exercise prescription. Therefore, the *ACSM® Exercise Guidelines for Cancer Survivors* are not being reviewed, but it is key to understand the processes that were used to determine and categorize the noncancerous outcomes into strong, moderate, and insufficient levels of evidence. Since the landmark 2010 *ACSM® Exercise Recommendations for Cancer Survivors*, exercise randomized trials have increased exponentially (1, 2). This astounding increase in research prompted ACSM®, in 2018, to convene an international, multidisciplinary group of exercise oncology leaders to discuss the next guidelines. Forty representatives from 20 different organizations (Box 8.1) were invited to participate on the basis of their scientific and clinical expertise to contribute to knowledge related to exercise for cancer: 1. prevention and control; 2. management of acute, long-term, and later side effects; and 3. translation of the evidence into clinical and community settings.

Box 8.1 2018 ACSM® International Multidisciplinary Roundtable Discussion of Next Oncology Exercise Guidelines: Participating Organizations

- American College of Sports Medicine®
- American Cancer Society
- Exercise Sports Science Australia
- Oncology Nursing Society
- American Association of Physical Medicine and Rehabilitation
- National Comprehensive Cancer Network
- German Union for Health Exercise and Exercise Therapy
- American Physical Therapy Association
- Sunflower Wellness
- Alberta Health Services
- Canadian Society for Exercise Physiology
- Royal Dutch Society for Physical Therapy
- Society of Surgical Oncology
- National Cancer Institute (U.S.)
- American College of Rehabilitative Medicine
- American College of Lifestyle Medicine
- Commission on Accreditation of Rehabilitation Facilities
- MacMillan
- Centers for Disease Control
- Society for Behavioral Medicine

Data from Schmitz KH, Courneya KS, Matthews C, et al. American College of Sports Medicine® roundtable on exercise guidelines for cancer survivors. *Med Sci Sports Exerc.* 2010;42(7):1409–26. doi:10.1249/MSS.0b013e3181e0c112 [Erratum in: *Med Sci Sports Exer.* 2011;43(1):195]; Campbell KL, Winters-Stone KM, Wiskemann J, et al. Exercise guidelines for cancer survivors: consensus statement from international multidisciplinary roundtable. *Med Sci Sports Exerc.* 2019;51(11):2375–90. doi:10.1249/mss.0000000000002116.

EVALUATING THE EVIDENCE

The expert group made several important decisions at the Roundtable meeting: 1. to determine cancer-related health outcomes with clinical relevance for which exercise may have a therapeutic benefit (Box 8.2) and 2. focus literature searches on traditional modalities of exercise (aerobic, resistance, or a combination of aerobic and resistance). A final decision was to develop a recommendation relevant to all PLWC, from which even the sickest and weakest could benefit.

Collectively, the experts reviewed thousands of studies (1). The studies that were used to determine the strength of the evidence included PLWBC who had primarily breast and prostate cancer. In time, as the research expands to include people with different types of cancer receiving different types of treatments, the recommendations may become more specific.

Mechanisms. Chain of events in a specific process.
Outcomes. A general term for the results of an intervention or process.

Box 8.2 Common Cancer-Related Health Outcomes for Review of Evidence for Therapeutic Efficacy of Exercise and Subsequent Exercise Prescriptions

- Anxiety
- Bone health
- Cardiotoxicity
- Chemotherapy-induced peripheral neuropathy
- Cognitive function
- Depressive symptoms
- Falls
- Fatigue
- Health-related quality of life
- Lymphedema
- Nausea
- Pain
- Physical function
- Sexual function
- Sleep
- Treatment tolerance

STRONG EVIDENCE

The following outcomes all have strong evidence to support recommending exercise to improve the side effects of anxiety, depression, fatigue, health-related quality of life (HRQoL), lymphedema, and physical function. **Strong evidence** for noncancer outcomes is defined as studies that include: 1. frequency, intensity, time, and type (FITT) prescription; 2. at least 5 RCTs with a sample of at least 150 people; 3. a strong exercise effect; and 4. consistent results across studies. The results for each outcome needed to be consistent to develop a FITT prescription for each outcome. Detailed FITT prescriptions for each outcome are provided in Chapter 11.

Anxiety

Anxiety is the feeling of unease, fear, worry, and dread caused by stress—in this case related to cancer. PLWBC experience anxiety when waiting to learn test and biopsy results, cancer staging, and treatment plans (pretreatment) with rates as high as 27% (3) and beginning and ending treatments (18%) (4). After cancer treatment, people experience anxiety about lingering side effects, fear of recurrence, regaining their QoL, relationships, and financial concerns.

Anxiety is caused by an interaction of biopsychosocial factors that cause a physiologic response. The central nervous system, especially the autonomic nervous system, activates norepinephrine, serotonin, dopamine, and gamma-aminobutyric acid (GABA) that heighten feelings of fear and anxiety (5). For example, a person starting chemotherapy may feel anxious before their first treatment and have an increased heart rate, feel nervous, and be fearful and afraid. Some people, if they have poorly controlled nausea, may experience anticipatory nausea when they come to the chemotherapy suite. This behavioral anxiety may be mitigated with better symptom management and education.

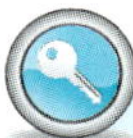

Strong evidence. For noncancer outcomes, studies that include: 1. FITT prescription; 2. at least 5 RCTs with a sample of at least 150 people; 3. a strong exercise effect; and 4. consistent results across studies.

Depressive Symptoms

Depressive symptoms include changes in affect, depressed mood, sleep disturbance, and changes in appetite and thought patterns. Depression occurs equally among men and women with cancer and affects approximately 15% to 25% of cancer patients (6-10). All PLWBC are confronted with fear of death, disruption of life, body image and self-esteem changes, changes in social role and lifestyle, and financial and legal concerns. For some these issues cause serious anxiety, depression, posttraumatic stress disorder, and, within the 2 months following diagnosis, an elevated risk of suicide (6, 9). Depression is more common among people who are receiving palliative care and are younger, have lower performance status, a smaller network of friends and family, and those who do not participate in organized religions (11).

Depression can be caused by medical conditions. Disruption in the serotonin/dopamine pathways can lead to depression. Depression can be a side effect of cancer treatment caused by the same physiological pathway or a tumor in the central nervous system, uncontrolled pain, and poor sleep. Many medications can also cause depression (Table 8.1) (12-14). Steroids can lower serotonin levels, causing depression. Steroids (eg, prednisone and dexamethasone) are routinely given during treatment with chemotherapy and immunotherapy to prevent side effects to the medications. Many treatment regimens, particularly for Hodgkin's lymphoma and non-Hodgkin's lymphoma, include high doses of steroids.

Fatigue

CRF is defined as a distressing, persistent, subjective sense of physical, emotional, and/or cognitive tiredness or exhaustion related to cancer or cancer treatment that is

Table 8.1 Medical Causes of Depression

CAUSES	EXAMPLES
Uncontrolled pain	
Chronic illness	
Metabolic abnormalities	Hypercalcemia Sodium/potassium imbalance Anemia Vitamin B12 or folate deficiency Fever
Endocrine abnormalities	Hyper/hypothyroidism Adrenal insufficiency
Medications	Steroids Endogenous and exogenous cytokines (eg, interferon-α, interleukin-2) Methyldopa Reserpine Propranolol Some antibiotics (eg, amphotericin B) Some chemotherapy drugs (eg, procarbazine, L-asparaginase

Data from PDQ® Supportive and Palliative Care Editorial Board. PDQ Depression Bethesda, MD: National Cancer Institute. [Internet]. 2021. Available from https://www.cancer.gov/about-cancer/coping/feelings/depression-hp-pdq#cit/section_1.13.

not proportional to recent activity and that significantly interferes with usual functioning. Cancer-related fatigue is the most common side effect of cancer and its treatment. It affects up to 90% of patients during treatment and can linger over the years after treatment ends (15). For as many as 30% of PLWC, fatigue continues to linger 5 to 10 years after treatment ends (16). Fatigue is associated with chemotherapy, radiation therapy, immunotherapy, biologic response modifiers, and BMT. There are different patterns of fatigue associated with type and frequency of treatment. A typical pattern of fatigue during chemotherapy is for fatigue to peak 3 to 5 days after treatment and slowly improve until the next treatment. Fatigue accumulates with each treatment so that with each treatment, the fatigue gets progressively worse. Radiation therapy causes a different pattern of fatigue that gradually increases over the course of treatment. Prolonged treatments with interferon-α for melanoma can cause profound fatigue that continues to increase over time. This fatigue can be so severe that patients may be unable to work or continue with school or other usual activities. Fatigue is measured subjectively. It can be measured simply by asking the patient to rate their fatigue on a 10-point scale or by using psychometrically sound scales. There are many different scales that are used to measure fatigue, including the Schwartz Cancer Fatigue Scale, the Cancer Fatigue Scale, the Brief Fatigue Inventory, the Functional Assessment of Cancer Therapy-Fatigue (FACT-F) Scale, and the Multidimensional Fatigue Inventory.

The exact mechanisms of fatigue are unknown and believed to be multifactorial (17-19). Fatigue may be influenced by demographic, medical, psychological, social behavioral, and biologic factors. Biological causes of fatigue include anemia, dysregulation of cytokines, 5 hydroxy tryptophan (5-HT), HPA axis, and changes in muscle metabolism because of alterations in adenosine triphosphate. Oxidative stress associated with cancer treatment is another potential biological cause of cancer-related fatigue. There is preliminary research to suggest that cell damage from radiation therapy may upregulate certain genes related to oxidative stress (20).

Cytokine dysregulation affects the inflammatory process. Tumors may stimulate an inflammatory response. Treatment also activates cytokines in response to damage to cells and tissues from radiation therapy and chemotherapy (21-23). The cytokine inflammatory response can persist after treatment as the body tries to heal and return to homeostasis. Studies propose that the inflammatory mechanism is caused by elevations in CRP, changes in IL-1 and IL-6, and potential reactivation of viral diseases, such as herpesviruses and cytomegalovirus, which may be induced by immune suppression (24). The inflammatory process is also associated with depression, sleep disturbance, physical inactivity, increased body mass (overweight and obesity), and stress, all of which compound inflammation.

Psychological factors may also contribute to fatigue. Depression, sleep disturbance, one's coping skills, and loneliness may all contribute to fatigue (25). When depression and insomnia are treated and fatigue persists, exercise oncology professionals speculate that inactivity and physical deconditioning cause fatigue. At this point, there is limited research to support the hypothesis that CRF is solely caused either by a biological or psychological factor. Undoubtedly there are a variety of factors that affect fatigue, but at this time, the lack of exercise and propensity to rest during cancer treatment may be the most plausible cause. When people are diagnosed with cancer, they tend to rest and take care of themselves. Resting more and being inactive leads to muscle weakness, decline in aerobic function, and physical debilitation (Figure 8.1). When one is debilitated, greater physical effort is required to work and perform one's usual activities, and an individual gets easily fatigued. Lower levels of physical activity after cancer treatment ends predict persistent fatigue in breast cancer survivors (26, 27). When one engages in regular physical activity, one's fatigue is reduced (2).

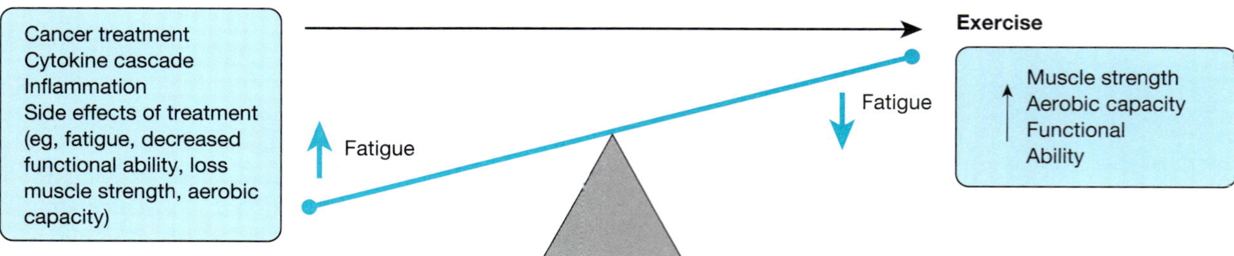

FIGURE 8.1. Balance of cancer, treatment and side effects with cancer-related fatigue.

Health-Related Quality of Life

QoL is the degree to which an individual is healthy, comfortable, and able to participate in or enjoy life events. The goal for PLWC is a cure, but equally important is the quality of their life during and after treatment. **HRQoL** is a **multidimensional** concept that measures physical and mental health, social support, and functional status. HRQoL is lower in PLWBC than in healthy people or those with other chronic illnesses (28). It is a measure of the impact of health on QoL of an individual or a group. Physical symptoms and psychological aspects (eg, fatigue, anxiety, and depression) associated with cancer treatment are recognized as critical components of HRQoL because they have a significant impact on QoL. HRQoL is even associated with risk of mortality (29). In cancer research, it is an important variable to assess the effects of an intervention. An example would be testing an exercise program to determine the effects on HRQoL of PLWBC.

Lymphedema

If lymph nodes are compressed by a tumor, removed during surgery, or damaged during radiation therapy, the lymph fluid may not drain properly from an extremity (arm or leg) (Figure 8.2). The abnormal accumulation of protein-rich lymph fluid causes swelling, which is called lymphedema (Figure 8.3). Lymphedema can develop rapidly, or it may occur slowly over time. While lymphedema usually occurs within 3 years of surgery, it can develop at any time. Lymphedema makes a limb feel tight and heavy, and when it is severe, it can make performing routine activities difficult and painful.

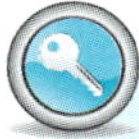

Health-Related Quality of Life (HRQoL). A multidimensional concept that measures physical and mental health, social support, and functional status.

Multidimensional. Something that has many different parts or aspects. For example, scales that measure HRQoL often include dimensions of physical, mental, social, and functional health.

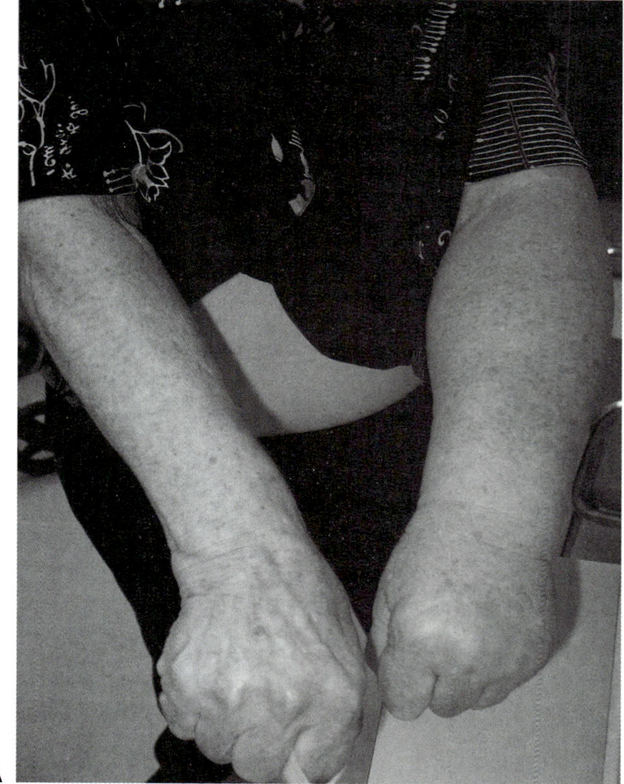

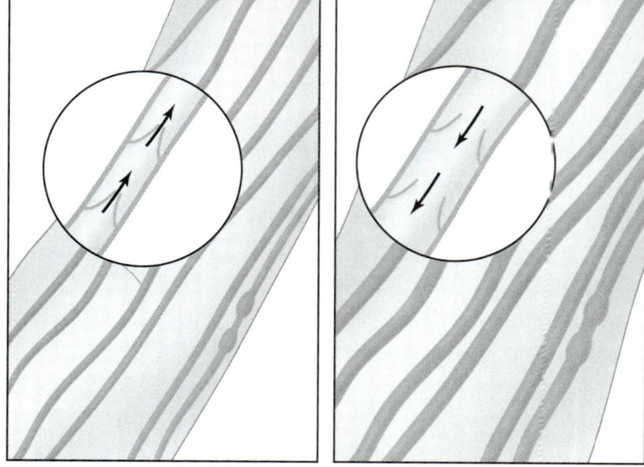

FIGURE 8.2. Normal lymphatic drainage and interrupted drainage causing lymphedema. (A, from Timby BK, Smith NE. *Introductory Medical-Surgical Nursing*, 11th ed. Philadelphia (PA): Wolters Kluwer; 2014. B, from The Barankin Collection: Wolters Kluwer; 2005.)

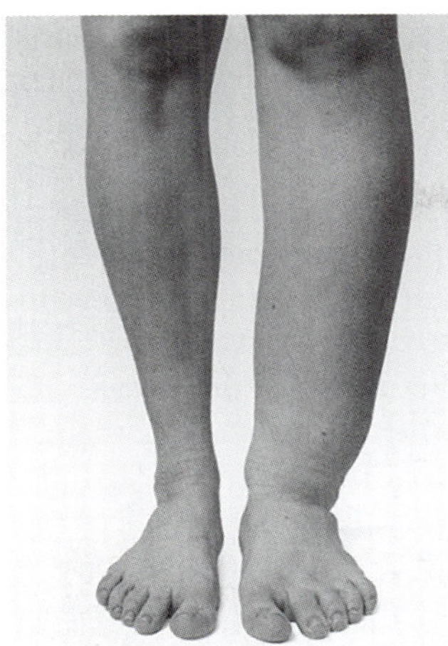

FIGURE 8.3. Lymphedema of left leg. (From Centers for Disease Control and Prevention. *Lymphedema.* [Internet]. 2021. Available from https://www.cdc.gov/cancer/survivors/patients/lymphedema.htm.)

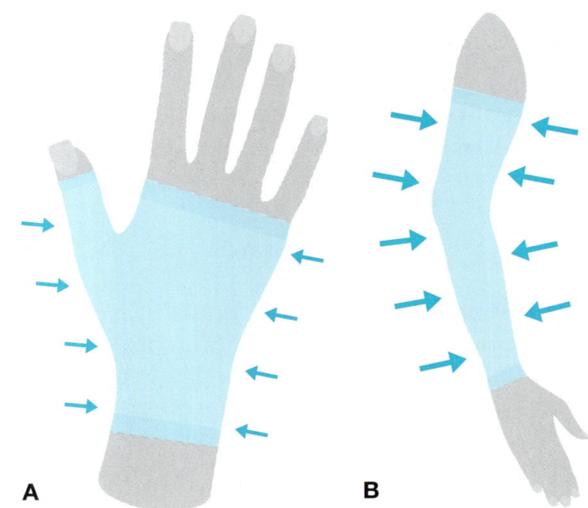

FIGURE 8.4. Lymphedema glove (A) and sleeve (B). (A, from Shutterstock, Vector ID 2322354101; B, from Shutterstock, Vector ID: 2322350541, both by Brsznca.)

Lymphedema occurs on the affected side of the body after surgery lymph nodes are removed. For example, breast cancer that involves removal of axillary (armpit) lymph nodes, lymphedema may occur in that arm. Lymphedema may occur in the leg(s) after surgery for prostate cancer, uterine cancer, lymphoma, or melanoma. It is diagnosed clinically by comparing differences in arm or leg size. A difference of greater than 2 cm in circumferential measurements of the affected compared with the unaffected limb often indicates lymphedema. Box 8.3 lists common signs of lymphedema. Lymphedema tends to be a chronic problem that predisposes people to infection in the limb because circulation is limited.

Lymphedema may be managed with exercise, compression garments, lymphatic drainage with massage, elevation of the limb, and pneumatic pumps to move the fluid out (Figure 8.4). Compression garments work by having different graduated pressure points to move the lymph fluid back to the central body. For example, an arm compression sleeve has higher pressure at the fingers to help move the lymphatic fluid back up the arm toward the torso (30, 31, 32).

Box 8.3 Signs of Lymphedema

Following are signs of lymphedema:

- Swelling in an arm or leg
- Heaviness in the affected limb
- Skin tightness
- Swelling that may interfere with movement (eg, fingers, hand, arm, toes, and leg)
- Skin that may become thick
- Affected area my itch or burn
- Difficult to wear rings, watch, bracelet, and socks

Historically, people at risk for upper limb lymphedema associated with breast cancer were told to avoid lifting anything heavier than their purse and to avoid aerobic and resistance exercise. This protective recommendation potentiated lymphedema because the affected arm became weak, and when used to a degree that exceeded its capacity, it could trigger lymphedema. Slowly progressive resistance exercise is associated with a reduction in the number of flare-ups of lymphedema among breast cancer survivors who already have the condition and reduces the onset of lymphedema by 70% among breast cancer survivors at elevated risk for lymphedema but who have not yet been diagnosed with lymphedema (33, 34).

Physical Function

Physical function is the ability to perform activities of daily living and participate in activities that are meaningful personally and socially. It is a broad concept that includes not only physical and emotional concepts but also how an individual relates to their family and community. It encompasses physical limitations, psychological conditions, cognition, and environmental issues that affect an individual. Examples of physical function include cooking, walking, climbing stairs, or being able to participate socially in life.

Declines in physical function occur with inactivity. In the past, the advice given to patients was to go home and rest or take care of themselves, certainly not to exercise or maintain their physical function. Following this advice may further reduce muscle mass as cancer, and its treatments may result in muscle wasting and muscle loss, as well as possibly increased fat mass, and certainly reduced physical function. It is now known that this advice caused more harm than good because of the disability that occurs with prolonged rest and inactivity. For example, it has been documented that women surviving breast cancer have cardiorespiratory fitness levels (a measure of physical function) that are similar to women who have never had cancer who are a decade older (35). PLWBC need to engage in both aerobic and resistance exercise to maintain muscle strength and cardiovascular function.

MODERATE EVIDENCE

Outcomes were deemed to have moderate evidence if there were more than 5 randomized clinical trials with a sample of greater than 150 and findings that were congruent with outcomes in a healthy (noncancer) population. In these situations, the strength of the evidence was judged to be moderate, and a FITT prescription was developed. The effect of exercise on bone health and sleep at this time is only moderate. There is robust research in people without cancer demonstrating the benefit of exercise on bone health and sleep, but additional research is needed in PLWBC (36, 37).

Bone Health

Bone health is important because our bones play many roles in the body: they provide structure, protect organs, anchor muscles, and store calcium. There are many factors that influence bone health, including calcium in the diet, physical activity, tobacco and alcohol use, gender (women have weaker bones), body size (people with a BMI of 19 kg/m^2 or less have weaker bones), age, race, hormone levels, eating disorders, and certain medications. Bone health is fundamentally connected to the metabolism of calcium and phosphorus. Calcium is critical for normal physiologic function, such as the muscle contraction, nerve conduction, and the function of blood vessels (constriction and relaxation). Calcium is needed for these essential functions. The concentration of calcium is controlled by the parathyroid hormone (PTH) and vitamin D, which influences bone health. When calcium intake is inadequate, the body uses calcium from bones to maintain circulating calcium in the normal range (8.9-10.1 mg/dL) to preserve normal heart, nerve, and muscle functions. Skeletal bone must be maintained to preserve bone density and mitigate bone turnover and loss to prevent osteopenia and osteoporosis. Mechanical forces, like exercise, help to maintain bone health by applying stress to the bones when the muscles contract. Calcium in combination with muscle contraction and physical activity stimulates the bone to maintain strength, density, and resilience.

Sleep

Sleep is an essential function that allows the body and mind to recharge, leaving one refreshed and alert upon awaking. Healthy sleep also helps the body remain healthy and stave off diseases. Sleep disturbance can exacerbate psychological distress, increase fatigue, impair healing, increase risk for infection, decrease cognitive functioning, impair ability to work, and increase health care costs. Cancer treatments can also interrupt sleep because of stress, depression, and drugs, for example, steroids. Pharmacological agents have side effects and may pose a risk for dependency (38). Aerobic exercise causes the body to release endorphins that arouse the brain and also increases core body temperature (39). Therefore, it is recommended to avoid exercise 2 to 3 hours before bed. Among adults not diagnosed with cancer, exercise reduces sleep disturbances (40). A systematic review found that approximately 50% of people living with or beyond cancer report sleep benefits from exercise (41). Exercise helps PLWBC fall asleep and stay asleep (39, 42). It appears that exercise has the potential to improve sleep for PLWBC, but more research is needed to conclusively determine this outcome.

INSUFFICIENT EVIDENCE

Outcomes that were deemed to have **insufficient evidence** were those that at this time do not have enough research to support providing a FITT recommendation. This should be distinguished from evidence of no effect. For the outcomes reviewed below, there is some, but insufficient evidence of a consistent beneficial effect of exercise. At this time, there is a gap in the research, but there is a growing body of research that will be useful to possibly determine a FITT recommendation for these outcomes in the future.

Cardiotoxicity

As discussed in Chapter 5, many cancer treatments cause cardiotoxicities that potentially lead to direct damage to the heart, often called cardiotoxicity. These treatments include surgery, radiotherapy, chemotherapy, molecularly targeted therapy (eg, imatinib [Gleevec], and rituximab [Rituxan]), and immunotherapy (eg, ipilimumab [Yervoy] and CAR T-cell therapy). Cardiac dysfunction may include atherosclerosis, hypertension, myocardial infarction, bradycardia, tachycardia, coronary vasospasm, heart failure, thromboembolism, and heart block (43). Box 8.4 shows common cardiac dysfunctions and associated cancer drugs. Cancer and CVD are common diseases that respond to exercise. Exercise has a strong cardioprotective role in the reduction of cancer-treatment-associated cardiotoxicity that not only improves the physiologic function but also the functional ability of PLWC (44). There is no reason to believe that the benefits of exercise for the cardiovascular system do not extend to PLWBC. However, more research is

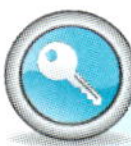

Insufficient evidence. Outcomes that at this time do not have enough research to support providing a FITT recommendation.

Box 8.4 Cardiac Side Effect Related to Cancer Drug

CARDIAC SIDE EFFECT	CANCER DRUG
Hypertension	Bevacizumab, sunitinib, sorafenib, pazopanib
Myocardial infarction	Sunitinib, sorafenib, pazopanib
Bradycardia	Taxanes (eg, taxol)
Tachycardia	Taxanes
Coronary vasospasm	Antimetabolites
Heart failure (late and irreversible)	Anthracyclines, trastuzumab and cyclophosphamide, sunitinib, sorafenib, pazopanib
Thromboembolism	Bevacizumab
Heart block	Taxanes
Acute coronary syndromes	Platinum drugs (eg, Adriamycin)

Data from Walls GM, Lyon AR, Harbinson MT, Hanna GG. Cardiotoxicity following cancer treatment. *Ulster Med J*. 2017;86(1):3–9.

needed to learn the optimal exercise approach for PLWBC to provide a FITT recommendation.

Chemotherapy-Induced Peripheral Neuropathy

CIPN is a nerve-damaging side effect of antineoplastic agents in the common cancer treatment, chemotherapy. CIPN afflicts between 30% and 40% of patients undergoing chemotherapy. CIPN is a common treatment-related side effect associated with taxanes, platinum, and vinca alkaloid-based chemotherapy. There is no standard treatment for the prevention of CIPN (45). Approximately half of the patients who receive these drugs experience CIPN that causes numbness, tingling, pain, cold sensitivity, and impaired function in their hands and feet, which often does not completely resolve after treatment (46). CIPN is a chronic condition that can persist longer than 6 years after treatment ends and can pose a significant fall risk (47, 48). There are a few studies that show benefits of exercise for CIPN symptoms, but too few to draw compelling conclusions at this time (49).

Cognitive Function

The signs of cancer-related cognitive impairment are more often minimized than those seen in people with Alzheimer disease or mild cognitive impairment. They include memory-related deficits, such as having difficulty concentrating to learn new things or organize tasks and being slower to process information. Cancer-related cognitive impairment, often called "chemo-brain," is a common side effect of many chemotherapy treatments. As many as 85% of people receiving cancer treatment self-report mild-to-severe cognitive complaints that can last months to years after treatment ends. The mechanism of changes may be linked to surgery; radiation; hormonal therapy; chemotherapy; immunotherapy; and side effects, such as fatigue, stress, anxiety, depress, sleep dysfunction, and other moderating or mediating factors (50-56). Although there is insufficient research to support recommending exercise for cognitive improvement for PLWBC, the body of literature is rapidly growing (57).

Falls

A fall is defined as the act of falling or collapsing and is most likely to cause problems when the person falls all the way to the floor. Studying falls is challenging because falls do not occur every day, so it takes time to accumulate data. People have to fall and remember to report that they fell down, and the number of reported falls is small. However, PLWBC fall more often because of muscle weakness, poor balance, CIPN, fatigue, and other causes that may include dizziness because of dehydration, a decrease in blood pressure, or electrolyte imbalances. It is important to remind people who are receiving cancer treatment to stay hydrated. Exercise is important to helping people maintain balance, strength, and flexibility to stay upright. Simple things such as keeping rooms well lit and removing possible obstacles are key to avoiding falls (Box 8.5) (58).

Nausea

Nausea is defined as a feeling of sickness with an inclination to vomit. This symptom is common in cancer patients receiving chemotherapy and radiation. An early breast cancer exercise trial observed that nausea during chemotherapy was reduced with vigorous exercise (59). More recently, a large trial in the Netherlands confirmed this finding (60). However, since

Box 8.5 Common Reasons for Fall Risk

- Poor balance
- Weak legs
- Dizziness
- Dehydration
- Low blood pressure
- Poor lighting
- Poor vision or hearing
- Obstacles, for example, slippery surfaces, throw rugs, stairs, toys, and pets
- Change in medications
- Shoes: Wear nonskid, rubber-soled, low-heeled, or lace-up

this trial, **antiemetic drugs** and nausea management have improved to such an extent that there are no differences in nausea between exercise intervention and control groups. Theoretically, future research could examine differences in well-controlled exercise interventions in highly emetogenic regimens to determine if there is an effect, but this would be difficult as the new drugs are highly efficacious drugs and it would be unethical to withhold these drugs in a clinical trial.

Pain

Pain is defined as physical suffering or discomfort caused by illness or injury. Physical pain is the result of the firing of nerve endings called nociceptors. For many years pain, much like fatigue, has been treated with rest. However, since the late 1980s, physical activity has been recognized as an important mechanism to reduce the severity of chronic pain and deconditioning, depression, insomnia, and often obesity that accompanies chronic pain and debilitation (56, 57). Physical activity and exercise have minimal adverse effects when adapted to the individual and help the person to feel independent and mentally and physically stronger. A single bout of exercise increases the production of endogenous opioids and increases antinociception. Repeating exercise yields long-lasting antinociception effects. Weight loss from aerobic exercise helps chronic pain management by reducing joint pain, and resistance exercise can improve strength to relieve stiffness and pain (61). Exercise training improves the emotional and physical balance and flexibility, which further reduces the risk of falls and risks for injury and bone fractures (58, 62).

Sexual Function

Sexual functioning is characterized by the absence of difficulty moving through the stages of sexual desire, arousal, and orgasm, as well as subjective satisfaction with the frequency and outcome of individual and partnered sexual behavior. Sexual function is threatened with cancer treatment for men and women. Men with prostate cancer receiving ADT face a rapid and profound decrease in testosterone, muscle mass, strength, endurance, and sexual function. There are mixed results on the effects of exercise on sexual function (63-65). However, there are limited studies that suggest that resistance exercise can prevent and restore some of the deleterious effects of ADT on a man's strength and endurance, which in turn improves his emotional outlook. For women, many cancer treatments provoke early menopause, either surgically or medically (ie, chemotherapy-induced). Early menopause increases risks for changes in body composition, such as bone loss and body fat distribution. Women with breast cancer who are taking antiestrogen therapy must cope with hot flashes, arthralgias, and bone loss that are common side effects of many drugs (eg, aromatase inhibitors) (66). For young women and men, infertility is a concern after radiation to the pelvis and certain chemotherapy, immunotherapy, targeted therapy, BMT, and CAR T-cell therapy (67).

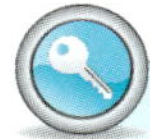

Antiemetics. Drugs that control nausea and vomiting.

Treatment Tolerance

Treatment tolerance is the ability of a person actively receiving treatment to get the planned dose of treatment on schedule. Receiving the planned dose of treatment on schedule is important because it theoretically increases the likelihood that the person with cancer receiving treatment will achieve an optimal outcome. When treatments need to be delayed because of side effects, there may be an opportunity for cellular growth. However, there are times when treatment must be delayed or doses of medications need to be reduced because of low blood cell counts (myelosuppression), infection or other, unexpected events. There is one randomized trial that suggests that exercise may have some selective benefits during treatment, such as improved tolerance for full dose treatment, prevention of weight gain, dose reduction because of neutropenia, and less fatigue in the exercise group (68). In addition, there are several other trials that have examined this as a secondary outcome and showed benefit of exercise on the chemotherapy completion rate among breast and colon cancer patients (60, 69). Clearly, at this point, there is insufficient research to recommend exercise to improve treatment tolerance.

SUMMARY

Review of the mechanisms underlying noncancer outcomes has clearly documented the beneficial effects of exercise on anxiety, depressive symptoms, fatigue, HRQoL, lymphedema, and physical function. In addition, there is growing evidence that exercise may be beneficial for bone health and sleep. Exercise is safe and effective for PLWBC. Although there is still a great deal we do not know about the mechanisms of exercise during and following cancer treatment, as the research and knowledge base expands, many of these questions will be answered. We do know that exercise needs to be individualized to each person to accommodate not only to their personal goals but also to their abilities, current state of health, and physical condition and comorbidities. The chapters of Section 3 will delve into greater detail about exercise prescription during and following cancer treatment. Chapter 11 will specifically address exercise prescription for the outcomes discussed in this chapter.

Case Study

Sarah is a 28-year-old woman with Stage III non-Hodgkin's lymphoma. Her treatment included mantle field radiation and R-CHOP (rituximab, cyclophosphamide, hydroxydaunorubicin, vincristine, and prednisone). Sarah's treatments ended 1 month ago, but she still feels tired, weak, and complains of chemo brain (particularly an inability to focus). She is concerned about working with her extremely low energy and fatigue. She can barely walk up the stairs. Sarah is talking to an exercise professional and wants to know how an exercise program will affect her fatigue, physical function, cognitive function, sexual function and overall QoL.

Questions

1. What will the exercise professional tell her about exercise and the side effects she is experiencing?
2. Sarah still complains of nausea. Will exercise reduce her nausea?
3. Sarah wants to know how the exercise recommendations were developed and if she can really benefit from them given how weak and fatigued she is.

Meet the Expert

FEATURED PROFESSIONAL

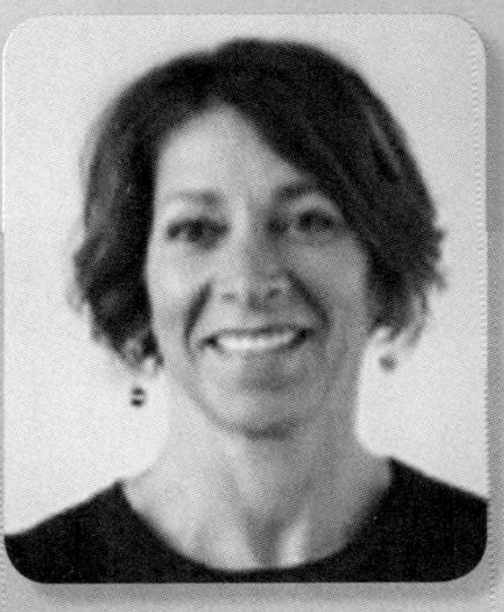

Kerri Winters-Stone, PhD, FACSM

Professor and Section Head, Cancer Population Sciences, Division of Oncological Sciences
Co-Program Leader, Cancer Prevention & Control
Co-Director, Community Partnership Program
Knight Cancer Institute, Oregon Health & Science University, Portland, Oregon

Q: "Where did you grow up?"

I was born in Oakland, CA, and grew up in the San Francisco Bay Area.

Q: "Where did you train?"

I'm trained as an exercise physiologist and graduated with a PhD in Human Performance from Oregon State University in 2000.

Q: "What are you best known for?"

My research now focuses on exercise and musculoskeletal health in cancer survivors, particularly older adults. I have done studies to understand how cancer treatment affects bone integrity, muscle health, postural stability, and frailty, and use this information to design exercise trials to identify the optimal exercise prescription to lower the risk of fractures by slowing bone loss and preventing falls.

Q: "What are you currently working on?"

In our trials we learned from patients that their spouses/partners were also suffering from the physical and mental toll of caregiving. We are currently conducting research to test new team-based exercise programs for couples coping with cancer and see if these programs can be implemented into cancer care.

Q: "Anything else you want to include?"

My initial interests were in skeletal exercise physiology, and with Dr. Christine Snow we were among the first to develop and test-specific bone loading programs to prevent osteoporosis in women. Then a chance of meeting with Dr. Anna Schwartz changed my career trajectory when she invited me to come work with her at Oregon Health & Science University. I had never worked with cancer patients before and I felt unprepared, but Anna's mentorship along with other oncology nurse scientists helped me learn what I needed to move into the field. A couple of studies with breast and prostate cancer survivors made such a positive impact on me personally that soon I realized that I wanted to stay in this field for the rest of my career. Since that "lateral pirouette" in my research program, I have focused in the area of exercise and musculoskeletal health in cancer survivors.

One lesson I have learned during my career is to be willing to go in new directions because that may be the next innovation that the field is looking for and it will keep you excited. Keep your ears and eyes open and think outside of the box!

Favorite Quote:

"If at first you don't succeed, try, try again."
—*Idiom*

STUDY QUESTIONS

1. The recommendations were designed for:
   a. The weakest and youngest
   b. The healthiest and eldest
   c. The sickest and weakest
   d. The youngest and strongest
2. Select the 3 outcomes that have demonstrated strong beneficial evidence of exercise.
3. What is lymphedema?
4. What is a lymphedema sleeve?
5. True or false. Fatigue affects 30% of people during treatment.
6. What is health-related QoL and why is it important?
7. What is chemotherapy-induced peripheral neuropathy (CIPN)?
8. What is treatment tolerance?
9. Define multidimensional.
10. List 5 of the 7 signs of lymphedema

REFERENCES

1. Schmitz KH, Courneya KS, Matthews C, et al. American College of Sports Medicine® roundtable on exercise guidelines for cancer survivors. *Med Sci Sports Exerc.* 2010;42(7):1409–26. doi:10.1249/MSS.0b013e3181e0c112 [Erratum in: *Med Sci Sports Exerc.* 2011;43(1):195]
2. Campbell KL, Winters-Stone KM, Wiskemann J, et al. Exercise guidelines for cancer survivors: consensus statement from international multidisciplinary roundtable. *Med Sci Sports Exerc.* 2019;51(11):2375–90. doi:10.1249/mss.0000000000002116
3. Watts S, Leydon G, Birch B, et al. Depression and anxiety in prostate cancer: a systematic review and meta-analysis of prevalence rates. *BMJ Open.* 2014;4(3):e003901. doi:10.1136/bmjopen-2013-003901
4. Watts S, Prescott P, Mason J, McLeod N, Lewith G. Depression and anxiety in ovarian cancer: a systematic review and meta-analysis of prevalence rates. *BMJ Open.* 2015;5(11):e007618. doi:10.1136/bmjopen-2015-007618
5. Chand SP, Marwaha R. Anxiety. *StatPearls.* [Internet]. Treasure Island (FL): StatPearls Publishing; 2021.
6. Liu Q, Wang, L, Kong K, et al. Subsequent risk of suicide among 9,300,812 cancer survivors in US: a population-based cohort study covering 40 years of data. *EClinicalMedicine.* 2022;44:101295. https://doi.org/10.1016/j.eclinm.2022.101295
7. Bodurka-Bevers D, Basen-Engquist K, Carmack CL, et al. Depression, anxiety, and quality of life in patients with epithelial ovarian cancer. *Gynecol Oncol.* 2000;78(3):302–8. doi:10.1006/gyno.2000.5908
8. Lloyd-Williams M, Friedman T. Depression in palliative care patients: a prospective study. *Eur J Cancer.* 2001;10(4):270–4. doi:10.1046/j.1365-2354.2001.00290.x
9. Zhang L, Liu X, Tong F, et al. The prevalence of psychological disorders among cancer patients during the COVID-19 pandemic: a meta-analysis. *Psychooncology.* 2022;31(11):1972–87.
10. Miaskowski C. Gender differences in pain, fatigue, and depression in patients with cancer. *J Natl Cancer Inst Monogr.* 2004;(32):139–43. doi:10.1093/jncimonographs/lgh024
11. Wilson KG, Chochinov HM, Graham Skirko M, et al. Depression and anxiety disorders in palliative cancer care. *J Pain Symptom Manage.* 2007;33(2):118–29. doi:10.1016/j.jpainsymman.2006.07.016
12. Weber D, O'Brien K. Cancer and cancer-related fatigue and the interrelationships with depression, stress, and inflammation. *J Evid Based Complementary Altern Med.* 2017;22(3):502–12. doi:10.1177/2156587216676122
13. Ji YB, Bo CL, Xue XJ, et al. Association of inflammatory cytokines with the symptom cluster of pain, fatigue, depression, and sleep disturbance in Chinese patients with cancer. *J Pain Symptom Manage.* 2017;54(6):843–52. doi:10.1016/j.jpainsymman.2017.05.003
14. Capuron L, Ravaud A, Neveu PJ, Miller AH, Maes M, Dantzer R. Association between decreased serum tryptophan concentrations and depressive symptoms in cancer patients undergoing cytokine therapy. *Mol Psychiatry.* 2002;7(5):468–73. doi: 10.1038/sj.mp.4000995
15. Fosså SD, Dahl AA, Loge JH. Fatigue, anxiety, and depression in long-term survivors of testicular cancer. *J Clin Oncol.* 2003;21(7):1249–54. doi:10.1200/jco.2003.08.163
16. Bower JE, Ganz PA, Desmond KA, et al. Fatigue in long-term breast carcinoma survivors: a longitudinal investigation. *Cancer.* 2006;106(4):751–8. doi:10.1002/cncr.21671
17. Saligan LN, Olson K, Filler K, et al. The biology of cancer-related fatigue: a review of the literature. *Support Care Cancer.* 2015;23(8):2461–78. doi:10.1007/s00520-015-2763-0
18. Berger AM, Mooney K, Alvarez-Perez A, et al. Cancer-related fatigue, version 2.2015. *J Natl Compr Canc Netw.* 2015;13(8):1012–39. doi:10.6004/jnccn.2015.0122
19. Bower JE, Wiley J, Peterson L, Irwin MR, Cole SW, Ganz PA. Fatigue after breast cancer treatment: biobehavioral predictors of fatigue trajectories. *Health Psychol.* 2018;37(11):1025–34. doi:10.1037/hea0000652
20. Dickinson K, Case AJ, Kupzyk K, Saligan L. Exploring biologic correlates of cancer-related fatigue in men with prostate cancer: cell damage pathways and oxidative stress. *Biol Res Nurs.* 2020;22(4):514–19. doi:10.1177/1099800420933347
21. Cohen RA, Gullett JM, Woods AJ, et al. Cytokine-associated fatigue prior to, during, and post-chemotherapy for breast cancer. *J Neuroimmunol.* 2019;334:577001. doi:10.1016/j.jneuroim.2019.577001
22. Clevenger L, Schrepf A, Christensen D, et al. Sleep disturbance, cytokines, and fatigue in women with ovarian cancer. *Brain Behav Immun.* 2012;26(7):1037–44. doi:10.1016/j.bbi.2012.04.003
23. Bower JE, Ganz PA, Tao ML, et al. Inflammatory biomarkers and fatigue during radiation therapy for breast and prostate cancer. *Clin Cancer Res.* 2009;15(17):5534–40. doi: 10.1158/1078-0432.Ccr-08-2584
24. Kuo CP, Wu CL, Ho HT, Chen CG, Liu SI, Lu YT. Detection of cytomegalovirus reactivation in cancer patients receiving chemotherapy. *Clin Microbiol Infect.* 2008;14(3):221–7. doi:10.1111/j.1469-0691.2007.01895.x
25. Bower JE. Cancer-related fatigue: mechanisms, risk factors, and treatments. *Nat Rev Clin Oncol.* 2014;11(10):597–609. doi:10.1038/nrclinonc.2014.127
26. Donovan KA, Small BJ, Andrykowski MA, Munster P, Jacobsen PB. Utility of a cognitive-behavioral model to predict fatigue following breast cancer treatment. *Health Psychol.* 2007;26(4):464–72. doi:10.1037/0278-6133.26.4.464

27. Gunnell AS, Joyce S, Tomlin S, et al. Pyshcial activity and survival among long-term cancer survivor and non-cancer cohorts. *Front Public Health*, 2017;5:19. https://doi.org/10.3389/fpubh.2017.00019
28. Annunziata MA, Muzzatti B, Flaiban C, et al. Long-term quality of life profile in oncology: a comparison between cancer survivors and the general population. *Support Care Cancer*. 2018;26(2):651–6. doi:10.1007/s00520-017-3880-8
29. Sitlinger A, Zafar SY. Health-related quality of life: the impact on morbidity and mortality. *Surg Oncol Clin*. 2018;27(4):675–84. doi:10.1016/j.soc.2018.05.008
30. Enerskin. Compression sleeves for lymphedema treatment Oct 1, 2019. [Internet]. 2021. Available from https://www.enerskin.com/blogs/blogs/compression-sleeves-for-lymphedema-management
31. Rescue Legs. *Lymphedema Sleeve Garments*. [Internet]. 2021. Available from https://www.rescuelegs.com/the-natural-brand/lymphedema-garments/
32. Luna Medical Inc. *Reidsleeve Compression Garments*. [Internet]. 2021. Available from https://www.lunamedical.com/products/reidsleeve/
33. Schmitz KH, Ahmed RL, Troxel A, et al. Weight lifting in women with breast-cancer–related lymphedema. *N Engl J Med*. 2009;361(7):664–73. doi:10.1056/NEJMoa0810118
34. Schmitz KH, Ahmed RL, Troxel AB, et al. Weight lifting for women at risk for breast cancer-related lymphedema: a randomized trial. *JAMA*. 2010;304(24):2699–705. doi:10.1001/jama.2010.1837
35. Lakoski SG, Barlow CE, Koelwyn GJ, et al. The influence of adjuvant therapy on cardiorespiratory fitness in early-stage breast cancer seven years after diagnosis: the Cooper Center Longitudinal Study. *Breast Cancer Res Treat*. 2013;138(3):909–16. doi:10.1007/s10549-013-2478-1
36. Dolezal BA, Neufeld EV, Boland DM, Martin JL, Cooper CB. Interrelationship between sleep and exercise: a systematic review. *Adv Prev Med*. 2017;2017:1364387. doi:10.1155/2017/1364387
37. Santos L, Elliott-Sale KJ, Sale C. Exercise and bone health across the lifespan. *Biogerontology*. 2017;18(6):931–46. doi:10.1007/s10522-017-9732-6
38. Wilt TJ, MacDonald R, Brasure M, et al. Pharmacologic treatment of insomnia disorder: an evidence report for a clinical practice guideline by the American College of Physicians. *Ann Intern Med*. 2016;165(2):103–12. doi:10.7326/m15-1781
39. Kline CE. The bidirectional relationship between exercise and sleep: implications for exercise adherence and sleep improvement. *Am J Lifestyle Med*. 2014;8(6):375–9. doi:10.1177/1559827614544437
40. Yang P-Y, Ho K-H, Chen H-C, Chien M-Y. Exercise training improves sleep quality in middle-aged and older adults with sleep problems: a systematic review. *J Physiother*. 2012;58(3):157–63. doi:10.1016/S1836-9553(12)70106-6
41. Mercier J, Savard J, Bernard P. Exercise interventions to improve sleep in cancer patients: a systematic review and meta-analysis. *Sleep Med Rev*. 2017;36:43–56. doi:10.1016/j.smrv.2016.11.001
42. Takemura N, Cheung DST, Smith R, et al. Effectiveness of aerobic exercise and mind-body exercise in cancer patients with poor sleep quality: a systematic review and meta-analysis of randomized controlled trials. *Sleep Med Rev*. 2020;53:101334. doi:10.1016/j.smrv.2020.101334
43. Walls GM, Lyon AR, Harbinson MT, Hanna GG. Cardiotoxicity following cancer treatment. *Ulster Med J*. 2017;86(1):3–9.
44. Kang DW, Wilson RL, Christopher CN, et al. Exercise cardio-oncology: exercise as a potential therapeutic modality in the management of anthracycline-induced cardiotoxicity. *Front Cardiovasc Med*. 2021;8:805735 doi:10.3389/fcvm.2021.805735
45. Hershman DL, Lacchetti C, Dworkin RH, et al. Prevention and management of chemotherapy-induced peripheral neuropathy in survivors of adult cancers: American Society of Clinical Oncology Clinical Practice Guideline. *J Clin Oncol*. 2014;32(18):1941–67. doi:10.1200/JCO.2013.54.0914
46. Gordon BS, Gbadamosi B, Jaiyesimi IA. The relationship between chemotherapy-induced neuropathy and quality of life in breast cancer survivors. *J Clin Oncol*. 2018;36(suppl 15):e22111. doi:10.1200/JCO.2018.36.15_suppl.e22111
47. Byrne LM, Rodrigues FB, Blennow K, et al. Neurofilament light protein in blood as a potential biomarker of neurodegeneration in Huntington's disease: a retrospective cohort analysis. *The Lancet Neurol*. 2017;16(8):601–9. doi:10.1016/S1474-4422(17)30124-2
48. Winters-Stone KM, Horak F, Jacobs PG, et al. Falls, functioning, and disability among women with persistent symptoms of chemotherapy-induced peripheral neuropathy. *J Clin Oncol*. 2017;35(23):2604–12. doi:10.1200/JCO.2016.71.3552
49. Duregon F, Vendramin B, Bullo V, et al. Effects of exercise on cancer patients suffering chemotherapy-induced peripheral neuropathy undergoing treatment: a systematic review. *Crit Rev Oncol Hematol*. 2018;121:90–100. doi:10.1016/j.critrevonc.2017.11.002
50. Ahles TA, Root JC, Ryan EL. Cancer- and cancer treatment-associated cognitive change: an update on the state of the science. *J Clin Oncol*. 2012;30(30):3675–86. doi:10.1200/JCO.2012.43.0116
51. Wigmore P. The effect of systemic chemotherapy on neurogenesis, plasticity and memory. In: Belzung C, Wigmore P, editors. *Neurogenesis and Neural Plasticity*. Berlin, Heidelberg: Springer Berlin Heidelberg; 2013, pp. 211–40. https://doi.org/10.1007/7854_2012_235
52. Seigers R, Fardell JE. Neurobiological basis of chemotherapy-induced cognitive impairment: a review of rodent research. *Neurosci Biobehav Rev*. 2011;35(3):729–41. doi:10.1016/j.neubiorev.2010.09.006
53. Wefel JS, Schagen SB. Chemotherapy-related cognitive dysfunction. *Curr Neurol Neurosci Rep*. 2012;12(3):267–75. doi:10.1007/s11910-012-0264-9
54. Vardy J, Wefel JS, Ahles T, Tannock IF, Schagen SB. Cancer and cancer-therapy related cognitive dysfunction: an international perspective from the Venice cognitive workshop. *Ann Oncol*. 2008;19(4):623–9. doi:10.1093/annonc/mdm500
55. Hermelink K, Bühner M, Sckopke P, et al. Chemotherapy and post-traumatic stress in the causation of cognitive dysfunction in breast cancer patients. *J Natl Cancer Inst*. 2017;109(10). doi:10.1093/jnci/djx057
56. Ahles TA, Hurria A. New challenges in psycho-oncology research IV: cognition and cancer: conceptual and methodological issues and future directions. *Psychooncology*. 2018;27(1):3–9. doi:10.1002/pon.4564
57. Campbell KL, Zadravec K, Bland KA, Chesley E, Wolf F, Janelsins MC. The effect of exercise on cancer-related cognitive impairment and applications for physical therapy: systematic review of randomized controlled trials. *Phys Ther*. 2020;100(3):523–42. doi:10.1093/ptj/pzz090
58. Stevens J, Burns E. *A CDC Compendium of Effective Fall Interventions: What Works for Community-Dwelling Adults*. Atlanta (GA): Centers for Disease Control and Prevention, National Center for Injury Prevention and Control; 2015.
59. Winningham ML, MacVicar MG. The effect of aerobic exercise on patient reports of nausea. *Oncol Nurs Forum*. 1988;15(4):447–50.
60. van Waart H, Stuiver MM, van Harten WH, et al. Effect of low-intensity physical activity and moderate- to high-intensity physical exercise during adjuvant chemotherapy on physical fitness, fatigue, and chemotherapy completion rates: results of the PACES randomized clinical trial. *J Clin Oncol*. 2015;33(17):1918–27. doi:10.1200/jco.2014.59.1081
61. Messier SP, Mihalko SL, Legault C, et al. Effects of intensive diet and exercise on knee joint loads, inflammation, and clinical outcomes among overweight and obese adults with knee osteoarthritis: The IDEA randomized clinical trial. *JAMA*. 2013;310(12):1263–73. doi:10.1001/jama.2013.277669
62. Better balance: mental and physical fitness are both essential. *Harvard Men's Health Watch*. 2013;17(11):5.
63. Galvão DA, Taaffe DR, Chambers SK, et al. Exercise intervention and sexual function in advanced prostate cancer: a randomised controlled trial. *BMJ Support Palliat Care*. 2020. doi:10.1136/bmjspcare-2020-002706

64. Cormie P, Chambers SK, Newton RU, et al. Improving sexual health in men with prostate cancer: randomised controlled trial of exercise and psychosexual therapies. *BMC Cancer.* 2014;14(1):199. doi:10.1186/1471-2407-14-199
65. Cormie P, Newton RU, Taaffe DR, et al. Exercise maintains sexual activity in men undergoing androgen suppression for prostate cancer: a randomized controlled trial. *Prostate Cancer Prostatic Dis.* 2013;16(2):170–5. doi:10.1038/pcan.2012.52
66. Wong SM, Freedman RA, Sagara Y, Aydogan F, Barry WT, Golshan M. Growing use of contralateral prophylactic mastectomy despite no improvement in long-term survival for invasive breast cancer. *Ann Surg.* 2017;265(3):581–9. doi:10.1097/SLA.0000000000001698
67. Poorvu PD, Frazier AL, Feraco AM, et al. Cancer treatment-related infertility: a critical review of the evidence. *JNCI Cancer Spectr.* 2019;3(1):pkz008. doi:10.1093/jncics/pkz008
68. Kirkham AA, Gelmon KA, Van Patten CL, et al. Impact of exercise on chemotherapy tolerance and survival in early-stage breast cancer: a nonrandomized controlled trial. *J Natl Compr Canc Netw.* 2020;18(12):1670–7. doi:10.6004/jnccn.2020.7603
69. Courneya KS, McKenzie DC, Mackey JR, et al. Effects of exercise dose and type during breast cancer chemotherapy: multicenter randomized trial. *J Natl Cancer Inst.* 2013;105(23):1821–32. doi:10.1093/jnci/djt297

SECTION 3

Assessing and Prescribing Exercise Before, During, and After Cancer

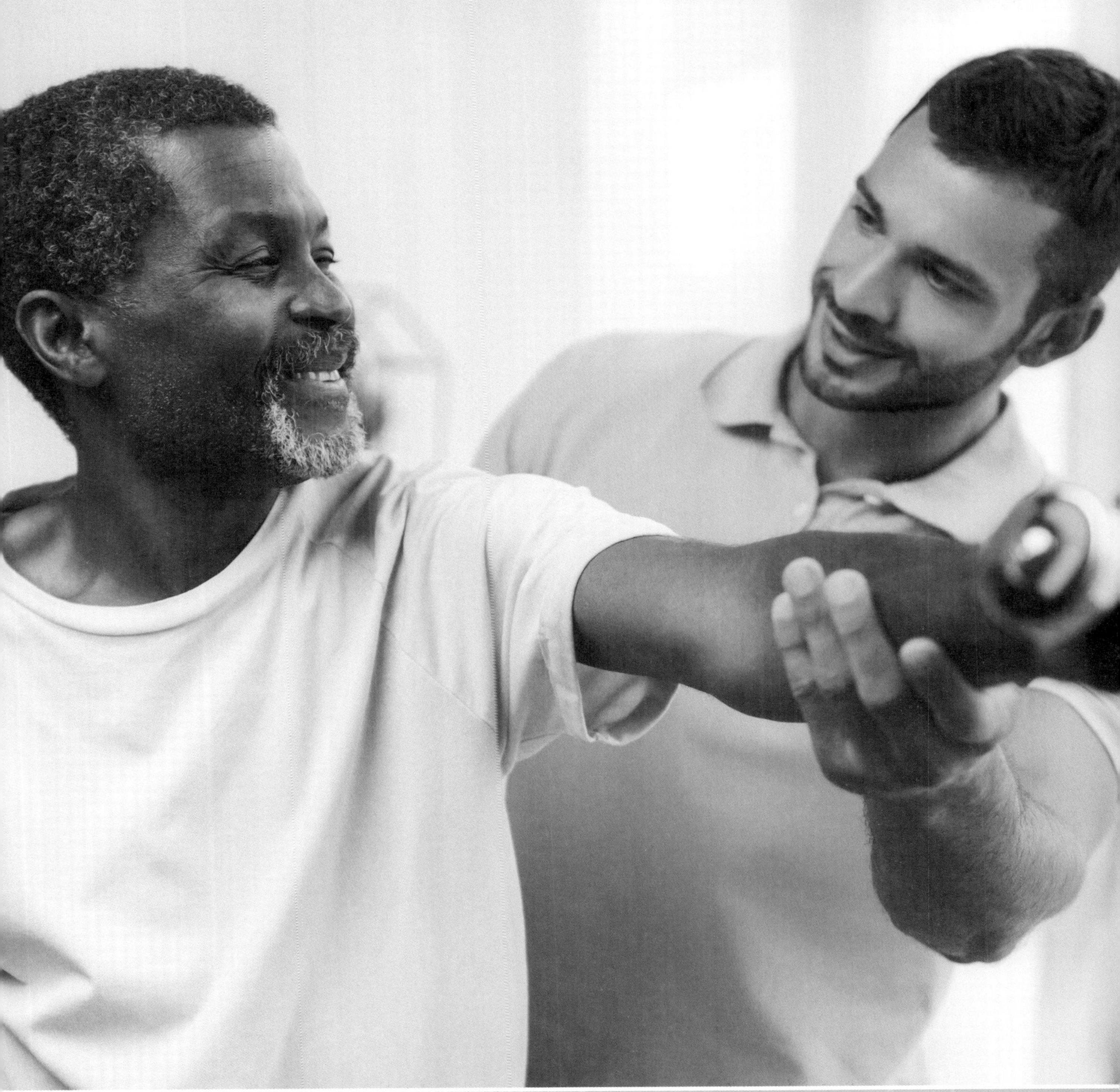

CHAPTER

9

Prescribing Exercise for Cancer Risk Reduction

OUTLINE

1. Introduction
2. Physical Activity Recommendations for Cancer Risk Reduction
3. Pre-exercise Assessments
   a. Screening Process
4. Achieving the Recommendations
   a. Active: Symptomatic or With Known Disease
   b. Sedentary: Healthy or With Symptoms or Known Disease
   c. Active: Healthy
5. Maintaining the Physical Activity Recommendations
6. The Role of Resistance Exercise in Cancer Risk Reduction
7. Mechanisms by Which Physical Activity Reduces Cancer Risk
8. A Word About Secondary Prevention (Prescribing Exercise for Cancer Survivors)
9. Summary
10. Case Study
11. Meet the Expert
12. Study Questions
13. References

OBJECTIVES

After completing review of this chapter, students will be able to:

1. Know the physical activity recommendations for cancer risk reduction.
2. Understand which pre-exercise assessments to apply according to risk and the activity level.
3. Create (prescribe) a program to achieve and maintain physical activity recommendations according to the baseline activity level.
4. Understand the role of resistance exercise in the context of physical activity and cancer risk reduction.
5. Comprehend what the physical activity recommendations are for secondary cancer risk reduction.

INTRODUCTION

For physical activity to be useful in the context of cancer risk reduction, the recommendation for all Americans is to meet the current physical activity guidelines. The magnitude of risk reduction varies by cancer type, as shown in Table 9.1 (1). Also provided in the table is the overall evidence grade for the association of physical activity and the specific cancer and an indication of whether there is evidence for a dose-response relationship (1). A dose-response relationship indicates that a greater amount of exposure (eg, more physical activity) is associated with a greater amount of change in risk (eg, the amount of physical activity is directly related to the magnitude of cancer risk reduction). Evidence of a dose-response relationship increases our confidence that the association is causal.

This chapter is focused on helping the exercise oncology professional to follow evidence-based guidelines for pre-exercise screening and prescribe exercise that meets participants' level of activity and fitness and ensures cancer risk reduction. By doing so, we believe that we are ensuring both the safety and success of exercise oncology clinical practice.

PHYSICAL ACTIVITY RECOMMENDATIONS FOR CANCER RISK REDUCTION

Current physical activity recommendations for cancer risk reduction arise from 3 major sources: 1. ACSM®, 2. ACS, and 3. the U.S. Department of Health and Human Services (US DHHS) (1, 2, 3). The recommendations are presented in Box 9.1. In summary, the current recommendations are to achieve 150 to 300 minutes per week of moderate-intensity aerobic physical activity (the metabolic equivalent or MET level of 3-5.99; equivalent to brisk walking) or 75 to 150 minutes per week of vigorous-intensity aerobic physical activity (the MET level of 6 or higher; equivalent to jogging, vigorous cycling, or swimming), as well as resistance exercise twice weekly. In addition, it is recommended that people should limit their sedentary behavior, and, in context of this chapter,

Table 9.1 2018 US DHHS Physical Activity Guidelines Advisory Committee Evidence on the Relationship Between Physical Activity and Risk of Developing Invasive Cancer

CANCER	OVERALL EVIDENCE GRADE	APPROXIMATE % RR REDUCTION	DOSE-RESPONSE GRADE
Bladder	Strong	15	Yes, moderate
Breast	Strong	12-21	Yes, strong
Colon	Strong	19	Yes, strong
Endometrium	Strong	20	Yes, moderate
Esophagus (adenocarcinoma)	Strong	21	No, limited
Gastric	Strong	19	Yes, moderate
Renal	Strong	12	Yes, limited
Lung	Moderate	21-25	Yes, limited
Hematologic	Limited	Variable effect sizes	Not assignable
Head & neck	Limited	Variable effect sizes	Not assignable
Ovary	Limited	8	Yes, limited
Pancreas	Limited	11	No, limited
Prostate	Limited	Variable effect sizes	Not assignable
Brain	Grade not assignable	Variable effect sizes	Not assignable
Thyroid	Limited	0	Not assignable
Rectal	Limited	0	Not assignable

US DHHS, U.S. Department of Health and Human Services.
Reprinted from McTiernan A, Friedenreich CM, Katzmarzyk PT, et al; 2018 Physical Activity Guidelines Advisory Committee. Physical activity in cancer prevention and survival: a systematic review. *Med Sci Sports Exerc.* 2019;51(6):1252–61, Table 1.

Box 9.1 Recommendations for Cancer Risk Reduction: Be Physically Active

- Adults should engage in 150 to 300 minutes of moderate-intensity physical activity per week, or 75 to 150 minutes of vigorous-intensity physical activity, or an equivalent combination; achieving or exceeding the upper limit of 300 minutes is optimal.
- Perform muscle strengthening activities at least 2 days a week.
- Limit sedentary behavior, such as sitting, lying down, and watching television, and other forms of screen-based entertainment.

watch the tendency to increase sitting time as they increase their physical activity levels.

PRE-EXERCISE ASSESSMENTS

When prescribing exercise, the *ACSM® Guidelines for Exercise Testing and Prescription* (4) recommends pre-exercise evaluations to ensure that exercise is safe, particularly with regard to cardiovascular risk. These guidelines remain intact in the setting of prescribing exercise for the purpose of cancer risk reduction. Overarching goals of pre-exercise evaluation include balancing safety with avoidance of unnecessary barriers to achieving and maintaining recommendations for physical activity. The goal of pre-exercise assessments is to triage participants into 3 possible categories: 1. ready to exercise in an unsupervised community or home-based setting, 2. requires supervision to exercise safely, or 3. requires further medical evaluation before proceeding with exercise.

Screening Process

There are 3 steps in the **screening process**:

1. The first step is to ask questions to identify signs and symptoms of underlying cardiovascular, metabolic, and kidney disease (eg, for CVD, the signs and symptoms include chest discomfort with exertion, unreasonable breathlessness, dizziness, fainting, blackouts, ankle swelling, unpleasant awareness of a forceful, rapid, or irregular heart rate, burning, or cramping sensations in lower legs when walking a short distance, or known heart murmur).

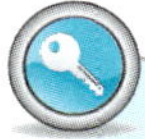

Screening process. The pre-exercise screening process involves 3 steps. First is to discern signs and symptoms of chronic diseases that may pose a risk for exercise. Second is to discern current activity levels. Third is to evaluate prior diagnoses of chronic illnesses that may alter exercise prescription.

2. The second step is to ask questions to evaluate whether the participant is currently regularly active, defined as engaging in at least 30 minutes of moderate-intensity exercise on at least 3 days per week for at least the past 3 months.
3. The third step is to evaluate whether the participant has currently or has previously had any cardiovascular or metabolic disease diagnosed (eg, a heart attack, heart surgery, cardiac catheterization, or coronary angioplasty, pacemaker/implantable cardiac defibrillator/rhythm disturbance, heart valve disease, heart failure, heart transplantation, congenital heart disease, diabetes, and renal disease).

Upon completion of these steps, there is a need to triage participants for safety reasons. Those who mark "no" to all items in all steps should proceed to slowly increase physical activity toward recommendations. Those who mark "no" to all items in Steps 1 and 3 (signs and symptoms and cardiovascular and metabolic diagnoses) and "yes" to all items in Step 2 should increase activity levels to recommended levels. Those who answer "yes" to any signs and symptoms (Step 1 of Figure 9.1) should receive medical clearance before increasing their activity level. Those who answer "yes" to Step 2 (adequately physically active) and marked "yes" to any of the cardiovascular or metabolic diseases in Step 3 should start with light-to-moderate physical activity and should receive medical clearance prior to proceeding with vigorous-intensity activity. Those who answer "no" to Step 2 (not currently physically active) and marked "yes" to any of the cardiovascular or metabolic diseases in Step 3 should be asked to obtain medical clearance prior to increasing their physical activity levels. Table 9.2 summarizes when medical clearance is needed.

It is possible that there will be settings when participants will need to self-direct (make a personal decision) as to whether they need medical clearance. In these settings, ACSM® recommends the use of the Physical Activity Readiness Questionnaire (PARQ+) survey as shown in Figure 9.2. This survey starts with 7 questions that allow the participant to self-determine whether medical clearance is advisable prior to starting an exercise program, including multiple follow-up questions. If exercise oncology professionals choose to use this survey with participants, it should be checked carefully to see that it was completed thoroughly.

Finally, all of the instructions above regarding screening make the assumption that the exercise oncology professional is working with the general public. Preparticipation evaluation for participants with complicated clinical conditions may need to be more extensively evaluated (eg, neurologic conditions, symptomatic cardiovascular diagnoses, and recent cardiovascular events). These issues are covered by the screening guidelines above, but the level of medical clearance and supervision advisable will vary according to the risk level for a given participant. Students interested in more details on this topic are advised to review chapter 2 in *ACSM's® Guidelines for Exercise Testing and Prescription* (4).

Assess your client's health needs by marking all statements.

Step 1

SIGNS AND SYMPTOMS

Does your client experience:

___ chest discomfort with exertion
___ unreasonable breathlessness
___ dizziness, fainting, blackouts
___ ankle swelling
___ unpleasant awareness of a forceful, rapid or irregular heart rate
___ burning or cramping sensations in your lower legs when walking short distance
___ known heart murmur

If you **did** mark any of these statements under the symptoms, **STOP**, your client should seek medical clearance before engaging in or resuming exercise. Your client may need to use a facility with a **medically qualified staff**.

If you **did not** mark any symptoms, continue to steps 2 and 3.

Step 2

CURRENT ACTIVITY

Has your client performed planned, structured physical activity for at least 30 min at moderate intensity on at least 3 days per week for at least the last 3 months?

Yes ☐ No ☐

Continue to Step 3.

Step 3

MEDICAL CONDITIONS

Has your client had or do they currently have:

___ a heart attack
___ heart surgery, cardiac catheterization, or coronary angioplasty
___ pacemaker/implantable cardiac defibrillator/rhythm disturbance
___ heart valve disease
___ heart failure
___ heart transplantation
___ congenital heart disease
___ diabetes
___ renal disease

Evaluating Steps 2 and 3:

- If you **did not mark any of the statements in Step 3**, medical clearance is not necessary.
- If you marked Step 2 "**yes**" and **marked any of the statements in Step 3**, your client may continue to exercise at light to moderate intensity without medical clearance. However, medical clearance is recommended before engaging in vigorous exercise.
- If you marked Step 2 "**no**" and **marked any of the statements in Step 3**, medical clearance is recommended. Your client may need to use a facility with a **medically qualified staff**.

FIGURE 9.1. Exercise Preparticipation Health Screening Questionnaire for Exercise Professionals. (From American College of Sports Medicine®. In: Liguori G, editor. *ACSM's® Guidelines for Exercise Testing and Prescription.* 11th ed. Philadelphia (PA): Wolters Kluwer; 2021, Figure 2.3.)

Table 9.2 When Medical Clearance Is Needed for the Prescription of Moderate-Intensity Exercise

	MEDICAL STATUS				
	SYMPTOMATIC, ACTIVE OR SEDENTARY (YES/NO)	SEDENTARY, KNOWN DISEASE (YES/NO)	ACTIVE, KNOWN DISEASE (YES/NO)	SEDENTARY HEALTHY (YES/NO)	ACTIVE, HEALTHY (YES/NO)
Signs or symptoms (Step 1)	Yes	No	No	No	No
Currently adequately active (Step 2)	Yes or No	No	Yes	No	Yes
Known cardiovascular or metabolic disease?	Yes or No	Yes	Yes	No	No
Group name	Symptomatic, active or sedentary	Sedentary, known disease	Active, known disease	Sedentary healthy	Active, healthy

2023 PAR-Q+

The Physical Activity Readiness Questionnaire for Everyone

The health benefits of regular physical activity are clear; more people should engage in physical activity every day of the week. Participating in physical activity is very safe for MOST people. This questionnaire will tell you whether it is necessary for you to seek further advice from your doctor OR a qualified exercise professional before becoming more physically active.

GENERAL HEALTH QUESTIONS

Please read the 7 questions below carefully and answer each one honestly: check YES or NO.	YES	NO
1) Has your doctor ever said that you have a heart condition ☐ OR high blood pressure ☐?	☐	☐
2) Do you feel pain in your chest at rest, during your daily activities of living, **OR** when you do physical activity?	☐	☐
3) Do you lose balance because of dizziness **OR** have you lost consciousness in the last 12 months? Please answer **NO** if your dizziness was associated with over-breathing (including during vigorous exercise).	☐	☐
4) Have you ever been diagnosed with another chronic medical condition (other than heart disease or high blood pressure)? **PLEASE LIST CONDITION(S) HERE:** ______	☐	☐
5) Are you currently taking prescribed medications for a chronic medical condition? **PLEASE LIST CONDITION(S) AND MEDICATIONS HERE:** ______	☐	☐
6) Do you currently have (or have had within the past 12 months) a bone, joint, or soft tissue (muscle, ligament, or tendon) problem that could be made worse by becoming more physically active? Please answer **NO** if you had a problem in the past, but it **does not limit your current ability** to be physically active. **PLEASE LIST CONDITION(S) HERE:** ______	☐	☐
7) Has your doctor ever said that you should only do medically supervised physical activity?	☐	☐

If you answered NO to all of the questions above, you are cleared for physical activity.
Please sign the PARTICIPANT DECLARATION. You do not need to complete Pages 2 and 3.

- Start becoming much more physically active – start slowly and build up gradually.
- Follow Global Physical Activity Guidelines for your age (https://www.who.int/publications/i/item/9789240015128).
- You may take part in a health and fitness appraisal.
- If you are over the age of 45 yr and NOT accustomed to regular vigorous to maximal effort exercise, consult a qualified exercise professional before engaging in this intensity of exercise.
- If you have any further questions, contact a qualified exercise professional.

PARTICIPANT DECLARATION

If you are less than the legal age required for consent or require the assent of a care provider, your parent, guardian or care provider must also sign this form.

I, the undersigned, have read, understood to my full satisfaction and completed this questionnaire. I acknowledge that this physical activity clearance is valid for a maximum of 12 months from the date it is completed and becomes invalid if my condition changes. I also acknowledge that the community/fitness center may retain a copy of this form for its records. In these instances, it will maintain the confidentiality of the same, complying with applicable law.

NAME ______ DATE ______

SIGNATURE ______ WITNESS ______

SIGNATURE OF PARENT/GUARDIAN/CARE PROVIDER ______

If you answered YES to one or more of the questions above, COMPLETE PAGES 2 AND 3.

Delay becoming more active if:

- You have a temporary illness such as a cold or fever; it is best to wait until you feel better.
- You are pregnant - talk to your health care practitioner, your physician, a qualified exercise professional, and/or complete the ePARmed-X+ at www.eparmedx.com before becoming more physically active.
- Your health changes - answer the questions on Pages 2 and 3 of this document and/or talk to your doctor or a qualified exercise professional before continuing with any physical activity program.

 1 / 4
01-11-2022

FIGURE 9.2. The Physical Activity Readiness Questionnaire for Everyone (PAR-Q+). (Reprinted with permission from the PAR-Q+ Collaboration and the authors of the PAR-Q+. Available from http://eparmedx.com/ for the most current annual update of the PAR-Q+.)

Table 9.3 Plan to Achieve Physical Activity Recommendations for Active Patients With Symptoms or Known Disease

EXERCISE	WK 1	WK 2	WK 3	WK 4	WK 5	WK 6	WK 7	WK 8	WK 9	WK 10	WK 11	WK 12
Aerobic	30 min 3×; MET level 3-5.99	35 min 3×; MET level 3-5.99	40 min 3×; MET level 3-5.99	45 min 3×; MET level 3-5.99	50 min 3×; MET level 3-5.99	50 min 3×; MET level 3-5.99	50 min 3×; MET level 3-5.99	50 min 3×; MET level 3-5.99	50 min 3×; MET level 3-5.99	50 min 3×; MET level 3-5.99	50 min 3×; MET level 3-5.99	50 min 3×; MET level 4-5.99
Resistance	Nothing	Nothing	Nothing	Nothing	Nothing	2 sessions 1 exercise per 9 muscle groups[a]: 1× each 10 repetitions, initial resistance set low to allow learning biomechanics	2 sessions 1 exercise per 9 muscle groups[a]: 2× each 10 repetitions, no increase in resistance	2 sessions 1 exercise per 9 muscle groups[a]: 2× each 10 repetitions, 10%-20% increase in resistance	2 sessions 1 exercise per 9 muscle groups[a]: 2× each 10 repetitions, no increase in resistance	2 sessions 1 exercise per 9 muscle groups[a]: 2× each 10 repetitions, 10%-20% increase in resistance	2 sessions 1 exercise per 9 muscle groups[a]: 2× each 10 repetitions, no increase in resistance	2 sessions 1 exercise per 9 muscle groups[a]: 2× each 10 repetitions, 10%-20% increase in resistance
Sitting time	Advice to sit less throughout the day and, in particular, to watch for and avoid increases in sitting time as physical activity goes up.											

MET, metabolic equivalent.
[a]Chest, back, deltoids, biceps, triceps, quadriceps, hamstrings, gluteus maximus, calves.

ACHIEVING THE RECOMMENDATIONS

All recommendations below follow the FITT-VP principle: Frequency, Intensity, Time, and Type of exercise are specified in each section, as well as volume and progression. This is the standard for exercise prescription. Plan that every exercise prescription made will include each of these elements, to ensure that it is clear for the participant what they are being asked to do, and so that progress can be documented with specificity.

Active: Symptomatic or With Known Disease

The first step with symptomatic participants is to obtain medical clearance prior to proceeding. The remainder of this section assumes that clearance has been obtained from a clinician. No clearance is required for currently active participants with a known disease.

Here we are describing participants who are already active. Therefore, this participant population is starting with at least 90 minutes per week of moderate-intensity physical activity. The screening query does not ask about resistance exercise. We start here with the assumption that the participant is currently achieving 90 minutes per week of moderate-intensity physical activity and no resistance exercise. Given the risk of adverse clinical events with vigorous activity in this population, it is advisable to continue to prescribe continued moderate-intensity activity until or unless the participant specifically asks to do vigorous activity. Our goal is for the participant to be fully adherent to physical activity recommendations by the end of 12 weeks. Table 9.3 is a plan to get there. Note that the weekly increases are modest (10%-20%) or add only to the resistance exercise plan, not both at the same time, to avoid overwhelming the participant (behaviorally and physiologically).

FITT-VP. Frequency, intensity, time, type, volume, and progression. This is the abbreviation to denote the dose and progression of exercise to be prescribed in a manner that can document all aspects of the activities to be performed.

Sedentary: Healthy or With Symptoms or Known Disease

The first step for sedentary participants with symptoms or known disease is to obtain medical clearance prior to proceeding. The remainder of this section assumes that clearance has been obtained from a clinician. It is recommended that those who are currently sedentary increase their activity first by performing activities of light-to-moderate intensity (MET levels of 2-3), gradually increasing the duration of activities to 150 to 300 minutes per week and to moderate intensity (MET levels of 3-5 on the 0-10 scale). A 12-week plan to achieve the recommendations for aerobic exercise is provided in Table 9.4.

We do acknowledge that the delay to starting resistance exercise is not ideal from a physiologic benefits standpoint. However, from the viewpoint of behavior change, it may be preferable to get the aerobic exercise habit established before adding resistance exercise. It is possible that some participants may prefer/be able to proceed more quickly than what is outlined above, and exercise oncology professionals should set goals appropriate to the specific participant. It is also possible that a particular participant might prefer to do more resistance training than aerobic exercise. Asking a participant to proceed too slowly can be just as detrimental as suggestions to proceed faster than is comfortable or safe. A balance should be obtained between evaluating what is safe for the participant and what will keep the participant's engaged. We review behavioral issues in Chapter 15 of this book.

Active: Healthy

This population has no symptoms or known disease and are already doing moderate-intensity aerobic exercise at least 3 times weekly, 30 minutes per session. The amount of activity in such a population is determined by asking the

Table 9.4 Exercise Progression for Sedentary Participants, Regardless of Disease History (From No Exercise to Meeting the Aerobic Guidelines in 12 Weeks)

EXERCISE	WK 1	WK 2	WK 3	WK 4	WK 5	WK 6	WK 7	WK 8	WK 9	WK 10	WK 11	WK 12
Aerobic	15 min 3×; MET levels 2-3	20 min 3×; MET levels 2-3	25 min 3×; MET levels 2-3	30 min 3×; MET levels 2-3	30 min 3×; MET levels 3-4	35 min 3×; MET levels 3-4	40 min 3×; MET levels 3-4	40 min 3×; MET levels 4-5	45 min 3×; MET levels 4-5	50 min 3×; MET levels 4-5	50 min 3×; MET levels 4-5.99	50 min 3×; MET levels 4-5.99
Resistance	None. Add resistance exercise after aerobic exercise is maintained for several months.											
Sitting time	Advice to sit less throughout the day and, in particular, to watch for and avoid increases in sitting time as physical activity goes up.											

MET, metabolic equivalent.

Table 9.5 **Achieving the Physical Activity Recommendations by the End of 12 Weeks, Starting Active and Healthy**

EXERCISE	WK 1	WK 2	WK 3	WK 4	WK 5	WK 6	WK 7	WK 8	WK 9	WK 10	WK 11	WK 12
Aerobic	30 min 3×; MET levels 3-5.99	35 min 3×; MET levels 3-5.99	40 min 3×; MET levels 3-5.99	45 min 3×; MET levels 3-5.99	50 min 3×; MET levels 3-5.99	50 min 3×; MET levels 4-6	50 min 3×; MET levels 4-6	50 min 3×; MET levels 5-7	50 min 3×; MET levels 5-7	50 min 3×; MET levels 6-8	50 min 3×; MET levels 6-8	50 min 3×; MET levels 6-8
Resistance	2 sessions 1 exercise per 9 muscle groups[a]: 1× each 10 repetitions, initial resistance set low to allow learning biomechanics	2 sessions 1 exercise per 9 muscle groups[a]: 2× each 10 repetitions, no increase in resistance	2 sessions 1 exercise per 9 muscle groups[a]: 2× each 10 repetitions, 10%-20% increase in resistance	2 sessions 1 exercise per 9 muscle groups[a]: 2× each 10 repetitions, no increase in resistance	2 sessions 1 exercise per 9 muscle groups[a]: 2× each 10 repetitions, 10%-20% increase in resistance	2 sessions 1 exercise per 9 muscle groups[a]: 2× each 10 repetitions, no increase in resistance	2 sessions 1 exercise per 9 muscle groups[a]: 2× each 10 repetitions, 10%-20% increase in resistance	2 sessions 1 exercise per 9 muscle groups[a]: 2× each 10 repetitions, no increase in resistance	2 sessions 1 exercise per 9 muscle groups[a]: 2× each 10 repetitions, 10%-20% increase in resistance	2 sessions 1 exercise per 9 muscle groups[a]: 2× each 10 repetitions, no increase in resistance	2 sessions 1 exercise per 9 muscle groups[a]: 2× each 10 repetitions, 10%-20% increase in resistance	2 sessions 1 exercise per 9 muscle groups[a]: 2× each 10 repetitions, no increase in resistance
Sitting time	Advice to sit less throughout the day and, in particular, to watch for and avoid increases in sitting time as physical activity goes up.											

MET, metabolic equivalent.

[a]chest, back, deltoids, biceps, triceps, quadriceps, hamstrings, gluteus maximus, calves.

Table 9.6 Examples and Explanation of Intensity for Several Ranges of Metabolic Equivalent Levels

MET LEVEL	EXAMPLES	BREATHING/HEART RATE	HOW IT FEELS (RPE ON A 1-10 SCALE)
2-3 (light-to-moderate intensity)	Walking 2-2.9 miles per hour, stationary cycling at 50 watts, leisurely canoeing, croquet, bowling, slow ballroom dancing, golf with a cart, playing catch, playing piano, stretching exercises or yoga	Minimal increase, can continue singing (holding a note)	Feels easy (RPE: 1-3)
3-5.99 (moderate intensity)	Walking 3-4.5 miles per hour; biking outside; leisurely, stationary biking 100 watts; low-impact aerobic dance; badminton, baseball, or softball; basketball, shooting hoops; dancing fast; golf, walking with bag; horseback riding; ice skating; kayaking; skateboarding; swimming at moderate pace; table tennis; tai chi; doubles tennis	Noticeable increase, can continue singing for shorter periods (holding a note)	Feels between easy and somewhat hard (RPE: 4-6)
5-7 (moderate-to-vigorous intensity)	Jogging 4.5-4.7 miles per hour, stationary cycling 100 watts, baseball or softball, ballet dancing, fencing, hiking, ice skating, kayaking, shoveling snow, downhill skiing, surfing, aerobic dance, backpacking, singles tennis	Noticeable to large increase in breathing and heart rate, ability to speak in full sentences, but not sing	Feels somewhat hard (RPE: 5-7)
6-8 (vigorous intensity)	Jogging up to 5 miles per hour, bicycling 12-13 miles per hour, aerobic dance, basketball game, touch football, ultimate frisbee, ice or field hockey, lacrosse, racquetball, skipping rope, cross-country skiing, snow shoeing, soccer, swimming laps at a moderate pace, tennis, water jogging, walking up stairs	Large increase in breathing and heart rate, but not breathlessness, inability to speak full sentences	Feels somewhat hard to hard (RPE: 7-10)

RPE, Rated Perceived Exertion.

participant. This active or healthy group can expand their exercise dose to meet the guidelines with moderate- or vigorous-intensity exercise, and they should be doing resistance exercise as well. To delineate from other populations, the example for this population seeks to meet the upper end of the guidelines, using vigorous-intensity activities and adding resistance exercise (Table 9.5). The principles of progression are the same, however, with increases in the 10% to 20% range weekly. A key difference in this example is that there is a focus on increasing intensity.

Examples of Exercises at Various Metabolic Equivalent Levels

Throughout the examples above there are references to MET levels for specific exercise prescriptions. But what are the exercises to recommend to those who should be doing the exercise of MET levels of 2 to 3, 3 to 5.99, or 6 to 8? In Table 9.6, we present examples of exercises at each of these ranges of METs.

MAINTAINING THE PHYSICAL ACTIVITY RECOMMENDATIONS

Once a participant has reached the recommended level of physical activity for cancer risk reduction, there is a new goal—maintaining that level of activity for the long term. The benefits of regular physical activity for cancer risk reduction are mostly enjoyed by those who exercise regularly for many years, not just for a few weeks. Behavioral science has empirically tested multiple strategies to help people to maintain a physical activity program for the long term. These include making physical activity fun and interesting, making it part of a daily routine, developing a reward system for those who perform regular exercise, writing down activity sessions (logging), setting SMART (specific, measurable, attainable, relevant, and time-bound) goals for activity, finding someone to exercise with, and maintaining flexibility.

By making activity fun and interesting, we address the potential pitfall of becoming bored with our routine. Some people enjoy the routine of the same walk on the same route day after day. But if a participant reports being bored by their activity routine, suggest some variety. Make activity more like play. Set up games and/or make activity more of a social event. By making activity part of a daily routine, we tap into a very well established human tendency for habit defined as a settled, regular practice that is hard to give up,

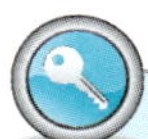

SMART. SMART stands for specific, measurable, attainable, relevant, and time-bound. The recommendation is to set goals with these attributes to promote increased exercise adherence.

that is, something that we do automatically, without thinking. The behavioral literature about habit formation suggests that it takes between 18 and 254 days to form a habit, with an average of 66 days (5). Tips to build the habit of staying with a physical activity routine include attaching the behavior to something else (eg, making coffee leads to physical activity), do it every day, set things up to make it easy (eg, put out exercise clothes and shoes in the evening to be ready for a morning workout), and build a reward system (eg, massage after 6 weeks of consistent exercise).

By setting SMART goals and documenting our activity sessions in a logging system, we create the opportunity to establish accountability. A SMART goal for maintaining the recommended physical activity levels might be to specify the goals themselves, which are measurable (logging helps), and to ensure that time and resources are managed to make this long-term goal attainable. The element of being relevant could be a connection to family risk for cancer, or it could be a goal that a person sets for her/himself, which is specifically relevant to her/his life (eg, a father who sets a goal to climb Mt. Rainier in Washington State with his son, a year from now). Time-bound goals are helpful as well, such as our example of training to climb a mountain. The goal of "I will maintain the physical activity recommendations for cancer risk reduction because it is good for me" is not likely to work for most people. Work to identify something specifically relevant and time-bound to increase the likelihood of physical activity maintenance success. Along the way, in order for the SMART goal approach to work, it is useful to measure progress by writing down every activity session along the way. There are any number of electronic trackers on the market that may assist with this process.

By finding someone to exercise with, we address an important construct of social support for exercise. People vary with regard to their willingness and need for having someone to exercise with, and this may change over time. But if someone is struggling to stay with a routine that is solo (running alone), suggest finding another person to keep them accountable, provide company, and to motivate to keep going. This is a well-established contributor to exercise adherence (6).

By maintaining flexibility to our exercise adherence successes, we avoid the all-or-nothing thinking that can lead to abandoning the goal based on normal, expected fluctuations in success along the path. Behavioral scientists refer to behavioral shaping as a process of establishing a behavior that is not learned or performed at present (7). This process requires trial and error and may require many attempts for achieving the success. Well-established elements of successful behavioral shaping include starting with rewarding anything that is remotely similar to the desired behavior (eg, getting to 75 minutes of moderate-intensity exercise in a week), shifting rewards to behaviors that are closer to the goal (eg, getting to 125 minutes of moderate-intensity exercise in a week), and only rewarding achieving the goal itself (eg, getting 150 minutes of moderate-intensity exercise and twice weekly resistance exercise in a week).

For more about behavioral strategies to increase and maintain higher physical activity levels, see Chapter 15.

THE ROLE OF RESISTANCE EXERCISE IN CANCER RISK REDUCTION

The *US DHHS Physical Activity Guidelines* are to achieve 150 to 300 minutes per week of moderate-intensity aerobic exercise or 75 to 150 minutes per week of vigorous-intensity aerobic exercise, as well as twice weekly strengthening exercise. These guidelines were developed to address risk for all chronic diseases, including CVD, diabetes, cognitive disorders, obesity, and cancer. The physical activity recommendations for cancer risk reduction from the ACS and ACSM® focus on aerobic exercise, with limited to no mention of the strengthening exercises referred to by the US DHHS recommendations. This can be explained by reviewing the scientific evidence base available for generating such recommendations. The large epidemiologic cohort studies and case control studies that are the sources of the evidence leading to the physical activity recommendations for cancer risk reduction have largely collected data about leisure-time physical activity, most of which is aerobic activity. In contrast, there is limited research on the role of resistance exercise in cancer risk reduction. One excellent example examined data from the National Institutes of Health American Association of Retired Persons Diet and Health Study follow-up to evaluate whether resistance exercise was associated with reduced risk for 10 different cancers (8). In this study of 215,122 older adults, the association of resistance exercise with 10 types of cancers was assessed: colon, kidney, bladder, breast, lung, non-Hodgkin's lymphoma, pancreatic, prostate, rectum, and melanoma. About 25% of the sample reported some resistance exercise. Resistance exercise was associated with reduced risk of colon and kidney cancers, but after adjusting for aerobic activity, the association only remained for colon cancer. There was no association noted for the other cancers aforementioned. The authors hypothesized that the lack of association with the other cancers may result from a modest number of incident cancers as compared with the large studies of associations with aerobic exercise.

This may well be a situation of a "lack of evidence" as opposed to the "evidence of a lack of effect." Evidence supports the use of resistance exercise for promoting greater muscle gain and strength, improving and maintaining blood glucose homeostasis, lowering blood pressure, improving ability to perform activities of daily living, walking, and climbing stairs. All of these could underlie the observed association with the reduced incidence of colon and kidney cancers. The effect of resistance exercise on body composition could be of particular interest for reducing the risk of cancer through mechanisms reviewed in Chapter 6.

MECHANISMS BY WHICH PHYSICAL ACTIVITY REDUCES CANCER RISK

Being more physically active on a regular basis and avoiding sedentary behavior has a number of salutary physiologic

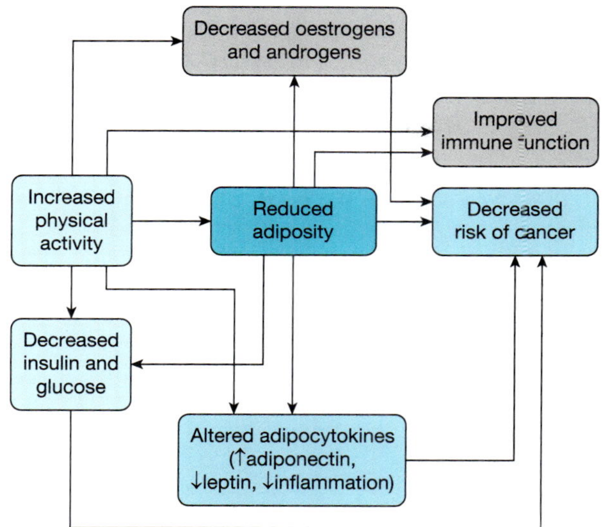

FIGURE 9.3. Hypothesized mechanisms linking physical activity to cancer risk. Denotations: ↑, increased; ↓, decreased. (Redrawn from McTiernan A. Mechanisms linking physical activity with cancer. *Nat Rev Cancer.* 2008;8(3):205–11, Figure 1.)

effects that are hypothesized to underlie the observed association of reduced cancer incidence. Central to these mechanisms is the reduction of body fat that contributes to all of the other mechanisms through which physical activity is thought to reduce cancer risk, as shown in Figure 9.3. In addition to effects secondary to reduced body fatness, regular physical activity also has direct effects on hormones (estrogens and androgens), improved immune (and inflammatory) function, reduced insulin and glucose (and improve insulin sensitivity), as well as altered adipocytokines (increased adiponectin and decreased leptin and inflammation) (9).

A WORD ABOUT SECONDARY PREVENTION (PRESCRIBING EXERCISE FOR CANCER SURVIVORS)

The ACS and ACSM® physical activity recommendations for cancer risk reduction are the same for those who have never had cancer and those who have had a prior cancer diagnosis. There is strong epidemiologic support for reduced risk for cancer-specific and all-cause mortality from breast, colon, and prostate cancers among those who are more physically active, compared with sedentary survivors. The magnitude of risk reduction is larger for secondary than primary prevention. As shown in Table 9.7, the evidence grade for these associations varies from limited to moderate, but the approximate risk reduction ranges from 37% to 48%, much larger than the primary prevention ranges documented in Table 9.1. The authors of the *US DHHS Physical Activity Guidelines* noted that the lack of evidence for a secondary prevention benefit for the other cancers for which there is a primary benefit may result from the need for additional cohorts examining physical activity in survivors. This may be another example of a "lack of evidence" rather than "evidence of lack of an association."

Table 9.7 2018 US DHHS Physical Activity Guidelines Advisory Committee Evidence on Relationship between Physical Activity and Mortality in Cancer Survivors

CANCER	EVIDENCE GRADE	APPROXIMATE % RELATIVE RISK REDUCTION
All-cause mortality		
Breast	Moderate	48
Colorectal	Moderate	42
Prostate	Limited	37-49
Cancer-specific mortality		
Breast	Moderate	38
Colorectal	Moderate	38
Prostate	Moderate	38

US DHHS, U.S. Department of Health and Human Services.
Reprinted from McTiernan A, Friedenreich CM, Katzmarzyk PT, et al; 2018 Physical Activity Guidelines Advisory Committee. Physical activity in cancer prevention and survival: a systematic review. *Med Sci Sports Exerc.* 2019;51(6):1252–61, Table 2.

SUMMARY

Physical activity has a well-established effect of cancer risk reduction in the primary prevention setting and a growing evidence base for secondary prevention. There are multiple national organizations in the US (and beyond) that recommend regular physical activity for cancer risk reduction. To apply these recommendations, the exercise oncology professional must be familiar with ACSM® pre-exercise evaluations and risk stratification strategies. Strategies to increase physical activity to the recommended levels should follow standard guidelines to increase activity levels by 10% to 20% per week. Strategies to promote the long-term maintenance of physical activity recommendations are largely behavioral in nature. Resistance exercise has been documented to make changes in body composition and other physiologic changes relevant to cancer risk reduction, despite minimal epidemiologic evidence that resistance exercise alone reduces cancer risk. We have reiterated the mechanisms through which physical activity is hypothesized to reduce cancer risk. Physical activity works through reducing body fat and altering a number of physiological pathways to exert its documented effects on cancer risk reduction.

Case Study

Dorothy is 72 years old. She lives alone; her husband died of colon cancer a year ago. Her husband's death has led to her thinking more about what she can do to reduce her risk of additional cancer diagnoses or dying of cancer. She is also interested in reducing her fall risk, increasing her ability to perform activities of daily living, climb the stairs in her home, and reduce residual adverse effects of the chronic diseases with which she has been diagnosed. Her BMI is 27, she has high blood pressure, a heart murmur, and type II diabetes. Her current activity includes walking her dog every day for about 10 minutes. She does no resistance exercise. She is asking for your help in planning an exercise program that will reduce her cancer risk.

Questions

1. What information do we have to help us screen Dorothy?
2. What exercise prescription would be provided to Dorothy to get her to the recommended levels of physical activity?

Meet the Expert

FEATURED PROFESSIONAL

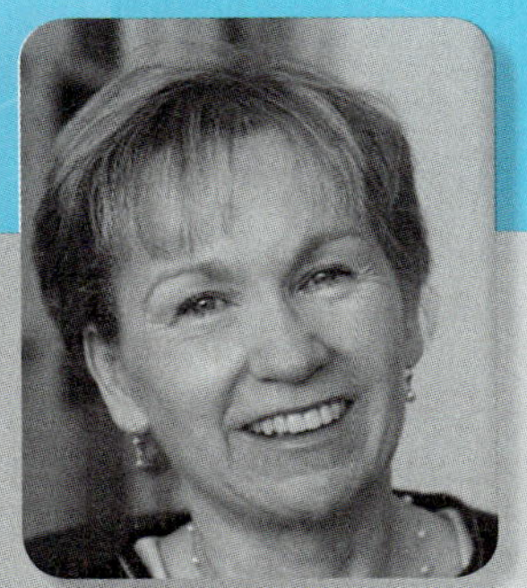

Anne McTiernan, MD, PhD

Professor, Epidemiology Program, Division of Public Health Sciences
Fred Hutchinson Cancer Research Center
Seattle, Washington DC, USA

Q: "Where did you grow up?"

I grew up in a working-class section of Boston, MA, and I was the first person in my family to finish college. I received a BA in Sociology in 1974 from Boston University, an MA in Medical Sociology with epidemiology training at the State University of New York Buffalo, and a PhD in Epidemiology at the University of Washington in 1982. During this time, I married and had 2 children, and then I attended medical school at New York Medical College. In 1989 I was awarded an MD degree. I finally finished residency training in Internal Medicine in 1992.

Q: "What are you best known for?"

I'm known for my work looking at the effects of exercise on cancer risk and prognosis in large clinical trials and observational studies, such as the Women's Health Initiative and other randomized clinical trials. Throughout my career I have focused on mentoring scientists and physicians to become leaders in exercise oncology.

Q: "What are you currently working on?"

Currently, I am funded by the Breast Cancer Research Foundation to test the acute effects of moderate-intensity aerobic exercise on biomarkers related to breast cancer.

Q: "Anything else you want to include?"

I have published 2 memoirs (Cured: A Doctor's Journey from Panic to Peace; https://www.amazon.com/Cured-Doctors-Journey-Panic-Peace/dp/1949481387/ *and Starved: A Nutrition Doctor's Journey from Empty to Full;* http://www.amazon.com/Starved-Nutrition-Doctors-Journey-Empty/dp/1942094280). *In my spare time, I enjoy hiking with my husband and family, and caring for my grandchildren. Sports I currently view is my grandchildren's soccer games and track and field events.*

Favorite Quote:

I had a circuitous route to becoming an exercise researcher. It matters less how you get there than what you do to improve people's health and lives.

—*Anne McTiernan*

STUDY QUESTIONS

1. What are the current physical activity recommendations for cancer risk reduction?
2. Risk for developing cancers for which of the organs is reduced by being more physically active? Name 4.
3. What is the goal of a pre-exercise assessment?
   a. To understand what the client wants from the program
   b. To clarify how much the participant can pay
   c. To triage participants into risk levels
   d. To discern whether they are going to be a long-term client
4. What are the 3 steps involved in pre-exercise assessment?
   a. VO_2 max test, 1-repition maximum test, and a sit-and-reach test
   b. Sit-and-reach test, balance test, and a 6-minute walk test
   c. Behavioral assessment, sit-and-reach test, and a 6-minute walk test
   d. Assess physical activity, assess signs and symptoms, and assess known diseases/diagnoses and histories
5. True or false. The pre-exercise assessment can be self-administered.
6. The FITT principle of exercise prescription refers to:
   a. Frequency, intensity, time, and type of exercise
   b. Frequency, inherent skills, time, and type of exercise
   c. Frequency, intensity, type of resistance exercise (isometric vs isotonic), and time
7. True or false. As a general rule of thumb, we seek to increase time or intensity by about 10% to 20% per week as we increase the activity level.
8. Name 4 examples of light- to moderate-intensity activity (2-3 METs).
9. Behavioral strategies for the maintenance of the recommended levels of physical activity include:
   a. Keeping a log, setting up rewards, setting goals
   b. Making exercise a daily routine and making exercise fun and interesting
   c. Making exercise a daily routine, making exercise fun and interesting
   d. a and b
   e. b and c
   f. All of the above
10. True or false. Resistance exercise may change cancer risk through changes in body composition.
11. True or false. The primary mechanism through which exercise is thought to reduce cancer risk involves changed hormone status.
12. The magnitude of risk reduction for cancer mortality after breast, colon, and prostate cancer is ____________ the magnitude of risk reduction for primary prevention of these cancers.
    a. Greater than
    b. Less than
    c. The same as
    d. Unknown for

REFERENCES

1. McTiernan A, Friedenreich CM, Katzmarzyk PT, et al. Physical activity in cancer prevention and survival: a systematic review. *Med Sci Sports Exerc.* 2019;51(6):1252–61. doi:10.1249/MSS.0000000000001937
2. Patel AV, Friedenreich CM, Moore SC, et al. American College of Sports Medicine® roundtable report on physical activity, sedentary behavior, and cancer prevention and control. *Med Sci Sports Exerc.* 2019;51(11):2391–402. doi:10.1249/MSS.0000000000002117
3. Rock CL, Thomson C, Gansler T, et al. American Cancer Society guideline for diet and physical activity for cancer prevention. *CA Cancer J Clin.* 2020;70(4):245–71. doi:10.3322/caac.21591
4. American College of Sports Medicine®. In: Liguori G, editor. *ACSM's® Guidelines for Exercise Testing and Prescription.* 11th ed. Philadelphia (PA): Wolters Kluwer; 2021.
5. Lally P, Van Jaarsveld CHM, Potts HWW, Wardle J. How are habits formed: modelling habit formation in the real world. *Eur J Soc Psychol.* 2010;40(6):998–1009.
6. Courneya KS, Plotnikoff RC, Hotz SB, Birkett NJ. Social support and the theory of planned behavior in the exercise domain. *Am J Health Behav.* 2000;24(4):300–8.
7. Ferster CB, Skinner, BF. *Schedules of Reinforcement.* New York (NY): Appleton-Century-Crofts; 1957.
8. Mazzilli KM, Matthews CE, Salerno EA, Moore SC. Weight training and risk of 10 common types of cancer. *Med Sci Sports Exerc.* 2019;51(9):1845–51. doi:10.1249/MSS.0000000000001987
9. McTiernan A. Mechanisms linking physical activity with cancer. *Nat Rev Cancer.* 2008;8(3):205–11. doi:10.1038/nrc2325

CHAPTER

10

Prehabilitation

OUTLINE

1. Introduction
2. Definition of Prehabilitation
3. Measurement and Impact of Poor Fitness Levels on Surgery Outcomes
4. Benefits of Cancer Prehabilitation
    a. Lung Cancer
    b. Abdominal Cancer
    c. Prostate Cancer
    d. Breast Cancer
5. Prehabilitation in the Cancer Care Pathway
6. Prehabilitation Exercise Prescription
    a. Screening
    b. Assessment
    c. Intervention
    d. Monitoring and Evaluation
7. Summary
8. Case Study
9. Meet the Expert
10. Study Questions
11. References

OBJECTIVES

After completing review of this chapter, students will be able to:

1. Define of prehabilitation.
2. Understand the rationale for exercise-based prehabilitation.
3. Describe the impact of poor fitness on surgery outcomes.
4. Comprehend the evidence on the benefits of prehabilitation.
5. Be aware of the process for providing exercise-based prehabilitation.

INTRODUCTION

The phase before a surgical procedure is said to be the ideal time to prepare patients for an optimal surgical outcome by carrying out prehabilitation (1). Interest in prehabilitation started in the field of sports medicine in the 1980s (2). In 2002, a theoretical model of prehabilitation (3, 4) proposed that presurgical exercise to improve functional capacity prior to a surgical procedure would lead to a shorter postoperative recovery period compared with patients who remain physically inactive through the preoperative period (Figure 10.1).

In the field of exercise oncology, the concept of prehabilitation is relatively new. Newly diagnosed cancer patients usually experience a wide range of emotional responses while waiting for treatment and are uncertain what they are allowed to do. This can result in unfavorable physical, psychological, and social issues at the start of cancer treatment and have a detrimental long-term effect in domains such as activities of daily living, family relationships, work, and, generally, QoL (5, 6). Prehabilitation interventions start at cancer diagnosis and continue during the pretreatment/presurgery period to provide strategies to support and prepare patients to cope with the impacts of cancer treatments. Currently, referral to prehabilitation is the responsibility of the perioperative team (eg, anesthetists and surgeons) and other physicians (eg, medical or radiation oncologists), who may also direct their patients to prehabilitation while undergoing neoadjuvant treatments.

DEFINITION OF PREHABILITATION

Cancer prehabilitation has been defined by Silver and Baima (7) as

> a process on the continuum of care that occurs between the time of cancer diagnosis and the beginning of acute treatment, includes physical and psychological assessments that establish a baseline functional level, identifies impairments, and provides targeted interventions that improve a person's health to prevent or reduce the incidence and the severity of current and future impairments.

As outlined in Figures 10.1 and 10.2, prehabilitation should not replace posttreatment rehabilitation but complement it.

Prehabilitation interventions can be either unimodal or multimodal. One unimodal approach is the exclusive application of different forms of exercise. To date, many prehabilitation interventions reported are unimodal probably because there is already a strong level of evidence for the benefits of exercise on cancer-related health outcomes. The second approach is the multimodal cancer prehabilitation regimen—an interdisciplinary and multiprofessional combination of exercise with further components, such as patient education and information, nutrition, psychological counseling and support, smoking cessation, and reduction of alcohol consumption. Multimodal prehabilitation focuses on issues such as limitations on active daily living,

Prehabilitation regimes vary in their composition, with some interventions seen in literature and service example *always*, some seen *often* and others *sometimes*.

Prehabilitation interventions	Always	Often	Sometimes	Rare
Physical Activity*	■			Other rare but possible interventions in a multimodal prehabilitation may include: • Balance gait • Joint range of movement • Swallowing • Sleep hygiene • Fatigue • Pulmonary function • Behavior change • Urinary incontinence • Mindfulness • Social coping
Dietary Support*		■		
Psychological Wellbeing*		■		
Anemia Management			■	
Smoking Cessation			■	
Alcohol Reduction			■	
Respiratory Exercises			■	
Lymphoedema Management			■	
Medication and Comorbidities Review			■	
Other (See Appendix A)			■	

*Based on current evidence, it is suggested that patients should have access to physical activity, dietary and psychological support as a minimum.

FIGURE 10.1. Prehabilitation interventions.

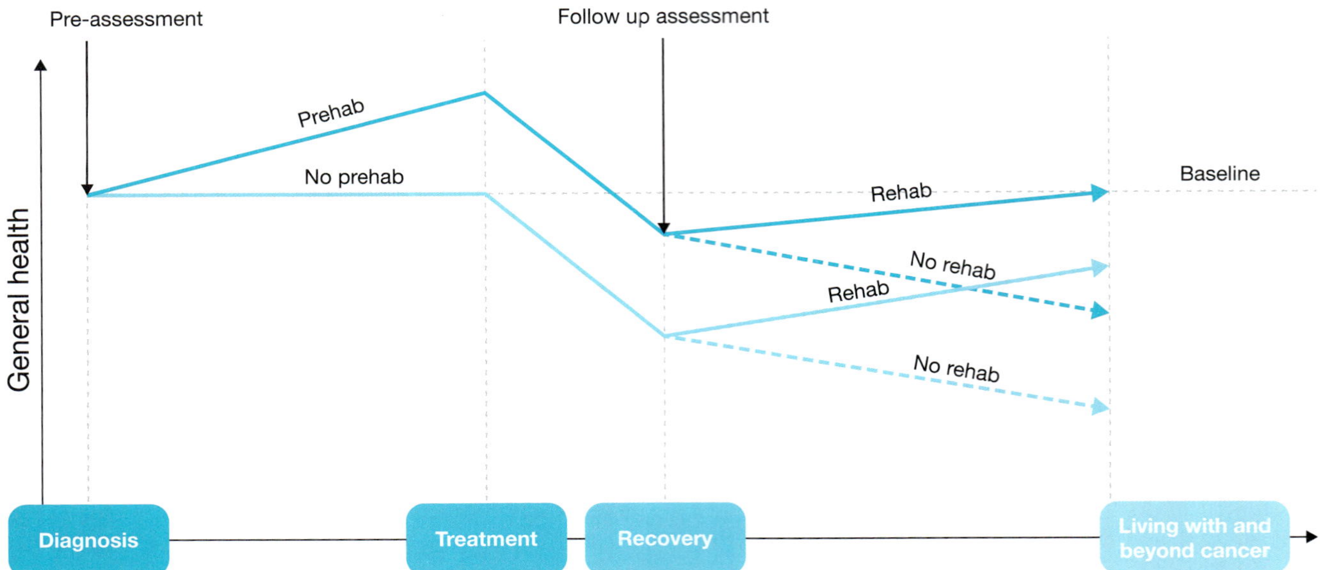

FIGURE 10.2. Possible outcomes with or without prehabilitation and rehabilitation on general health. (From Selvaraju K, Bates A. *Prehabilitation*. Centre for Perioperative Medicine, London: UCL Press; 2020. doi:10.14324/111.444.9781787356917.08; adapted from Principles and guidance for prehabilitation within the management and support of people with cancer, 2020. © Macmillan Cancer Support, 2023.)

nutritional concerns, and anxiety about future cancer treatments. Most experts in a clinical setting prefer this approach, although it may be more difficult to establish and undertake in the short time available presurgery. See Figures 10.1 and 10.3 for various examples of prehabilitation interventions.

There are consistent elements across prehabilitation services. A physical activity is always present, whereas other elements vary in frequency. In this chapter, we will concentrate on the evidence and guidelines with unimodal exercise-based prehabilitation interventions.

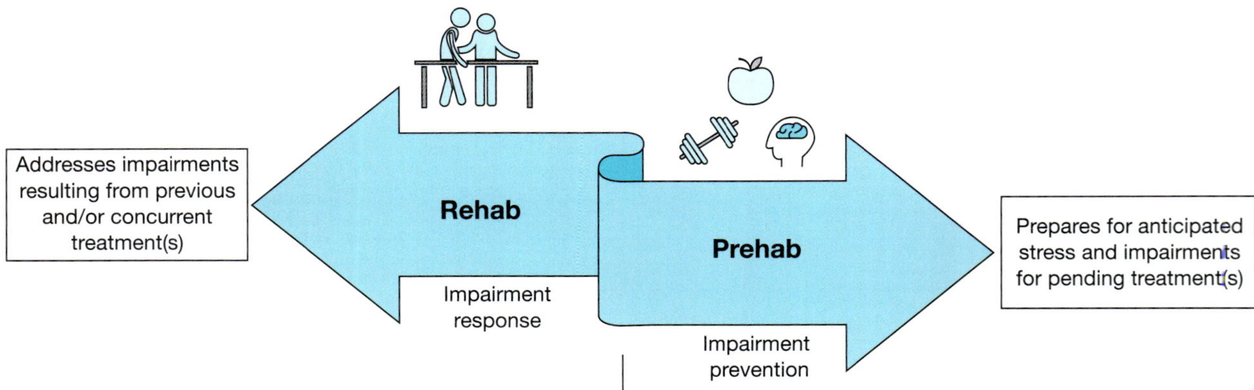

Interventions addressing impairments resulting from treatment. Rehabilitation modalities are focused on the recovery of function for activities of daily living, occupational tasks, and recreational activities. Example for patient undergoing tumor resection: affected limb/joint mobilization and functional recovery; psychosocial support to address changes in occupational/recreational/social activities; dietetic strategies to resolve malnutrition and ingestion/digestion function.

Interventions to prepare patients for a stressful event and buffer against declines in physiologic and psychosocial function known to be associated with pending treatment(s). Prehabilitation modalities must accommodate impairments resulting from previous treatments while maximizing the tolerable dose of health-optimizing behaviors. Examples for patients receiving adjuvant radiation or chemotherapy: aerobic conditioning to attenuate cardiorespiratory deconditioning and fatigue, protein supplementation to support an anabolic state, and psychosocial strategies to manage symptoms and challenges of systemic therapy.

FIGURE 10.3. Comparison of prehabilitation and rehabilitation. (Redrawn from Santa MD, van Rooijen SJ, Minnella EM, et al. Multiphasic prehabilitation across the cancer continuum: a narrative review and conceptual framework. *Front Oncol.* 2020;10:598425, Figure 1.)

MEASUREMENT AND IMPACT OF POOR FITNESS LEVELS ON SURGERY OUTCOMES

As mentioned in Chapter 1, those who are overweight or obese and do not reach the weekly recommended level of physical activity for health benefits have a higher risk of a diagnosis of cancer. In addition, older and frail cancer patients are likely to have comorbidities, such as diabetes, cardiorespiratory disease, and arthritis. Patients diagnosed with cancer are often deconditioned because of their underlying disease or neoadjuvant treatments (8). The resulting state of low physical fitness and reduced physiological reserve at the point of diagnosis/surgery can have a negative impact on surgical candidacy and postoperative outcomes. The gold standard method to objectively evaluate functional capacity and preoperative risk stratification is cardiopulmonary exercise testing (CPET), with gas-exchange-derived variables, such as oxygen consumption at anerobic threshold and oxygen consumption at peak exercise (peak VO_2), identified as good predictors of postoperative morbidity (Figure 10.4). CPET evaluates physical fitness under stress, mimicking major surgery, and is used to accurately stratify risk before major thoracic and abdominal surgery (9).

Studies have demonstrated a statistically significant association between CPET variables and in-hospital morbidity following major colon and rectal cancer surgery. In a study of 703 colorectal cancer patients, the analysis of CPET data showed that a low VO_2 peak and O_2 pulse was associated with increased odds of in-hospital morbidity, and those with low values were more likely to endure in-hospital complications, such as a leak to an **anastomosis** or treatment with intravenous antibiotics, and more likely to develop further morbidity and have their discharge from hospital delayed (10).

Neoadjuvant chemotherapy and **chemoradiotherapy** *prior* to surgery usually reduce physical fitness and physiological reserve further. This reduction is also associated with poor surgical outcomes, that is, postoperative morbidity and mortality. In addition, poor cardiorespiratory fitness at time of cancer diagnosis is associated with a higher prevalence of acute cardiovascular issues and often results in a reduction in the recommended dose of a cardiotoxic chemotherapy drug (11, 12).

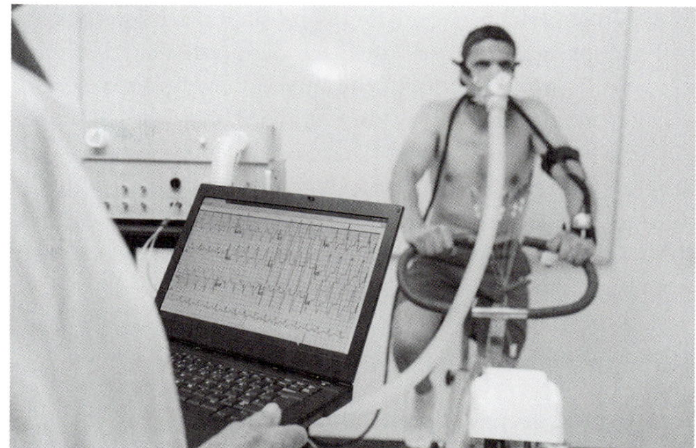

FIGURE 10.4. Example of a hospital-based cardiopulmonary exercise test. (From https://anaesthesiajournalclub.co.uk/2017/09/02/journal-club-29th-august-2017/.)

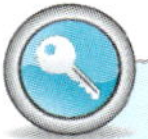

Anastomosis. Surgical connection between 2 structures. It usually means a connection that is created between tubular structures, such as blood vessels or loops of intestine. For example, when part of an intestine is surgically removed, the 2 remaining ends are sewn or stapled together (anastomosed).

Neoadjuvant chemotherapy. Neoadjuvant treatment is given as a first step to shrink a tumor before the main treatment—which is usually surgery—is undertaken. Examples of neoadjuvant therapy include chemotherapy, radiation therapy, and hormone therapy. It is a type of induction therapy.

Chemoradiotherapy. Treatment that combines chemotherapy with radiation therapy.

BENEFITS OF CANCER PREHABILITATION

All evidence to date suggests that it is safe and feasible to undertake exercise in the weeks prior to surgery and during neoadjuvant treatment (13). There are several systematic reviews of exercise-based interventions prior to cancer surgery that demonstrate that prehabilitation reduces postoperative stress and complications, enhances early discharge from hospital, and improves clinical outcomes by optimizing cardiopulmonary reserve prior to surgery (13-20). Most prehabilitation studies were undertaken with patients undergoing surgery for abdominal (eg, colon, rectal, esophageal, and gastric) cancers or lung cancer because these surgical procedures are challenging, complex, and normally entail a significant time period under general anesthetic. The post-surgery benefits would most likely be similar these instead of the other cancer types. In some cases, specific prehabilitation interventions, for example, pelvic floor muscle exercises (PFMEs) or shoulder range-of-motion exercises, have been implemented and assessed to address treatment-specific issues relevant to prostate and breast cancer, respectively.

Lung Cancer

In a Cochrane review of 5 RCTs involving 167 lung cancer patients, the exercise intervention reduced the risk of developing a postoperative pulmonary complication by 67%; also, postoperative length of hospital stay in the exercise group was lowered by 4.24 days. An intercostal drain (also known as a chest drain or pleural drain) is sometimes required following lung cancer surgery. The catheter is inserted through the chest wall into the pleural space to drain pneumothoraxes or effusions from the intrathoracic space. The mean number of days that patients needed an intercostal catheter in the control groups ranged from 7.4 to 8.8 days, whereas the number of days that patients in the intervention groups needed an intercostal catheter was, on average, 3.33 fewer days (95% CI 5.35 to 1.3 fewer days) (21). Pooled data from 2 of the lung cancer studies demonstrated that compared with the nonexercise group, the postintervention 6-minute walk test (6MWT) distance and postintervention forced vital capacity were higher in the exercise group (22, 23).

Abdominal Cancer

A systematic review of prehabilitation before abdominal surgery included 15 RCTs in the analysis with 457 prehabilitation patients and 450 control group patients. A significant reduction in overall and pulmonary morbidity was observed in the prehabilitation group (19). Two systematic reviews show that walking or cycling programs in patients before undergoing abdominal surgery resulted in significant cardiorespiratory fitness improvements using the 6MWT (24). There was a statistically significant decrease in the 6MWT distance of 27.9 meters postoperatively only in the control group and improvements in 6MWT distance of 58 meters 4 to 8 weeks postoperatively in the prehabilitation group compared with the control group (13).

Prostate Cancer

In patients with prostate cancer, prehabilitation that concentrates on pelvic floor strengthening exercises appears to lead to a reduction in postoperative urinary incontinence following prostatectomy (25). In a systematic review of 11 studies that included 739 men undergoing prostatectomy, preoperative PFMEs improved postoperative urinary incontinence after radical prostatectomy by 36% (26).

Breast Cancer

While there is substantial data supporting the use of range of movement exercises after breast cancer surgery to facilitate shoulder function recovery, few studies to date have implemented this type of protocol preoperatively. A recent study showed that a breast cancer prehabilitation intervention that includes upper quadrant-specific resistance training consisting of standing rows, shoulder external rotation, front raise, lateral raise, bicep curls, triceps extensions, wall push-ups, and chest press led to better shoulder girdle mobility which is important for future radiotherapy treatment and long-term range of movement (27). This study demonstrated that patients continued to exercise after surgery, which facilitated the recovery of shoulder function.

Breast cancer patients with higher baseline (prechemotherapy) cardiovascular fitness and muscular strength were associated with better chemotherapy dose tolerance and higher chemotherapy completion rates and therefore better outcomes. In a study of 543 patients with breast cancer, those in the top 20% of the VO_2 peak category were significantly more likely to complete >85% of the recommended dose of prechemotherapy (28). Adverse chemotherapy drug reactions, such as neutropenia or peripheral neuropathy, can result in chemotherapy dose reductions (ie, amount of dose administered), dose delays (ie, timing of administration), or a combination of both. RDI is the ratio of delivered dose intensity versus the planned dose intensity, and an RDI <85% is a the clinical threshold whereby adjuvant chemotherapy effectiveness and patient prognosis, including disease recurrence and survival, significantly worsen (29, 30). Accordingly, identifying strategies to improve chemotherapy dosing and tolerability is a priority. Thus, exercise interventions prior to chemotherapy treatment may have clinical implications in that exercise may improve the patient's tolerability of the planned chemotherapy dose.

In summarizing the research to date, there is an emerging body of evidence suggesting that exercise-based prehabilitation programs can result in reduced morbidity, better tolerance to subsequent cancer treatments, and a potential reduction of health care costs because of a reduction in complications and length of hospital stay. Prehabilitation may also foster a sense of control during this stressful phase and provide an opportunity to reflect on the role of healthy lifestyle practices following a cancer diagnosis and promote positive health behavior change, thereby enhancing longer-term health-related QoL (7, 20, 31, 32).

Overall, these findings suggest that exercise-based prehabilitation improves the physical and psychological health of cancer patients; however, the benefits are more likely to be enhanced by including the 2 other cornerstones of prehabilitation: providing nutritional support/advice and addressing psychological concerns (33).

PREHABILITATION IN THE CANCER CARE PATHWAY

Patients are less vulnerable to the side effects of cancer treatments if they are as fit and healthy as possible. Therefore, cancer prehabilitation should be initiated during the waiting period for testing and/or treatment before the onset of the necessary cancer treatment. It is an intervention that aims to prevent or reduce cancer treatment-related functional decline and any acute and chronic consequences. In the period after cancer diagnosis, a prehabilitation plan should be offered to help patients with cancer to reach a better level of endurance capacity and muscular strength to maximize resilience to treatment. Prehabilitation is mainly a presurgical intervention (which may include during neoadjuvant chemotherapy treatment), and most prehabilitation exercise interventions aim to improve endurance capacity (cardiovascular health) and include muscle strength exercises. This is because prehabilitation aims to optimize physiological reserve and address modifiable risk factors prior to surgery to improve postoperative outcomes, such as postsurgery complications and stay in the hospital (14).

PREHABILITATION EXERCISE PRESCRIPTION

A challenge to providing prehabilitation is that cancer patients may be deconditioned because of their underlying disease and are highly likely to have comorbidities that complicate treatment delivery and reduce physical fitness. With an aging demographic, where more than 60% of cancer patients are over 65 years of age, comorbidity and poor physical and functional health can have an impact on cancer treatment delivery and outcomes. This provides a further strong rationale for providing prehabilitation to maximize cancer treatment outcomes. It is important to remember that each patient will have unique physical performance capacity and possibly one or more comorbidities, so screening and assessments should be performed prior to the provision of an exercise program to ensure it is targeted and tailored to meet their specific needs.

Screening

Screening should take place as soon as possible after diagnosis. It has 2 functions:

- to ensure that the participant is safe to exercise and
- to identify the baseline physical activity level of the patient.

Screening for underlying unstable and stable cardiac, respiratory, and metabolic comorbidities should be implemented using a validated tool such as the PARQ+ (http://eparmedx.com/). Physical activity levels can be measured using a validated tool such as the International Physical Activity Questionnaire (IPAQ) (34). The screening approaches outlined in Chapter 11 are appropriate for this population.

Regarding screening, the following patients would be identified as high-risk patients and require more assessments and interventions by specialists:

- complex acute/chronic needs,
- severe physical impairment and/or disability,
- very low functioning levels,
- unstable or stable cardiac/respiratory issues,
- very low confidence, and
- severe psychological disabilities.

Assessment

Individualized assessment should encompass a comprehensive identification and evaluation of the specific needs of the patient, as this will inform the individualized prescription. Assessment requires conducting specific functional and fitness tests. Tests such as "sit to stand" and "sit and reach" can be used to assess basic functioning (35). Wearable technology monitors are also increasingly being used to obtain objective measures of the physical activity level and can help identify whether a person meets a specific threshold for specific physical activity/exercise interventions.

Physical fitness screening tests such as the 6MWT, incremental shuttle test, timed get up and go, or the 60-second chair stand test can be used (36). However, for the patients with a higher level of fitness, there will be a ceiling effect, and therefore the 12-minute Cooper test, a submaximal test, or CPET would be more appropriate assessments of aerobic fitness. There is also a need to know the baseline functions of specific parts of the body likely to be affected by the cancer treatment, for example, pelvic floor and shoulder range of movement, so that deficits are quantified and prehabilitation and rehabilitation targets can be appropriately set.

Intervention

The primary aim of prehabilitation for patients is to increase their physical activity levels, within the relatively short time frame, toward meeting current guideline recommendations (Table 10.1). This is the crucial goal and the dose of exercise will determine the level of cardiorespiratory improvement that can be obtained, most effectively preparing the patient for the stress of surgery. When prescribing an exercise program, always consider the patient's needs/preferences for supervision (ie, in the hospital, gym, or home-based program), type of program (ie, group classes or individual training—remote or face to face) and modality (type of exercise). Other factors, such as parking and transportation, are also important to consider for the patient's adherence to the program in this short time before surgery. Unaccustomed exercise intensity or a program in which the patient does not feel confident that they can accomplish can result in poor adherence. A patient-centric approach enhances adherence and maximizes the opportunity to achieve positive clinical outcomes in the presurgical time frame. Regardless of the degree of supervision preferred by the patient, adequate supervision by a trained professional is imperative to ensure that the exercises are being performed properly/safely and that there is sufficient progression to support a training effect. Given the relatively condensed period in which prehabilitation is being performed, careful monitoring of the program is critical.

Improving aerobic fitness levels plays a fundamental role in prehabilitation. Increasing evidence suggests that aerobic HIIT may be superior or equal to established moderate-continuous-intensity interventions. HIIT is defined as a discontinuous mode of endurance exercise characterized by relatively short bouts of high-intensity workloads interspersed by periods of rest or low-intensity activity during recovery. The rationale behind interval training programs is that the total accumulated time of vigorous exercise is higher than what could be achieved during a single bout of continuous exercise at the same intensity before getting exhausted. This time-efficient and effective method might be particularly relevant in the period from diagnosis to surgery when the time frame for a potential training intervention is limited. Nevertheless, patients might benefit from cardiovascular improvements, for example, lung cancer patients awaiting lung resection surgery. Adams and colleagues (37) found

Table 10.1 Example of the Physical Activity and Exercise Goals in the Prehabilitation Period

GOAL	GUIDELINE	HOW OFTEN? INTENSITY?	EXAMPLES
1. Reduce sitting/ sedentary time	Provide strategies for patient to break up sitting time by standing or walking	All day, every day. Very light intensity	Every 20 minutes, individual should get up; strategize how to stand up on regular basis, work standing when possible
2. Increase health benefits	Achieve 30 minutes of physical activity daily (can be broken into 3× 10 minutes) or can be expressed as 10,000 steps daily	30 minutes, every day RPE: 1-3	Housekeeping, light gardening, walk to mailbox, walk dog
3. Improve cardiovascular fitness benefits	Accumulate a minimum of 150 minutes of moderate to vigorous exercise daily, if possible	150 minutes can be spread out over week (ie, 5 exercise sessions per week; 30 minutes per session); RPE: 3-6 (moderate) and 7+(vigorous)	Brisk walk, swimming, dancing, team sports, bicycling, jogging, running, fitness classes. Activities are dependent on the abilities of the patient.
4. Improve skeletal muscle fitness benefits	Exercise all major muscle groups; at least 1 set of 8-12 repetitions	Every second day to allow for adequate recovery; intensity	Resistance bands, hand weights, barbells. Activities are dependent on the abilities of the patient.
5. Improve flexibility	Slow stretches (at least 20 seconds) of muscles exercised or problem muscle groups	Light intensity, stretch to point of tightening (but not more); to be performed at least after every exercise training session, if not more often	Lunges, attempt to touch toes, attempt to "scratch back." Activities are dependent on the abilities of the patient.

RPE: rate of perceived exertion on a 1-10 scale.
From Carli F, Gillis C, Scheede-Bergdahl C. Promoting a culture of prehabilitation for the surgical cancer patient. *Acta Oncol.* 2017;56(2): 128–33, Table 1.

that HIIT increased the muscular function and significantly reduced breathlessness and fatigue symptoms in testicular cancer patients. Meta-analysis of 8 HIIT studies in the cancer prehabilitation period revealed a significant improvement of VO_2 peak achieved with HIIT compared with usual care (15). Furthermore, HIIT was feasible and safe, showing low risk of adverse events and positive effects on health-related outcomes in prehabilitative settings even with a short duration of average of 4-weeks aerobic capacity. Three of the 8 HIIT studies presented postoperative outcomes, and 1 study reported a significant reduction in (pulmonary) complications and a shorter stay in the postanesthesia care unit (38).

Monitoring and Evaluation

Monitoring of the interventions can be self-monitoring by the patient or using appropriate validated measures. It is only by monitoring adherence to the intervention and recording efficacy and experience outcomes that the effectiveness from a personal and program level can be evaluated. It will help to develop a prehabilitation service by providing information on why some patients decline to engage or partly adhere to the prescribed intervention and to determine the factors that influence/optimize the response to a prehabilitation intervention.

SUMMARY

Cancer prehabilitation should begin between the time cancer is diagnosed and the onset of acute cancer treatments. Cancer prehabilitation programs involving exercise interventions have been shown to be able to improve functional status, physical and psychological health outcomes, and reduce overall disease burden (Figure 10.5). Significant improvements in physical fitness can be achieved in a short period of time. Prehabilitation could be readily integrated into the surgical and oncological patient pathways, particularly for those people who are identified at high risk for postoperative complications at cancer diagnosis.

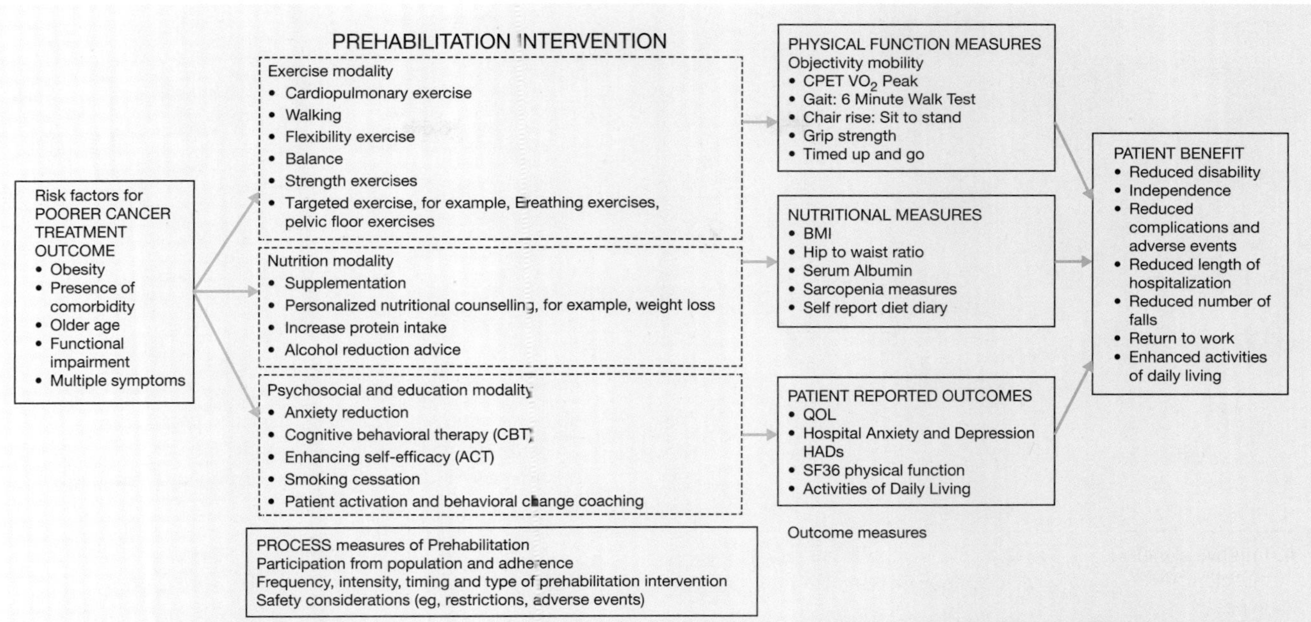

FIGURE 10.5. Summary of multimodal prehabilitation including outcomes and assessments. (Redrawn from Faithfull S, Turner L, Poole K, et al. Prehabilitation for adults diagnosed with cancer: a systematic review of long-term physical function, nutrition and patient-reported outcomes. *Eur J Cancer Care (Engl)*. 2019 Jul;28(4):e13023. doi:10.1111/ecc.13023, Figure 2.)

Case Study

Sylvia, a 79-year-old woman, has Stage I lung cancer and presented at diagnosis with several comorbidities, including osteoarthritis, limited mobility, and dyspnea (shortness of breath). The patient had previous surgeries for knee and back pain and was deconditioned. After assessment, her surgeon concluded that the patient would likely experience poor outcomes from surgery and would likely need to go to a nursing facility post procedure.

The patient was sent to an exercise professional for a 6-week prehabilitation program. After a 6 minute walk test and some balance and strength tests, Sylvia was given a progressive balance training, functional strengthening, and aerobic endurance program—some supervised and some home-based. Once comfortable and confident with the exercises (mostly walking and functional exercises), the program was progressed on a weekly basis.

Initially Sylvia was asked to try walk for 10 minutes 3 times a week. The duration, distance, and frequency of this walk were increased gradually each week, and at the end of the 6-week prehabilitation, Sylvia was walking for 20 minutes 5 times a week at a higher intensity. She was also given some simple balance and strengthening exercises, such as heel raises, toe raises, heel toe stand, one leg stand, heel toe walking, and sit to stand with chair for support. Once comfortable and confident with the exercises, she was provided with a video showing her how to do these exercises at home (https://www.youtube.com/watch?v=n8s-8KtfgFM). At the end of this 6-week prehabilitation program, Sylvia was reassessed, and there was a 53% increase in her 6MWT. Specifically, the patient improved her walking distance, her dyspnea had resolved, and she was deemed fit for surgery. After a lung resection, she returned home after only 3 days in the hospital because her functional ability had increased so much from the prehabilitation program. She then received 4 weeks of physical therapy before transitioning to a local exercise program.

Questions

1. Why was Sylvia's cardiorespiratory fitness assessed with a 6-minute walk test? (6MWT)
2. Give examples of the functional strengthening and progressing balance training that Sylvia was taught.
3. At the start of her prehabilitation, Sylvia walked 320 meters in 6 minutes. What was the distance she achieved at the end of the prehabilitation program?
4. The average hospitalization after lung resection is 6 days. How does this compare to Sylvia's stay in hospital after her lung resection?

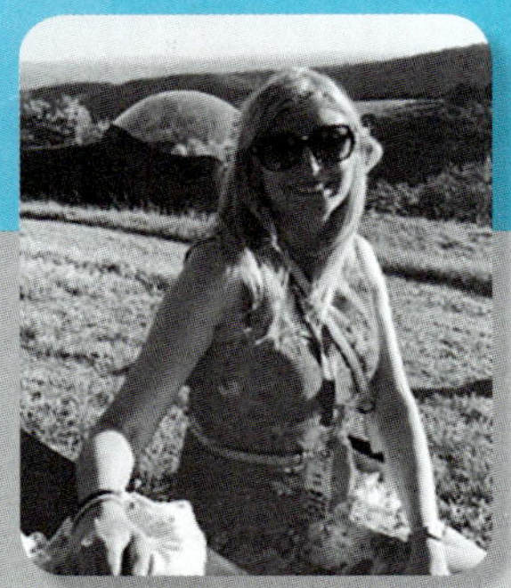

Meet the Expert

FEATURED PROFESSIONAL

Sandy Jack, BSc, MSc, PhD

Professor, Prehabilitation Medicine
Faculty of Medicine
University of Southampton
Southampton, England, United Kingdom

Q: "Where did you grow up?"

Southport, England, United Kingdom

Q: "Where did you train? What is your training?"

I trained in Liverpool and Manchester in England, UK. I have a BSc, MSc (1998) and PhD (2004) in Physiological Measurement and Medical Physics and in Biomedical Sciences from University of Salford, Scotland. I worked in the Cardiorespiratory Department at the Aintree University Hospitals Foundation Trust in Liverpool for a number of years. In 2012, I moved South to work at the University Hospital Southampton, Hampshire, UK as a Consultant Clinician Scientist in the Critical Care Research Department and within the NIHR Biomedical Research Centre. I was appointed as an Honorary Associate Professor in 2016 and an Honorary Professor of Prehabilitation Medicine in 2018. In 2021, this post was made substantive; I am very proud to say that I am now the first Professor in Prehabilitation Medicine globally.

Q: "What are you best known for?"

I am probably best known for focusing my research on patients undergoing neoadjuvant cancer treatments and surgery. I was the first to show that cancer treatments caused harm as well as good and that this could be reversed or ameliorated with a prescribed high-intensity responsive exercise-training program in hospital originally and now in community gyms. I was also one of the first to show the positive effects HIIT training on tumor outcomes. Perhaps what I feel I am best known for is my consistent messaging and fight for the national rollout of Prehabilitation Medicine service as standard care for all patients with cancer. I have spent the past 15 years working toward this goal and have recently succeeded in securing a recurrently funded service in my hospital and am now working toward implementation regionally.

Q: "What are you currently working on?"

I am now working on 2 funded pilot services for prehabilitation in patients with advanced cancer near end of life and those undergoing cardiac surgery. I am also working as Prehabilitation Lead for our Perioperative and Critical Care Theme for our £25m NIHR Southampton NIHR Biomedical Research Centre. My main interest is mechanistic experimental studies in immunotherapy to elucidate mechanisms of action (pheno-genotype and the immune-ecology of patients and tumors) of exercise and nutritional interventions and cancer outcomes.

Q: "Anything else you want to include?"

I feel so incredibly lucky to have worked with and continue to work with the most knowledgeable, humble, and wonderful people who just want to improve patient care and their lives. My work has never felt like a job; it is an absolute honor and privilege to work in this field and have firsthand evidence of how we can improve and extend patients' lives by listening.

Favorite Quote:

"Nature has given us all the pieces required to achieve exceptional wellness and health but has left us to put it together."
—*Diane McLaren*

STUDY QUESTIONS

1. When should prehabilitation begin?
   a. Immediately after adjuvant chemotherapy
   b. Immediately after neoadjuvant chemotherapy
   c. Immediately after surgery
   d. Immediately after diagnosis

2. Which of these interventions is NOT usually a component of a multimodal prehab program?
   a. Nutritional advice
   b. Financial support
   c. Psychological support
   d. Behavior-change advice

3. What is the gold standard means of measuring functional capacity presurgery?
   a. Cooper test
   b. Forced vital capacity test
   c. Cardiopulmonary exercise test
   d. 6-minute walk test
4. Which of the following statements is true about cancer patients with low fitness levels precancer surgery?
   a. Cancer patients are often deconditioned because of their underlying disease.
   b. Many have comorbidities that also contribute to deconditioning.
   c. Low fitness levels are associated with in-hospital morbidity and delayed hospital discharge.
   d. All of the above
5. True or false. Poor cardiorespiratory fitness at the time of cancer diagnosis often results in a reduction in the recommended dose of a cardiotoxic chemotherapy drug.
6. Most exercise prehabilitation studies have been undertaken with which cancer types? Why is that?
   a. Breast and abdominal
   b. Abdominal and lung: these surgical procedures are challenging, complex, and normally entail a significant time period under general anesthetic
   c. Breast and prostate
   d. Lung and prostate
7. What specific exercises should be prescribed in a prehabilitation program for men undergoing a prostatectomy?
   a. Pelvic floor exercises
   b. Grip strength exercises
   c. Abdominal range of movement exercises
   d. Intercostal muscle exercises
8. Why is it possible that prehabilitation may result in a potential reduction of health care costs?
   a. Less travel expenses
   b. Shorter hospital stay
   c. Better quality of life
   d. Less depression
9. What is the first stage when planning a cancer prehabilitation program for a patient?
   a. Assessment
   b. Monitor
   c. Screen
   d. Prescribe

REFERENCES

1. Santa Mina D, Clarke H, Ritvo P, et al. Effect of total-body prehabilitation on postoperative outcomes: a systematic review and meta-analysis. *Physiotherapy*. 2014;100(3):196–207.
2. Spain J. Prehabilitation. *Clin J Sports Med*. 1985;4(3):575–85.
3. Topp R, Ditmyer M, King K, Doherty K, Hornyak J, III. The effect of bed rest and potential of prehabilitation on patients in the intensive care unit. *AACN Adv Crit Care*. 2002;13(2):263–76.
4. Ditmyer MM, Topp R, Pifer M. Prehabilitation in preparation for orthopaedic surgery. *Orthop Nurs*. 2002;21(5):43–54.
5. Herschbach P, Book K, Brandl T, et al. Psychological distress in cancer patients assessed with an expert rating scale. *Br J Cancer*. 2008;99(1):37–43.
6. Lukez A, Baima J. The role and scope of prehabilitation in cancer care. *Semin Oncol Nurs*. 2020;36(1):150976.
7. Silver JK, Baima J. Cancer prehabilitation: an opportunity to decrease treatment-related morbidity, increase cancer treatment options, and improve physical and psychological health outcomes. *Am J Phys Med Rehabil*. 2013;92(8):715–27.
8. Mallard J, Hucteau E, Schott R, et al. Early skeletal muscle deconditioning and reduced exercise capacity during (neo)adjuvant chemotherapy in patients with breast cancer. *Cancer*. 2023;129(2):215–25.
9. Junejo MA, Mason JM, Sheen AJ, et al. Cardiopulmonary exercise testing for preoperative risk assessment before pancreaticoduodenectomy for cancer. *Ann Surg Oncol*. 2014;21(6):1929–36.
10. West MA, Asher R, Browning M, et al. Validation of preoperative cardiopulmonary exercise testing-derived variables to predict in-hospital morbidity after major colorectal surgery. *Br J Surg*. 2016;103(6):744–52.
11. Moller T, Lillelund C, Andersen C, et al. The challenge of preserving cardiorespiratory fitness in physically inactive patients with colon or breast cancer during adjuvant chemotherapy: a randomised feasibility study. *BMJ Open Sport Exerc Med*. 2015;1(1):e000021.
12. Groen WG, Naaktgeboren WR, van Harten WH, et al. Physical fitness and chemotherapy tolerance in patients with early-stage breast cancer. *Med Sci Sports Exerc*. 2022;54(4):537–42.
13. Michael CM, Lehrer EJ, Schmitz KH, Zaorsky NG. Prehabilitation exercise therapy for cancer: a systematic review and meta-analysis. *Cancer Med*. 2021;10(13):4195–205.
14. Waterland JL, McCourt O, Edbrooke L, et al. Efficacy of prehabilitation including exercise on postoperative outcomes following abdominal cancer surgery: a systematic review and meta-analysis. *Front Surg*. 2021;8:628848.
15. Palma S, Hasenoehrl T, Jordakieva G, Ramazanova D, Crevenna R. High-intensity interval training in the prehabilitation of cancer patients-a systematic review and meta-analysis. *Support Care Cancer*. 2021;29(4):1781–94.
16. Meneses-Echavez JF, Loaiza-Betancur AF, Triana-Reina HR, Diaz-Lopez VA, Echavarria-Rodriguez AM. Prehabilitation programs for cancer patients: a systematic review of randomized-controlled trials (protocol). *Med Sci Sports Exerc*. 2021;53(8S):471.
17. Meneses-Echavez JF, Loaiza-Betancur AF, Diaz-Lopez V, Echavarria-Rodriguez AM. Prehabilitation programs for cancer patients: a systematic review of randomized controlled trials (protocol). *Syst Rev*. 2020;9(1):34.
18. Bundred JR, Kamarajah SK, Hammond JS, Wilson CH, Prentis J, Pandanaboyana S. Prehabilitation prior to surgery for pancreatic cancer: a systematic review. *Pancreatology*. 2020;20(6):1243–50.
19. Hughes MJ, Hackney RJ, Lamb PJ, Wigmore SJ, Christopher Deans DA, Skipworth RJE. Prehabilitation before major abdominal surgery: a systematic review and meta-analysis. *World J Surg*. 2019;43(7):1661–8.
20. Faithfull S, Turner L, Poole K, et al. Prehabilitation for adults diagnosed with cancer: a systematic review of long-term physical function, nutrition and patient-reported outcomes. *Eur J Cancer Care (Engl)*. 2019;28(4):e13023.

21. Cavalheri V, Granger C. Preoperative exercise training for patients with non-small cell lung cancer. *Cochrane Database Syst Rev.* 2017; 6(6):CD012020.
22. Lai Y, Huang J, Yang M, Su J, Liu J, Che G. Seven-day intensive preoperative rehabilitation for elderly patients with lung cancer: a randomized controlled trial. *J Surg Res.* 2017;209:30–6.
23. Morano MT, Araujo AS, Nascimento FB, et al. Preoperative pulmonary rehabilitation versus chest physical therapy in patients undergoing lung cancer resection: a pilot randomized controlled trial. *Arch Phys Med Rehabil.* 2013;94(1):53–8.
24. Hijazi Y, Gondal U, Aziz O. A systematic review of prehabilitation programs in abdominal cancer surgery. *Int J Surg.* 2017;39:156–62.
25. Santa Mina D, Hilton WJ, Matthew AG, et al. Prehabilitation for radical prostatectomy: a multicentre randomized controlled trial. *Surg Oncol.* 2018;27(2):289–98.
26. Chang JI, Lam V, Patel MI. Preoperative pelvic floor muscle exercise and postprostatectomy incontinence: a systematic review and meta-analysis. *Eur Urol.* 2016;69(3):460–7.
27. Brahmbhatt P, Sabiston CM, Lopez C, et al. Feasibility of prehabilitation prior to breast cancer surgery: a mixed-methods study. *Front Oncol.* 2020;10:571091.
28. An KY, Arthuso FZ, Kang DW, et al. Exercise and health-related fitness predictors of chemotherapy completion in breast cancer patients: pooled analysis of two multicenter trials. *Breast Cancer Res Treat.* 2021; 188(2):399–407.
29. Lyman GH, Dale DC, Crawford J. Incidence and predictors of low dose-intensity in adjuvant breast cancer chemotherapy: a nationwide study of community practices. *J Clin Oncol.* 2003;21(24):4524–31.
30. Wildiers H, Reiser M. Relative dose intensity of chemotherapy and its impact on outcomes in patients with early breast cancer or aggressive lymphoma. *Crit Rev Oncol Hematol.* 2011;77(3):221–40.
31. Boereboom CL, Williams JP, Leighton P, Lund JN. Exercise prehabilitation in colorectal cancer Delphi study G: forming a consensus opinion on exercise prehabilitation in elderly colorectal cancer patients: a Delphi study. *Tech Coloproctol.* 2015;19(6):347–54.
32. Shun SC. Cancer prehabilitation for patients starting from active treatment to surveillance. *Asia Pac J Oncol Nurs.* 2016;3(1):37–40.
33. Tsimopoulou I, Pasquali S, Howard R, et al. Psychological prehabilitation before cancer surgery: a systematic review. *Ann Surg Oncol.* 2015;22(13):4117–23.
34. Craig CL, Marshall AL, Sjostrom M, et al. International physical activity questionnaire: 12-country reliability and validity. *Med Sci Sports Exerc.* 2003;35(8):1381–95.
35. Simmonds M. Physical function in patients with cancer: psychometric characteristics and clinical usefulness of a physical performance test battery. *J Pain Symptom Manage.* 2002;24(4):404–14.
36. Liguori G, Medicine ACoS. *ACSM's® Guidelines for Exercise Testing and Prescription.* Philadelphia (PA): Lippincott Williams & Wilkins; 2020.
37. Adams SC, DeLorey DS, Davenport MH, et al. Effects of high-intensity aerobic interval training on cardiovascular disease risk in testicular cancer survivors: a phase 2 randomized controlled trial. *Cancer.* 2017;123(20):4057–65.
38. Karenovics W, Licker M, Ellenberger C, et al. Short-term preoperative exercise therapy does not improve long-term outcome after lung cancer surgery: a randomized controlled study. *Eur J Cardiothorac Surg.* 2017;52(1):47–54.

CHAPTER

11

Prescribing Exercise During Active Treatment

OUTLINE

1. Introduction
2. Evaluating the Exercise Evidence
3. Strong Evidence
    a. Anxiety
    b. Depressive Symptoms
    c. Fatigue
    d. Health-Related Quality of Life
    e. Lymphedema
    f. Physical Function
4. Moderate Evidence
    a. Bone Health
    b. Sleep
    c. Insufficient Evidence
    d. Cardiotoxicity
    e. Chemotherapy-Induced Peripheral Neuropathy
    f. Cognitive Function
    g. Falls
    h. Nausea
    i. Pain
    j. Sexual Function
    k. Treatment Tolerance
5. Limitations to FITT Exercise Prescriptions
6. Other Exercise Modes
7. Effect of Cancer Treatment and Adverse Effects Related to Exercise
    a. Cardiovascular Changes
    b. Endocrine Changes
    c. Gastrointestinal Changes
    d. Immunologic Changes
    e. Metabolic Changes
    f. Neurological Changes
    g. Pulmonary Changes
    h. Skin Changes
    i. Fatigue
    j. Lymphedema
    k. Pain
8. Medical Clearance and Exercise Testing
9. Exercise Safety and Training Tolerance
10. Implementing FITT Prescriptions in Practice
11. Summary
12. Case Study
13. Meet the Expert
14. Study Questions
15. References

OBJECTIVES

After completing review of this chapter, students will be able to:

1. Describe the *ACSM® Exercise Guidelines for Cancer Survivors.*
2. Understand the effects of cancer treatment and the adverse effects related to exercise.
3. List steps to ensure that people in active treatment can exercise safely.
4. Explain how a FITT prescription could be implemented in practice.

INTRODUCTION

This chapter focuses on the *American College of Sports Medicine (ACSM) Exercise Guidelines for Cancer Survivors.* We will review the strength of the evidence for the outcomes to support recommending exercise during active treatment and build on the definitions of terms described in Chapter 9. Also included will be information about how to apply the guidelines to prescribe exercise during active cancer treatment. Common effects of cancer treatment, adverse effects of treatment, and how they may affect exercise will be presented. The exercise professional will be provided the knowledge to work with PLWC during treatment to safely prescribe exercise.

EVALUATING THE EXERCISE EVIDENCE

As discussed in Chapter 10, the ACSM® international multidisciplinary expert group made 2 important decisions at the Roundtable meeting: (A) to determine cancer-related health outcomes with clinical relevance that exercise may have a therapeutic benefit (Box 11.1) and (B) to concentrate literature searches on traditional modalities of exercise (aerobic, resistance, or a combination of aerobic and resistance). These decisions were made because there is a plethora of high-quality research using these modalities, and there is a consistent manner in the application of the exercise, whereas there may not be consistent quantifiable application of other forms of exercise movement therapy, such as yoga. Additional decisions were made that included the following: (A) an exercise prescription would only be created for a specific outcome if there were adequate high-quality evidence to allow for the description of the components of frequency, intensity, time, and type (a FITT prescription) and (B) the fitness components, such as aerobic capacity, muscular strength, endurance, and body composition, would not be considered **fidelity measures** because they are not cancer-health-related outcomes. The final decision was to recommend the lowest dose of exercise that was documented to have a beneficial effect. This last decision was made to ensure that the sickest and weakest person with cancer could still benefit from the recommendations.

The majority of studies have been conducted with people living with and beyond breast and prostate cancer. In time, as research expands, evidence will be inclusive of PLWBC with a broad spectrum of cancers. There are studies with people diagnosed with colon cancer, gynecologic cancer, melanoma, leukemia, and lymphoma, but the number of studies is limited and insufficient to make a recommendation specific to these diagnoses, so the recommendations are for cancer in general. As you will learn, there are specific considerations for people living with and beyond different types of cancer and receiving different types of treatment. As evidence and clinical experience grow, the recommendations may become more specific.

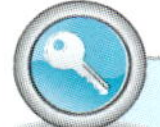

Fidelity measures. Ways to ensure that the treatment in a study is applied consistently and reliably. Fidelity measures are the changes along the way in a program or an intervention (eg, muscle strength and endurance increase), which show that the FITT prescription is working.

Box 11.1 Common Cancer-Related Health Outcomes for Review of Evidence for Therapeutic Efficacy of Exercise and Subsequent Exercise Prescriptions

- Anxiety
- Bone health
- Cardiotoxicity
- Chemotherapy-induced peripheral neuropathy
- Cognitive function
- Depressive symptoms
- Falls
- Fatigue
- Health-related quality of life
- Lymphedema (specifically breast cancer-related lymphedema)
- Nausea
- Pain
- Physical function
- Sexual function
- Sleep
- Treatment tolerance

STRONG EVIDENCE

The cancer-related outcomes that have strong evidence to provide a FITT prescription are anxiety, depression, fatigue, HRQoL, lymphedema, and physical function. The term strong evidence was used if there were (A) at least 5 RCTs that evaluated the efficacy of exercise to improve the outcome, (B) there were at least 150 people in those trials, (C) the effect of the exercise intervention was not close to zero, and (D) there was consistency in the results across the studies. There also needed to be sufficient information to allow a consistent FITT prescription to be proposed for each outcome. Figure 11.1 provides a summary of the exercise recommendations for each outcome.

The outcomes with strong evidence to support an exercise prescription are improved with low levels of aerobic, resistance, and sometimes a combination of aerobic and

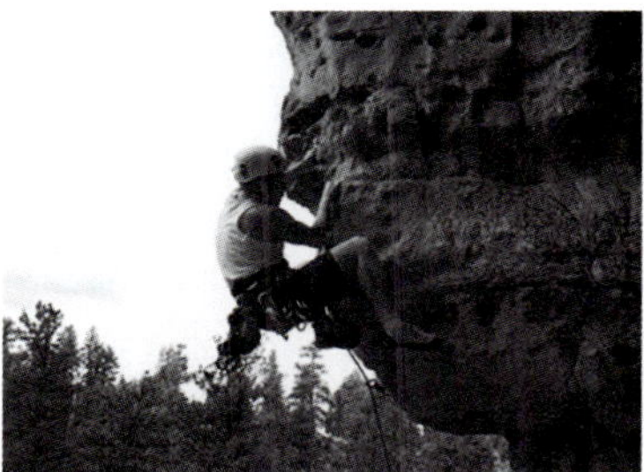

FIGURE 11.1. Rock climber.

resistance exercise. The effects of these outcomes are related and overlap to effect other areas in a person's life. For example, as a person increases her or his physical function, it could be assumed that the increased strength and fitness might help her or him to feel better about her or his health and physical abilities to pursue activities that are meaningful, and thereby reduce anxiety and depression. It is also reasonable to predict that as patients' physical function improves and they get stronger, they will have less fatigue because they now require less energy to complete routine tasks because of their increased functional ability.

Anxiety

Anxiety, the feeling of unease, fear, worry, and dread caused by the stress of cancer (or a test or just about anything that is stressful and causes unease) can be reduced by exercise. Evidence demonstrates that exercise can reduce anxiety during and after treatment (1-5). The dose of exercise to reduce anxiety is of moderate intensity. Aerobic exercise is performed 3 times per week for 12 weeks, or a combination of aerobic and resistance exercise is performed 2 times a week for 6 to 12 weeks (Table 11.1). At present, research does not support the use of resistance exercise alone to reduce anxiety. There is insufficient evidence to know if there is a dose-response relationship between exercise intensity and changes in anxiety. More research is needed to determine this relationship. Supervised exercise programs appear to have a better effect than unsupervised home-based programs.

Table 11.1 Exercise Dose to Reduce Anxiety and Depression[a]

FREQUENCY	INTENSITY	TIME	TYPE
3 days per week	Moderate	12× weeks	Aerobic
3 days per week	Moderate	12× weeks	Aerobic + Resistance

[a]There appears to be a dose-response relationship with aerobic exercise with longer periods of aerobic exercise reducing depression. Supervised exercise also appears to be more effective for reducing depression. Note that more research is needed to validate these findings.

Depressive Symptoms

Depression is highly responsive to exercise. Moderate-intensity aerobic exercise preformed 3 days per week for at least 12 weeks or aerobic and resistance exercise performed twice a week for 6 to 12 weeks can significantly reduce depression (see Table 11.1) (6, 7). At present, research does not support the use of resistance exercise alone to reduce depression. Evidence suggests that there may be a dose-response relationship of exercise and depression. A longer duration of aerobic exercise, about 90 to 180 minutes per week, leads to greater reductions in depression. Supervised exercise programs appear to more effectively reduce depression than unsupervised or home-based exercise programs.

Fatigue

CRF—which makes PLWBC feel too tired to move, think, or pursue their usual activities—can be alleviated with exercise. It seems counterintuitive to many people, but regular physical activity reduces fatigue (8). Moderate-intensity aerobic exercise performed 3 times per week significantly reduces fatigue during and after treatment (9, 10). A combination of moderate-intensity aerobic exercise and resistance training 2 to 3 times a week, or moderate-intensity resistance training performed twice a week also reduces fatigue (Table 11.2). It appears that there is a dose-response relationship with longer durations of exercise conferring less fatigue. However, there are limited data for aerobic exercise duration beyond 150 minutes per week. The dose-response relationship appears to show a benefit for moderate-to-vigorous exercise compared with low-intensity training. There is no apparent benefit by type of training setting (eg. supervised or unsupervised) (11-13).

Health-Related Quality of Life

Quality of life is improved with physical activity. The minimum exercise to have a beneficial effect on health-related quality of life is aerobic and resistance exercise combined. This prescription, performed two to three days per week for at least 12 weeks, improves health-related quality of life (HRQoL) during and after treatment (Table 11.3) (5). The combination of aerobic and resistance training is more

Table 11.2 Exercise Prescription for Fatigue

FREQUENCY	INTENSITY	TIME	TYPE
3 days	Moderate	30 minutes	Aerobic
2 days	Moderate	30 minutes	Resistance
2-3 days	Moderate	30 minutes	Aerobic + Resistance

Table 11.3 Health-Related Quality of Life Exercise Prescription

FREQUENCY	INTENSITY	TIME	TYPE
2-3 days	Moderate	At least 12 weeks	Aerobic + Resistance

beneficial than either aerobic or resistance training alone. The exercise setting makes a difference and supervised programs have better outcomes than programs that are unsupervised or home-based (14, 15).

Lymphedema

Current research demonstrates that exercise is safe and may reduce the risk for developing lymphedema (16, 17). Resistance exercise does not increase the risk for lymphedema if performed in a safe and gradual manner. Resistance exercise does not exacerbate lymphedema; it can actually help to reduce the intensity of flares if the initial resistance is low and the progression of resistance is slow.

Perhaps the most important recommendation to reduce the risk of lymphedema is to focus on safety and to keep in mind the need to progress slowly with exercise. Recommendations for exercise with lymphedema include a supervised program that focuses on large muscle groups, using very light weights, and progresses slowly (Table 11.4). Progressing to heavier weights quickly may predispose the person to lymphedema or a lymphedema flare. It is unclear if exercise has the same benefit for lower limb lymphedema. The majority of studies have been in supervised settings, which, particularly when starting resistance exercise, may be beneficial to ensure that the person living with or beyond cancer adheres to a slow, progressive program. While there have been no studies that have examined whether aerobic exercise would help lymphedema, the lack of lymphedema-related adverse events from the hundreds of aerobic exercise studies that have been conducted in women living with and beyond breast cancer leads to the conclusion that aerobic exercise is safe with regard to lymphedema risk. Aerobic exercise may be performed at a vigorous intensity for up to 5 days per week for 30 minutes per session.

Table 11.4 Exercise Prescription for Breast-Cancer-Related Lymphedema

FREQUENCY	INTENSITY	TIME	TYPE
Up to 5 days	Moderate-to-vigorous	30 minutes/session	Aerobic
2 days	Start very light, progress slowly		Resistance

Table 11.5 Exercise Prescription for Physical Function

FREQUENCY	INTENSITY	TIME	TYPE
3 days	Moderate	8-12 weeks	Aerobic
2 days	Moderate	8-12 weeks	Resistance
3 days	Moderate	8-12 weeks	Aerobic + Resistance

Physical Function

PLWBC need to move, and movement is key to maintaining physical function. Exercise is essential to preventing decline and even improving physical function for PLWBC. Aerobic exercise or resistance exercise alone or in combination, when performed at a moderate intensity for 8 to 12 weeks, improves physical function (Table 11.5). Supervised exercise programs appear to yield better results than unsupervised programs, but home-based exercise, especially for older adults, is effective (11, 18, 19).

MODERATE EVIDENCE

Moderate evidence is available to support a FITT recommendation for 2 exercise outcomes: bone health and sleep. These outcomes need additional research to determine if there is strong evidence for a FITT prescription. However, given the robust evidence for the benefits of exercise in preserving bone health in people without cancer, it is reasonable to speculate that as the body of evidence increases, these benefits will be observed in PLWBC. The same expectation is anticipated to hold true for sleep.

Bone Health

There is moderate evidence to recommend exercise to improve bone health in PLWBC, and there is growing evidence to support it. A year-long, supervised, moderate-to-vigorous intensity resistance and high-impact training performed for 2 to 3 days a week improves bone health by slowing down the loss of bone density and increasing bone density at the lumbar spine (20-23). High-impact training includes exercises that increase the ground reaction force—4 times that of a person's body weight. Examples of high-impact exercises are jumping and burpees. These exercises may not be safe for people with osteoporosis, bone metastasis at the hip or spine, or people with stability or orthopedic problems. For any of these individuals, the risk of falling must be considered when developing an exercise plan. There is moderate evidence to suggest that a FITT recommendation of 2 to 3 days of moderate-to-vigorous intensity resistance exercise plus high-impact training can increase bone density at the lumbar spine.

Current thought leaders in oncology, physical therapy, exercise physiology, and research determined in a series of surveys that medical guidance is recommended prior to beginning a structured exercise program for all people living with bone metastasis who are beginning a structured exercise program (24-26). Medical guidance is required if an individual is having bone pain or has a history of disease-related fracture.

The goal for the exercise professional is to seek medical guidance to obtain medical information (ie, bone scan reports) to guide decision-making related to exercise prescription and to develop a collaborative relationship with the oncology team (24, 26). A review of clinical trials suggests that exercise, both aerobic and resistance, may be safe for people living with bone metastasis, but the dose of exercise is unknown, and there are not enough studies to determine if there may be strong evidence for this recommendation (25). At this time, there is not enough evidence to suggest that either aerobic or resistance exercise alone or aerobic and resistance exercise in combination may be beneficial.

Sleep

We know that in a general healthy population, sleep is important to recharge the mind and the body and that sleep helps to avoid weight gain, heart disease, and stress. There is mixed evidence for the benefits of exercise and sleep quality for PLWC. Some studies demonstrate a benefit, whereas others show no effect (27-30). However, there is strong evidence in studies of people without cancer that moderate-to-vigorous intensity aerobic exercise improves sleep quality. Therefore, to improve sleep, moderate-intensity aerobic exercise, such as walking, 3 to 4 days a week for 30 to 40 minutes, is recommended for PLWBC. Studies among PLWBC observed improvements in sleep after 12 weeks.

Insufficient Evidence

The following outcomes have insufficient evidence to provide an exercise recommendation. This means that not enough research has been conducted on these outcomes to conclusively recommend that exercise is beneficial. It does not mean that there will never be sufficient evidence to make FITT prescriptions for these outcomes. Currently, the gaps in the knowledge related to these outcomes require more research to determine whether or not a consistent, meaningful effect can be established for aerobic exercise, resistance exercise, or their combination.

Cardiotoxicity

Many cancer treatments, such as chemotherapy treatments with anthracyclines, can cause cardiac dysfunction. This is an emerging area of research. There is promising research, in both animal models and some limited evidence with humans, that suggests that exercise may have beneficial effects on left ventricular function and exercise capacity (31-34). Larger controlled clinical trials are needed to determine exercise effects on cardiac end points during and following cancer treatments to have a better understanding of exercise on cardiac function during and following cancer treatments. That said, there is more than sufficient evidence to document the benefits of exercise training for heart health in general (Box 11.2). This is relevant to cancer populations in that there is published evidence that cardiovascular mortality is elevated in those who have received treatment for cancer (35). Therefore, although exercise may not have a specifically defined effect on the cardiotoxic effects of cancer therapies, the vast evidence base demonstrates that exercise improves cardiovascular health and also benefits to those living with and beyond cancer.

Box 11.2 End Points and Outcomes

Throughout this chapter, the terms *end point* and *outcome* have been used. The word **end point** refers to a parameter that is measured over a precise time period (eg, baseline, 6 months, and 1 year) in order to detect changes. By contrast, **outcomes** are measurable changes in health or function that result from doing something.

However, sometimes **end point** is used with **outcomes** when discussing the target outcome and primary end point. For example, cognitive function was not the primary end point or outcome measure. Outcomes and end points can each be the primary variable of interest.

Chemotherapy-Induced Peripheral Neuropathy

CIPN causes nerve damage in the fingers and toes that can extend up to affect the hands, feet, and extremities. CIPN can make simple tasks like buttoning a shirt or picking up a piece of paper difficult and can deaden the nerve endings so that balance is affected and even holding a coffee cup requires conscious effort. Few rigorous studies have examined (36) the effects of exercise on CIPN. Although several studies have concluded that exercise reduces symptoms of CIPN, there is insufficient evidence to conclude empirically that exercise definitively improves CIPN (37-40). More research is needed to determine whether there is a particular dose of exercise required for meaningful decreases in the effects of CIPN.

Cognitive Function

Cognitive impairment, often called "chemo brain," is a side effect of treatment that can affect word finding and thought processing and can cause difficulty concentrating. Research has demonstrated that exercise has positive effects on the cognitive function of older adults, but there is limited research on cognitive impairment as the primary outcome among PLWBC (41, 42). However, an emerging body of research suggests that there may be positive effects of exercise for chemotherapy-related cognitive impairment (41). Cognitive impairment in exercise studies, which was measured by self-report, was not the primary end point. Although these studies noted that exercise improved cognitive function, additional research is needed specific to PLWBC where cognitive function is the primary outcome.

Falls

No one likes to fall, especially as one gets older. Combined muscle weakness, CIPN, poor balance, and general debilitation increase the risk of falls for PLWBC. However, there are an insufficient number of studies on the effects of exercise training on the number of falls and fall-risk reduction, specifically for PLWBC, to recommend exercise(s) specifically for fall prevention. Despite this lack of research, it is logical to surmise that exercise in general and specifically, fall-prevention exercises, should be recommended to reduce the risks of falls among PLWBC (43). Fall-prevention exercises for the general population of older adults should focus on strength, balance, and flexibility.

Nausea

Nausea is a dreadful feeling that often preceeds to vomiting, a common side effect of many cancer treatments. An early breast cancer exercise trial observed that nausea during chemotherapy was reduced with vigorous exercise; a more recent large trial in the Netherlands confirmed this finding (44, 45). It would be unethical to withhold current highly efficacious antiemetic drugs to determine the effect of exercise on nausea with and without antiemetics. In addition, it would be unlikely that any person receiving chemotherapy with a highly emetogenic regimen would want to enroll in such a trial.

Pain

Pain is physical suffering caused by a bodily disorder, such as, after surgery, an injury, or CIPN as a result of chemotherapy. Pain is a secondary outcome in exercise trials and MAY not BE specific to cancer pain. However, there are 2 different clinical trials that studied pain as the primary end point and demonstrated the benefit of exercise. Women with breast cancer who participated in a home-based aerobic and resistance exercise training program demonstrated reduced aromatase inhibitor-related arthralgia (46). The second study demonstrated reduced shoulder pain in people with head and neck cancer who participated in a supervised upper extremity resistance exercise training program (47). Many more studies are needed with pain as the primary outcome before it can be determined that exercise reduces pain. If pain is not well controlled, many PLWBC may not be able to exercise.

Sexual Function

Sexual function of men with prostate cancer is ablated with cancer treatment. ADT has rapid and profound negative effects on a man's libido, testosterone, and body composition. There are mixed results on the effects of exercise on sexual function (48-50). However, there are limited studies that suggest that resistance exercise can prevent and restore some of the deleterious effects of ADT on a man's strength and endurance, which in turn improves his emotional outlook. For women with cancer, exercise can improve body image, and sexual function and satisfaction can be improved with pelvic floor exercises (51, 52). Even though there is strong evidence that exercise has a positive effect on sexual function in the healthy population of men and women, the effect of cancer treatment on hormone and anatomical function is significant (eg, nerve damage in prostate cancer surgery) and overpowers the effects of exercise on PLWC (53, 54). Therefore, at this time, there is insufficient evidence to recommend an exercise intervention to improve sexual function of men or women.

Treatment Tolerance

Although there is observational and anecdotal evidence to suggest that treatment tolerance may be improved with exercise, there are no rigorously designed clinical trials that have a primary goal to demonstrate this effect of exercise. Intuitively, however, it makes sense that if side effects are less intense, then one would have a greater tolerance for treatment, but at this time, there are no conclusive studies that have tested this as a primary outcome. Promising preliminary evidence in this area arises from several studies that included treatment tolerance as a secondary outcome in breast and colon cancer, and there is ongoing research that examines this issue as a primary outcome in colon cancer (45, 55). In addition, NCI is planning to fund a new initiative to address this outcome specifically. A nonrandomized clinical trial noted some positive benefits with exercise compared with historical controls, but further research is needed to confirm these findings (56). Evidence on this outcome is expected to grow in the next 5 to 10 years as more rigorous research is conducted testing this outcome.

LIMITATIONS TO FITT EXERCISE PRESCRIPTIONS

There are limitations to these FITT prescriptions. These prescriptions are intended to serve as general guidelines for fitness and health care professionals working with PLWBC. Most of the research that is available is limited to the most common cancers (eg, breast and prostate cancers) and to early-stage disease, which limits our ability to extrapolate to other diseases and more advanced stages of disease. It is important to remember that there is limited research on the dose response for people of all ages, types and stages of disease, types of treatment, and time beyond diagnosis. More research is needed to understand how exercise dose modifications may affect exercise tolerance for individuals receiving different types of treatment or with different types of comorbidities. There are many questions that remain unanswered. In the future, we will have a far greater understanding of how to modify exercise for different types of cancer, stages of cancer, types of treatment, and many more combinations and permutations of comorbidities, and limitations that PLWBC may face.

OTHER EXERCISE MODES

Other exercise modes, such as yoga, climbing, and dragon boat racing are of great interest to PLWBC and their friends and family; an insufficient volume of systematic research has been conducted to quantify the dose of exercise to determine if these exercises are safe or effective. PLWBC report that they experience many benefits from yoga, climbing (Figure 11.2), dragon boat racing, triathlon, and other exercise modes, but there is insufficient evidence to provide an exercise prescription at this time. There is simply a lack of information on the dose, side effects, safety, and efficacy of these types of exercises (57-63). It is particularly challenging to quantify the FITT dose of exercise for activities, such as yoga, tai chi, or qigong, which are slow and focus on balance and breathing. These activities, while beneficial, may not actually meet the minimal exercise recommendations for PLWBC.

EFFECT OF CANCER TREATMENT AND ADVERSE EFFECTS RELATED TO EXERCISE

Cancer treatments cause many adverse effects that can have an impact on exercise. It is critical for the exercise professional to have a solid understanding of the person's type and stage of cancer, treatments, side effects to expect during or following treatment, and how they may impact the individual's ability to exercise (Table 11.6). During active treatment, the exercise professional must anticipate and be comfortable working closely with the oncology team. Often the exercise professional spends more time with the person on active treatment than any other person on the oncology team, so they must be prepared to talk about issues related to life expectancy, employment, family matters, and other personal and emotional concerns.

Cardiovascular Changes

Cardiovascular changes can be affected by chemotherapy, radiation, hormonal therapy, and targeted therapy or immunotherapy. During treatment with cardiotoxic drugs, the oncologist monitors left ventricular function (eg, ejection fraction) to ensure that adequate heart function is retained. If ejection fraction is reduced, the dose of trastuzumab, or other cardiotoxic drug, is decreased or stopped. During active treatment, changes in blood pressure (BP) can be a concern with as many as 17% to 80% experiencing hypertension (high BP) (64). Some drugs cause hypertension (eg, trastuzumab and bevacizumab). Paclitaxel is a common drug that can cause hypotension (low BP) or hypertension. These are 3 common drugs that provide examples of the need to take a person's BP before exercise, or to have the ability to take their BP, if an individual is not feeling well during exercise. Encouraging people on active treatment to stay well hydrated before and after exercise can help minimize episodes of hypotension.

Endocrine Changes

Endocrine changes can occur because of any form of cancer treatment (see Table 11.6) and may negatively affect bone health and body composition, predisposing the person receiving cancer treatment to gain weight, lose muscle mass, and lose bone density. There is also a risk of endocrine damage from immunotherapy to the thyroid leading to hypothyroid, requiring the need for thyroid replacement. Most of these changes occur after treatment has ended.

Gastrointestinal Changes

GI consequences of cancer treatment are common with all treatments except hormonal therapies. Nausea, vomiting, and constipation are common acute effects of cancer treatments and can be managed with medications. These side effects should be managed early before they become significant and limit activities of daily living. Some research suggests that exercise reduces nausea and vomiting (44, 45). Aerobic exercise clearly helps to reduce constipation and move food through the large intestine.

Immunologic Changes

Immunologic changes can be acute or for long term. We will discuss the long-term changes in Chapters 14 and 15. In both phases, acute and long term, they are related to radiation, chemotherapy, immunotherapy, or targeted therapies that reduce white blood cells, RBCs, and/or platelets. These drugs may affect all or one specific cell line to cause neutropenia (low white blood cell count), anemia (low red blood cell count), thrombocytopenia (low platelet count), or myelosuppression (low blood cell count). Some drugs affect the blood counts to a greater degree than others. Most drugs cause a decrease in blood counts approximately 5 to 7 days after the infusion or conclusion of oral ingestion. This low point is called the nadir. This is the time when a person is most at risk for infection. From an exercise perspective, it is important to ensure that the individual does not have a fever and that exercise personnel are healthy, the exercise environment is

Moving Through Cancer

ExeRcise is Medicine® | AMERICAN COLLEGE of SPORTS MEDICINE

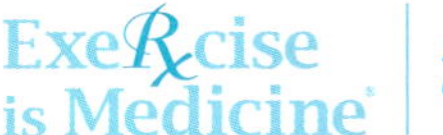

Name: ______________________________ Date: ______________

Aerobic Activity 3 or more days/week

Intensity: ❑ Light (casual walk) ❑ Moderate (brisk walk) ❑ Vigorous (like jogging)

Time (minutes/day): Build up to 30 minutes/day

Type: ❑ Walk ❑ Run ❑ Bike ❑ Swim/Water Exercise ❑ Other ______________

Steps/day: ❑ 2,500 ❑ 5,000 ❑ 7,000 ❑ 9,000 or more ❑ Other ________________

What about aerobic activity?

- Moderate activity is at a pace where you can talk but cannot "sing." Examples: *brisk walking, light biking, water exercise* and *dancing.*
- Vigorous activity is at a pace where you have trouble talking and may be out of breath. Examples: *jogging, tennis* and *fast bicycling.*
- While the recommendation is to build up to 30 minutes/day, at least 3 days/week, you can exercise for any length of time. For example, you might walk:
  - 5 minutes here, 10 minutes there
  - 15 minutes daily
  - Just work your way up to 30 minutes 3 days/week
- Gradually build up to a daily step count of 7,000-9,000 steps/day.

Muscle Strength Training 2 days/week

What about strength training?

- You don't have to go to a gym. You can use elastic bands, do body weight exercises (kitchen counter push-ups, chair sit-to-stands) or lift dumbbells. Heavy work around your home also builds strength.
- Strengthen your legs, back, chest and arms. To start, try 10-15 repetitions using light effort. Build up to medium or hard effort for 8-12 repetitions. Repeat 2-4 times, 2-3 days/week.
- Give yourself a rest day between each strength training session.

Notes (local programming, specific risks or instructions):

See www.exerciseismedicine.org/movethruca for a registry of local programs.

Referrer's Signature:

How will you get started **this week?**

FIGURE 11.2. Moving through cancer exercise prescription. (From American College of Sports Medicine®. *Exercise Is Medicine®: Moving Through Cancer.* [Internet]. 2021. Available from https://www.exerciseismedicine.org/wp-content/uploads/2021/04/EIM-moving-through-cancer-form-web.pdf.)

Table 11.6 Potential Impact of Cancer Treatments on Exercise Tolerance and Safety (8)

		SURGERY	CHEMOTHERAPY[a]	RADIATION	ANTIHORMONAL THERAPY (SURGICAL OR PHARMACEUTICAL)	TARGETED THERAPY OR IMMUNOTHERAPY[a]
Cardiovascular changes	Cardiac damage or increased risk of CVD		√	√	√	√
Endocrine changes						
	Worsening bone health		√	√	√	
	Changes in body composition (weight gain)		√		√	
	Changes in body composition (weight loss/muscle mass loss)	√	√	√	√	√
Gastrointestinal changes						
	Nausea		√			√
	Diarrhea		√	√		√
	Altered GI function	√	√	√		√
Immune changes	Impaired immune function and/or anemia		√	√	√	√
Metabolic changes						
	Development/worsening of metabolic syndrome		√		√	√[b]
Neurological changes	Peripheral neuropathy		√			
	Cognitive changes	√ (brain surgery)	√	√	√	
Pulmonary changes	Altered lung function or pneumonitis	√ (lung surgery)	√	√		
Skin changes						
	Redness, irritation			√		
	Rashes			√		√
	Reduced ROM	√ (by healing at surgical site)		√		
Fatigue		√	√	√	√	√
Lymphedema[c]		√		√		
Pain	General	√	√	√	√	√
	Myalgia/Arthralgia		√		√	√

CVD, cardiovascular disease; GI, gastrointestinal.
[a]Depends on type or target of agent.
[b]Especially common with PI3kinase inhibitors.
[c]Can occur in any type of cancer when and where lymph nodes are surgically resected and/or radiation over lymph nodes.
From Campbell KL, Winters-Stone KM, Wiskemann J, et al. Exercise guidelines for cancer survivors: consensus statement from international multidisciplinary roundtable. *Med Sci Sports Exerc.* 2019;51(11):2375–90. doi:10.1249/mss.0000000000002116.

clean, and the equipment is wiped down when used between individuals to decrease the spread of infection.

Metabolic Changes

Metabolic changes can be induced with chemotherapy, hormonal therapy, and targeted therapies. These drugs tend to cause endocrine imbalances, a predisposition to weight gain, and central obesity. Exercise considerations for these individuals are to start slowly and be aware that their weight gain may impair their balance and **kinesthetic awareness**. People who may have been athletic before cancer may be downhearted about the changes in their physical ability and physique.

Neurological Changes

Neurological changes can occur in several ways. Chemotherapy may cause CIPN. Cognitive changes may be caused by surgery to the brain, radiation to the brain, chemotherapy, and hormonal therapy. Exercise considerations for patients with CIPN will depend, to a great extent, on the severity of the CIPN, but must focus on safety. Balance and an individual's risk for falling are concerns if the CIPN affects their feet. Use of a treadmill should be avoided; a stationary bicycle would be a safer option. If the CIPN mostly affects their fingers and hands, using exercise machines or bands would be safer than using free weights, which the person may drop if they do not have much feeling in their hands.

Pulmonary Changes

Pulmonary changes can be caused by lung surgery (removal of part or all of a lung), damage from radiation, and chemotherapy. The damage from radiation and chemotherapy is usually permanent and leads to the reduction in lung function. Exercise tolerance may be impaired owing to lung damage or removal. Exercise prescription may need to be altered to accommodate the individual's pulmonary capacity and exercise tolerance. Aerobic exercise may need to start at a lower level and increase more gradually to accommodate the individual's pulmonary status.

Skin Changes

Skin changes can occur from surgery, radiation (eg, radiation dermatitis), and some immunotherapies and targeted therapies. Surgery can also cause the reduced ROM of the skin and underlying structures. Surgical sites with decreased ROM may benefit from stretching or referral to physical therapy for a supervised exercise regimen to maximize recovery and ROM. Many immunotherapy and targeted treatment drugs can cause skin toxicities. Depending on the drug, as many as 42% to 80% of patients will develop skin toxicities that range from mild to severe and require dose modification. Developing skin toxicity often looks like a red rash (red, raised, and pimply) that is sometimes itchy. Often skin toxicities indicate that the medication is working. Exercise implications of each of these complications vary.

People with surgical scars or radiation dermatitis and people receiving cancer drugs should protect their skin from the sun by wearing sunscreen or protective clothing and a hat. A scar that develops a sunburn will become more pigmented than the surrounding skin. Radiation dermatitis affects 95% of people receiving radiation therapy. It is a reddening of the skin from radiation. The skin often blisters and peels and can be painful. During exercise the skin should be covered and protected from perspiration that may cause irritation and additional pain. When people are receiving radiation or immunotherapy or a targeted treatment, their skin tends to be photosensitive (they can get sunburned more easily). Therefore, sun precautions are important, and individuals should avoid the sun or at least wear clothing that covers the skin, large brimmed hat, sunscreens with high sun protection factor, and sun glasses.

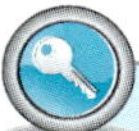

Kinesthetic awareness. The ability to move in space with an awareness of joint position, balance, and movement.

Fatigue

Fatigue is experienced by nearly all patients (98%) during active treatment. Fatigue is more severe during chemotherapy than with radiation therapy, but for all people receiving treatment, it disrupts their normal daily life. Fatigue is not relieved by rest or sleep and has a profoundly negative effect on QoL. Exercise is the one intervention that consistently reduces fatigue. The exercise dose may need to be attenuated when people receiving active treatment are profoundly fatigued, but an exact formula for that is unknown at this time. However, fatigue is usually reduced when people exercise at least every other day.

Lymphedema

Lymphedema may occur shortly after surgery, radiation therapy, during chemotherapy, or many years later. When lymphedema occurs at any time, it requires follow-up by the surgeon, oncologist, and a physical therapist. A physical therapist is important to help the person learn exercises to regain and maintain ROM and learn to manage the lymphedema with massage, wrapping, or bandaging. They may fit with a compression sleeve too. As an exercise professional, it is important to be aware of the signs of lymphedema (Box 11.4) and be alerted to changes a patient may report, such as heaviness in their arm. Patients with, or at risk of, lymphedema have no restrictions in an aerobic exercise program but need to begin a resistance exercise program with very light weights (eg, 1 lb) and progress in small increments (eg, 0.5 lb) to prevent a flare or actually trigger the onset of lymphedema.

Pain

Pain can be caused by surgery, chemotherapy, radiation therapy, hormonal treatment, immunotherapy, and targeted therapy. The pain of surgery may be brief related to nerve damage and scars that form adhesions (thickening of the tissues) that limit ROM. Surgical pain usually resolves over time. Chemotherapy, immunotherapy, and targeted therapy may cause a variety of pains, including CIPN, dermatitis (rashes), stomatitis (mouth sores caused by infection) that occur when people have very low blood counts (neutropenia), and sometimes from other infections. Radiation therapy often causes radiation dermatitis that can be painful and is addressed in the "Skin Changes" section. Pain must be managed before engaging in exercise. Very often, when pain is present, people move in a way to protect the painful body part. In doing so, their normal movement pattern is changed; for example, their walking gait is changed. This will put compensatory pressure on their other leg and hip, which can cause undue stress and pain and injury. For this reason, it is important for pain to be controlled, movement is at ease, and exercise can be as pleasurable as possible.

MEDICAL CLEARANCE AND EXERCISE TESTING

Safety is of utmost importance when working with anyone living with or beyond cancer. Guidance for when to obtain medical clearance is provided in Table 11.7. Given that many cancer treatments increase the risk for CVD, the need for medical clearance or medical evaluation prior to starting an exercise program may be relevant. If the exercise professional is concerned about a patient's condition, it is prudent to seek consultation from the oncology team and clearly document the correspondence or answer. Table 11.7, from the National Comprehensive Cancer Network Survivorship Guidelines, provides a framework to determine when medical clearance or further medical evaluation is necessary, or when a higher level of supervised exercise training to ensure safety is indicated (65).

A comprehensive assessment of health-related physical fitness components (eg, cardiorespiratory fitness, muscle strength, endurance, body composition, and flexibility) should be considered for all PLWBC who are beginning an exercise program (Box 11.3). However, if this is not possible, this should not be used as a reason not to prescribe light-intensity activities. Exercise professionals must be aware of cancer-specific considerations to safely and optimally individualize an exercise prescription. No physical assessments are required to start a low-intensity exercise program, such as walking, which gradually increases in intensity. There is also no assessment required for a resistance or flexibility exercise program that begins slowly and progresses gradually. The goal is to avoid creating barriers to initiating exercise. However, medical clearance may be indicated for patients with a history of exercise intolerance, presence of cardiovascular (heart and/or lung), and renal (kidney) or metabolic symptoms (Box 11.4). It may be helpful to review the Exercise Preparticipation Health Screening Questionnaire for Exercise Professionals in Chapter 9 (Figure 9.1).

Table 11.7 Adapted National Comprehensive Cancer Network Triage Approach Based on Risk of Exercise-Induced Adverse Events

DESCRIPTION OF PATIENTS	EVALUATION, PRESCRIPTION, AND PROGRAMMING RECOMMENDATIONS
No comorbidities	• No further medical evaluation • Follow general exercise recommendations
Peripheral neuropathy, arthritis/musculoskeletal issues, poor bone health (eg, osteopenia or osteoporosis), lymphedema	• Recommend pre-exercise medical evaluation • Modify general exercise recommendations based on assessments • Consider referral to trained personnel[b]
Lung or abdominal surgery, ostomy, cardiopulmonary disease, ataxia, extreme fatigue, severe nutritional deficiencies, worsening/changing physical condition (ie, lymphedema exacerbation), bone metastases	• Pre-exercise medical evaluation and clearance by physician prior to exercise[a] • Referral to trained personnel[b]

[a]Depends on type of treatment.
[b]Physical and occupational therapists, certified exercise professionals, and rehabilitation specialists.
From Campbell KL, Winters-Stone KM, Wiskemann J, et al. Exercise guidelines for cancer survivors: consensus statement from international multidisciplinary roundtable. *Med Sci Sports Exerc*. 2019;51(11): 2375–90. doi:10.1249/mss.0000000000002116.

EXERCISE SAFETY AND TRAINING TOLERANCE

Exercise is well established to be safe and beneficial for PLWBC (66). However, it should be recognized that studies are required to have eligibility requirements that often result in participants who are healthier and have higher physical function and motivation to exercise than many people in the general population. For this reason, some people in the community may be more infirm, debilitated, and less motivated to exercise. However, most people, when faced with serious illness that threatens their well-being and mortality, become interested in what they can do to maintain their independence. Even the most sedentary individuals may become more inclined to exercise.

Box 11.3 Exercise Testing Recommendations

Standard exercise testing methods are generally appropriate for patients with cancer who do not require medical clearance or who have been medically cleared for exercise with the following considerations:

- Be aware of a survivor's health history, comorbid chronic diseases, and health conditions, and any general exercise contraindications before commencing health-related fitness assessments or designing the exercise prescription.
- Be familiar with the most common toxicities associated with cancer treatments, including increased risk for fractures and cardiovascular events, along with neuropathies or musculoskeletal morbidities related to specific types of treatment.
- Health-related fitness assessments may be valuable for evaluating the degree to which components of fitness have been affected by CRF or other commonly experienced symptoms that impact function.
- In principle, there is no evidence that the level of medical supervision required for symptom-limited or maximal CPET need to be different for patients with cancer than for other populations.
- The evidence-based literature indicates 1-RM testing is safe among survivors of breast and prostate cancer without bony metastases.
- Among patients with bony metastases or known or suspected osteoporosis, routine assessments of muscle strength and/or endurance involving musculature that attaches to and/or acts on a skeletal site that contains bone lesions should be avoided (67). For example, 1-RM testing for leg strength (eg, leg press) should be avoided in patients who have bony metastases in the proximal femur (ie, hip) or vertebrae. Other sites where lesions are absent could be tested. In this example, if the patient had no lesions in the upper body, 1-RM for a chest press or 1-RM for a seated row might be feasible, given no other contraindications. Medical clearance from a physician (ie, orthopedic or radio-oncology) may be mandatory depending on the scope of practice or protocols at a specific site/facility.
- Older survivors and/or survivors treated with neurotoxic chemotherapy (typical for breast, colon, lung, and ovarian cancers) may especially benefit from a standard assessment of balance and mobility to assess fall risk.
- CVD has become a competing cause of morbidity and mortality for survivors of cancer with a favorable prognosis. Given the potential for underlying CVD, cancer survivors should be screened for evidence or underlying CVD using the ACSM® preparticipation guidelines, and if implicated, have a cardiopulmonary exercise test prior to beginning an exercise program.

From Campbell KL, Winters-Stone KM, Wiskemann J, et al. Exercise guidelines for cancer survivors: consensus statement from international multidisciplinary roundtable. *Med Sci Sports Exerc.* 2019; 51(11):2375–90. doi:10.1249/mss.0000000000002116.

PLWBC respond to exercise training by increasing cardiorespiratory fitness, muscular strength, endurance, and body composition (68-71). However, the effects of active treatment may have a significant impact on exercise tolerance by affecting physiology (eg, anemia), side effects of treatment (eg, fatigue), or demographic factors (eg, age) (72-74). Side effects during treatment can be variable, and patients need to learn the patterns of their side effects (eg, fatigue, pain, and nausea) from their treatments so that they can optimize their good days.

Box 11.4 Common Signs of Lymphedema

Following are the common signs of lymphedema:

- Swelling in an arm or leg
- Limb feels heavy
- Skin feels tight
- Swelling may interfere with movement (eg, fingers, hand, arm, toes, and leg)
- Skin may become thick
- Affected area my itch or burn
- Difficult to wear rings, watch, bracelet, and socks

Cardiorespiratory fitness declines during chemotherapy because of inactivity and can be maintained with aerobic exercise, especially in patients with low baseline fitness levels. Aerobic exercise should begin and progress slowly so that it is tolerated and the individual can see their progression and success. An abrupt loss of muscle strength and endurance is common, especially among men receiving ADT for prostate cancer (75, 76). ADT causes rapid and profound declines in androgens, which causes a decline in muscle mass, lean body mass, strength, endurance, sex drive, and QoL. Resistance exercise training helps to build a small but statistically significant amount of lean mass (77). It is critical to assess baseline strength and develop a resistance program that progressively increases the strength with a focus on the major muscle groups.

We have presented side effects and symptoms individually as outcomes of exercise. However, symptoms rarely occur in isolation. In PLWBC, symptoms occur in clusters. During treatment, there are a cascade of changes that occur. During chemotherapy and immunotherapy, the change is more rapid than it is during radiation therapy where the onset is more gradual. Nonetheless, the symptoms do not occur in isolation; they occur in groups or what are called **symptom clusters**. The example of rapid changes caused by ADT are also accompanied by fatigue, weakness, and often depression (78).

Many people expect that cancer treatment will lead to weight loss, but many treatments actually cause weight gain and unfavorable changes in body composition, including increases in body fat, loss of muscle mass, and declines in bone density. Weight gain can be a common side effect of chemotherapy and antiestrogen therapy for breast and antiandrogen therapy for prostate cancer. For cases where weight gain and obesity are a concern, exercise should focus on orthopedic limitations and protection and CVD-risk reduction (65, 79). Weight loss and loss of lean body mass concern with advanced lung, colon, and pancreatic cancer (80). When loss of lean body mass is a problem, exercise focus should be on building muscle mass with resistance exercise and not on creating an energy deficit that will aggravate the weight loss and fatigue (79, 81, 82).

IMPLEMENTING FITT PRESCRIPTIONS IN PRACTICE

The exercise recommendation for cancer-related side effects includes moderate-intensity aerobic exercise at least 3 days a week for at least 30 minutes, for 8 to 12 weeks. Combining resistance training with aerobic training, at least 2 days per week, using at least 2 sets of 8 to 15 repetitions of weights that are at least 60% of 1 repetition maximum, appears to result in similar benefits (Table 11.8).

The FITT prescription should clearly describe the frequency, intensity, time or duration, and type of exercise. Measuring exercise intensity may be done subjectively by the patient using the rating of perceived exertion on a scale of 0 to 10, or objectively, using devices (eg, wearables) that measure METs, heart rate, or the amount of oxygen consumed. The intensity of exercise is often hard to quantify during active treatment because, for example, side effects of treatment, including fatigue, may increase a person's perception of fatigue and weakness and make exercise more difficult, or anemia may cause increased heart rate and require a decreased intensity of exercise. Patients should be monitored regularly, and the FITT prescription should be modified based on the individual's response to their cancer treatment, progress with the exercise prescription, physical condition, endurance, fatigue, and strength.

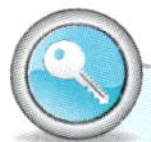

Symptom clusters. Side effects (which occur as a result of treatment) and symptoms (which occur from a disease) related to cancer and cancer treatment rarely occur in isolation. More commonly, they occur in groups or clusters. For example, fatigue, weakness, depression, and anxiety may occur together. This symptom cluster decreases QoL. There is an interrelationship between side effects and symptoms.

Table 11.8 Expected Patient Benefits from Exercise Training by Mode (8)

AEROBIC	RESISTANCE	AEROBIC + RESISTANCE
Reduced anxiety	Less fatigue	Reduced anxiety
Fewer depressive symptoms	Better QoL	Fewer depressive symptoms
Less fatigue	No risk of exacerbating lymphedema	Less fatigue
Better QoL	Improved perceived physical function	Better QoL
Improved perceived physical function		Improved perceived physical function

PLWBC have individual preferences regarding supervised and unsupervised exercise programs. Some studies suggest that they prefer supervised exercise over unsupervised home-based exercise programs, whereas others suggest home-based over supervised. It is unclear if this is because it is easier to achieve a higher dose of exercise in a supervised training setting or if there are other attributes to a supervised setting (eg, more attention, motivation, reinforcement, and access to equipment). Many PLWBC anecdotally report that they enjoy the camaraderie they experience being with other people who have a shared experience and can support each other along their journey. A supervised setting offers the opportunity for people who are debilitated or who have other comorbidities or cardiovascular risk factors to begin an exercise program in a supervised setting with physical therapists or other exercise professionals before transitioning to a community-based or a home-based program. This offers people an opportunity to develop confidence and motivation, and learn exercise techniques in a safe environment. For many patients, a blend of supervised exercise that transitions to unsupervised exercise in a gym or home-based setting may be ideal and preferred.

The fitness professional should be prepared to create individualized exercise programs to meet their patients' needs and goals. Customized programs should meet the patients where they are in their cancer journey. Exercise programs also need to consider the effects specific to cancer,

Table 11.9 Exercise Programming Considerations for Specific Cancer Survivors

CONSIDERATION	RECOMMENDATIONS
Ostomy	• Empty ostomy bag before engaging in exercise • Weight lifting/resistance exercises should start with low resistance and progress slowly under the guidance of trained exercise professionals • Avoid contact sports and exercises that result in excessive intra-abdominal pressure

Peripheral neuropathy	• Stability, balance, and gait should be assessed before engaging in exercise; consider balance training as indicated
	• Consider alternative aerobic exercise (stationary biking and water exercise) rather than walking if neuropathy affects stability or use treadmill with safety handrails
	• Resistance training recommendations:
	  • Monitor discomfort in hands when using handheld weights
	  • Consider using dumbbells with soft/rubber coating, and/or wear padded gloves
	  • Consider resistance machines over free weights (Streckmann F, et al., 2014).

Bone loss/bone metastases	• Avoid contraindicated movements that place an excessively high load on fragile skeletal sites. These include the following: high-impact loads, hyperflexion or hyperextension of the trunk, flexion or extension of the trunk with added resistance, and dynamic twisting motion • Specific guidance on how to modify exercise programs based on the site of bony lesions is provided elsewhere (71, Rief H, et al., 2014) • Preventing falls must also be a goal of therapy, since falls play an important role in fracture etiology (83) • Be aware of signs and symptoms of bone metastases in survivors, as well as common locations where these occur (ie, spinal vertebrae, ribs, humerus, femur, and pelvis). Bone pain can be an initial sign of skeletal metastases thus, exercise trainers should refer survivors who report pain back to the medical team for clinical evaluation prior to continuing exercise
Older adults	• Physical problems reported by cancer survivors, such as cognitive difficulty, neuropathy, sarcopenia, muscle weakness slowing, and fatigue, may be similar to those of older people without cancer, but cancer treatment can accelerate these declines (84, 85; Maccormick RE, 2006). • Exercise professionals will need to combine ACSM® guidelines on exercise programming for older adults (86) with the recommendations in this publication. • Integrate fitness and functional assessments prior to beginning an exercise program to more accurately determine baseline functional abilities.
Symptom clusters	• Symptoms and side effects of cancer treatment rarely appear in isolation rather symptom clusters are the norm (ie, frailty, depression, and anxiety), especially in those with advanced disease or complicated medical histories (87; Fan et al., 2007). • Exercise professionals must be aware of this complexity and be prepared to refer patients back to the medical team (ie, rehabilitation or oncology physician, general practitioner, or nurse) for review and management of symptoms when safety concerns develop.
Lymphedema	• To date, there is insufficient evidence to support or refute this clinical advice to wear a compression garment during exercise to prevent or reduce symptoms of breast cancer-related upper body lymphedema. Therefore, it is recommended that exercise professionals provide this information as part of patient education and defer to an individual's preference regarding use of a compression sleeve. • Being overweight or deconditioned have been associated with a higher risk of developing cancer-related lymphedema in observational studies. At this time, there is insufficient evidence that weight loss or improving aerobic fitness can lower the risk of developing cancer-related lymphedema (87).
Stem cell transplantation	• Home-based exercise encouraged • A full recovery of the immune system recommended before return to gym facilities with the general public • Start with light intensity, short durations but high frequency, and progress slowly • Exercise volume (intensity and duration) should be adapted on a daily basis based on the individual's presentation

Data from Schmitz KH, Courneya KS, Matthews C, et al. American College of Sports Medicine® roundtable on exercise guidelines for cancer survivors. *Med Sci Sports Exerc.* 2010;42(7):1409–26. doi:10.1249/MSS.0b013e3181e0c112. [Erratum in: *Med Sci Sports Exerc.* 2011;43(1):195]; Paskett ED, Dean JA, Oliveri JM, Harrop JP. Cancer-related lymphedema risk factors, diagnosis, treatment, and impact: a review. *J Clin Oncol.* 2012;30(30):3726–33. doi:10.1200/jco.2012.41.8574; Fan G, Filipczak L, Chow E. Symptom clusters in cancer patients: a review of the literature. *Curr Oncol.* 2007;14(5):173–9. doi:10.3747/co.2007.145; Esper P. Symptom clusters in individuals living with advanced cancer. *Semin Oncol Nurs.* 2010;26(3):168–74. doi:10.1016/j.soncn.2010.05.002; Chodzko-Zajko WJ, Proctor DN, Fiatarone Singh MA, et al. American College of Sports Medicine® position stand. Exercise and physical activity for older adults. *Med Sci Sports Exerc.* 2009;41(7):1510–30. doi:10.1249/MSS.0b013e3181a0c95c; Clough-Gorr KM, Stuck AE, Thwin SS, Silliman RA. Older breast cancer survivors: geriatric assessment domains are associated with poor tolerance of treatment adverse effects and predict mortality over 7 years of follow-up. *J Clin Oncol.* 2010;28(3):380–6. doi:10.1200/jco.2009.23.5440; Klepin HD, Geiger AM, Tooze JA, et al. Physical performance and subsequent disability and survival in older adults with malignancy: results from the health, aging and body composition study. *J Am Geriatr Soc.* 2010;58(1):76–82. doi:10.1111/j.1532-5415.2009.02620.x; Maccormick RE. Possible acceleration of aging by adjuvant chemotherapy: a cause of early onset frailty? *Med Hypotheses.* 2006;67(2):212–15. doi:10.1016/j.mehy.2006.01.045; Frost HM. Should future risk-of-fracture analyses include another major risk factor? The case for falls. *J Clin Densitom.* 2001;4(4):381–3. doi:10.1385/jcd:4:4:381; Galvão DA, Taaffe DR, Spry N, et al. Exercise preserves physical function in prostate cancer patients with bone metastases. *Med Sci Sports Exerc.* 2018;50(3):393–9. doi:10.1249/mss.0000000000001454; Rief H, Petersen LC, Omlor G, et al. The effect of resistance training during radiotherapy on spinal bone metastases in cancer patients: a randomized trial. *Radiother Oncol.* 2014;112(1):133–9. doi:10.1016/j.radonc.2014.06.008; Streckmann F, Zopf EM, Lehmann HC, et al. Exercise intervention studies in patients with peripheral neuropathy: a systematic review. *Sports Med.* 2014;44(9):1289–304. doi:10.1007/s40279-014-0207-5.

Oncology Clinician's Guide to Referring Patients to Exercise

Step 1: ASSESS

Question #1: *How many days during the past week have you performed physical activity where your heart beats faster and your breathing is harder than normal for 30 minutes or more?*

Question #2: *How many days during the past week have you performed physical activity to increase muscle strength, such as lifting weights?*

Question #3: *Would this patient be safe exercising without medical supervision (eg, walking, hiking, cycling, weight lifting)*

Question #3 answer is Yes. (Patient is ambulatory, ECOG score 0-2)	**Question #3 answer is No** *Or* **I'm not sure and I don't have the capacity to evaluate.** **(ECOG score 3+ or other complications present)**

• **Step 2: ADVISE**
  • EIM ExRx for Oncology, based on current report of activity to increase to:
    • Moderate intensity aerobic exercise (talk but not sing) for up to 30 minutes, 3 times/week
    • Resistance exercise 2x weekly 20-30 min
• **Step 3: REFER** to best available community program
	• **Step 2: ADVISE**
	  • Advise patient to follow-up with outpatient rehabilitation health care professional for further evaluation
	• **Step 3: REFER**
	  • Outpatient rehabilitation health care professional will recommend best available program

REPEAT AT REGULAR INTERVALS AT CLINICAL ENCOUNTERS DURING AND AFTER ACTIVE TREATMENT

FIGURE 11.3. Assess, advise, and refer. (From Schmitz KH, Campbell AM, Stuiver MM, et al. Exercise is medicine in oncology: engaging clinicians to help patients move through cancer. *CA Cancer J Clin.* 2019;69(6):468–84, Figure 1.)

if an individual has a **port** or an **ostomy**, has peripheral neuropathy, bone metastasis, and age. Table 11.9 provides adaptations of some of the NCCN guidelines and recommendations for modifications to exercise programs.

Connecting patients to exercise during active therapy is a particular challenge, and the FITT prescription must be individualized to each patient. Recommendations from ACSM® are to adopt the Exercise is Medicine® approach, which starts with assessing physical activity levels, followed by advising patients that exercise would be useful for symptoms and side effects, followed by referral to appropriate exercise programming given the clinical profile of the patient (Figure 11.3). Sometimes referral would need to be to a more medically supervised setting (eg, physical therapy). Other times the referral could be to an exercise professional or a community-based program such as Livestrong at the YMCA.

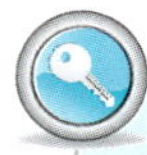

Port or Port-a-Cath. Type of catheter that is placed under the skin in the chest or upper arm. It reduces the need for repeated needle sticks, stays in place for a long time, and reduces the risk that the chemotherapy drug might leak outside of the vein (extravasate).

Ostomy. A surgically made opening in the body that collects urine or feces in a bag that needs to be emptied several times a day. It can be temporary or permanent.

A key piece of the ACSM® guidelines includes asking oncologists to assess, advise, and refer (Figure 11.4). This critical piece of the exercise oncology framework asks oncologists to assess if patients are doing any physical exercise, advise patients to exercise, and refer patients to an appropriate exercise oncology rehabilitation program (Figure 11.4).

SUMMARY

ACSM® provides clear guidelines to develop safe and effective FITT prescriptions for people with cancer who are actively receiving treatment. It is critical for exercise professionals to be aware of the potential impact of cancer treatments on exercise tolerance and safety and how to adapt exercise and a FITT prescription to each individual. The goal is to keep PLWBC physically active and moving, but to do so safely and to avoid causing harm. Therefore, it is of utmost importance that exercise professionals have strong ties with the oncology team to seek advice and ask questions. There are still many gaps in the science about exercise and cancer during treatment, but we do know that exercise needs to be individualized to each person.

Effects of Exercise on Health-Related Outcomes in Those with Cancer

What can exercise do?

- **Prevention of 7 common cancers***
  Dose: 2018 Physical Activity Guidelines for Americans: 150-300 min/week moderate or 75-150 min/week vigorous aerobic exercise
- **Survival of 3 common cancers****
  Dose: Exact dose of physical activity needed to reduce cancer-specific or all-cause mortality is not yet known; Overall more activity appears to lead to better risk reduction

**bladder, breast, colon, endometrial, esophageal, kidney and stomach cancers*
***breast, colon and prostate cancers*

Overall, avoid inactivity, and to improve general health, aim to achieve the current physical activity guidelines for health (150 min/week aerobic exercise and 2x/week strength training).

Outcome	Aerobic Only	Resistance Only	Combination (Aerobic + Resistance)
Strong Evidence	Dose	Dose	Dose
Cancer-related fatigue	**3x**/week for **30** min per session of moderate intensity	**2x**/week of **2** sets of **12-15** reps for major muscle groups at moderate intensity	**3x**/week for **30** min per session of moderate aerobic exercise, plus**2x**/week of resistance training **2** sets of **12-15** reps for major muscle groups at moderate intensity
Health-related quality of life	**2-3x**/week for **30-60** min per session of moderate to vigorous	**2x**/week of **2** sets of **8-15** reps for major muscle groups at a moderate to vigorous intensity	**2-3x**/week for **20-30** min per session of moderate aerobic exercise plus **2x**/week of resistance training **2** sets of **8-15** reps for major muscle groups at moderate to vigorous intensity
Physical Function	**3x**/week for **30-60** min per session of moderate to vigorous	**2-3x**/week of **2** sets of **8-12** reps for major muscle groups at moderate to vigorous intensity	**3x**/week for **20-40** min per session of moderate to vigorous aerobic exercise, plus **2-3x**/week of resistance training **2** sets of **8-12** reps for major muscle group at moderate to vigorous intensity
Anxiety	**3x**/week for **30-60** min per session of moderate to vigorous	Insufficient evidence	**2-3x**/week for **20-40** min of moderate to vigorous aerobic exercise plus **2x**/week of resistance training of **2** sets, **8-12** reps for major muscle groups at moderate to vigorous intensity
Depression	**3x**/week for **30-60** min per session of moderate to vigorous	Insufficient evidence	**2-3x**/week for **20-40** min of moderate to vigorous aerobic exercise plus **2x**/week of resistance training of **2** sets, **8-12** reps for major muscle groups at moderate to vigorous intensity
Lymphedema	Insufficient evidence	**2-3x**/week of progressive, supervised, program for major muscle groups does not exacerbate lymphedema	Insufficient evidence
Moderate Evidence			
Bone health	Insufficient evidence	**2-3x**/week of moderate to vigorous resistance training plus high impact training (sufficient to generate ground reaction force of **3-4** time body weight) for at least **12** months	Insufficient evidence
Sleep	**3-4x**/week for **30-40** min per session of moderate intensity	Insufficient evidence	Insufficient evidence

Citation: bit.ly/cancer_exercise_guidelines

Moderate intensity (40%-59% heart rate reserve or VO_2R) to vigorous intensity (60%-89% heart rate reserve or VO_2R) is recommended.

ExeRcise is Medicine® | AMERICAN COLLEGE of SPORTS MEDICINE.

FIGURE 11.4. Exercise guidelines cancer-related health outcomes. (From American College of Sports Medicine®. *Effects of Exercise on Health-Related Outcomes in Those with Cancerr.* [Internet]. 2021. Available from https://www.exerciseismedicine.org/wp-content/uploads/2021/04/exercise-guidelines-cancer-infographic.pdf.)

Case Study

Mark is a 58-year-old man with Stage III colorectal cancer. His treatment included a colon resection with temporary colostomy. He is currently receiving adjuvant FOLFOX chemotherapy (5-fluorouracil and oxaliplatin). Mark has received 8 treatments and is feeling tired; has pain and numbness in his fingers, toes, hands, and feet; and his eyes are constantly watering. He is still working full time. Mark is having problems with his ostomy bag because he has flatulence and watery diarrhea. He wants to join the cancer exercise program that includes aerobic and resistance exercise. He is embarrassed about his colostomy bag and is uncertain about his ability because of his treatment schedule.

Questions

1. What are the exercise recommendations for people living with colorectal cancer?
2. How will the resistance exercise program be adapted for Mark's ostomy?
3. Chemotherapy-induced peripheral neuropathy is a significant concern when working with Mark. How will this be addressed?
4. How will the exercise program help Mark?
5. There is an interrelationship between side effects and symptoms.

Meet the Expert

FEATURED PROFESSIONAL

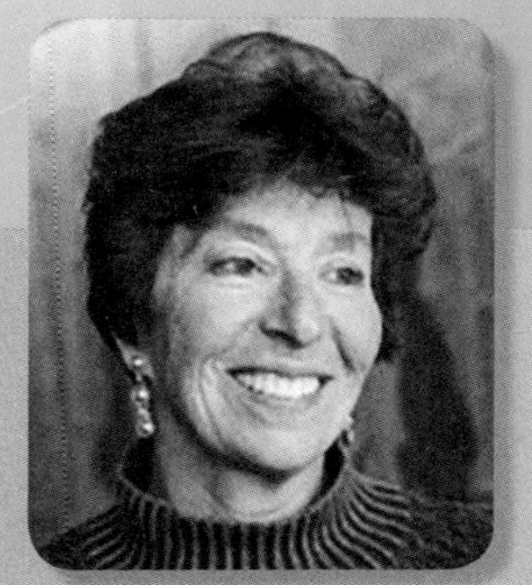

Anna L. Schwartz, PhD, FNP-BC, FAAN

Professor & Charlotte Peck Lienemann & Alumni Distinguished Chair
University of Nebraska Medical Center
College of Nursing
Omaha, NE, USA

Q: "Where did you grow up?"

All over the U.S. and for a few years in Victoria, Canada.

Q: "Where did you train? What is your training?"

I got a BS Physical Education and a BSN Nursing from University of Florida. Right out of school I worked in the Bone Marrow Transplant Unit at Shand's Hospital, University Florida. My observations there, along with my own personal experiences with cancer and as a world record setting bicycle racer, sparked my interest in studying cancer and exercise and sent me on a journey to find a mentor to support my work: MS Health Education, Florida State University, MS Nursing and Nursing Practitioner Certification at Arizona State University and finally a mentor who believed my idea at University of Utah (PhD).

Q: "What are you best known for?"

Initially, my exercise trials studied the effect of exercise on cancer-related fatigue and other side effects during cancer treatment. Since then, my research has expanded to program implementation and cultural adaptation of exercise interventions for Native Americans. Throughout my career, I mentored students and faculty across disciplines to become successful researchers.

Q: "What are you currently working on?"

Developing a cancer exercise app to deliver individualized exercise programs on handheld devices for people living with and beyond cancer.

Q: "Anything else you want to include?"

Be patient with yourself as you seek to figure out what your calling is. Finding what you love and have a passion for will give your life and work meaning. Believe in yourself and your dreams no matter what others may think. Only you know what you can do. So, put the stones in place to reach your goals and change the world.

Favorite Quote:

"The most certain way to succeed is always to try just one more time."
—*Thomas Edison*

STUDY QUESTIONS

1. What is the ACSM® exercise recommendation for reducing cancer-related side effects for cancer PLWBC?
2. Why is it important to adapt exercise and a FITT prescription to each person living with cancer?
3. True or false. PLWBC appear to prefer supervised exercise over unsupervised home-based exercise programs.
4. Why were only aerobic and resistance exercises included in the 2019 *ACSM® Exercise Guidelines for Cancer Survivors*?
5. True or false. Triathlon and dragon boat racing are considered safe and effective exercises.
6. What are the 3 different exercise prescriptions for fatigue?
7. Why is "do no harm" important for lymphedema?
8. True or false. Symptoms occur in isolation.
9. True or false. A supervised slowly progressive resistance exercise program is safe for a woman living with or beyond breast cancer.
10. What are the 3 key pieces of an oncologist referral to exercise?
11. List 3 of the 7 signs of lymphedema.

REFERENCES

1. Mishra SI, Scherer RW, Geigle PM, et al. Exercise interventions on health-related quality of life for cancer survivors. *Cochrane Database Syst Rev*. 2012(8):CD007566. doi:10.1002/14651858.CD007566.pub2
2. Mishra SI, Scherer RW, Snyder C, Geigle PM, Berlanstein DR, Topaloglu O. Exercise interventions on health-related quality of life for people with cancer during active treatment. *Cochrane Database Syst Rev*. 2012(8):CD008465. doi:10.1002/14651858.CD008465.pub2
3. Tlusty GC, Alonso WW, Berger AM. Exercise interventions during hospitalization for stem cell transplantation: an integrative review. *West J Nurs Res*. 2022;44(12):1167–82. doi:10.1177/01939459221124433
4. Zhou Y, Zhu J, Gu Z, Yin X. Efficacy of exercise interventions in patients with acute leukemia: a meta-analysis. *PLoS One*. 2016;11(7):e0159966. doi:10.1371/journal.pone.0159966
5. Lahart IM, Metsios GS, Nevill AM, Carmichael AR. Physical activity for women with breast cancer after adjuvant therapy. *Cochrane Database Syst Rev*. 2018(1):CD011292. doi:10.1002/14651858.CD011292.pub2
6. Marconcin P, Marques A, Ferrari G, Gouveia ÉR, Peralta M, Ihle A. Impact of exercise training on depressive symptoms in cancer patients: a critical analysis. *Biology (Basel)*. 2022;11(4):614. doi:10.3390/biology11040614
7. Singh B, Olds T, Curtis R, et al. Effectiveness of physical activity interventions for improving depression, anxiety and distress: an overview of systematic reviews. *Br J Sports Med*. doi:10.1136/bjsports-2022-106195
8. Campbell KL, Winters-Stone KM, Wiskemann J, et al. Exercise guidelines for cancer survivors: consensus statement from international multidisciplinary roundtable. *Med Sci Sports Exerc*. 2019;51(11):2375–90. doi:10.1249/mss.0000000000002116
9. Liu Y-C, Hung T-T, Konara Mudiyanselage SP, Wang C-J, Lin M-F. Beneficial exercises for cancer-related fatigue among women with breast cancer: a systematic review and network meta-analysis. *Cancers*. 2023; 15(1):151. https://doi.org/10.3390/cancers15010151
10. Meneses-Echávez JF, González-Jiménez E, Ramírez-Vélez R. Effects of supervised multimodal exercise interventions on cancer-related fatigue: systematic review and meta-analysis of randomized controlled trials. *BioMed Res Int*. 2015;2015:328636. doi:10.1155/2015/328636
11. Swartz MC, Lewis ZH, Lyons EJ, et al. Effect of home- and community-based physical activity interventions on physical function among cancer survivors: a systematic review and meta-analysis. *Arch Phys Med Rehabil*. 2017;98(8):1652–65. doi:10.1016/j.apmr.2017.03.017
12. Cataldi S, Greco G, Mauro M, Fischetti F. Effect of exercise on cancer-related fatigue: a systematic review. *J Hum Sport Exerc*. 2021;16(3):476–92. doi:10.14198/jhse.2021.163.01
13. Kelley GA, Kelley KS. Exercise and cancer-related fatigue in adults: a systematic review of previous systematic reviews with meta-analyses. *BMC Cancer*. 2017;17(1):693. doi:10.1186/s12885-017-3687-5
14. Sweegers MG, Altenburg TM, Chinapaw MJ, et al. Which exercise prescriptions improve quality of life and physical function in patients with cancer during and following treatment? A systematic review and meta-analysis of randomised controlled trials. *Br J Sports Med*. 2018;52(8):505. doi:10.1136/bjsports-2017-097891
15. Buffart LM, Sweegers MG, May AM, et al. Targeting exercise interventions to patients with cancer in need: an individual patient data meta-analysis. *J Natl Cancer Inst*. 2018;110(11):1190–200. doi:10.1093/jnci/djy161
16. Schmitz KH, Ahmed RL, Troxel AB, et al. Weight lifting for women at risk for breast cancer-related lymphedema: a randomized trial. *JAMA*. 2010;304(24):2699–705. doi: 10.1001/jama.2010.1837
17. Schmitz KH, Ahmed RL, Troxel A, et al. Weight lifting in women with breast-cancer-related lymphedema. *N Engl J Med*. 2009;361(7):664–73. doi:10.1056/NEJMoa0810118
18. Kilbreath SL, Refshauge KM, Beith JM, et al. Upper limb progressive resistance training and stretching exercises following surgery for early breast cancer: a randomized controlled trial. *Breast Cancer Res Treat*. 2012;133(2):667–76. doi:10.1007/s10549-012-1964-1
19. Katz E, Dugan NL, Cohn JC, Chu C, Smith RG, Schmitz KH. Weight lifting in patients with lower-extremity lymphedema secondary to cancer: a pilot and feasibility study. *Arch Phys Med Rehabil*. 2010;91(7):1070–6. doi:10.1016/j.apmr.2010.03.021
20. Dalla Via J, Daly RM, Fraser SF. The effect of exercise on bone mineral density in adult cancer survivors: a systematic review and meta-analysis. *Osteoporos Int*. 2018;29(2):287–303. doi:10.1007/s00198-017-4237-3
21. Fornusek CP, Kilbreath SL. Exercise for improving bone health in women treated for stages I–III breast cancer: a systematic review and meta-analyses. *J Cancer Surviv*. 2017;11(5):525–41. doi:10.1007/s11764-017-0622-3
22. Benedetti MG, Furlini G, Zati A, Letizia Mauro G. The effectiveness of physical exercise on bone density in osteoporotic patients. *Biomed Res Int*. 2018;2018:4840531. doi:10.1155/2018/4840531

23. Watson SL, Weeks BK, Weis LJ, Harding AT, Horan SA, Beck BR. High-intensity exercise did not cause vertebral fractures and improves thoracic kyphosis in postmenopausal women with low to very low bone mass: the LIFTMOR trial. *Osteoporos Int.* 2019;30(5):957–64. doi:10.1007/s00198-018-04829-z
24. Campbell KL, Weller S, Cormie P, Lane KN, Rauw JM, Goulart J. Enhancing safety of exercise for individuals with bone metastases: screening recommendations developed through Delphi consensus process. *J Clin Oncol.* 2020;38(suppl 15):e24042. doi:10.1200/JCO.2020.38.15_suppl.e24042
25. Weller S, Hart NH, Bolam KA, et al. Exercise for individuals with bone metastases: a systematic review. *Crit Rev Oncol Hematol.* 2021;166:103433. doi:10.1016/j.critrevonc.2021.103433
26. Rief H, Bruckner T, Schlampp I, et al. Resistance training concomitant to radiotherapy of spinal bone metastases: survival and prognostic factors of a randomized trial. *Radiat Oncol.* 2016;11:97. doi:10.1186/s13014-016-0675-x
27. Stout NL, Baima J, Swisher AK, Winters-Stone KM, Welsh J. A systematic review of exercise systematic reviews in the cancer literature (2005–2017). *PM R.* 2017;9(9S2):S347–84. doi:10.1016/j.pmrj.2017.07.074
28. Mercier J, Savard J, Bernard P. Exercise interventions to improve sleep in cancer patients: a systematic review and meta-analysis. *Sleep Med Rev.* 2017;36:43–56. doi:10.1016/j.smrv.2016.11.001
29. Rogers LQ, Courneya KS, Oster RA, et al. Physical activity and sleep quality in breast cancer survivors: a randomized trial. *Med Sci Sports Exerc.* 2017;49(10). doi:10.1249/MSS.0000000000001327
30. Steindorf K, Wiskemann J, Ulrich CM, Schmidt ME. Effects of exercise on sleep problems in breast cancer patients receiving radiotherapy: a randomized clinical trial. *Breast Cancer Res Treat.* 2017;162(3):489–99. doi:10.1007/s10549-017-4141-8
31. Yang H-L, Hsieh P-L, Hung C-H, et al. Early moderate intensity aerobic exercise intervention prevents doxorubicin-caused cardiac dysfunction through inhibition of cardiac fibrosis and inflammation. *Cancers (Basel).* 2020;12(5):1102. doi:10.3390/cancers12051102
32. Lee Y, Kwon I, Jang Y, Cosio-Lima L, Barrington P. Endurance exercise attenuates doxorubicin-induced cardiotoxicity. *Med Sci Sports Exerc.* 2020;52(1):25–36. doi:10.1249/mss.0000000000002094
33. Murray J, Bennett H, Bezak E, Perry R. The role of exercise in the prevention of cancer therapy-related cardiac dysfunction in breast cancer patients undergoing chemotherapy: systematic review. *Eur J Prev Cardiol.* 2022;29(3):463–72. doi:10.1093/eurjpc/zwab006
34. Scott JM, Nilsen TS, Gupta D, Jones LW. Exercise therapy and cardiovascular toxicity in cancer. *Circulation.* 2018;137(11):1176–91. doi:doi:10.1161/CIRCULATIONAHA.117.024671
35. Ramin C, Schaeffer ML, Zheng Z, et al. All-cause and cardiovascular disease mortality among breast cancer survivors in CLUE II, a long-standing community-based cohort. *J Natl Cancer Inst.* 2021;113(2):137–45. doi:10.1093/jnci/djaa096
36. Guo S, Han W, Wang P, Wang X, Fang X. Effects of exercise on chemotherapy-induced peripheral neuropathy in cancer patients: a systematic review and meta-analysis. *J Cancer Surviv.* 2023;17(2):318–31. doi:10.1007/s11764-022-01182-3
37. Kleckner IR, Kamen C, Gewandter JS, et al. Effects of exercise during chemotherapy on chemotherapy-induced peripheral neuropathy: a multicenter, randomized controlled trial. *Support Care Cancer.* 2018;26(4):1019–28. doi:10.1007/s00520-017-4013-0
38. Duregon F, Vendramin B, Bullo V, et al. Effects of exercise on cancer patients suffering chemotherapy-induced peripheral neuropathy undergoing treatment: a systematic review. *Crit Rev Oncol Hematol.* 2018;121:90–100. doi:10.1016/j.critrevonc.2017.11.002
39. Kleckner I, Gewandter JS, Heckler CE, et al. The effect of structured exercise during chemotherapy on chemotherapy-induced peripheral neuropathy (CIPN): a role for interoceptive brain circuitry. *J Clin Oncol.* 2019;37(suppl 15):11590. doi:10.1200/JCO.2019.37.15_suppl.11590
40. Kanzawa-Lee GA, Larson JL, Resnicow K, Smith EML. Exercise effects on chemotherapy-induced peripheral neuropathy: a comprehensive integrative review. *Cancer Nurs.* 2020;43(3):E172–E85. doi:10.1097/ncc.0000000000000801
41. Campbell KL, Zadravec K, Bland KA, Chesley E, Wolf F, Janelsins MC. The effect of exercise on cancer-related cognitive impairment and applications for physical therapy: systematic review of randomized controlled trials. *Phys Ther.* 2020;100(3):523–42. doi:10.1093/ptj/pzz090
42. Northey JM, Cherbuin N, Pumpa KL, Smee DJ, Rattray B. Exercise interventions for cognitive function in adults older than 50: a systematic review with meta-analysis. *Br J Sports Med.* 2018;52(3):154. doi:10.1136/bjsports-2016-096587
43. Stevens J, Burns E. *A CDC Compendium of Effective Fall Interventions: What Works for Community-Dwelling Adults.* 4th ed. Atlanta (GA): Centers for Disease Control and Prevention, National Center for Injury Prevention and Control; 2023.
44. Winningham ML, MacVicar MG. The effect of aerobic exercise on patient reports of nausea. *Oncol Nurs Forum.* 1988;15(4):447–50.
45. van Waart H, Stuiver MM, van Harten WH, et al. Effect of low-intensity physical activity and moderate- to high-intensity physical exercise during adjuvant chemotherapy on physical fitness, fatigue, and chemotherapy completion rates: results of the PACES randomized clinical trial. *J Clin Oncol.* 2015;33(17):1918–27. doi:10.1200/jco.2014.59.1081
46. Irwin ML, Cartmel B, Gross CP, et al. Randomized exercise trial of aromatase inhibitor-induced arthralgia in breast cancer survivors. *J Clin Oncol.* 2015;33(10):1104–11. doi:10.1200/JCO.2014.57.1547
47. Midgley AW, Lowe D, Levy AR, Mepani V, Rogers SN. Exercise program design considerations for head and neck cancer survivors. *Eur Arch Otorhinolaryngol.* 2018;275(1):169–79. doi:10.1007/s00405-017-4760-z
48. Galvão DA, Taaffe DR, Chambers SK, et al. Exercise intervention and sexual function in advanced prostate cancer: a randomised controlled trial. *BMJ Support Palliat Care.* 2020;12(1):29–32. doi:10.1136/bmjspcare-2020-002706
49. Cormie P, Chambers SK, Newton RU, et al. Improving sexual health in men with prostate cancer: randomised controlled trial of exercise and psychosexual therapies. *BMC Cancer.* 2014;14(1):199. doi:10.1186/1471-2407-14-199
50. Galvão DA, Taaffe DR, Chambers SK, et al. Exercise intervention and sexual function in advanced prostate cancer: a randomised controlled trial. *BMJ Support Palliat Care.* 2022;12(1):29–32.
51. Carter J, Lacchetti C, Andersen BL, et al. Interventions to address sexual problems in people with cancer: American Society of Clinical Oncology clinical practice guideline adaptation of cancer care ontario guideline. *J Clin Oncol.* 2018;36(5):492–511. doi:10.1200/jco.2017.75.8995
52. Barbera L, Zwaal C, Elterman D, et al. Interventions to address sexual problems in people with cancer. *Curr Oncol.* 2017;24(3):192–200. doi:10.3747/co.24.3583
53. Stanton AM, Handy AB, Meston CM. The effects of exercise on sexual function in women. *Sex Med Rev.* 2018;6(4):548–57. doi:10.1016/j.sxmr.2018.02.004
54. Gerbild H, Larsen CM, Graugaard C, Areskoug Josefsson K. Physical activity to improve erectile function: a systematic review of intervention studies. *Sex Med.* 2018;6(2):75–89. doi:10.1016/j.esxm.2018.02.001
55. Caan BJ, Meyerhardt JA, Brown JC, et al. Recruitment strategies and design considerations in a trial of resistance training to prevent dose-limiting toxicities in colon cancer patients undergoing chemotherapy. *Contemp Clin Trials.* 2021;101:106242. doi:10.1016/j.cct.2020.106242
56. Kirkham AA, Gelmon KA, Van Patten CL, et al. Impact of exercise on chemotherapy tolerance and survival in early-stage breast cancer: a nonrandomized controlled trial. *J Natl Compr Canc Netw.* 2020;18(12):1670–7. doi:10.6004/jnccn.2020.7603
57. Danhauer SC, Addington EL, Cohen L, et al. Yoga for symptom management in oncology: a review of the evidence base and future directions for research. *Cancer.* 2019;125(12):1979–89. doi:10.1002/cncr.31979

58. Harris SR. "We're all in the same boat": a review of the benefits of dragon boat racing for women living with breast cancer. *Evid Based Complement Alternat Med.* 2012;2012:167651. doi:10.1155/2012/167651
59. McDonough MH, Patterson MC, Weisenbach BB, Ullrich-French S, Sabiston CM. The difference is more than floating: factors affecting breast cancer survivors' decisions to join and maintain participation in dragon boat teams and support groups. *Disabil Rehabil.* 2019;41(15):1788–96. doi:10.1080/09638288.2018.1449259
60. Uth J, Hornstrup T, Christensen JF, et al. Efficacy of recreational football on bone health, body composition, and physical functioning in men with prostate cancer undergoing androgen deprivation therapy: 32-week follow-up of the FC prostate randomised controlled trial. *Osteoporos Int.* 2016;27(4):1507–18. doi:10.1007/s00198-015-3399-0
61. Crawford JJ, Vallance JK, Holt NL, Bell GJ, Steed H, Courneya KS. A pilot randomized, controlled trial of a wall climbing intervention for gynecologic cancer survivors. *Oncol Nurs Forum.* 2017;44(1):77–86. doi:10.1188/17.ONF.77-86
62. Ng AV, Cybulski AN, Engel AA, et al. Triathlon training for women breast cancer survivors: feasibility and initial efficacy. *Support Care Cancer.* 2017;25(5):1465–73. doi:10.1007/s00520-016-3531-5
63. Dolan LB, Campbell K, Gelmon K, Neil-Sztramko S, Holmes D, McKenzie DC. Interval versus continuous aerobic exercise training in breast cancer survivors: a pilot RCT. *Support Care Cancer.* 2016;24(1):119–27. doi:10.1007/s00520-015-2749-y
64. Cohen J, Geara A, Hogan J, et al. Hypertension in cancer patients and survivors. *J Am Coll Cardiol CardioOnc.* 2019;1(2):238–51. doi:10.1016/j.jaccao.2019.11.009
65. American College of Sports Medicine®, Reibe D, Ehrman JK, Liguori G, Magal M. *ACSM's® Guidelines for Exercise Testing and Prescription.* 10th ed. Philadelphia (PA): Wolters Kluwer; 2018.
66. Schmitz KH, Courneya KS, Matthews C, et al. American College of Sports Medicine® roundtable on exercise guidelines for cancer survivors. *Med Sci Sports Exerc.* 2010;42(7):1409–26. doi:10.1249/MSS.0b013e3181e0c112 [Erratum in: *Med Sci Sports Exerc.* 2011 Jan;43(1):195]
67. Galvão DA, Taaffe DR, Spry N, et al. Exercise preserves physical function in prostate cancer patients with bone metastases. *Med Sci Sports Exerc.* 2018;50(3):393–9. doi:10.1249/mss.0000000000001454
68. Scott JM, Zabor EC, Schwitzer E, et al. Efficacy of exercise therapy on cardiorespiratory fitness in patients with cancer: a systematic review and meta-analysis. *J Clin Oncol.* 2018;36(22):2297–305. doi:10.1200/jco.2017.77.5809
69. Fuller JT, Hartland MC, Maloney LT, Davison K. Therapeutic effects of aerobic and resistance exercises for cancer survivors: a systematic review of meta-analyses of clinical trials. *Br J Sports Med.* 2018;52(20):1311. doi:10.1136/bjsports-2017-098285
70. Hasenoehrl T, Palma S, Ramazanova D, et al. Resistance exercise and breast cancer-related lymphedema: a systematic review update and meta-analysis. *Support Care Cancer.* 2020;28(8):3593–603. doi:10.1007/s00520-020-05521-x
71. Padilha CS, Marinello PC, Galvão DA, et al. Evaluation of resistance training to improve muscular strength and body composition in cancer patients undergoing neoadjuvant and adjuvant therapy: a meta-analysis. *J Cancer Surviv.* 2017;11(3):339–49. doi:10.1007/s11764-016-0592-x
72. Dolan LB, Gelmon K, Courneya KS, et al. Hemoglobin and aerobic fitness changes with supervised exercise training in breast cancer patients receiving chemotherapy. *Cancer Epidemiol Biomarkers Prev.* 2010;19(11):2826–32. doi:10.1158/1055-9965.Epi-10-0521
73. Stout NL, Santa Mina D, Lyons KD, Robb K, Silver JK. A systematic review of rehabilitation and exercise recommendations in oncology guidelines. *CA Cancer J Clin.* 2021;71(2):149–75. https://doi.org/10.3322/caac.21639
74. Sweegers MG, Altenburg TM, Brug J, et al. Effects and moderators of exercise on muscle strength, muscle function and aerobic fitness in patients with cancer: a meta-analysis of individual patient data. *Br J Sports Med.* 2019;53(13):812. doi:10.1136/bjsports-2018-099191
75. Galvão DA, Spry NA, Taaffe DR, et al. Changes in muscle, fat and bone mass after 36 weeks of maximal androgen blockade for prostate cancer. *BJU Int.* 2008;102(1):44–7. doi:10.1111/j.1464-410X.2008.07539.x
76. Galvão DA, Taaffe DR, Spry N, Joseph D, Turner D, Newton RU. Reduced muscle strength and functional performance in men with prostate cancer undergoing androgen suppression: a comprehensive cross-sectional investigation. *Prostate Cancer Prostatic Dis.* 2009;12(2):198–203. doi:10.1038/pcan.2008.51
77. Chen Z, Zhang Y, Lu C, Zeng H, Schumann M, Cheng S. Supervised physical training enhances muscle strength but not muscle mass in prostate cancer patients undergoing androgen deprivation therapy: a systematic review and meta-analysis. *Front Physiol.* 2019;10:843. doi:10.3389/fphys.2019.00843 [Erratum published in *Front Physiol.* 2019;10:1126]
78. Lund CM, Vistisen KK, Olsen AP, et al. The effect of geriatric intervention in frail older patients receiving chemotherapy for colorectal cancer: a randomized trial (GERICO). *Br J Cancer.* 2021;124(12):1949–58. doi:10.1038/s41416-021-01367-0
79. Garcia CK, Renteria LI, Leite-Santos G, et al. Exertional heat stroke: pathophysiology and risk factors. *BMJ Med.* 2022;1:e000239. doi:10.1136/bmjmed-2022-000239
80. Fearon K, Arends J, Baracos V. Understanding the mechanisms and treatment options in cancer cachexia. *Nat Rev Clin Oncol.* 2013;10(2):90–9. doi:10.1038/nrclinonc.2012.209
81. Arends J, Bachmann P, Baracos V, et al. ESPEN guidelines on nutrition in cancer patients. *Clin Nutr.* 2017;36(1):11–48. doi:10.1016/j.clnu.2016.07.015
82. Lopes-Júnior LC, Ferrarini T, Pires LBC, Rodrigues JG, Salaroli LB, Nunes KZ. Cancer symptom clusters in adult patients undergoing chemotherapy: a systematic review and meta-analysis protocol. *PLoS ONE.* 2022;17(9):e0273411. doi:10.1371/journal.pone.0273411
83. Frost HM. Should future risk-of-fracture analyses include another major risk factor? The case for falls. *J Clin Densitom.* 2001;4(4):381–3. doi:10.1385/jcd:4:4:381
84. Clough-Gorr KM, Stuck AE, Thwin SS, Silliman RA. Older breast cancer survivors: geriatric assessment domains are associated with poor tolerance of treatment adverse effects and predict mortality over 7 years of follow-up. *J Clin Oncol.* 2010;28(3):380–6. doi:10.1200/jco.2009.23.5440
85. Klepin HD, Geiger AM, Tooze JA, et al. Physical performance and subsequent disability and survival in older adults with malignancy: results from the health, aging and body composition study. *J Am Geriatr Soc.* 2010;58(1):76–82. doi:10.1111/j.1532-5415.2009.02620.x
86. Chodzko-Zajko WJ, Proctor DN, Fiatarone Singh MA, et al. American College of Sports Medicine® position stand: exercise and physical activity for older adults. *Med Sci Sports Exerc.* 2009;41(7):1510–30. doi:10.1249/MSS.0b013e3181a0c95c
87. Paskett ED, Dean JA, Oliveri JM, Harrop JP. Cancer-related lymphedema risk factors, diagnosis, treatment, and impact: a review. *J Clin Oncol.* 2012;30(30):3726–33. doi:10.1200/jco.2012.41.8574

CHAPTER

12

Prescribing Exercise in the Survivorship Phase

OUTLINE

1. Introduction
2. Definition of the Cancer Survivorship Phase
   a. Reentry Phase
   b. Early Survivorship
   c. Long-Term Survivorship
3. Cancer Survivorship and Physical Activity Levels
4. General Exercise Recommendations for Cancer Survivors
5. Role of Exercise in Treating Specific Chronic and Late-appearing Treatment Side Effects
   a. Cancer-Related Fatigue (CRF) and Sleep Issues
   b. Anxiety and Depression
   c. Lymphedema
   d. Sarcopenia
   e. Endocrine Treatment Side Effects
   f. Cardiac Issues
6. Disease Prevention/Health Promotion
7. Summary
8. Case Study
9. Meet the Expert
10. Study Questions
11. References

OBJECTIVES

After completing review of this chapter, students will be able to:

1. Define and explain the cancer survivorship phase.
2. Identify current levels of physical activity in cancer survivors worldwide.
3. Comprehend the general exercise guidelines for cancer survivors.
4. Understand the evidence-based role of exercise in treating chronic and late-appearing treatment side effects.

INTRODUCTION

Following the guidelines on exercise during cancer treatment presented in Chapter 11, this chapter focuses on the evidence and guidelines for exercise prescription once active/neoadjuvant treatment has been completed and the survivorship phase starts. The treatment time period can be difficult to define when considering some of the long-term, less intensive treatments. Nevertheless, the focus of the treatment time period is usually on the "primary" cancer treatments, such as surgery, radiation therapy, chemotherapy, and some targeted therapies. Once this stage is completed, the person moves into the survivorship mode as described by Courneya (1) (Figure 12.1), and the focus is on restorative/rehabilitation programs. Although this is described as posttreatment, the cancer patient may still be receiving some long-term medications such as hormone treatment (eg, many women diagnosed with breast cancer will take daily hormone treatment such as tamoxifen for 5 years or longer) or biological therapies, and many will still be experiencing chronic/late-appearing treatment side effects. This chapter will provide evidence on the benefits of staying active and the guidelines on how to abate or prevent the most comment chronic side effects experienced by cancer survivors.

DEFINITION OF THE CANCER SURVIVORSHIP PHASE

The cancer survivorship phase is defined by the United States (US) Institute of Medicine as "the period following first diagnosis and treatment and prior to the development of a recurrence of cancer or death" (2). This period can be distinguished into the following 3 stages (which may overlap) (3):

- reentry
- early survivorship
- long-term survivorship phase

Reentry Phase

The reentry phase, immediately after treatment, can be described as the transition from a person with cancer to a person with a *history* of cancer. This phase can be very distressing to a cancer survivor because of the loss of their clinical safety net, the resumption or adaptation to their previous work and social roles and responsibilities, and often caused by the presence of remaining or emerging cancer-treatment-related side effects: "What I reacted to when it was over, and I'd become cancer free, were people's expectations. They were probably thinking, 'Now that you've recovered you can move on with your life.' However, you can't just move on" (4).

Early Survivorship

The early survivorship period is from the reentry phase to approximately 5 years after cancer diagnosis. During this phase, cancer survivors often experience periods of loneliness, elevated levels of fear at follow-up appointments, and suspicion that any new pain or deconditioning is a sign that the cancer has recurred. For most cancer survivors, if appropriate support is provided during these years, many treatment-related physical and psychological morbidities can be resolved.

Long-Term Survivorship

Long-term survivorship is defined by any time after 5 years (the oncology time marker of survival and when most follow-up appointments cease). By this stage, the quality of life (QoL) of most cancer survivors is, on average, indistinguishable from that of the general population (5). However, it is important to acknowledge that a minority of cancer survivors will still be struggling with specific

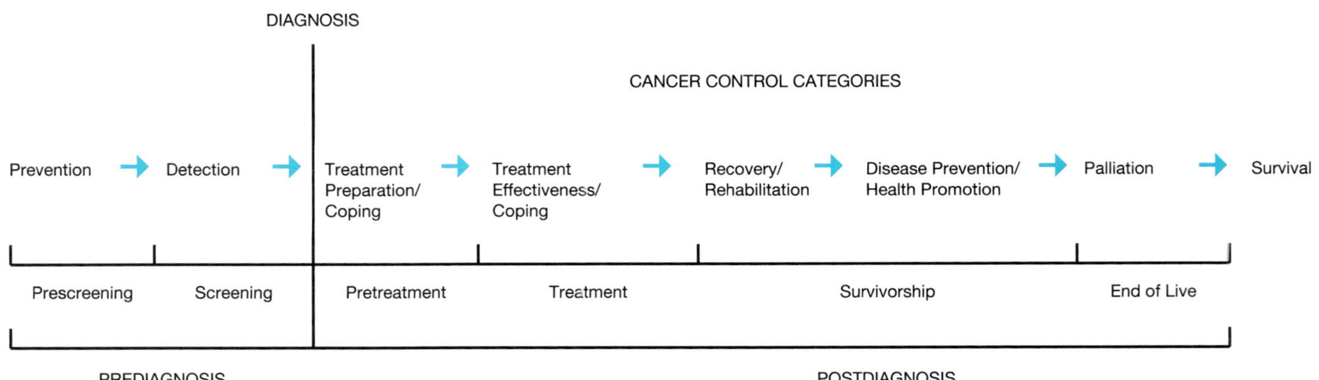

FIGURE 12.1. Physical activity and cancer control framework. (From Courneya KS, Friedenreich CM. Physical activity and cancer control. *Semin Oncol Nurs.* 2007;23(4):242–52.)

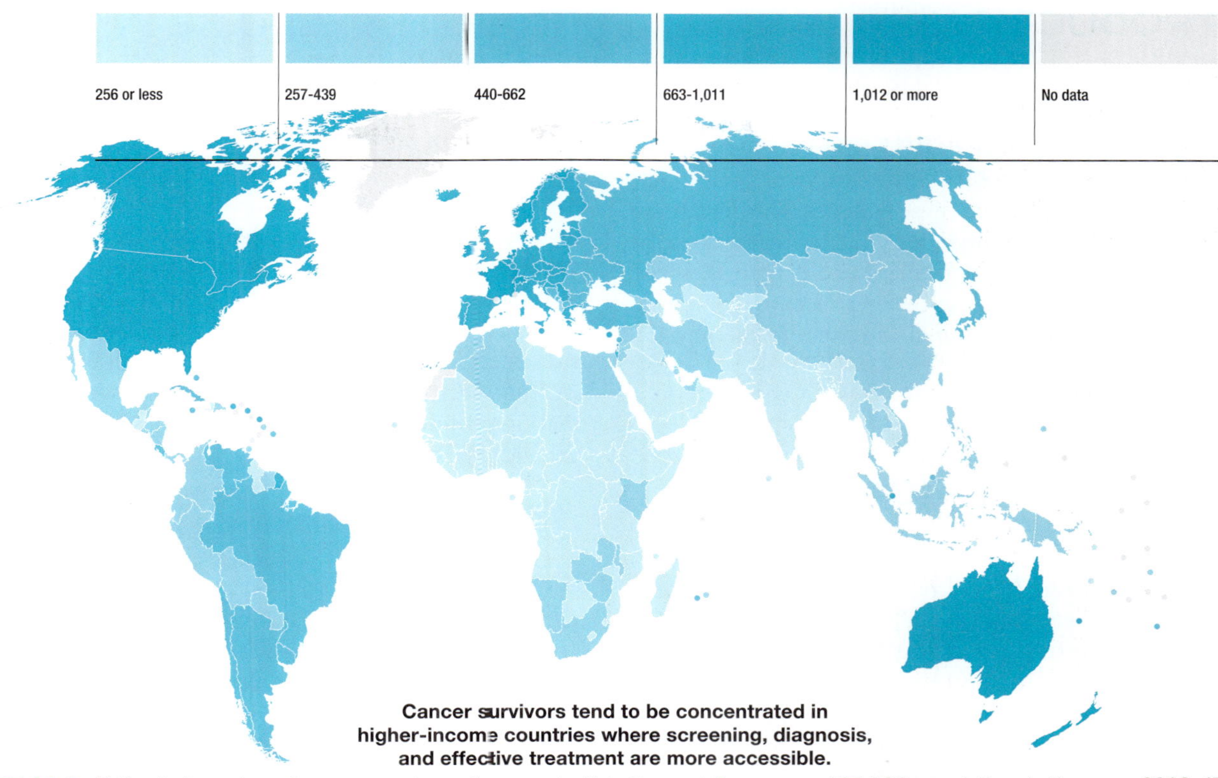

FIGURE 12.2. Estimated number of cancer survivors diagnosed within the past 5 years per 100,000 population, both sexes, 2018. (From The Cancer Atlas, Cancer Survivorship. *American Cancer Society, Inc.* 2019, MAP 25.1. Available from https://canceratlas.cancer.org/the-burden/cancer-survivorship/.)

physical and psychological side effects many years after diagnosis. From a health promotion perspective, many studies demonstrate that compared with adults with no cancer diagnosis, long-term cancer survivors have more physical activity limitations, poorer health status, higher medical expenditures, and greater indirect costs because of morbidities (6). Strategies to improve overall health are important at this stage.

CANCER SURVIVORSHIP AND PHYSICAL ACTIVITY LEVELS

In 2018, there were approximately 43.8 million cancer survivors worldwide. Owing to advances in early detection and treatment and an aging population, that number continues to increase exponentially, for example, in the US, from 15.5 million in 2016 to 26.1 million in 2040 (Figures 12.2 and 12.3).

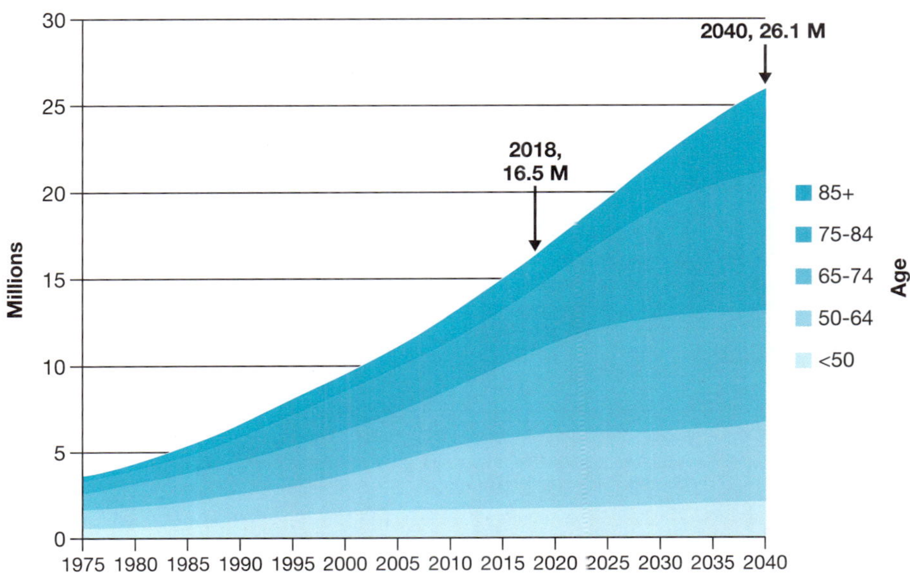

FIGURE 12.3. Estimated and projected numbers of US cancer survivors by age at prevalence. (From Feuerstein M, Nekhlyudov L. *Handbook of Cancer Survivorship*. 2nd ed. New York (NY): Springer; 2018, Chapter 2.)

Many cancer survivors report chronic cancer-related side effects, such as fatigue, weight gain, lymphedema, cardiac issues, impaired functional status, sarcopenia, endocrine symptoms, anxiety, and depression.

Despite many evidence-based health benefits of physical activity, only 17% to 47% cancer survivors participate in sufficient exercise to gain these benefits. The percentage of adherence to the recommended guidelines decreases the further out timewise from treatment and diagnosis, - with those at the reentry stage and having recently completed treatment being more motivated to adhere to the physical activity guidelines (7).

GENERAL EXERCISE RECOMMENDATIONS FOR CANCER SURVIVORS

Based on the current literature, the general exercise prescription for cancer survivors should include moderate-intensity aerobic training at least 3 times per week, for at least 30 minutes. In addition, the prescription should include resistance training at least 2 times per week, using at least 2 sets of 8 to 15 repetitions at least 60% of 1 repetition maximum. Exercise programs that are supervised appear to be more effective than strictly unsupervised or home-based programs (8). See Table 12.1 and Figure 12.4.

ROLE OF EXERCISE IN TREATING SPECIFIC CHRONIC AND LATE-APPEARING TREATMENT SIDE EFFECTS

This section will concentrate on the most common chronic or late-appearing cancer-related side effects found in the cancer survivorship phase. With each one, we will look at the prevalence of this side effect and suggest validated tools that can be used in most settings to assess the specific side effect, the evidence of the benefit with physical activity, the specific guidelines, and finally any specific information or modifications when working with patients with this side effect.

Cancer-Related Fatigue (CRF) and Sleep Issues

CRF is the most reported and also the most distressing side effect of cancer treatments. Although CRF will resolve for some survivors after the completion of treatments, there are still approximately 30% to 40% of cancer survivors who will still have persistent CRF up to 10 years following treatment (9) There are over 40 tools available to detect CRF, but the use of a simple tool such as FACT-F (10) or a unidimensional measure that includes a severity rating such as the visual analogue scale (11) are recommended for identifying

Table 12.1 FITT Recommendations for Cancer Survivors

	AEROBIC	RESISTANCE	FLEXIBILITY
Frequency	3-5 d wk^{-1}	2-3 d wk^{-1} with a minimum of 48 h between sessions	2-3 d wk^{-1} up to daily
Intensity	40%-<60% $\dot{V}O_2R$ or HRR. Survivors may find RPE useful to gauge exercise intensity.	60%-80% 1-RM or allow for 6-15 repetitions. Increase weight as tolerated and when repetitions >15. RPE is correlated with % 1-RM in cancer survivors ([a]).	Stretch within limits of pain to the point of tightness or slight discomfort.
Time	≥30 min d^{-1}. No lower limit on bout length. During treatment, exercise length may need to be modified due to chemotherapy or radiation-related toxicities.	≥1 set, ≥8 repetitions per set; ≥60 s rest between sets	Hold each stretch for 10-30 s.
Type	Walking, cycling, swimming. Swimming should not be prescribed for survivors with central lines, those with ostomies, those in an immunocompromised state or who are currently receiving radiation therapy.	8-10 exercises of major muscle groups; machines or free weights	Static stretches (passive and/or active), for all major muscle tendon groups. Tai chi and yoga may be preferred.

[a]1-RM, one repetition maximum; HRR, heart rate reserve; RPE, rating of perceived exertion; $\dot{V}O_2R$, oxygen uptake reserve.

From Fairman CM, LaFountain RL, Lucas AR, Focht BC. Monitoring resistance exercise intensity using ratings of perceived exertion in previously untrained patients with prostate cancer undergoing androgen deprivation therapy. *J Strength Cond Res.* 2018;32(5):1360–5; Campbell KL, Winters-Stone KM, Wiskemann J, May AM, Schwartz AL, Courneya KS, et al. Exercise guidelines for cancer survivors: consensus statement from international multidisciplinary roundtable. *Sci Sports Exerc.* 2019;51(11):2375–90.

Effects of Exercise on Health-Related Outcomes in Those with Cancer

What can exercise do?

- Prevention of 7 common cancers*
  Dose: 2018 Physical Activity Guidelines for Americans: 150-300 min/week moderate or 75-150 min/week vigorous aerobic exercise
- Survival of 3 common cancers**
  Dose: Exact dose of physical activity needed to reduce cancer-specific or all-cause mortality is not yet known; Overall more activity appears to lead to better risk reduction

*bladder, breast, colon, endometrial, esophageal, kidney and stomach cancers
**breast, colon and prostate cancers

Overall, avoid inactivity, and to improve general health, aim to achieve the current physical activity guidelines for health (150 min/week aerobic exercise and 2x/week strength training).

Outcome	Aerobic Only	Resistance Only	Combination (Aerobic + Resistance)
Strong Evidence	Dose	Dose	Dose
Cancer-related fatigue	**3x**/week for **30** min per session of moderate intensity	**2x**/week of **2** sets of **12-15** reps for major muscle groups at moderate intensity	**3x**/week for **30** min per session of moderate aerobic exercise, plus **2x**/week of resistance training 2 sets of 12-15 reps for major muscle groups at moderate intensity
Health-related quality of life	**2-3x**/week for **30-60** min per session of moderate to vigorous	**2x**/week of **2** sets of **8-15** reps for major muscle groups at a moderate to vigorous intensity	**2-3x**/week for **20-30** min per session of moderate aerobic exercise plus **2x**/week of resistance training **2** sets of **8-15** reps for major muscle groups at moderate to vigorous intensity
Physical Function	**3x**/week for **30-60** min per session of moderate to vigorous	**2-3x**/week of **2** sets of **8-12** reps for major muscle groups at moderate to vigorous intensity	**3x**/week for **20-40** min per session of moderate to vigorous aerobic exercise, plus **2-3x**/week of resistance training **2** sets of **8-12** reps for major muscle group at moderate to vigorous intensity
Anxiety	**3x**/week for **30-60** min per session of moderate to vigorous	Insufficient evidence	**2-3x**/week for **20-40** min of moderate to vigorous aerobic exercise plus **2x**/week of resistance training of **2** sets, **8-12** reps for major muscle groups at moderate to vigorous intensity
Depression	**3x**/week for **30-60** min per session of moderate to vigorous	Insufficient evidence	**2-3x**/week for **20-40** min of moderate to vigorous aerobic exercise plus **2x**/week of resistance training of **2** sets, **8-12** reps for major muscle groups at moderate to vigorous intensity
Lymphedema	Insufficient evidence	**2-3x**/week of progressive, supervised program for major muscle groups does not exacerbate lymphedema	Insufficient evidence
Moderate Evidence			
Bone health	Insufficient evidence	**2-3x**/week of moderate to vigorous resistance training plus high impact training (sufficient to generate ground reaction force of **3-4** time body weight) for at least **12** months	Insufficient evidence
Sleep	**3-4x**/week for **30-40** min per session of moderate intensity	Insufficient evidence	Insufficient evidence

Citation: bit.ly/cancer_exercise_guidelines

Moderate intensity (40%-59% heart rate reserve or VO_2R) to vigorous intensity (60%-89% heart rate reserve or VO_2R) is recommended.

MOVING THROUGH CANCER — Exercise is Medicine — AMERICAN COLLEGE of SPORTS MEDICINE

FIGURE 12.4. Effects of exercise on health-related outcomes in those with cancer. (From Campbell KL, Winters-Stone KM, Wiskemann J, et al. Exercise guidelines for cancer survivors: consensus statement from international multidisciplinary roundtable. *Med Sci Sports Exerc.* 2019;51(11):2375–90. doi:10.1249/MSS.0000000000002116.)

the presence of CRF among survivors (12). When looking specifically at a **subanalysis** of exercise studies undertaken solely in the survivorship phase, aerobic exercise has been shown to have a moderate effect on fatigue compared with a control group (standardized mean difference [SMD] = −0.63) (13). A review of posttreatment breast cancer patients consisting of 9 RCTs and 581 participants showed significantly reduced fatigue in the experimental group at the immediate follow-up (SMD = 1.20) and 12 weeks later (SMD = 3.37) (14). Current guidelines suggest that a 12-week training program of moderate-to-vigorous aerobic training plus resistance training sessions (with or without stretching) 3 times per week will reduce CRF after treatment (8). Low-intensity exercise training does not appear to reduce fatigue. A study with prostate cancer survivors showed that supervised aerobic exercise for 50 minutes per session, 2 sessions per week for 8 weeks, had a moderate effect on CRF, whereas the same dose of exercise using shorter sessions occurring more frequently, that is, 20 to 30 minutes per session, 3 sessions per week, only had a small effect on CRF when it was performed (13). Therefore, greater reductions in fatigue appear to be provided with exercise sessions longer than 30 minutes and programs longer than 12 weeks.

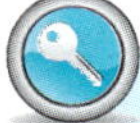

Subanalysis. Evaluation of the effect of an intervention for a specific endpoint in a subgroup of patients defined by a baseline characteristic (eg, treatment stage).

Sleep disturbances, a common issue during treatment, often do not disappear immediately after cancer treatment but can persist for several years. Aerobic exercise, particularly walking, 3 to 4 times per week, for 30 to 40 minutes per

Box 12.1 Considerations When Working With a Person With Fatigue

One consideration when selecting a specific mode of exercise to combat fatigue is that many prostate cancer survivors may prefer resistance training only to aerobic training, and it has been shown that twice weekly moderate-intensity resistance training is equally effective at reducing fatigue with this cancer group.

Data from Keogh JWL, MacLeod RD. Body composition, physical fitness, functional performance, quality of life, and fatigue benefits of exercise for prostate cancer patients: a systematic review. *J Pain Symptom Manage.* 2012;43(1):96–110.

session over 12 weeks has been shown to have a strong positive effect on sleep quality with cancer survivors (15). See Box 12.1 (16).

Anxiety and Depression

The prevalence of depression has been found to be highest during cancer treatment (14%), reducing to 9% in the first year after treatment and to 8% in more than a year posttreatment (17). However, for many cancer survivors, once treatment is over, they feel as if they have fallen into a black hole, and the trauma of the treatment phase causes feelings of depression. In contrast, a systematic review on anxiety in ovarian cancer patients found that anxiety tended to be the highest following treatment (27%) compared with during treatment (26%) and pretreatment (19%) (18). This heightened anxiety in the survivorship phase is partly caused by the fear of recurrence—one of the most commonly reported issues and an important area of unmet need for cancer survivors. In a recent study of long-term survivors (5-10 years post diagnosis), moderate-to-severe depression and anxiety were reported in 17% and 9% of the survivors, respectively. There were no significant differences between the 5 years and 10 years after diagnosis, and depression and anxiety were more commonly reported in women than in men. Cancer survivors younger than 60 years of age were more depressed and anxious than older cancer survivors and more than the general population (19). A validated screening questionnaire commonly used for anxiety and depression is the Hospital Anxiety and Depression Scale (HADS) (20).

A review of exercise interventions (8) shows that depressive symptoms in cancer survivors after treatment can be reduced with moderate-intensity aerobic training 3 times per week for at least 12 weeks or aerobic and resistance training combined twice weekly for 6 to 12 weeks. For reducing anxiety, moderate-intensity aerobic training 3 times per week for 12 weeks or aerobic and resistance training combined twice weekly for 6 to 12 weeks is required after treatment. Based on current evidence, it does not appear that resistance training alone reduces anxiety, and supervised training programs are more effective than those that are predominantly unsupervised or home-based.

Lymphedema

The incidence of Breast cancer related lymphedema (BCRL) posttreatment is 21%. The incidence of BCRL mostly occurs in the first 2 years postsurgery of breast cancer (21), with new cases continuing to appear beyond this time but at a slower rate. A simple tool to assess if upper limb lymphedema is affecting active daily living is to use the Disabilities of the Arm, Shoulder and Hand (DASH) outcome questionnaire (22). Historically, patients with breast cancer were advised to refrain from exercise, particularly resistance training, in order to avoid the onset or exacerbation of lymphedema. The evidence is now strong that staying active is safe and does not increase the risk of lymphedema or make it worse. Now, most lymphedema advisory groups, including the National Lymphedema Network in the US, stress that exercise (aerobic, strength, and flexibility) is an essential part of a healthy lifestyle and essential for effective lymphedema management. The National Lymphedema Network also points out that patients with or at risk of lymphedema should perform aerobic and weight-lifting exercise in a safe environment. Historically, there were concerns that resistance training may trigger or exacerbate lymphedema; however, in 2015, a review 2015 by Stuiver et al (23) showed that resistance training after breast cancer treatment does not increase the risk of developing BCRL. In order to be safe when providing a resistance program for cancer survivors with or at risk for lymphedema, it is important to focus on the large muscle group and progress with the principle "start low, progress slow." On a positive note, a 2019 review of the effects of weight lifting and resistance training on women at risk for or with BCRL showed that this mode of exercise did not alter arm volume change or increase swelling and did not cause lymphedema or adverse events. In fact, a review of 3 studies reported that arm volume was significantly reduced in the weight-lifting or resistance exercise group compared with those in the control group (24). See Box 12.2 for considerations when working with a patient with lymphedema.

Box 12.2 Considerations When Working With a Person With Lymphedema

- **Flexibility:** Swelling may make limb heavy and result in a limited range of movement.
- **Aerobic exercise:** Pumping movements are beneficial, but not for long repetitive periods.
- **Resistance training:** Start low, progress slow.
- **Compression sleeve:** Consider keeping compression sleeve on when exercising.
- **Good ventilation:** Good ventilation when exercising in order to prevent overheating.
- **Water exercise:** Water exercise is excellent because of buoyancy and resistive pressure of water on the limb.

Sarcopenia

Sarcopenia is characterized by a progressive and generalized loss of skeletal muscle mass and loss of muscle strength or physical functioning. The prevalence of secondary sarcopenia (ie, due to cancer and treatments) in cancer survivors ranges from 14% to 79% with the highest prevalence in patients with esophagogastric cancer (43%-79%), pancreatic cancer (56%-63%), liver cancer (28%-68%), and renal cell carcinoma (53%-54%) (25). Older cancer survivors are at a higher risk of both primary sarcopenia and secondary sarcopenia; therefore, it is vital to prevent and treat sarcopenia to reduce adverse health outcomes and improve their prognosis. The SARC-F questionnaire (26) is a screening test for sarcopenia that can be undertaken during a consultation. In addition, the assessment of muscle mass (using anthropometric measurements), muscle strength (hand grip or sit to stand), and physical performance (gait speed, timed up-and-go, 6MWT) can help define the presence and the extent of sarcopenia.

A review in 2022 (25) on the effects of exercise on sarcopenia among cancer survivors showed that exercise programs were able to increase skeletal muscle postintervention by 2.1% to 12.8% compared with that in the control groups, and in the 3 studies (25-29), the situation was reversed with an improvement of 18.2% to 42.9% decrease in sarcopenia in exercise groups compared with a 5.2% increase to 16.7% decrease in sarcopenia in control groups. There is no specific physical activity prescription for the management of cancer-related sarcopenia. However, a supervised progressive resistance training program for at least 12 weeks is the most effective for improving muscle strength, muscle mass, and physical performance in frailer, older people (30, 31).

Endocrine Treatment Side Effects

Many breast cancer survivors taking adjuvant endocrine medications report the following significant symptoms: low energy levels; bone loss and osteoporosis; arthralgia (joint pain and stiffness); weight gain and body image concerns; cognitive side effects such as difficulty concentrating and memory loss; sexual dysfunction and menopausal symptoms, including hot flashes; night sweats (resulting in poor sleep quality); and vaginal dryness (32). The presence and severity of these side effects have been identified as barriers to hormone treatment adherence. A review of 29 studies showed that the prevalence of adherence ranged from 41% to 72%, with 50% of women taking less than 80% of the prescribed dosage; and discontinuation by the fifth year of prescription ranged from 31% to 73% (33). A study that examined the prevalence of hormone treatment symptoms in prostate cancer survivors reported that the most common side effects were erectile dysfunction (56%), loss of libido (42%), urinary incontinence (15%), hot flushes (8%), and breast changes (5%) (34). A tool to use to assess endocrine symptoms in women undergoing hormone treatment for breast cancer is Functional Assessment Cancer Therapy-Endocrine Symptoms (FACT-ES) (35). For prostate cancer survivors taking ADT, the appropriate questionnaire is Functional Assessment of Cancer Therapy-Prostate (FACT-P) (36). These common hormone therapy side effects are reviewed individually as follows.

Bone Health

In a Swedish study of 180,000 older men, those men with prostate cancer undergoing ADT were 4 times more likely to develop significant bone deficiency. In a large study of men surviving 4 to 5 years after the diagnosis of prostate cancer, 19.4% of those who received ADT had a fracture compared with 12% in men who did not take hormone treatment (37). **Osteopenia** has been detected in 44% of breast cancer patients in complete remission, and **osteoporosis** was found in 16% (38).

With respect to exercise prescription, studies in breast and prostate cancer survivors (39, 40) indicate that a 1-year supervised program of combined moderate-to-vigorous intensity resistance plus high-impact training (ie, exercise that generates ground reaction forces above 3-4 times body weight) performed 2 to 3 days per week is the best mode of exercise to improve bone health (eg, slow loss or slightly improve BMD at the hip and lumbar spine). In contrast, aerobic training, particularly walking, does not appear to provide a sufficient stimulus to improve bone outcomes (8).

The American Society of Clinical Oncology (ASCO) recommendations for the management of osteoporosis in survivors of adult cancers with nonmetastatic disease state that patients on hormone treatment should be offered BMD testing every 2 years or, more frequently, if deemed medically necessary. These cancer survivors should be actively encouraged to engage in a combination of exercise types, including balance training, flexibility or stretching exercises, endurance exercise, and resistance and/or progressive strengthening exercises, to reduce the risk of fractures caused by falls. Whenever possible, exercise should be tailored according to the needs and abilities of the individual patient. Patients with an impairment hindering their gait or balance should be offered medical rehabilitation (41). In addition, the FITT recommendations and special considerations for individuals with osteoporosis in *ACSM® Guidelines for Exercise Testing and Prescription* (42) should be followed (Table 12.2).

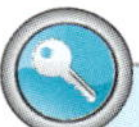

Osteopenia. A decrease in BMD below normal reference values, but not low enough to meet the diagnostic criteria for osteoporosis.

Osteoporosis. A BMD of 2.5 standard deviations below the mean peak mass (average of young healthy adults) as measured by DXA applied to the femoral neck and reported as a T-score.

Table 12.2 FITT Recommendations for Individuals With Osteoporosis

	AEROBIC	RESISTANCE	FLEXIBILITY
Frequency	4-5 d wk^{-1}	Start with 1-2 nonconsecutive d wk^{-1}; may progress to 2-3 d wk^{-1}	5-7 d wk^{-1}
Intensity	Moderate intensity (40%-59% $\dot{V}O_2R$ or HRR). Use of the CR-10 scale with ratings of 3-4 might be a more appropriate method of establishing intensity.	Adjust resistance so that last 2 repetitions are challenging to perform. High-intensity and high-velocity training can be beneficial in those who can tolerate it.	Stretch to the point of feeling tightness or mild discomfort.
Time	Begin with 20 min; gradually progress to a minimum of 30 min (with a maximum of 45-60 min). Increase time initially to a minimum of 10 min before increasing intensity. Progress to 30-60 min as tolerated.	Begin with 1 set of 8-12 repetitions; increase to 2 sets after ~2 wk; no more than 8-10 exercises per session.	Hold static stretch for 10-30 s; 2-4 repetitions of each exercise
Type	Walking, cycling, or other individually appropriate aerobic activity (weight bearing preferred). Impact loading exercises, such as jumping or bench stepping, can be used in those with low or moderate risk for fracture.	Standard equipment can be used with adequate instruction and safety considerations. Compound movement exercises are best.	Static stretching of all major joints

HRR, heart rate reserve; $\dot{V}O_2R$, oxygen uptake reserve.
Data from American College of Sports Medicine®, Chodzko-Zajko WJ, Proctor DN et al. American College of Sports Medicine® position stand: exercise and physical activity for older adults. *Med Sci Sports Exerc.* 2009;41(7):1510–30; Beck BR, Daly RM, Singh MAF, Taaffe DR. Exercise and Sports Science Australia (ESSA) position statement on exercise prescription for the prevention and management of osteoporosis. *J Sci Med Sport.* 2017;20(5):438–45; Giangregorio LM, McGill S, Wark JD, et al. Too fit to fracture: outcomes of a Delphi consensus process on physical activity and exercise recommendations for adults with osteoporosis with or without vertebral fractures. *Osteoporos Int.* 2015;26(3):891–910.

Arthralgia (Joint Pain)

Hormone-induced arthralgia can be defined as pain and/or stiffness in the joints. It typically occurs within 3 months after the initiation of hormone treatment and peaks at around the 6-month mark. It is bilateral with symmetric pain in the joints, together with early-morning stiffness and sleeping problems (43). To obtain specific information about pain and stiffness of affected joints and the duration of those symptoms throughout the day, the Rheumatoid Arthritis Disease Activity Index may be used (43). On a 4-point scale from "no" to "heavy," patients record for every joint how much pain and stiffness they experience, and on an 8-point scale, patients report the minutes/hours on a day that they experience pain and/or stiffness, ranging from 0 (no) to 7 (all day). A 10-point numerical rating scale is included to assess the level of pain experienced at this very moment and on average in the past week.

Predictors for the development of arthralgia include a BMI of 25 to 30 kg/m^2, taxane-based chemotherapy, Stage III cancer, and a duration of menopause of 5 to 10 years or >10 years (44). The incidence of arthralgias in breast cancer survivors using hormone therapy is between 5% and 50% and is more commonly reported with aromatase inhibitors than with tamoxifen (45). There are very few studies that specifically examine the role of exercise to reduce hormone-induced arthralgia. One RCT reported that a combined aerobic plus supervised resistance training intervention for breast cancer survivors taking an aromatase inhibitor decreased the worst joint pain scores by 1.6 points (29%) at 12 months, as well as significantly decreased pain severity and interference (46). Other forms of exercise shown to be beneficial in training cancer survivors with hormone therapy-induced arthralgia include aquatic exercise, which significantly reduced pain in the neck, hand, shoulder, and leg (47) and Nordic walking (48).

Sexual Dysfunction

Over 50% of female breast, gynecologic, and colorectal cancer survivors report long-term adverse impacts on sexual function after completing treatment (49). There are various direct and indirect factors that may contribute to **sexual dysfunction** in female cancer survivors, such as

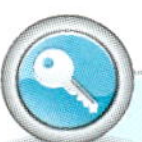

Sexual dysfunction. Difficulty experienced by an individual or partners during any stage of normal sexual activity, including physical pleasure, desire, preference, arousal, or orgasm.

breast/gynecological surgery and possible disfigurement, radiotherapy, hormone treatment, neuropathy, and the presence of a stoma, which can lead to a negative perception of body image and feelings of unattractiveness (50). The prevalence of sexual dysfunction in breast cancer survivors is between 40% and 80%, and it affects the QoL of patients through many years. The main symptoms of sexual dysfunction reported include difficulties in arousal or excitation, decreased sexual desire, insufficient lubrication, and penetration pain (51).

After prostate cancer treatments, such as prostatectomy, radiotherapy, and hormone treatment, many prostate cancer survivors report sexual dysfunction issues, in particular erectile dysfunction and libido loss (34). Questionnaires most commonly used to quantify the effect of exercise on sexual dysfunction in cancer survivors are the FACT-ES (Functional Assessment of Cancer Therapy-Endocrine Symptoms) which is a self-report 18-item questionnaire that accompanies the breast cancer QoL measure FACT-B (35) and FACT-P, which is a self-report 12-item questionnaire (36).

Three studies have examined exercise as a treatment for sexual dysfunction in breast cancer survivors (52). Only the 1-year-long strength training program had a positive effect (53). There are more promising results on the effect of exercise on sexual dysfunction among patients with prostate cancer, who were treated with ADT and radiotherapy (54). A recent review shows that exercise, particularly pelvic floor muscle exercise (PFMEs), resulted in significant positive effects on sexual dysfunction as a primary end point in favor of the intervention prostate cancer group (55).

Urinary Incontinence

Radical prostatectomy is the leading treatment option for men with prostate cancer, and the symptoms of urinary incontinence typically appear immediately post surgery and generally subside within the first few months following surgery. However, in some cases, patients may never regain urinary continence. One strategy to manage urinary incontinence pre- or postprostatectomy is PFME. PFME interventions provided preoperatively and postoperatively have been shown to reduce the duration of urinary incontinence in men with prostate cancer (56, 57). In addition, a meta-analysis of 20 RCTs involving 2,188 men demonstrated that supervised PFME is the most effective method in reducing short-term urinary incontinence (nonsupervised PFME has the same effect as no PFME). To reduce urinary incontinence long term a high volume of PFME needs to be undertaken in the initial 6 months following prostatectomy (58).

Hot Flashes

A **hot flash** has been defined as "a subjective sensation of heat that is associated with objective signs of cutaneous vasodilation and a subsequent drop in core temperature" (59). A recent review of interventions to reduce hot flashes in breast and prostate cancer survivors suggests that exercise does not decrease the frequency of hot flashes (60). However, it is important to be aware of this side effect that may negatively affect a cancer survivor's ability to comfortably exercise (see considerations in Box 12.3).

Box 12.3 Considerations When Working With a Person With Endocrine Treatment Side Effects

- **Resistance exercises:** Include resistance exercises to strengthen bones.
- **Pelvic floor exercises:** Include pelvic floor exercises.
- **Hot flashes:** Be aware that the client may have a hot flash, ensure exercise area is well ventilated, perhaps have a small fan for client, and suggest multiple layers of clothing to add or remove during exercise.
- **Night sweats:** Patient may potentially be suffering from fatigue and poor sleep quality.
- **Risk of low bone density:** Include resistance, weight bearing, and high-impact exercises UNLESS the person has already been informed that their BMD is significantly reduced owing to treatment, in which case, use guidelines for osteoporosis.
- **Rising cholesterol:** Evidence shows that exercise and diet can have impacts on the levels of HDL and LDL.

Cognitive Dysfunction

Reduced **cognitive function** is a commonly reported side effect of cancer and its treatment, including chemotherapy (chemobrain/chemofog) and hormone treatments (61). Cancer survivors can report and manifest this as difficulties with learning, memory, attention, concentration, processing speed, and executive function. Up to 85% of patients receiving cancer treatment have been found

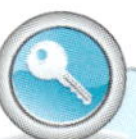

Hot flash. Spontaneous, sudden-onset, sporadic feelings of warmth usually felt on the chest, neck, and face and immediately followed by an outbreak of sweating.

Cognitive function. This is the mental processes involved in the acquisition of knowledge, processing of information, and reasoning examples, such as perception, memory, learning, attention, decision-making, and language abilities.

to report mild-to-severe cognitive complaints, which can last months and even years after treatment completion. Voluntary exercise can improve cognitive function by producing cerebral plasticity. Exercise such as choreographic dancing or learning new technical movements may also increase memory and attention (38). In a study with women with breast cancer who self-reported cognitive dysfunction following chemotherapy treatment they were randomized to either a 24-week aerobic exercise intervention or usual lifestyle control. Compared with the control group, the exercisers took significantly less time to complete a processing speed test (62), and there was a notable pattern of neural activation with the exercise group over 2 regions (the cingulate cortex and superior frontal gyrus), both of which are implicated in conflict monitoring. This suggests that following the exercise intervention, less mental effort was needed to maintain the same level of cognitive task performance, indicating greater cognitive efficiency to compensate for underlying cognitive deficits. A recent systematic review on the effect of exercise on cancer-related cognitive impairment (63) observed a statistically significant benefit on self-reported cognitive function in 12 RCTs. Two trials reported statistically significant effects of aerobic exercise or combined aerobic and resistance exercise on objective neuropsychological tests of cognitive function. Thus, although limited, emerging evidence suggests a possible positive impact of exercise on cancer-related cognitive dysfunction.

Cardiac Issues

Anthracyclines are particularly known to increase the risk of cardiomyopathy with **systolic dysfunction** and heart failure by generation of free radicals, leading to cardiac cell damage. More than 50% of all patients exposed to anthracycline chemotherapy will show some degree of cardiac dysfunction 10 to 20 years after chemotherapy, and 5% will develop overt heart failure with up to 60% mortality (64). The effect of exercise to prevent or ameliorate cardiotoxicity is an emerging field of research. Promising results for a protective effect of exercise in humans for cardiac function include better left ventricular and vascular endothelial function (65). Nagy et al (66) examined the effect of regular exercise in 55 women breast cancer survivors with no cardiovascular risk factors. Five years after anthracycline chemotherapy, symptoms of heart failure were less frequently reported in the active group than in the inactive one (19.45% vs 68.42%). An important cohort of cancer survivors with high risk of cardiovascular issues are survivors of childhood acute lymphoblastic leukemia. Smith et al (67) developed a 12-week home-based combined aerobic and resistance intervention with 5 survivors of childhood cancer (>10 years posttreatment) who had been diagnosed with subclinical anthracycline-induced cardiomyopathy. No adverse events were noted, and the survivors showed improvements in peak maximal oxygen uptake (VO_2 peak) (10.6%) and ejection fraction (12.6%). Oxygen pulse improved, increasing by a mean of 13.6%. Given that anthracyclines elevate the risk of cardiotoxicity and cardiovascular morbidity and mortality among cancer survivors, it is critical to be aware of the cardioprotective benefits of exercise and its ability to reduce anthracycline-induced cardiotoxicities while preserving the maximal heart rate response and the respiratory exchange ratio. See Box 12.4.

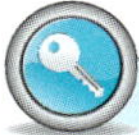

Systolic dysfunction. A defect in the function of cardiac myofibrils resulting in an inability of the left ventricle to eject blood at relatively high pressure into the aorta.

Box 12.4 Considerations When Working With a Person With Mild Cardiomyopathy

CPET may be required to assist in the stratification of patients into low-, moderate-, and high-risk groups on the basis of chemotherapy exposures. ASCO have identified patient subgroups considered at high risk of left ventricular dysfunction or heart failure. Unfortunately, available risk stratification models provide limited information with which to design targeted exercise prescriptions.

Data from Ligibel JA, Bohlke K, May AM, et al. Exercise, diet, and weight management during cancer treatment: ASCO guideline. *J Clin Oncol.* 2022;40(22):2491–507; Scott JM, Nilsen TS, Gupta D, Jones LW. Exercise therapy and cardiovascular toxicity in cancer. *Circulation.* 2018;137(11):1176–91.

DISEASE PREVENTION/ HEALTH PROMOTION

Weight gain can be a common side effect of chemotherapy and antiestrogen therapy for breast cancer or antiandrogen therapy for prostate cancer. When comparing obese versus nonobese a clinically relevant increase has been observed in all-cause and cancer-specific mortality in breast, prostate, and colorectal cancer survivors. Cancer survivors also have an increased risk of developing CVD (such as heart disease, hypertension, cerebrovascular disease, atherosclerosis, and aortic aneurysm), stroke, and diabetes. Shockingly, for cancer survivors (all sites) diagnosed before 55 years old, the risk of cardiovascular mortality is more than 10-fold greater than for the general population (68). To reduce these risks, lifestyle

Box 12.5 American Cancer Society Guideline on Diet and Activity for Cancer Survivors 2022

General recommendations for cancer survivors:

- Nutritional assessment and counseling should begin as soon as possible after diagnosis, with the goal of preventing or resolving nutrient deficiencies, preserving muscle mass, and managing side effects of treatments that may adversely affect nutritional status.
- Physical activity assessment and counseling should begin as soon as possible after diagnosis, with the goal of helping patients prepare for treatments, tolerate and respond to treatments, and manage some cancer-related symptoms and treatment-related side effects.

Recommendations to improve long-term health and increase the likelihood of survival:

- Avoid obesity and maintain and increase muscle mass through diet and physical activity.
- Engage in regular physical activity, with the consideration of type of cancer, patient health, treatment modalities, and symptoms and side effects.
- Follow a healthy eating pattern that meets nutrient needs and is consistent with recommendations to prevent chronic disease.
- Follow the general advice of the American Cancer Society *Guideline for Diet and Physical Activity for Cancer Prevention* to reduce risk of a new cancer.

From American Cancer Society *Guideline on Diet and Activity for Cancer Survivors 2022.*

modifications such as exercise/physical activity, weight loss, and appropriate diet for a healthy lifestyle have been recommended (69).

A recent review (70) shows that diet and exercise interventions for breast cancer survivors result in significant improvements in body weight, waist circumference, hip circumference, BMI, systolic BP, body fat, fat mass, and lean body mass. The ACS has published guidelines for physical activity and nutrition for cancer survivors (Box 12.5) (71). See Box 12.6 for considerations for working with a cancer survivor to reduce weight.

Box 12.6 Considerations When Working With a Person to Reduce Weight

Where survivors may be prone to weight gain and/or obesity be aware of the safety considerations related to exercise, including orthopedic limitations and metabolic/CVD risk. If weight loss is a specific goal for these individuals, it may be prudent for the exercise professional or the cancer survivor to link with a registered dietician.

SUMMARY

During the survivorship phase, many individuals will still be experiencing chronic/late-appearing side effects from the cancer and its treatment. The most prevalent side effects at this stage of the cancer trajectory irrespective of cancer type are fatigue/sleep problems, depression, sarcopenia, and cardiac issues. Prostate and breast cancer survivors also have problems with lymphedema, hormone treatment side effects, and weight gain. There is convincing evidence that exercise interventions can prevent or reduce these treatment issues and improve the QoL of cancer survivors. With significant evidence concerning some cancer-related outcomes, specific guidelines on how to abate or prevent some of the most common chronic side effects experienced by cancer survivors are available. It is important to always consider any specific issues in order to ensure the exercises and the programs are safe, individualized, and effective.

Case Study

Elizabeth is a 46-year-old woman and works as a project manager in a large finance company. Two years ago, she was diagnosed with Stage III invasive ductal breast cancer. She had 6 rounds of neoadjuvant chemotherapy called FEC every 3 weeks. FEC is named after the initials of the drugs used for this treatment "fluorouracil" (also called 5FU), epirubicin, and cyclophosphamide.

Then Elizabeth had a mastectomy and full lymph node clearance, followed by radiotherapy every weekday for 3 weeks. The scar tissue from the surgery and radiotherapy left her with a poor range of movement on her affected arm. Her treatment was completed approximately 1 year ago, and she is currently on 18 cycles of trastuzumab (Herceptin) and hormone treatment (20-mg tamoxifen). Since cancer diagnosis, she has gradually gained 9 kg and now has a BMI of 31 kg/m^2. She has also been found to have high levels of cholesterol and high BP and has been prescribed 10-mg Ramipril. She had a blood clot (located in the shoulder) during chemotherapy owing to a peripherally inserted central catheter (PICC) line insertion, but this was resolved on Apixaban, an anticoagulant twice a day. She is no longer on this medication.

Elizabeth has been complaining about general soreness in her back and headaches and recently had scans and blood tests with no evidence of cancer recurrence. She is really keen to get back to working full time, but is unable to work more than 2 days a week because of fatigue. She enjoys aerobics, yoga, and working with resistance bands and weights (1-16 kg).

Questions

1. List 4 reasons why Elizabeth is at high risk of developing lymphedema.
2. Lymphedema development is of significant concern when working with Elizabeth. List 3 ways that this will be addressed.
3. What 3 indicators are there that Elizabeth is at risk of cardiovascular disease?
4. Elizabeth's main side effect from the cancer treatment that she is really still suffering from low cardiorespiratory fitness, and she does not have the energy for her high-pressure job. Provide her with the evidence-based exercise prescription.
5. What other 3 treatment issues may Elizabeth have that would you consider when prescribing the exercise?

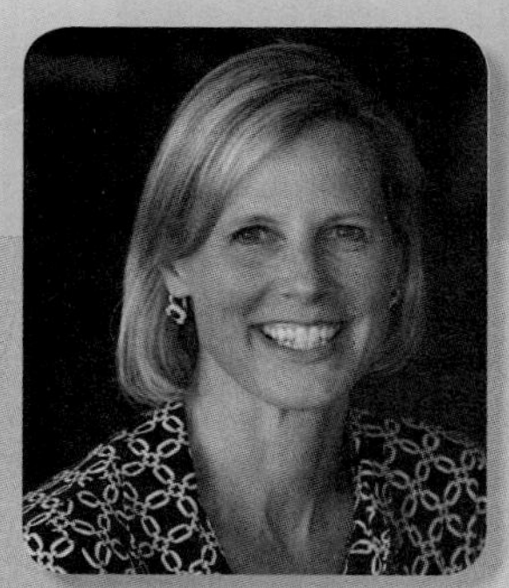

Meet the Expert

FEATURED PROFESSIONAL

Melinda Irwin, PhD, MPH

Associate Dean of Research and Susan Dwight Bliss Professor of Epidemiology
Associate Cancer Center Director, Population Sciences; Co-Leader, Cancer Prevention and Control, Yale Cancer Center; Deputy Director, Yale Center for Clinical Investigation
Yale University
New Haven, CT, USA
Epidemiologist

Q: "Where did you grow up?"

Wellesley, MA.

Q: "Where did you train? What is your training?"

William and Mary (BS: Kinesiology); UNC-Chapel Hill (MS: Exercise Physiology); University of South Carolina (PhD: Exercise Science); University of Washington (MPH: Epidemiology); Fred Hutch Cancer Center (Postdoctoral Fellowship: Cancer Prevention and Control).

Q: "What are you best known for?"

Trials of exercise and weight management on cancer biomarkers in women with breast cancer.

Q: "What are you currently working on?"

Trial of exercise and nutrition on treatment outcomes in women receiving chemotherapy for ovarian cancer.

Q: "Anything else you want to include?"

I am so thankful for my mentors, Drs. Barb Ainsworth and Anne McTiernan, who paved the way for examining physical activity from a public health approach and for cancer prevention.

Favorite Quote:

"Exercise oncology research keeps getting methodologically stronger and more clinically relevant. I am excited for the day when these research findings translate to the incorporation of exercise prescriptions as standard of oncology care."

—*Author*

STUDY QUESTIONS

1. True or False: Low-intensity exercise reduces fatigue.
2. Has anxiety been reported to increase or decrease with time postovarian cancer diagnosis?
3. True or False: Resistance training reduces anxiety.
4. What are the evidence-based exercise guidelines for treating depression?
5. What is sarcopenia?
6. Provide an exercise program that has been shown to reduce or prevent sarcopenia.
7. Which of the following is NOT a side effect of hormone treatment?
   a. Hot flushes
   b. Limited range of movement
   c. Lower bone density
   d. Arthralgia
8. Of the following hormone treatment side effects, for which one there is NO significant evidence of a benefit with exercise?
   a. Arthralgia
   b. Bone density
   c. Hot flashes
   d. Sexual dysfunction
9. What is the exercise prescription to help preserve bone density?
10. Cancer survivors can be at increased risk of cardiovascular disease. List some evidence-based benefits of the cardiovascular system that diet and exercise have been shown to provide for cancer survivors.

REFERENCES

1. Courneya KS, Friedenreich CM. Physical activity and cancer control. *Semin Oncol Nurs.* 2012;23(4):242–52.
2. Ganz PA. Quality of care and cancer survivorship: the challenge of implementing the institute of medicine recommendations. *J Oncol Pract.* 2009;5(3):101–5.
3. Williamson TJ, Stanton AL. Adjustment to life as a cancer survivor. In: Feuerstein M, Nekhlyudov L, editors. *Handbook of Cancer Survivorship.* 2nd ed. New York (NY): Springer; 2018, pp. 29–48.
4. Ueland V, Rortveit K, Dysvik E, Furnes B. Life after cancer treatment: existential experiences of longing. *Int J Qual Stud Health Well-being.* 2020;15(1):1838041.
5. Arndt V, Koch-Gallenkamp L, Jansen L, et al. Quality of life in long-term and very long-term cancer survivors versus population controls in Germany. *Acta Oncol.* 2017;56(2):190–7.
6. Guy GP, Jr., Ekwueme DU, Yabroff KR, et al. Economic burden of cancer survivorship among adults in the United States. *J Clin Oncol.* 2013;31(30):3749–57.
7. Troeschel AN, Leach CR, Shuval K, Stein KD, Patel AV. Physical activity in cancer survivors during "Re-Entry" following cancer treatment. *Prev Chronic Dis.* 2018;15:E65.
8. Campbell KL, Winters-Stone KM, Wiskemann J, et al. Exercise guidelines for cancer survivors: consensus statement from international multidisciplinary roundtable. *Med Sci Sports Exerc.* 2019;51(11):2375–90.
9. Mustian KM, Lin PJ, Loh KP, Kleckner IR. Fatigue. In: Feuerstein M, Nekhlyudov L, editors. *Handbook of Cancer Survivorship.* New York (NY): Springer; 2018, pp. 129–44.
10. Yellen SB, Cella DF, Webster K, Blendowski C, Kaplan E. Measuring fatigue and other anemia-related symptoms with the Functional Assessment of Cancer Therapy (FACT) measurement system. *J Pain Symptom Manage.* 1997;13(2):63–74.
11. Banthia R, Malcarne VL, Roesch SC, et al. Correspondence between daily and weekly fatigue reports in breast cancer survivors. *J Behav Med.* 2006;29(3):269–79.
12. Seyidova-Khoshknabi D, Davis MP, Walsh D. Review article: a systematic review of cancer-related fatigue measurement questionnaires. *Am J Hosp Palliat Care.* 2011;28(2):119–29.
13. Tian L, Lu HJ, Lin L, Hu Y. Effects of aerobic exercise on cancer-related fatigue: a meta-analysis of randomized controlled trials. *Support Care Cancer.* 2016;24(2):969–83.
14. Lin HP, Kuo YH, Tai WY, Liu HE. Exercise effects on fatigue in breast cancer survivors after treatments: a systematic review and meta-analysis. *Int J Nurs Pract.* 2022;28(4):e12989.
15. Fang YY, Hung CT, Chan JC, Huang SM, Lee YH. Meta-analysis: exercise intervention for sleep problems in cancer patients. *Eur J Cancer Care (Engl).* 2019;28(5):e13131.
16. Keogh JWL, MacLeod RD. Body composition, physical fitness, functional performance, quality of life, and fatigue benefits of exercise for prostate cancer patients: a systematic review. *J Pain Symptom Manage.* 2012;43(1):96–110.
17. Niedzwiedz CL, Knifton L, Robb KA, Katikireddi SV, Smith DJ. Depression and anxiety among people living with and beyond cancer: a growing clinical and research priority. *BMC Cancer.* 2019;19(1):943.
18. Watts S, Prescott P, Mason J, McLeod N, Lewith G. Depression and anxiety in ovarian cancer: a systematic review and meta-analysis of prevalence rates. *BMJ Open.* 2015;5(11):e007618.
19. Gotze H, Friedrich M, Taubenheim S, Dietz A, Lordick F, Mehnert A. Depression and anxiety in long-term survivors 5 and 10 years after cancer diagnosis. *Support Care Cancer.* 2020;28(1):211–20.
20. Zigmond AS, Snaith RP. The hospital anxiety and depression scale. *Acta Psychiatr Scand.* 1983;67(6):361–70.
21. DiSipio T, Rye S, Newman B, Hayes S. Incidence of unilateral arm lymphoedema after breast cancer: a systematic review and meta-analysis. *Lancet Oncol.* 2013;14(6):500–15.
22. Gummesson C, Atroshi I, Ekdahl C. The disabilities of the arm, shoulder and hand (DASH) outcome questionnaire: longitudinal construct validity and measuring self-rated health change after surgery. *BMC Musculoskelet Disord.* 2003;4:11–16.
23. Stuiver MM, ten Tusscher MR, Agasi-Idenburg CS, Lucas C, Aaronson NK, Bossuyt PM. Conservative interventions for preventing clinically detectable upper-limb lymphoedema in patients who are at risk of developing lymphoedema after breast cancer therapy. *Cochrane Database Syst Rev.* 2015;2015(2):CD009765.
24. Wanchai A, Armer JM. Effects of weight-lifting or resistance exercise on breast cancer-related lymphedema: a systematic review. *Int J Nurs Sci.* 2019;6(1):92–8.
25. Cao A, Ferrucci LM, Caan BJ, Irwin ML. Effect of exercise on sarcopenia among cancer survivors: a systematic review. *Cancers (Basel).* 2022;14(3):786.

26. Beaudart C, McCloskey E, Bruyere O, et al. Sarcopenia in daily practice: assessment and management. *BMC Geriatr.* 2016;16(1):170.
27. Adams SC, Segal RJ, McKenzie DC, et al. Impact of resistance and aerobic exercise on sarcopenia and dynapenia in breast cancer patients receiving adjuvant chemotherapy: a multicenter randomized controlled trial. *Breast Cancer Res Treat.* 2016;158(3):497–507.
28. Yamamoto K, Nagatsuma Y, Fukuda Y, et al. Effectiveness of a preoperative exercise and nutritional support program for elderly sarcopenic patients with gastric cancer. *Gastric Cancer.* 2017;20(5):913–18.
29. Dawson JK, Dorff TB, Todd Schroeder E, Lane CJ, Gross ME, Dieli-Conwright CM. Impact of resistance training on body composition and metabolic syndrome variables during androgen deprivation therapy for prostate cancer: a pilot randomized controlled trial. *BMC Cancer.* 2018;18(1):368.
30. Peterson MD, Sen A, Gordon PM. Influence of resistance exercise on lean body mass in aging adults: a meta-analysis. *Med Sci Sports Exerc.* 2011;43(2):249–58.
31. Lacroix A, Hortobagyi T, Beurskens R, Granacher U. Effects of supervised vs. unsupervised training programs on balance and muscle strength in older adults: a systematic review and meta-analysis. *Sports Med.* 2017;47(11):2341–61.
32. Cella D, Fallowfield LJ. Recognition and management of treatment-related side effects for breast cancer patients receiving adjuvant endocrine therapy. *Breast Cancer Res Treat.* 2008;107(2):167–80.
33. Murphy CC, Bartholomew LK, Carpentier MY, Bluethmann SM, Vernon SW. Adherence to adjuvant hormonal therapy among breast cancer survivors in clinical practice: a systematic review. *Breast Cancer Res Treat.* 2012;134(2):459–78.
34. Steentjes L, Siesling S, Drummond FJ, van Manen JG, Sharp L, Gavin A. Factors associated with current and severe physical side-effects after prostate cancer treatment: what men report. *Eur J Cancer Care (Engl).* 2018;27(1). doi:10.1111/ecc.12589
35. Fallowfield LJ, Leiatly SK, Howell A, Benson S, Cella D. Assessment of quality of life in women undergoing hormonal therapy for breast cancer: validation of an endocrine symptom subscale for the FACT-B. *Breast Cancer Res Treat.* 1999;55(2):189–99.
36. Esper P, Mo F, Chodak G, Sinner M, Cella D, Pienta K. Measuring quality of life in men with prostate cancer using the Functional Assessment of Cancer Therapy-Prostate instrument. *Adult Urology.* 1997;50(6):920–8.
37. Wallander M, Axelsson KF, Lundh D, Lorentzon M. Patients with prostate cancer and androgen deprivation therapy have increased risk of fractures: a study from the fractures and fall injuries in the elderly cohort (FRAILCO). *Osteoporos Int.* 2019;30(1):115–25.
38. Casla S, Hojman P, Marquez-Rodas I, et al. Running away from side effects: physical exercise as a complementary intervention for breast cancer patients. *Clin Transl Oncol.* 2015;17(3):180–96.
39. Dalla Via J, Daly RM, Fraser SF. The effect of exercise on bone mineral density in adult cancer survivors: a systematic review and meta-analysis. *Osteoporos Int.* 2018;29(2):287–303.
40. Fornusek CP, Kilbreath SL. Exercise for improving bone health in women treated for stages I-III breast cancer: a systematic review and meta-analyses. *J Cancer Surviv.* 2017;11(5):525–41.
41. Shapiro CL, Van Poznak C, Lacchetti C, et al. Management of osteoporosis in survivors of adult cancers with nonmetastatic disease: ASCO clinical practice guideline. *J Clin Oncol.* 2019;37(31):2916–46.
42. Liguori G. *ACSM's® Guidelines for Exercise Testing and Prescription.* 11 ed. Philadelphia (PA): Lippincott Williams & Wilkins; 2020.
43. Boonstra A, van Zadelhoff J, Timmer-Bonte A, Ottevanger PB, Beurskens CH, van Laarhoven HW. Arthralgia during aromatase inhibitor treatment in early breast cancer patients: prevalence, impact, and recognition by healthcare providers. *Cancer Nurs.* 2013;36(1):52–9.
44. Beckwee D, Leysen L, Meuwis K, Adriaenssens N. Prevalence of aromatase inhibitor-induced arthralgia in breast cancer: a systematic review and meta-analysis. *Support Care Cancer.* 2017;25(5):1673–86.
45. Mao JJ, Stricker C, Bruner D, et al. Patterns and risk factors associated with aromatase inhibitor-related arthralgia among breast cancer survivors. *Cancer.* 2009;115(16):3631–9.
46. Irwin ML, Cartmel B, Gross C, et al. Randomized exercise trial of aromatase inhibitor–induced arthralgia in breast cancer survivors. *J Clin Oncol.* 2015;33(10):1104–11.
47. Cantarero-Villanueva I, Fernández-Lao C, Caro-Morán E, et al. Aquatic exercise in a chest-high pool for hormone therapy-induced arthralgia in breast cancer survivors: a pragmatic controlled trial. *Clin Rehabil.* 2013;27(2):123–32.
48. Fields J, Richardson A, Hopkinson J, Fenlon D. Nordic walking as an exercise intervention to reduce pain in women with aromatase inhibitor-associated arthralgia: a feasibility study. *J Pain Symptom Manage.* 2016;52(4):548–59.
49. Smith T, Kingsberg SA, Faubion S. Sexual dysfunction in female cancer survivors: addressing the problems and the remedies. *Maturitas.* 2022;165:52–7.
50. Paterson CL, Lengacher CA, Donovan KA, Kip KE, Tofthagen CS. Body image in younger breast cancer survivors: a systematic review. *Cancer Nurs.* 2016;39(1):E39–58.
51. Taylor S, Harley C, Ziegler L, Brown J, Velikova G. Interventions for sexual problems following treatment for breast cancer: a systematic review. *Breast Cancer Res Treat.* 2011;130(3):711–24.
52. Castelo-Branco C, Anglès S, Cebrecos I, Mension E, Castillo H. Sexual function in breast cancer patients: a review of the literature. *Clin Exp Obstet Gynecol.* 2022;49(6):134.
53. Speck RM, Gross CR, Hormes JM, et al. Changes in the body image and relationship scale following a one-year strength training trial for breast cancer survivors with or at risk for lymphedema. *Breast Cancer Res Treat.* 2010;121(2):421–30.
54. Schumacher O, Galvao DA, Taaffe DR, et al. Effect of exercise adjunct to radiation and androgen deprivation therapy on patient-reported treatment toxicity in men with prostate cancer: a secondary analysis of 2 randomized controlled trials. *Pract Radiat Oncol.* 2021;11(3):215–25.
55. Reimer N, Zopf EM, Böwe R, Baumann FT. Effects of exercise on sexual dysfunction in patients with prostate cancer: a systematic review. *J Sex Med.* 2021;18(11):1899–914.
56. Sayner A, Nahon I. Pelvic floor muscle training in radical prostatectomy and recent understanding of the male continence mechanism: a review. *Semin Oncol Nurs.* 2020;36(4):151050.
57. Chang JI, Lam V, Patel MI. Preoperative pelvic floor muscle exercise and postprostatectomy incontinence: a systematic review and meta-analysis. *Eur Urol.* 2016;69(3):460–7.
58. Baumann FT, Reimer N, Gockeln T, et al. Supervised pelvic floor muscle exercise is more effective than unsupervised pelvic floor muscle exercise at improving urinary incontinence in prostate cancer patients following radical prostatectomy: a systematic review and meta-analysis. *Disabil Rehabil.* 2022;44(19):5374–85.
59. Boekhout AH, Vincent AD, Dalesio OB, et al. Management of hot flashes in patients who have breast cancer with venlafaxine and clonidine: a randomized, double-blind, placebo-controlled trial. *J Clin Oncol.* 2011;29(29):3862–8.
60. Hutton B, Hersi M, Cheng W, et al. Comparing interventions for management of hot flashes in patients with breast and prostate cancer: a systematic review with meta-analyses. *Oncol Nurs Forum.* 2020;47(4):E86–106.
61. Boykoff N, Moieni M, Subramanian SK. Confronting chemobrain: an in-depth look at survivors' reports of impact on work, social networks, and health care response. *J Cancer Surviv.* 2009;3(4):223–32.
62. Campbell KL, Kam JWY, Neil-Sztramko SE, et al. Effect of aerobic exercise on cancer-associated cognitive impairment: a proof-of-concept RCT. *Psychooncology.* 2018;27(1):53–60.
63. Campbell K, Zadravec K, Bland KA, Chesley E, Wolf F, Janelsins MC. The effect of exercise on cancer-related cognitive impairment and applications for physical therapy: systematic review of randomized controlled trials. *Phys Ther.* 2020;100(3):523–42.
64. Okwuosa TM, Anzevino S, Rao R. Cardiovascular disease in cancer survivors. *Postgrad Med J.* 2017;93(1096):82–90.
65. Tranchita E, Murri A, Grazioli E, et al. The beneficial role of physical exercise on anthracyclines induced cardiotoxicity in breast cancer patients. *Cancers (Basel).* 2022;14(9):2288.

66. Nagy AC, GulAcsi BP, CserEp Z, Hangody L, Forster T. Late cardiac effect of anthracycline therapy in physically active breast cancer survivors: a prospective study. *Neoplasma*. 2017;64(1):92–100.
67. Smith WA, Ness KK, Joshi V, Hudson MM, Robison LL, Green DM. Exercise training in childhood cancer survivors with subclinical cardiomyopathy who were treated with anthracyclines. *Pediatr Blood Cancer*. 2014;61(5):942–5. doi:10.1002/pbc.24850
68. Sturgeon KM, Deng L, Bluethmann SM, et al. A population-based study of cardiovascular disease mortality risk in US cancer patients. *Eur Heart J*. 2019;40(48):3889–97.
69. Demark-Wahnefried W, Platz EA, Ligibel JA, et al. The role of obesity in cancer survival and recurrence. *Cancer Epidemiol Biomarkers Prev*. 2012;21(8):1244–59.
70. Wang S, Yang T, Qiang W, Zhao Z, Shen A, Zhang F. Benefits of weight loss programs for breast cancer survivors: a systematic reviews and meta-analysis of randomized controlled trials. *Support Care Cancer*. 2022;30(5):3745–60.
71. Rock CL, Thomson CA, Sullivan KR, et al. American Cancer Society nutrition and physical activity guidelines for cancer. *CA Cancer J Clin*. 2022;72(3):230–62.

CHAPTER

13

Prescribing Exercise for Patients Receiving Ongoing Treatment

OUTLINE

1. Introduction
2. Role of Exercise During Ongoing Treatment
3. Exercise Considerations Based on the Individual
4. Exercise Modifications During Treatment
    a. Cardiotoxicity
    b. Endocrine Changes
    c. Metabolic Changes
    d. Pulmonary Metastasis
    e. Fatigue
    f. Lymphedema
    g. Pain
5. Summary
6. Case Study
7. Meet the Expert
8. Study Questions
9. References

OBJECTIVES

After completing review of this chapter, students will be able to:

1. Know the role of exercise during ongoing cancer treatment.
2. Explain exercise considerations related to comorbid conditions, type, and stage of cancer.
3. Comprehend the basics of exercise modification during cancer treatment.
4. Explain how different treatments and their side effects influence how people actively receiving treatment and exercise.
5. Identify severe side effects of ongoing treatment (eg, cardiotoxicity, lymphedema, pain, and ascites).

INTRODUCTION

The focus in this chapter will be on the person who is receiving ongoing treatment for advanced or metastatic cancer (Box 13.1). The care for such people is inherently more complicated than those who are receiving their initial treatment for cancer. People with metastatic cancer often present with fatigue, weakness, shortness of breath, loss of energy, new onset of lymphedema, and unintentional weight loss. People living with metastatic cancer are receiving ongoing treatment for recurrent cancer. Sites that cancer commonly metastasizes to are the liver, lungs, bones, and brain. For some people, there is hope that the treatment will put their disease in long-lasting remission, but for others the hope is that the treatment will provide long-lasting control of their disease. For the latter patients, cancer is treated like a chronic illness, and treatment will be long-term and ongoing. Exercise is important for all patients with advanced cancer to maintain QoL and independence, but modifications to an exercise program may need to be made during treatment. Side effects and their management can influence if and how a person with advanced cancer can engage in exercise and live their life. Physical activity should be a standard component of every metastatic care plan (1, 2).

ROLE OF EXERCISE DURING ONGOING TREATMENT

Exercise during ongoing treatment, whether treatment is for a locally advanced cancer recurrence or widespread metastatic disease, is feasible and important to improve mood, physical function, CIPN, body weight management, QoL, and reduce fatigue (3-8). When people are faced with recurrence and metastatic disease, their QoL and survival are threatened. Exercise becomes an ally in maintaining mobility and independence.

More research is needed to understand the FITT of exercise that is optimal. A supervised exercise or consultative exercise program that transitions to a home-based exercise program may be ideal given the advantage that it limits the amount of travel and time away from home. Wearable activity monitors, smartphone applications, and online interventions may prove to be optimal means of providing home-based exercise programs, but research will determine which of these methods of exercise delivery are preferred by people living with metastatic disease. Their preference may be driven by resources and access to broadband internet, or by their own historic enjoyment of exercising and sport. Supervised exercise programs are increasingly provided in hospice and supportive care settings.

Box 13.1 Describing the Spread of Cancer

- Locally advanced cancer, widespread recurrence, and metastatic disease are commonly used terms. They refer to any cancer that has spread outside of its original site. Locally advanced means that the cancer has started to spread but has not extended to other organs and can still be curable.
- Widespread cancer is the same as metastatic cancer and means that cancer has spread to distant organs. Some metastatic cancers, such as testicular cancer, are curable.

EXERCISE CONSIDERATIONS BASED ON THE INDIVIDUAL

People living with metastatic cancer who are receiving ongoing treatment to try and achieve control of their disease need to be assessed on an individual basis and regularly, especially if their treatment regimen changes. The 2023 PAR-Q+ (see Figure 9.2) is a validated tool that may be useful to assess comorbidities. Another measure is the American College of Cardiology screening tool, which provides specific guidelines for pre-exercise assessment for patients with cancer (Box 13.2) (9). This box delineates some situations that may necessitate stopping an exercise test and referring the patient back to their physician for follow-up evaluation and care prior to beginning an exercise program. The exercise professional should recognize that these patients already have complex medical disease(s). These patients' disease burdens will cause unique symptoms that necessitate obtaining medical clearance prior to working with them and then adapting a FITT prescription to the individual's situation.

Considerations such as age and previous exercise history are important to know in the general background of people with whom you are working, but these factors become less important when faced with advanced disease. For example, a 40-year-old person with metastatic lung cancer may be debilitated and frail enough to appear far older than their stated age. Therefore, knowing a person's current physical condition and their goals is important, and using a validated tool, such as the PAR-Q+ or the IPAQ, will help to provide initial guidance regarding the physical activity level and beginning an exercise prescription (10, 11). For some people living with metastatic cancer, the goal may be to maintain or improve their fitness. However, there are athletic people with advanced cancer who achieve remarkable athletic feats, for

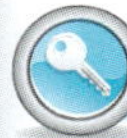

2023 PAR-Q+. A tool to determine comorbidities that a person may have in addition to cancer.
International Physical Activity Questionnaire (IPAQ). A tool to help determine estimates of physical activity.

Box 13.2 Pre-exercise Assessment of Patients With Cancer

Normal Testing

Cardiopulmonary Exercise Testing (CPET):

- Resting blood pressure (BP) ≤160/90 mmHg (If elevated, recheck after 5 minutes. If still elevated, then reschedule CPET after patient is seen by provider to adjust BP medications.)
- Normal BP response to exercise
- No inducible ischemia
- No atrial or ventricular arrhythmias
- Maintain normal O_2 saturations
- No symptoms (Symptoms such as dyspnea, chest pain, dizziness, or other cardiac symptoms during exercise deemed abnormal by supervising physician.)

6-Minute Walk Test:

- Resting BP ≤160/90 mmHg (If elevated, recheck after 5 minutes. If still elevated, then reschedule CPET after the patient is seen by the provider to adjust BP medications.)
- Maintain normal O_2 saturations

Note: In patients with bone metastases, consider whether testing is necessary or not. Tests should avoid the site of the actual bone lesion(s).

No Baseline Symptoms

- Acute nausea during exercise
- Vomiting within 24 hours
- Disorientation
- Blurred vision

Ongoing Cancer Complications

- Acute infection
- Acute metabolic disease (Examples include abnormal thyroid function, uncontrolled diabetes mellitus, and electrolyte abnormalities.)
- New onset lymphedema
- Mental or physical impairment to exercise
- Initial wound healing after surgery
- Bone or brain metastasis (For patients with bone or brain metastases, a plan needs to include a consultation with oncology rehabilitation and, in the case of bone metastasis, a clinically led risk assessment, supported by clinical imaging, to establish a patient-specific safe exercise plan.)

Displays Exercise Knowledge

- Understands how to perform aerobic and resistance exercises
- Demonstrates correct form on equipment
- Understands perceived exertion and heart rate goals; performs exercise accordingly

Data from Ellahham SH. *Exercise Before, During, and After Cancer Therapy.* American College of Cardiology; 2019, December 04. Available from: https://www.acc.org/latest-in-cardiology/articles/2019/12/04/08/22/exercise-before-during-and-after-cancer-therapy; originally from Gilchrist SC, Barac A, Ades PA, et al. Cardio-oncology rehabilitation to manage cardiovascular outcomes in cancer patients and survivors: a scientific statement from the American Heart Association. *Circulation.* 2019;139:e997–1012; and Campbell KL, Cormie P, Weller S, et al. Exercise recommendation for people with bone metastases: expert consensus for health care providers and exercise professionals. *JCO Oncol Pract.* 2022;18(5): e697–709.

example, backpacking, climbing mountains, and completing marathons and triathlons. But for the vast majority, the goal is to maintain function, independence, and the ability to pursue activities they enjoy and to live as fully as possible for as long as possible.

Exercise prescriptions must be designed based on the individual's ability at the time you meet them and on the basis of their goals, including their enjoyment and preferences, to maximize their likely adherence. Then the prescription needs to be shaped around the individuals' treatment schedule, work, family, and their dream (goal), in whatever order that fits, with the realization that cancer treatment, side effects, and disease severity may change over time and sometimes very rapidly. The role of the exercise professional is to be the steady advisor to help each individual reach, and for some, even surpass their goal(s). The exercise professional should know that most people set goals far below what they can achieve because they have no idea of what they are capable of, especially when they have the cloud of cancer hanging over them.

Some people diagnosed with metastatic disease will be treated with aggressive chemotherapy, immunotherapy, BMT, or CAR T-cell therapy, and may possibly get cured. These patients are generally diagnosed with cancers such as Hodgkin's lymphoma, non-Hodgkin's lymphoma, some leukemias, or multiple myeloma. They will be very sick from the treatment but will be given a second chance at life. These people benefit from a structured yet flexible exercise program during treatment and their recovery. Other people—for example, some people living with breast or prostate cancer who have bone metastasis—often live many years with their disease. These individuals have time to enjoy life, travel, pursue their interests, and spend quality time with their families and grandchildren. For these PLWC is an extension of life that requires frequent visits to the cancer center for check-ups, blood draws, infusions, medication monitoring, and sometimes scans. Exercise programs should be designed to work alongside the timing of treatment cycles. Life goes on, albeit with the stress of uncertainty. With good patient-provider communication, treatment schedules can be modified to accommodate lengthy vacations, sporting events, or treks to faraway places.

Exercise is critical in both examples, and the proper, individualized exercise prescription that adapts to variations in how the person feels on a day-to-day basis is important. The science, at this time, does not provide the exact formula for how to prescribe a FITT prescription for people with metastatic disease. However, at this point, it is reasonable to assume that people living with metastatic cancer can be trained to think like athletes and adjust their exercise programs in much the same way. They can learn to use a rating of perceived exertion scale to target the intensity of their workouts and find the right intensity to exert themselves (Figure 13.1). The RPE scale is used to self-score exercise intensity during exercise, not after the exercise bout. After a warm-up, patients should target their exercise in the 5 to 6 RPE (moderate) range, which means that they can talk but they cannot sing. They should be slightly breathless.

Once the patient learns to use the RPE scale, they should be taught to rate their most common side effect and use that to determine how much exercise to do each day. For most patients, this will be fatigue. It is important for the individual to track their level of fatigue and adjust their exercise on the basis of their fatigue. For example, measure fatigue on a scale of 0 to 10, with 1 being "very mild fatigue" and 10 being "extreme/worst possible fatigue" (Figure 13.2).

If fatigue is rated 8 to 10, the person needs to rest, hydrate, and assess why they feel bad. Are they 3 to 5 days past their last treatment? Are they getting sick? Do they have a fever? Are they experiencing undue stress? If their fatigue persists, it is advisable to refer them to talk to their health care provider. If pain is the main limiting factor for exercise, then pain can also be measured daily, and exercise can be adjusted in the same fashion (Figure 13.3). The exercise professional may seek guidance from the patient's oncology team or oncology physical therapist regarding pain, particularly around whether pain is an indictor to stop, or to push through.

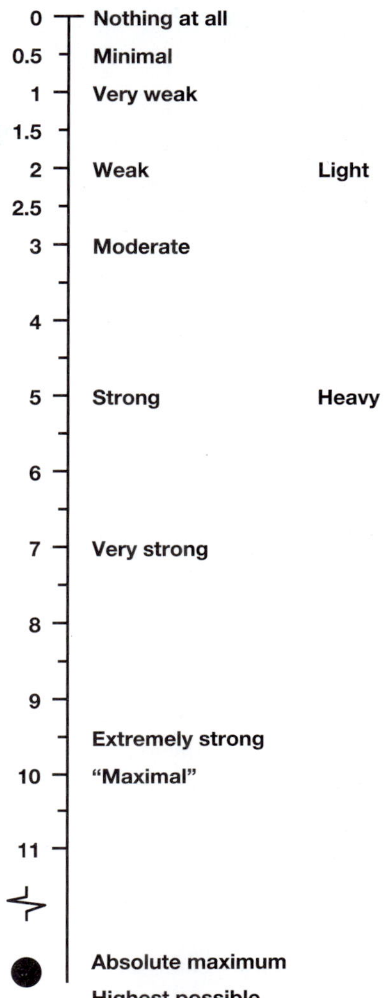

FIGURE 13.1. Rating of perceived exertion scale; Borg CR10 Scale. (Copyright Gunnar Borg, 1982, 2004, 2016. Available from https://borgperception.se/obtain-a-license/.)

As with any exercise program, a warm-up period should be built into exercise, and exercise should be symptom limited. Symptom-limited exercise means that the exercise bout is limited by the individual's symptoms (eg, fatigue, nausea, dizziness and shortness of breath). If the symptom persists, the individual should be told to stop exercising and sit down. If the symptom does not resolve, they should be advised to seek medical advice.

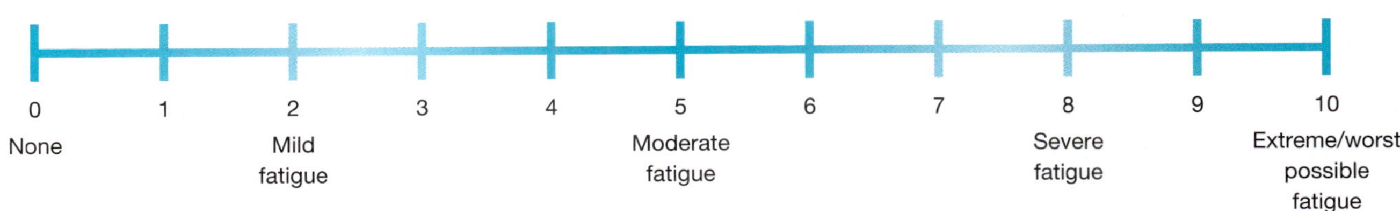

FIGURE 13.2. Fatigue scale from 0 to 10 to adjust exercise.

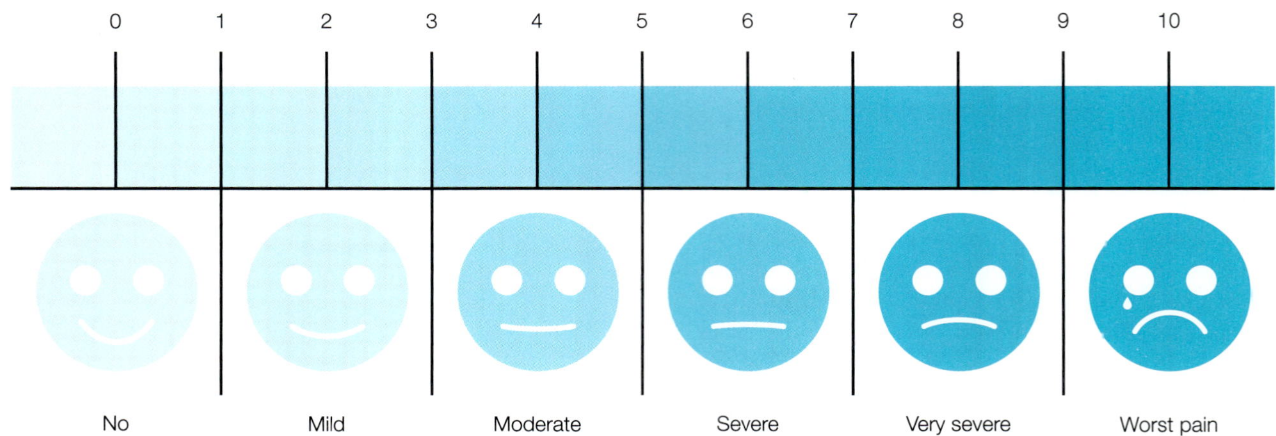

FIGURE 13.3. Pain rating scale to adjust exercise. (From iStock, Stock illustration ID:539684888, upload date: June 16, 2016. EgudinKa.)

EXERCISE MODIFICATIONS DURING TREATMENT

There are many considerations when working with people living with metastatic cancer, and it is critically important to conduct a pre-exercise assessment using the 2020 PAR-Q+ (see Figure 13.1). This assessment is key to safely develop an exercise prescription to help them maintain or improve their strength and fitness without causing complications. Table 13.1 lists the potential impact of different types of cancer treatments which when combined with previous treatments can create more intense (worse) side effects (12). When people receive multiple types of treatments over time, the side effects of treatment can be additive. Many of the exercise-related effects are described in Chapters 4, 5, and 8, but some side effects can cause physiologic effects years after cancer treatments have ended and are discussed here. Side effects that occur long after treatment has ended are called late effects. When a person living with cancer has a recurrence and also has a late effect of cancer, such as cardiotoxicity and CIPN, medical decisions are made regarding the treatment regimens. A treatment will be selected to minimize the cardiac side effects to try to avoid causing life-threatening cardiac problems such as heart failure.

The exercise professional must bear in mind that ongoing treatments cause an accumulation of side effects that can make exercise more of a challenge. As CIPN, because of drugs such as paclitaxel, worsens, it becomes harder to stand, get one's balance and walk, and even painful to push against an exercise band. Hand-foot syndrome (**palmar-plantar erythrodysesthesia**) is a painful, tingling, swelling, redness, blistering of the hands and feet that can make walking and using the hands difficult (Figure 13.4) (13). It can be so severe that it can cause the nails to lift off the nail beds and ulcers to develop on the soles of the feet and palms of the hands. Hand-foot syndrome can be caused by capecitabine, doxorubicin, and other drugs.

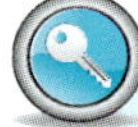

Palmar-plantar erythrodysesthesia. Certain chemotherapy agents can cause painful swelling, tingling, blisters, and peeling of the hands and feet.

Cardiotoxicity

Cardiotoxicity is observed is as many as 28% of people with cancer as a consequence of cancer treatment (14). The cardiotoxic effects include damage to the function of the heart, such as heart failure, heart block, bradycardia, tachycardia, and coronary vasospasm. People with cancer also face an increased risk of CVD that is caused by atherosclerosis, hypertension, and ultimately an increased risk for myocardial infarction. PLWC who have cardiac damage may require a medically supervised exercise oncology program, at least when they begin to exercise. Much like healthy individuals, PLWC benefit from exercise to reduce the risk of CVD. PLWC who are receiving cardiotoxic drugs, such as trastuzumab, are at risk of reduced left ventricular ejection fraction. The oncology team should communicate with the exercise professional if there are significant changes in cardiac function that could affect exercise ability. Left ventricular ejection fraction should be measured every 3 months when a patient is receiving trastuzumab, and the exercise professional can ask a patient when their test is scheduled and follow up with the patient or their oncology team regarding the results.

Endocrine Changes

Endocrine changes can occur owing to any form of cancer treatment (see Table 13.1) and may negatively affect bone health and body composition predisposing the person receiving cancer treatment to gaining weight losing muscle mass and losing bone density. There is also a

Table 13.1 Potential Impact of Cancer Treatments on Exercise Tolerance and Safety

		SURGERY	CHEMOTHERAPY	RADIATION	ANTI-HORMONAL THERAPY (SURGICAL OR PHARMACEUTICAL)	TARGETED THERAPY OR IMMUNOTHERAPY[a]
Cardiovascular changes	Cardiac damage or increased CVD risk		√	√	√	√
Endocrine changes						
	Worsening bone health		√	√	√	
	Changes in body composition (weight gain)		√		√	
	Changes in body composition (weight loss/muscle mass loss)	√	√	√	√	√
Gastrointestinal changes						
	Nausea		√			√
	Diarrhea		√	√		√
	Altered GI function	√	√	√		√
Immune changes	Impaired immune function and/or anemia		√	√	√	√
Metabolic changes						
	Development/worsening of metabolic syndrome		√		√	√
Neurological changes	Peripheral Neuropathy		√			
	Cognitive changes	√ (brain surgery)	√	√	√	
Pulmonary changes	Altered lung function or pneumonitis	√ (lung surgery)	√	√		
Skin changes						
	Redness, irritation			√		
	Rashes			√		√
	Reduced ROM	√ (by healing at surgical site)		√		
Fatigue		√	√	√	√	√
Lymphedema[b]		√		√		
Pain	General	√	√	√	√	√
	Myalgia/arthralgia		√		√	√

CVD, cardiovascular disease; GI, gastrointestinal; ROM, range of motion.
[a]Depends on type or target of agent.
[b]Can occur in any type of cancer when and where lymph nodes are surgically resected and/or radiation over lymph nodes.
Adapted from Campbell KL, Winters-Stone KM, Wiskemann J, et al. Exercise guidelines for cancer survivors: consensus statement from international multidisciplinary roundtable. *Med Sci Sports Exerc.* 2019;51(11):2375–90.

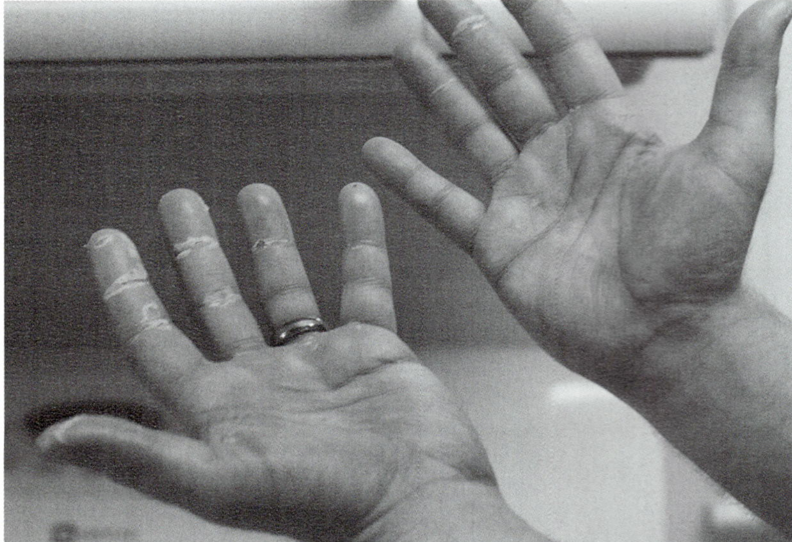
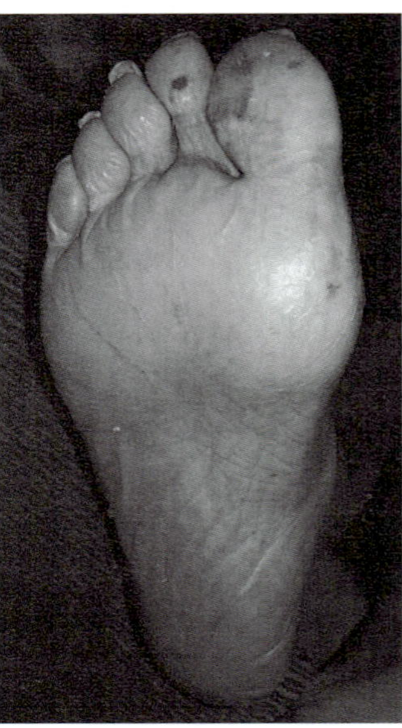

FIGURE 13.4. Hand-foot syndrome (erythrodysesthesia). (From Wehler TC, Cao Y, Galle PR, Theobald M, Moehler M, Schimanski CC. Combination therapies with oxaliplatin and oral capecitabine or intravenous 5-FU show similar toxicity profiles in gastrointestinal carcinoma patients if hand-food syndrome prophylaxis is performed continuously. *Oncol Lett.* 2012;3(6):1191–4.)

risk of endocrine damage from immunotherapy, which in mild cases can cause thyroid impairment leading to hypothyroidism, which requires the need for thyroid hormone replacement. In severe cases, the endocrine damage from immunotherapy can cause hypophysitis, which is an inflammation of the pituitary gland that can be life-threatening. Immunotherapy with immune checkpoint inhibitors (monoclonal antibodies) is used to treat solid tumors and hematologic malignances (15). Exercise will be difficult for patients who have imbalances in thyroid or pituitary function because of the profound fatigue that frequently accompanies these diseases.

Bones are a common site of metastasis. Exercise is recommended for people living with metastatic cancer. It is safe, reduces fatigue, and improves QoL and physical function (3, 16-21). The exercise recommendations for people with bone metastasis include:

- performing a clinical risk assessment of skeletal complications (eg, CT or MRI);
- consulting with a medical professional is strongly encouraged before the exercise professional provides structured exercise for a person with bone metastasis to obtain key medical information and develop bidirectional communication;
- physical therapists and exercise physiologists are best suited for working with people with bone metastasis;
- professional judgment should determine if baseline and follow-up exercise testing is necessary; and
- exercise testing should follow the International Exercise Guidelines for Cancer Survivors (1).

Metabolic Changes

Metabolic changes include **cachexia** (weakness, muscle wasting, and weight loss owing to cancer). Cachexia is defined as a weight loss of greater than 5% of body weight. Cancer cachexia is an imbalance of metabolic regulation and reduced food intake. Cachexia is highly prevalent and affects as many as 40% of patients with breast cancer, sarcoma, leukemia, and Hodgkin's lymphoma; 61% of patients with colon, lung, prostate, and non-Hodgkin's lymphoma; and 87% of patients with pancreatic and gastric cancer. It is a sign of poor prognosis and accounts for 30% of cancer-related deaths (22). There is no medical treatment for cachexia. Exercise counteracts some of the muscle wasting and helps to maintain strength, functional ability, and balance, and reduce fatigue (23, 24).

Another change that can occur is **ascites** that is a collection of fluid in the abdomen. It is caused either by cancer that spreads to the (A) peritoneum (the lining of the organs), which leaks fluid into the abdominal cavity and is called malignant ascites or (B) liver metastasis, which blocks the lymph channel or produces extra fluid and forces fluid to leak into the abdomen. Ascites makes the abdomen swell, and patients complain of tightness, feeling nauseated, and

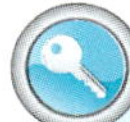

Cachexia. Muscle wasting and weight loss of at least 5% of initial body weight.

Ascites. Fluid that collects in the abdomen that contains cancer cells.

shortness of breath. The procedure to reduce the fluid volume uses a needle and syringe called paracentesis. The fluid is checked for cancer cells to determine if the ascites is related to metastasis or liver damage or another cause. Exercise has no beneficial effects on ascites, and when a patient has ascites, they will not want to exercise.

Pulmonary Metastasis

Pulmonary metastasis an occur with any cancer and can lead to shortness of breath and fluid in the lung. Similar to ascites, **pleural effusions** can be drained, and the fluid is sent to pathology to be reviewed for cancer, infection, or another cause of the fluid buildup. As discussed in Chapter 4, patients can have lung damage from surgery, radiation, or chemotherapy, but the changes seen in the metastatic setting are different and more severe and often necessitate changes to the exercise program when they occur. Patients with lung metastasis need to be reevaluated and their condition discussed with the oncology team so that a safe and effective exercise prescription can be adapted to the individual. Breathing exercises or pulmonary rehabilitation is important not only for improving breathing capacity and QoL but also for functional ability and muscular strength (25-27).

Fatigue

Fatigue is almost universal among people living with metastatic cancer. It is caused by their disease, the treatment, and the numerous side effects and symptoms they experience and struggle to manage. As shown previously, exercise reduces fatigue and is undoubtedly the most important intervention for fatigue management throughout the cancer trajectory. Resistance training specifically has been shown to increase functional capacity and to decrease fatigue in people with metastatic cancer (28).

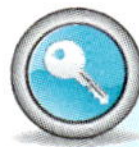

Pleural effusion. A collection of fluid in the lung(s) that when look at in a pathology lab contains cancer cells.

Lymphedema

Lymphedema may be a presenting sign of recurrent disease if a lymph node is compressing lymphatic flow. In women with breast cancer, lymphedema may present on the affected or unaffected side, if the cancer has spread or metastasized to involve a lymph node. In an individual with Hodgkin's lymphoma, for example, who initially presented with disease in the chest and now has lymphedema in a lower leg, it could recur in a pelvic lymph node. New onset lymphedema is concerning and should be a red flag that would prompt the exercise professional to advise the person living with cancer to seek follow-up care with their oncology team. Supervised resistance training, including the use of weights, has been shown conclusively to be both safe and advantageous for women at risk of breast cancer-related lymphedema (29).

Pain

Pain from metastasis can occur because of surgery, chemotherapy, radiation therapy, and other forms of treatment. It is also common that pain is associated with the tumor. The tumor may exert pressure on organs or nerves and cause pain that radiates along the path of the nerve. The pattern of pain may be unrelenting or shooting depending on how the area is affected.

Chemotherapy-induced neuropathy is another type of nerve pain that can become severe and completely debilitating with ongoing treatment. The pain can interfere with activities of daily living to the point that ambulation, dressing, picking up a pen, and even using a cell phone are impossible. Other sources of pain include skin changes, such as hand-foot syndrome, which can interfere with ambulation and daily activities. Some treatments can cause severe mouth and throat pain. Pain can limit QoL and certainly one's ambition to exercise, even when exercise is the key to maintaining independence and mobility. As an exercise professional, it is critical to encourage people living with metastatic cancer to manage their treatment side effects early before they get out of control so that they can optimize the benefits of an exercise program.

SUMMARY

People living with metastatic cancer and receiving ongoing treatment can safely exercise. Exercise is beneficial for them both physically and emotionally. There are specific considerations the exercise professional should take into account when developing an individualized exercise program for a person living with metastatic cancer, and a collaborative relationship with the treating oncology team is important. As an exercise professional, it is critical to encourage people living with metastatic cancer to manage treatment side effects early before they get out of control, in order to optimize the benefits of an exercise program.

Case Study

George is a 69-year-old gentleman with Stage IV pancreatic cancer. He had a complex abdominal surgery called a Whipple procedure and is now cleared by his oncology team to begin an exercise program. He is on several oral chemotherapy drugs, one of which is making his hands very sore and red. His abdomen is distended, and he is experiencing dyspnea (shortness of breath). George was a marathon runner until age 45, and since then he has not done much. He denies smoking, drug use, and drinks socially 1 to 2 times a week. He is a retired accountant and loves to count. He said that he would count his laps in the pool, around a track, repetitions with his weights. George is eager to resume exercise to get his strength back, but he is exhausted and has a lot of pain.

Questions

1. Why is George's abdomen distended?
2. True or false. George should not exercise because of his sore hands.
3. Why does George have dyspnea?

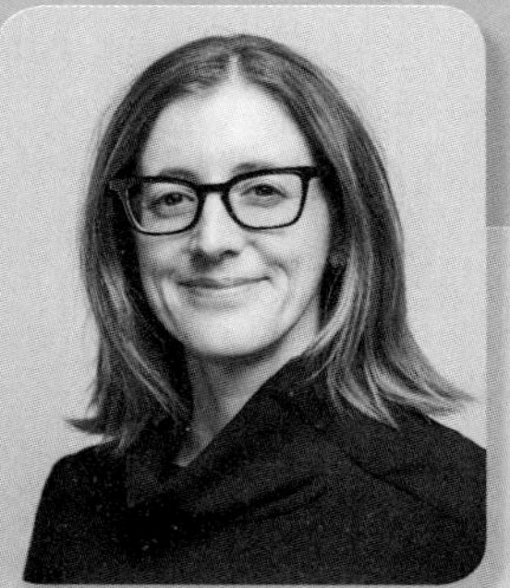

Meet the Expert

FEATURED PROFESSIONAL

Kristin Campbell, BSc PT, PhD

Professor, Department of Physical Therapy
Faculty of Medicine
University of British Columbia
Vancouver, British Columbia, Canada
Rehabilitation Researcher

Q: "Where did you grow up?"

Kingston, Ontario, Canada.

Q: "Where did you train? What is your training?"

I got my physical therapy degree from Queen's University in Canada, and after working as a physical therapist, I returned to graduate school. I got a PhD in Exercise Physiology from the University of Alberta and did a Postdoctoral Fellowship in Public Health at the Fred Hutchinson Cancer Research Centre.

Q: "What are you best known for?"

I think I am best known for the studies focusing on how to use exercise training principles to inform the design and reporting of exercise prescription in exercise oncology research and for co-leading the 2019 "Exercise Guidelines for Cancer Survivors: Consensus Statement from International Multidisciplinary Roundtable," which provided more insights into the dose of exercise needed to help with managing common symptoms and side effects of cancer and cancer treatments.

Q: "What are you currently working on?"

I am currently working on how to increase the reach of exercise programming for people with cancer, such as virtual supervised exercise programs, and continuing to test how different doses and types of exercise can improve common symptoms and side effects of cancer and cancer treatments, including the ability to receive the planned cancer treatment.

Q: "Anything else you want to include?"

Though understanding the potential of exercise after a cancer diagnosis to decrease the risk of cancer coming back is important, until we have better data on this, it is important to highlight that moving more and sitting less benefits nearly everyone in terms of improving overall health and well-being.

Favorite Quote:

"If exercise was a pill, doctors would prescribe it for every patient with cancer."
—*Anonymous*

STUDY QUESTIONS

1. What is Stage IV pancreatic cancer?
2. True or false. Pancreatic cancer is a risk factor for ascites?
3. How will the exercise for George's hands and feet be adapted?
4. How should George be advised to measure the intensity of his exercise?
5. How should George be advised to measure the intensity of his pain?
6. If George's pain increases (worsens), from whom would the health care professional seek guidance?
7. Why would George have pain?
8. Why would George have dyspnea?
9. What is the difference between locally advanced cancer, widespread recurrence, and metastatic disease?

REFERENCES

1. Campbell KL, Cormie P, Weller S, et al. Exercise recommendation for people with bone metastases: expert consensus for health care providers and exercise professionals. *JCO Oncol Pract*. 2022;18(5):e697–e709.
2. Wilk M, Kepski J, Kepska J, Casselli S, Szmit S. Exercise interventions in metastatic cancer disease: a literature review and a brief discussion on current and future perspectives. *BMJ Support Palliat Care*. 2020;10(4):404–10.
3. Dittus KL, Gramling RE, Ades PA. Exercise interventions for individuals with advanced cancer: a systematic review. *Prev Med*. 2017;104:124–32.
4. Do J, Cho Y, Jeon J. Effects of a 4-week multimodal rehabilitation program on quality of life, cardiopulmonary function, and fatigue in breast cancer patients. *J Breast Cancer*. 2015;18(1):87–96.
5. Gagnon B, Murphy J, Eades M, et al. A prospective evaluation of an interdisciplinary nutrition-rehabilitation program for patients with advanced cancer. *Curr Oncol*. 2013;20(6):310–18.
6. Peddle-McIntyre CJ, Singh F, Thomas R, Newton RU, Galvão DA, Cavalheri V. Exercise training for advanced lung cancer. *Cochrane Database Syst Rev*. 2019;2(2):CD012685.
7. Wu C, Zheng Y, Duan Y, et al. Nonpharmacological interventions for cancer-related fatigue: a systematic review and Bayesian network meta-analysis. *Worldviews Evid Based Nurs*. 2019;16(2):102–10.
8. Zimmer P, Trebing S, Timmers-Trebing U, et al. Eight-week, multimodal exercise counteracts a progress of chemotherapy-induced peripheral neuropathy and improves balance and strength in metastasized colorectal cancer patients: a randomized controlled trial. *Support Care Cancer*. 2018;26(2):615–24.
9. Ellahham SH. *Exercise Before, During, and After Cancer Therapy*. [Internet]. American College of Cardiology; 2019, December 04. Available from https://www.acc.org/latest-in-cardiology/articles/2019/12/04/08/22/exercise-before-during-and-after-cancer-therapy
10. Lee PH, Macfarlane DJ, Lam T, et al. Validity of the international physical activity questionnaire short form (IPAQ-SF): a systematic review. *Int J Behav Nutr Phys Act*. 2011;8:115. doi:10.1186/1479-5868-8-115
11. PAR-Q+ Collaboration. *The Physical Activity Readiness Questionnaire for Everyone: The International Standard for Pre-Participation Screening*. [Internet]. November 2023. Available from http://eparmedx.com/
12. Campbell KL, Winters-Stone KM, Wiskemann J, et al. Exercise guidelines for cancer survivors: consensus statement from international multidisciplinary roundtable. *Med Sci Sports Exerc*. 2019;51(11):2375–90.
13. Wehler TC, Cao Y, Galle PR, Theobald M, Moehler M, Schimanski CC. Combination therapies with oxaliplatin and oral capecitabine or intravenous 5-FU show similar toxicity profiles in gastrointestinal carcinoma patients if hand-food syndrome prophylaxis is performed continuously. *Oncol Lett*. 2012;3(6):1191–4.
14. Mouhayar E, Salahudeen A. Hypertension in cancer patients. *Tex Heart Inst J*. 2011;38(3):263–5.
15. Prete A, Salvatori R. Hypophysitis. In: Feingold K, Anawalt B, Boyce A, editors. *Endotext* [Internet]. South Dartmouth (MA): MDText.com, Inc; 2000.
16. Albrecht TA, Taylor AG. Physical activity in patients with advanced-stage cancer: a systematic review of the literature. *Clin J Oncol Nurs*. 2012;16(3):293–300.
17. Beaton R, Pagdin-Friesen W, Robertson C, Vigar C, Watson H, Harris SR. Effects of exercise intervention on persons with metastatic cancer: a systematic review. *Physiother Can*. 2009;61(3):141–53.
18. Chen YJ, Li XX, Ma HK, et al. Exercise training for improving patient-reported outcomes in patients with advanced-stage cancer: a systematic review and meta-analysis. *J Pain Symptom Manage*. 2020;59(3):734–49 e10.
19. Heywood R, McCarthy AL, Skinner TL. Safety and feasibility of exercise interventions in patients with advanced cancer: a systematic review. *Support Care Cancer*. 2017;25(10):3031–50.
20. Heywood R, McCarthy AL, Skinner TL. Efficacy of exercise interventions in patients with advanced cancer: a systematic review. *Arch Phys Med Rehabil*. 2018;99(12):2595–620.
21. Nadler MB, Desnoyers A, Langelier DM, Amir E. The effect of exercise on quality of life, fatigue, physical function, and safety in advanced solid tumor cancers: a meta-analysis of randomized control trials. *J Pain Symptom Manage*. 2019;58(5):899–908 e7.
22. Lim S, Brown JL, Washington TA, Greene NP. Development and progression of cancer cachexia: perspectives from bench to bedside. *Sports Med Health Sci*. 2020;2(4):177–85. doi:10.1016/j.smhs.2020.10.003
23. Arends J, Bachmann P, Baracos V, et al. ESPEN guidelines on nutrition in cancer patients. *Clin Nutr*. 2017;36(1):11–48.
24. Fearon K, Arends J, Baracos V. Understanding the mechanisms and treatment options in cancer cachexia. *Nat Rev Clin Oncol*. 2013;10(2):90–9.
25. Liu W, Pan YL, Gao CX, Shang Z, Ning LJ, Liu X. Breathing exercises improve post-operative pulmonary function and quality of life in patients with lung cancer: a meta-analysis. *Exp Ther Med*. 2013;5(4):1194–200.
26. Michaels C. The importance of exercise in lung cancer treatment. *Transl Lung Cancer Res*. 2016;5(3):235–8.
27. Rivas-Perez H, Nana-Sinkam P. Integrating pulmonary rehabilitation into the multidisciplinary management of lung cancer: a review. *Respir Med*. 2015;109(4):437–42.
28. Support MC. *Physical Activity for People with Metastatic Bone Disease 2020*. [Internet]. November 30, 2020. Available from https://www.macmillan.org.uk/healthcare-professionals/news-and-resources/guides/physical-activity-for-people-with-metastatic-bone-disease
29. Schmitz KH, Ahmed RL, Troxel AB, et al. Weight lifting for women at risk for breast cancer-related lymphedema: a randomized trial. *JAMA*. 2010;304(24):2699–705.

CHAPTER

14

Prescribing Exercise at End of Life

OUTLINE

1. Introduction
2. Palliative Care and Hospice Care
3. The Role of the Exercise Professional
4. Goals of Physical Activity and Exercise
5. Exercise Considerations Based on the Individual
6. Exercise Modifications
7. Summary
8. Case Study
9. Meet the Expert
10. Study Questions
11. References

OBJECTIVES

After completing review of this chapter, students will be able to:

1. Distinguish between palliative care and hospice care.
2. Understand the role of exercise at the end of life.
3. Explain exercise considerations related to mobility.
4. Comprehend the basics of exercise modification during cancer treatment.

INTRODUCTION

We now turn to a person who is receiving palliative or hospice care at the end of life. Both palliative and hospice care focus on achieving the best QoL and enabling one to live well for as long as possible with cancer. Palliative care may begin earlier in a patient's treatment, whereas hospice begins no sooner than 6 months before the expected end of life. Exercise plays an important role in helping a person to remain as functionally able and independent (able to dress themselves and ambulate) for as long as possible. The exercise approach will need to be individualized to each person as their condition changes and certainly as they transition through hospice and the final days and hours at the end of life. Because patients on palliative care may be anywhere along the cancer trajectory, this chapter will provide an in-depth discussion of palliative care and focus on people who are within the last 6 months of life or on hospice.

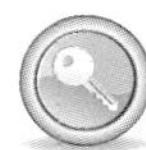

Palliative care. Symptom management provided by a specialized team of experts who focus on providing the optimal QoL for a person during and after cancer treatment.

Hospice. Comfort care provided in what is expected to be the last 6 months of a person's life.

PALLIATIVE CARE AND HOSPICE CARE

Palliative the end of life. However, there is a trend to implement palliative care earlier in the disease trajectory when patients could benefit from palliative interventions to improve their QoL. The International Association of Hospice and Palliative Care suggests that palliative care provided concurrently with other medical treatments throughout the course of illness can positively impact the course of disease (1). Box 14.1 provides the global consensus-based definition of palliative care and essential steps that should be taken to ensure that palliative care becomes integrated into the care of the person living with and beyond cancer so that all people have access to it (2).

The focus of hospice is care at the end of life. Like palliative care, the intent here is to provide the best QoL possible, but it is focused on the final 6 months of life. There is neither an intent to prolong life with treatment nor an intent to hasten death. Care is focused on helping people live life as fully

Box 14.1 Definition of Palliative Care

Palliative care is the active holistic care of individuals across all ages with serious health-related suffering[a] because of severe illness[b] and especially of those near the end of life. It aims to improve the QoL of patients, their families, and their caregivers.

Palliative Care

- Includes, prevention, early identification, comprehensive assessment, and management of physical issues, such as pain and other distressing symptoms, psychological distress, spiritual distress, and social needs. Whenever possible, these interventions must be evidence based.
- Provides support to help patients live as fully as possible until death by facilitating effective communication, helping them and their families determine goals of care.
- Is applicable throughout the course of an illness, according to the patient's needs.
- Is provided in conjunction with disease-modifying therapies whenever needed.
- May positively influence the course of illness.
- Intends neither to hasten nor postpone death, affirms life, and recognizes dying as a natural process.
- Provides support to the family and the caregivers during the patient's illness and in their own bereavement.
- Is delivered recognizing and respecting the cultural values and beliefs of the patient and the family.
- Is applicable throughout all health care settings (place of residence and institutions) and in all levels (primary to tertiary).
- Can be provided by professionals with basic palliative care training.
- Requires specialist palliative care with a multiprofessional team for referral of complex cases.

[a]Suffering is health related when it is associated with illness or injury of any kind. Health-related suffering is serious when it cannot be relieved without professional intervention and when it compromises physical, social, spiritual, and/or emotional functioning. Available from http://pallipedia.org/serious-health-related-suffering-shs/.

[b]Severe illness is any acute or chronic illness and/or health condition that carries a high risk of mortality, negatively impacts QoL and daily function, and/or is burdensome in symptoms, treatments, or caregiver stress. Available from https://pallipedia.org/severe-illness/.

From IAHPC. *Global Consensus Based Palliative Care Definition.* Houston (TX): The International Association for Hospice and Palliative Care; 2018. Available from https://hospicecare.com/what-we-do/projects/consensus-based-definition-of-palliative-care/definition/.

and comfortably as possible. Support is also provided for the patient's loved ones, which may include their immediate family and friends. Not all people in the last 6 months of life are on hospice. Many continue to take treatment in the hope of extending their life. These people are often interested in ways to improve their functional ability and independence.

THE ROLE OF THE EXERCISE PROFESSIONAL

The role of the exercise professional can vary greatly when working with people at the end of life depending on their degree of illness, debilitation, and interest in maintaining function. There are people at the end of life who persist in maintaining their independence and remaining as fully functional as possible. These individuals benefit from physical activity and exercise that is focused on improving one's ability to perform activities of daily living (eg, dressing, bathing, eating, ambulating, and cooking). Other people may be bedridden and on hospice and may face a protracted death with a desire to be able to sit up on their own, hold a pencil, or maintain their strength to stand. During this stage of the cancer trajectory, strong partnerships between the exercise professional and the outpatient rehabilitation team, palliative and hospice care, and other care providers are essential. Exercise professionals have an important role in the care of PLWC at the end of life, but that care must be in close coordination with the individual's medical professionals who are providing and leading that care, especially as the medical acuity of the individual becomes more complex (3). Although an exercise professional may work in this area, their scope of practice may be limited and will be dictated by the policies and procedures of their institution. As the person becomes severely compromised and enters the final days of life, maintaining physical function is no longer a goal, and the role of the exercise professional ends.

GOALS OF PHYSICAL ACTIVITY AND EXERCISE

Hospice generally begins when a person is expected to have fewer than 6 months to live. Not all PLWC will be on hospice, but many find the added benefits are helpful not only for themselves but also for their family members. The last 6 months can be a dynamic and fragile time when a person's health can rapidly deteriorate and then suddenly rebound for a period of weeks to months to once again take an unexpected and precipitous turn for the worse. PLWC at the end of life have different physical activity and exercise goals than people who are newly diagnosed with cancer or receiving ongoing treatment. Most often the primary goal of exercise at the end of life is to maintain physical function, independence, and QoL (Box 14.2). PLWC at the end of life may still be receiving some treatments to slow their disease progression or palliate (control) progressive effects of their disease (eg, pain or nausea), but they are not receiving treatment for a cure. Even when people at the end of life are physically getting worse, specific exercises can enable them to be actively involved in their own health and well-being in a positive way. Clinical experience demonstrates that exercise gives people a sense of control, an opportunity to socially interact with others, and a sense of achievement and purpose. People at the end of life report that exercise gives them greater confidence, self-esteem, and their life back (4).

Box 14.2 Examples of Functional Goals at the End of Life

- Open a jar
- Dress oneself
- Feed oneself
- Shower and toilet independently
- Stand from a chair unaided
- Play with grandchildren
- Take a walk
- Climb stairs
- Cook a meal
- Socialize with friends
- Attend an event
- Shop
- Carry groceries

Exercise is safe and feasible for people with cancer at the end of life and improves mood, fatigue, physical function, CIPN, body weight management, and QoL (5-12). Many of these people may have received several different types of cancer treatment, and they may be physically limited by severe side effects from cancer treatments, such as profound fatigue and pain, severe physical debilitation and functional decline, cachexia and muscle weakness, and CIPN and impaired balance. Nonetheless, they may benefit from exercise, and physical function may actually increase while disease progresses (Box 14.3). While the FITT of an exercise prescription may not be appropriate, some people may like general guidance on how to adjust their daily activity according to their individual, daily overall ratings of fatigue or pain (see Chapter 13). It is not uncommon that the activity or exercise plan will be reduced to accommodate fatigue or pain. People who are truly at the last days of life will not be able to follow an activity or exercise program, but those who are seeking to maintain their functional ability and independence can see steady progress. It must be recognized that there will be day-to-day variability in exercise

Box 14.3 Experiences of Exercise Within Hospice Care

Quantitative studies use objective outcome measures, that is, instruments that can determine progress and change with established reliability and validity. Qualitative studies interview people, either individually or in groups, about their experiences and use written transcripts of the discussions to distill out the major themes and concepts to describe an individual or groups' understanding of their reality.

This qualitative study asked patients with advanced cancer in hospice about their experience with exercise. The data were collected through a series of interviews. The researchers wanted to know what exercise meant to PLWC at the end of life and how exercise affected their lives. Nine people living with advanced cancer participated in the study.

Setting: Marie Curie Hospice Day Therapy Unit in Hampstead, London. The exercise program was tailored to each individual's goals, ability, and relevant contraindications. Sessions varied in length from 10 minutes to 1.5 hours with the majority of participants attending 1 or 2 days per week and exercising at home. There was no limit on the amount of home exercise. Once participants were confident in the supervised exercises, they could progress to exercising at a gym closer to their home.

Sampling: Fliers were placed in the gym to recruit participants. Informed consent was obtained prior to study participation.

Interviews: One-to-one interviews were conducted for data collection at the Day Therapy Unit in a quiet, comfortable room without interruption.

Interviews: The interviewer was trained in qualitative data collection and followed a semi-structured interview format to understand that patient's experience and perceptions. The first research question used was: "Can you explain to me whether participating in the gym sessions here has, in any way, affected your quality of life?" From this question, the interviewer would ask follow-up questions to further explore the physical, emotional, and social impacts of exercise.

Data analysis: Data were transcribed verbatim, and the transcripts were read multiple times to determine major themes, themes, and subthemes that emerged that were common to all participants.

Results: Ten patients consented to interviews, but 1 died before the interview. Results of 9 interviews are reported on participants who ranged in age from 55 to 82 years old. All had cancer. Three had attended the gym less than 10 times, 3 had attend 11 to 20 times, 2 more than 20 times, and 1 over 100 times.

Findings: Three major themes emerged, and each was further divided into themes and subthemes that are described in Table 14.1.

Data from Turner K, Tookman A, Bristowe K, Maddocks M. "I am actually doing something to keep well. That feels really good": experiences of exercise within hospice care. *Prog Palliat Care.* 2016;24(4):204–12. doi:10.1080/09699260.2015.1123441.

tolerance, given changes in symptoms. Any planned activity or exercise needs to be responsive to these changes and at times may be aborted in favor of rest or stretching. Extreme care should be taken to avoid making the person feel worse (eg, causing profound fatigue or pain), given that the overarching purpose of activity and exercise at the end of life is to promote a person's ability to engage in as full a life as possible. From the qualitative study described in Box 14.3, each of 3 major themes was further divided into themes and subthemes shown in Table 14.1.

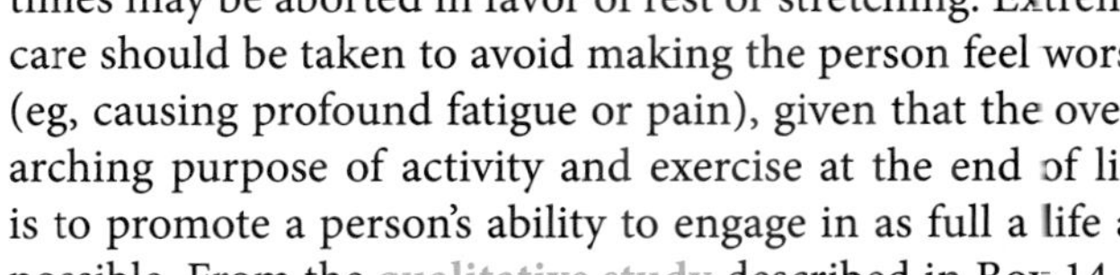

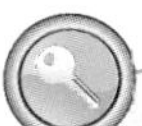

Qualitative study. Studies that collect nonnumerical data through talking with study participants and focusing on their words meanings and experiences. Researchers then take the data and categorize them into major themes, or ideas, and subthemes.

Quantitative study. Uses measures that can be counted, measured, and reported in the numerical form.

EXERCISE CONSIDERATIONS BASED ON THE INDIVIDUAL

PLWC at the end of life need to be assessed frequently, especially as their condition changes. For safety reasons, medical clearance to exercise is necessary. Exercise testing should be minimal and must not be exhaustive. The 3 best ways to assess changes in the person at the end of life are a combination of interviews, questionnaires, and short functional assessment tests. An interview should be focused on how they are feeling, what their current level of activity is, and if they have changes in their fatigue or pain or new symptoms that may interfere with their ability to perform certain planned exercises or functional activities. If the individual has given permission, the exercise professional should speak with the patient's health care team, as a regularly scheduled

Table 14.1 Themes That Emerged From Qualitative Interviews Regarding Patients' Experience of Exercise Within Hospice Care

MAJOR THEMES	THEMES	SUBTHEMES
Consequences of attending	Physical consequences	Strength and fitness Movement and function Physical cost of not attending
	Psychological impact	Positive emotional effects Positive outlook on self and life Sense of achievement
Impact of others	Influence of other patients	Encouragement/camaraderie Comparison with others Social aspect Loss
	Professional involvement	Support Expectations
Sense of meaning	Attitude towards exercise in the gym	Importance Toil
	Active in own well-being	Positive involvement in own health Reclaiming control Importance of choice
	Facing the future	Prolonging independence Confidence and hope Declining despite exercise Not giving up

From Turner K, Tookman A, Bristowe K, Maddocks M. "I am actually doing something to keep well. That feels really good": experiences of exercise within hospice care. *Prog Palliat Care.* 2016;24(4):204–12. doi:10.1080/09699260.2015.1123441.

update from the team will provide firsthand knowledge of changes in the patient's status. In previous chapters, we recommend using the 2023 PAR-Q+ to determine initial activity-level guidance; however, most PLWC at the end of life will be taking multiple medications and have comorbid medical conditions that will necessitate medical clearance prior to exercise. Therefore, we recommend the Paffenbarger Physical Activity Questionnaire (PPAQ) (Figure 14.1). The PPAQ measures physical activity in leisure time among adults (13). Questions are related to the duration and intensity of activity and if the respondent thinks that their level of activity is sufficient for health. Question 8 has demonstrated predictive validity compared with fitness measures in the healthy population (14, 15). A screening tool may provide specific guidelines if pre-exercise assessment is performed (Box 14.4). Regular assessment of fatigue and pain at each session may be the best guide for the individual at the end of life. The following section provides greater detail about modifying exercise based on the fatigue and pain levels. See Table 13.1 that delineates some situations that may necessitate stopping an exercise test and referring the patient back to their hospice or medical team for follow-up evaluation and care prior to continuing to exercise.

It is critical that the exercise professional must recognize that individuals at the end of life do not focus on pushing themselves too intensely. The idea is that a little exercise is good and QoL is best. For this reason, the 6-minute walk may not be appropriate, and shorter functional assessment tests—such as the Timed Up and Go test, the sit-to-stand test, or the Short Physical Performance Battery—may be more easily performed and less physically taxing. Given that these people are approaching the end of their life and they have asked to engage in exercise, a solid knowledge of how to develop a FITT prescription and adapt it to the individual's

Paffenbarger Physical Activity Questionnaire

1 How many city blocks or their equivalent do you normally walk each day? _____ blocks/day

Let (12 blocks = 1 mile)

2. What is your usual pace of walking? (Please check one.)

a. ___ Casual or strolling (less than 2 mph)   b. ___ Average or normal (2-3 mph)

c. ___ Fairly brisk (3-4 mph)   d. ___ Brisk or striding (4 mph or faster)

3. How many flights or stairs do you climb up each day? ___ flights/day (Let 1 flight = 10 steps)

4. List any sports or recreation you have actively participated in during the past year.

Please remember seasonal sports or events.

Sport, Recreation, or Other Physical Activity	Number of Times/Year	Average Time/Episode		Years Participation
		Hours	Minutes	
a.				
b.				
c.				
d.				
e.				
f.				

5. Which of these statements best expresses your view? (Please check one.)
   a. ___ I take enough exercise to keep healthy. b. ___ I ought to take more exercise. c. ___ Don't know.
6. At least once a week, do you engage in regular activity akin to brisk walking, jogging, bicycling, swimming, etc. long enough to work up a sweat, get your heart thumping, or get out of breath?
   ___ No Why not? ___________ ___ Yes How many times per week? ___ Activity: ______________
7. When you are exercising in your usual fashion, how would you rate your level of exertion (degree of effort)? (Please circle one number.)

0	0.5	1	2	3	4	5	6	7	8	9	10
Normal	Very very weak (just noticeable)	Very weak	Weak	Moderate	Somewhat strong	Strong (heavy)		Very strong		Very very strong (almost maximal)	Maximal

FIGURE 14.1. Paffenbarger Physical Activity Questionnaire. (Reproduced with permission from Lippincott Williams & Wilkins/Wolters Kluwer Health from Paffenbarger RS Jr, Blair SN, Lee IM, Hyde RT. Measurement of physical activity to assess health effects in free-living populations. *Med Sci Sports Exerc.* 1993;25(1):60–70.) (*Continued*)

8. On a usual weekday and a weekend day, how much time do you spend on the following activities?
   Total for each day should add to 24 hours.

	Usual Weekday Hours/Day	Usual Weekend Day Hours/Day
a. Vigorous activity (digging in the garden, strenuous sports, jogging, aerobic dancing, sustained swimming, brisk walking, heavy carpentry, bicycling on hills, etc)		
b. Moderate activity (housework, light sports, regular walking, golf, yard work, lawn mowing, painting, repairing, light carpentry, ballroom dancing, bicycling on level ground, etc)		
c. Light activity (office work, driving car, strolling, personal care, standing with little motion, etc)		
d. Sitting activity (eating, reading, desk work, watching TV, listening to radio, etc)		
e. Sleeping or reclining		

FIGURE 14.1. *(Continued)*

Box 14.4 Brief Pre-exercise Assessment of People Living With Cancer at End-of-Life Cancer Who Are Able to Undergo Testing

Brief Testing at End of Life

Timed Up and Go, sit-to-stand assuming the following:

- Resting BP ≤160/90 mmHg (If elevated, recheck after 5 minutes. If still elevated, then reschedule after patient is seen by the provider to adjust BP medications.)
- Normal blood pressure response to exercise
- No exercise induces ischemia
- No atrial or ventricular arrhythmias
- Maintain normal O_2 saturations
- No symptoms such as dyspnea, chest pain, dizziness, or other cardiac symptoms during exercise deemed abnormal by supervising physician.
- No blurred vision

Modify Activity/Exercise Related to End-of-Life Issues and Consult With Medical Team

- Acute infection
- Acute metabolic disease(s), for example, thyroid abnormalities, uncontrolled diabetes mellitus, and electrolyte abnormalities.
- Moderate-to-severe side effects, for example, fatigue, pain, dyspnea, and lymphedema.
- Depression, anxiety, nausea, chemotherapy-induced peripheral neuropathy, edema, cough, and confusion.
- Other comorbid conditions, for example, hypertension, heart disease, and chronic obstructive pulmonary disease.
- New onset lymphedema

Activity/Exercise Knowledge (Person at End of Life or Caregiver[s])

- Understands the purpose of physical activity and exercise
- Demonstrates the correct form
- Understands the use of rating fatigue and pain and how to modify exercise accordingly

Data from Gilchrist SC, Barac A, Ades PA, et al. Cardio-oncology rehabilitation to manage cardiovascular outcomes in cancer patients and survivors: a scientific statement from the American Heart Association. *Circulation*. 2019;139:e997–e1012.

situation as their disease progresses is critically important. A FITT prescription will not focus on building strength and endurance but on giving an individual a guide of activities to improve their daily function and independence and the direction to adapt their activity to their levels of fatigue and pain. The activity or exercise plan may be developed by physical therapists or other rehabilitation professionals, and the exercise professional's role may be to oversee the exercises and make sure that they are performed correctly at an appropriate intensity (easy) and to assist the individual if needed. The exercise professional needs to have a clear understanding of the person's disease burden and the unique symptoms that necessitate modifying the exercise prescription to optimize the outcomes for the person. This will require working in close collaboration with the rehabilitation, hospice, and medical team. When the individual reaches the last few days of life and becomes bedridden and too ill to have functional ability as a concern or when the person says that they no longer want to pursue functional ability as a goal, then the exercise routine is retired.

While knowing the background of a person is critical to making a personal connection, the initial physical assessment is made when you see the person, watch them move, and conduct some basic assessment tests (eg, 6MWT, sit-to-stand, and single-leg balance test).

Exercise prescriptions for people at the end of life are complex and must be designed based on the individual's physical condition that may change rapidly. Meeting the ACSM® exercise guidelines is *not* the goal of the exercise prescription. Rather, the prescription should be conservative so that there is a balance between expending energy in exercise and being able to accomplish the person's goals. Avoiding adverse events, worsening symptoms, and injury is paramount.

EXERCISE MODIFICATIONS

Reductions in physical function and increased symptom burden are common at the end of life and have a negative impact on QoL, especially as the person becomes more debilitated and dependent on caregivers. Exercise modifications need to account for progressive changes that may occur as the patient's disease progresses and physical state deteriorates. Modifying exercise based on the levels of fatigue and pain on a 1 to 10 scale (see Figures 13.2 and 13.3) is clinically relevant, easy to do, and the amount of change in fatigue and pain (see Table 13.1) is a safe way to adapt to the exercise prescription. A 1-point change in fatigue on a 10-point scale is a clinically important difference (Box 14.1). This means that fatigue is causing significant changes to an individual's QoL (15, 16). A change of 2 points on a 10-point pain scale represents a **clinically important difference** in pain (15, 16).

If an individual rates her fatigue 9 to 10, then the person needs to rest, hydrate, and assess why she feels so fatigued. Is the pain uncontrolled? Is she on new pain medications? Does she have a fever? If her fatigue persists at this level, then the hospice or medical team should be alerted. Pain ratings above 5 should trigger the exercise professional to notify the hospice team of the individual's uncontrolled pain.

Other complications associated with metastatic cancer that impede function include severe dyspnea, and CIPN and associated problems with ambulation, balance, or problems holding things with their hands. Progressive brain metastasis may cause significant problems with balance and even impaired memory and cognition. When memory and cognition become impaired, exercise may need to be closely supervised to avoid accidental injury. Cancer cachexia is a wasting syndrome that includes loss of muscle and fat that leads to profound weakness and fatigue and may require changes in an exercise program to accommodate the rapid declines in strength that may also affect balance and pose a safety hazard (17). Cachexia causes a loss of appetite that can also lead to poor hydration. When a person becomes dehydrated, she is more likely to feel weak, unstable, dizzy, or even have cardiac arrythmias because of the electrolyte imbalances. Clearly, end of life is a complex time of rapid change in physiologic and physical function that necessitates astute exercise modifications be made on short notice as a patient's condition can change quickly even when they have been stable for an extended time. Reviewing the exercise modifications presented in Chapters 13 and 15 will help to prepare the reader for working with people at the end of life.

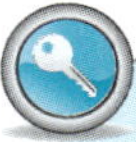

Clinically important difference. The smallest amount of change that is clinically meaningful to a patient.

SUMMARY

People with end-stage cancer can engage in physical activity and exercise and derive both physical and psychological benefits. Exercise at end of life provides people with the opportunity to maintain a degree of independence for as long as possible and may improve some symptoms such as fatigue, weakness, or shortness of breath. The goal is to develop an optimal and safe exercise program to maintain functional ability and independence as long as possible to help the individual meet their goals, not to achieve the ACSM® exercise goals for cancer survivors. The role of the exercise professional is limited in this setting and necessitates working collaboratively with the palliative, hospice, or medical care team.

Case Study

Ellie is a 46-year-old woman with Stage IV breast cancer. She has been receiving palliative care but has transitioned to hospice. Ellie has metastasis to the lungs, bones (femur and ribs bilaterally [both sides]), and brain. She had radiation to palliate (ease) the pain from the bone metastasis in her left femur and ribs. Cranial radiation ended 2 months ago, and she is on low-dose dexamethasone (a steroid) to control the ongoing brain edema (swelling). This has led to muscle weakness, wasting, poor balance, and a loss of functional ability. The lung metastasis causes dyspnea (shortness of breath). Ellie is hopeful that exercise can help her to improve her ambulation and balance, and alleviate some of her dyspnea.

Questions

1. Ellie's goal is to improve ambulation. How will her baseline physiologic assessment be made?
2. True or false. Brain metastasis can cause poor balance.
3. True or false. Modify exercise based on fatigue levels.
4. Circle the correct answer: Brain metastasis and steroids can cause changes in body composition that:
   a. Increases body fat, decreases muscle mass, and causes loss of balance
   b. Decreases body fat and muscle mass and causes loss of balance
   c. There are no body composition changes, but there is loss of balance

Meet the Expert

FEATURED PROFESSIONAL

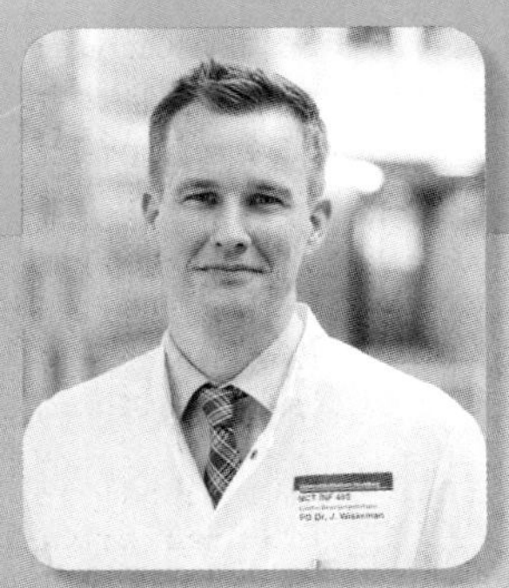

Joachim Wiskemann, PhD, FACSM

Working Group Exercise Oncology
Division of Medical Oncology
National Center for Tumor Diseases Heidelberg
Heidelberg, Germany

Q: "Where did you grow up?"

In a small German village with just 300 habitants in the green and rural heart in the middle of Germany. Meaning, in an extremely physical activity-friendly and supporting environment (eg, playing football on the Framer's meadow beyond our house, climbing large trees in the garden, and endless mountain bike tours through the woods).

Q: "Where did you train? What is your training?"

I was trained as an exercise physiologist in the field of preventive, clinical, and rehabilitative care at Ruprecht Karls University Heidelberg with a special additional education in sports psychology.

Q: "What are you best known for?"

In Germany, I guess for the network OnkoAktiv that is a quality-assured network of cancer centers building up local exercise facility networks of physiotherapist, rehabilitations centers, fitness centers, and sport clubs to deliver exercise oncology care to cancer patients close to their homes. Internationally, I guess for my work in the field of allogeneic stem cell transplantation and for my work with heavily treated or severely ill cancer patients.

Q: "What are you currently working on?"

Political perspective: I am currently leading and coordinating the first clinical guideline for exercise care in cancer patients in Germany, which is the first guideline on the same level and with the same methodological standard like all cancer-specific guidelines in Germany. Implementation perspective: Developing and evaluating an embedded multidisciplinary exercise oncology pathway for cancer centers in three different regions (56 clinical partners included) in Germany. Interventions perspective: Investigations on responders' and nonresponders' patterns in exercise oncology interventions.

Q: "Anything else you want to include?"

I am so grateful for the support of my wife Lea and my four kids Vincent, Johann, Phileas, and Joditha. They provide me with every freedom for this time-consuming job and energize me when we are together.

Favorite Quote:

"Walk the dog every day, even if you don't have a dog."
—*My mentor*

STUDY QUESTIONS

1. What is the difference between palliative and hospice care?
2. What concerns would there be regarding exercise with bone metastasis, and what modifications would be made?
3. Can dyspnea be alleviated with exercise?
4. How will the exercise be adapted for the individual's balance, muscle weakness, and shortness of breath?
5. True or false. Exercise should be done to exhaustion.
6. True or false. Exercise testing should always be done with hospice patients.
7. True or false. Meeting the ACSM® exercise guidelines is the goal of the hospice exercise prescription.

REFERENCES

1. Radbruch L, De Lima L, Knaul F, et al. Redefining palliative care: a new consensus-based definition. *J Pain Symptom Manage.* 2020;60(4): 754–64. doi:10.1016/j.jpainsymman.2020.04.027
2. International Association for Hospice & Palliative Care. *Global Consensus Based Palliative Care Definition.* [Internet]. Houston (TX): The International Association for Hospice and Palliative Care; 2018. Available from https://hospicecare.com/what-we-do/projects/consensus-based-definition-of-palliative-care/definition/
3. Alfano CM, Cheville AL, Mustian K. Developing high-quality cancer rehabilitation programs: a timely need. *Am Soc Clin Oncol Educ Book.* 2016;35:241–9. doi:10.14694/EDBK_156164
4. Turner K, Tookman A, Bristowe K, Maddocks M. "I am actually doing something to keep well. That feels really good": experiences of exercise within hospice care. *Prog Palliat Care.* 2016;24(4):204–12. doi:10.1080/09699260.2015.1123441
5. Dittus KL, Gramling RE, Ades PA. Exercise interventions for individuals with advanced cancer: a systematic review. *Prev Med.* 2017;104: 124–32. doi:10.1016/j.ypmed.2017.07.015
6. McGrillen K, McCorry NK. A physical exercise programme for palliative care patients in a clinical setting: observations and preliminary findings. *Prog Palliat Care.* 2014;22(6):352–7. doi:10.1179/1743291X14Y.0000000091
7. Peddle-McIntyre CJ, Singh F, Thomas R, Newton RU, Galvão DA, Cavalheri V. Exercise training for advanced lung cancer. *Cochrane Database Syst Rev.* 2019;2(2):CD012685. doi:10.1002/14651858.CD012685.pub2
8. Wu C, Zheng Y, Duan Y, et al. Nonpharmacological interventions for cancer-related fatigue: a systematic review and Bayesian network meta-Analysis. *Worldviews Evid Based Nurs.* 2019;16(2):102–10. doi:10.1111/wvn.12352
9. Do J, Cho Y, Jeon J. Effects of a 4-week multimodal rehabilitation program on quality of life, cardiopulmonary function, and fatigue in breast cancer patients. *J Breast Cancer.* 2015;18(1):87–96. doi:10.4048/jbc.2015.18.1.87
10. Zimmer P, Trebing S, Timmers-Trebing U, et al. Eight-week, multimodal exercise counteracts a progress of chemotherapy-induced peripheral neuropathy and improves balance and strength in metastasized colorectal cancer patients: a randomized controlled trial. *Support Care Cancer.* 2018;26(2):615–24. doi:10.1007/s00520-017-3875-5
11. Gagnon B, Murphy J, Eades M, et al. A prospective evaluation of an interdisciplinary nutrition-rehabilitation program for patients with advanced cancer. *Curr Oncol.* 2013;20(6):310–18. doi:10.3747/co.20.1612
12. Salakari MR, Surakka T, Nurminen R, Pylkkänen L. Effects of rehabilitation among patients with advances cancer: a systematic review. *Acta Oncol.* 2015;54(5):618–28. doi:10.3109/0284186x.2014.996661
13. Paffenbarger RS Jr, Blair SN, Lee IM, Hyde RT. Measurement of physical activity to assess health effects in free-living populations. *Med Sci Sports Exerc.* 1993;25(1):60–70.
14. Simpson K, Parker B, Capizzi J, et al. Validity and reliability of Question 8 of the Paffenbarger physical activity questionnaire among healthy adults. *Human Kinetics J.* 2013;12(1):116–23. doi:10.1123/jpah.2013-0013
15. Farrar JT, Young JP Jr, LaMoreaux L, Werth JL, Poole MR. Clinical importance of changes in chronic pain intensity measured on an 11-point numerical pain rating scale. *Pain.* 2001;94(2):149–58. doi:10.1016/S0304-3959(01)00349-9
16. Schwartz AL, Meek PM, Nail LM, et al. Measurement of fatigue: determining minimally important clinical differences. *J Clin Epidemiol.* 2002;55(3):239–44.
17. Roeland EJ, Bohlke K, Baracos VE, Bruerra E, del Fabbro E, Dixon S. Management of cancer cachexia: ASCO guideline. *J Clin Oncol.* 2020;38(21):2438–53.

SECTION 4

Behavioral and Logistical Considerations

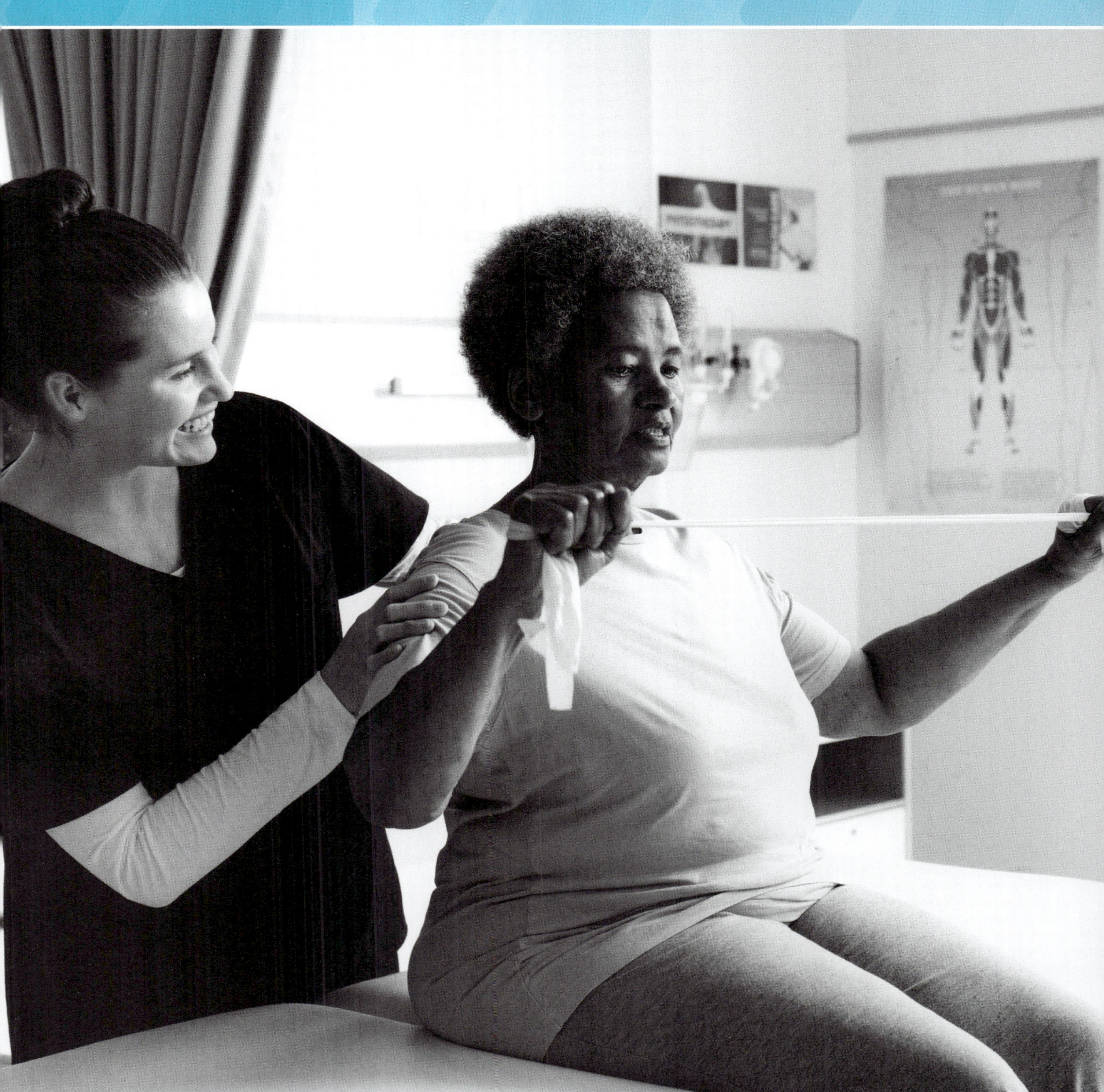

CHAPTER

15

Behavioral Considerations When Working With People Diagnosed With Cancer

OUTLINE

1. Introduction
2. Behavior Change Theories
   a. The Transtheoretical Model
   b. Self-Determination Theory
   c. Theory of Planned Behavior
   d. Affective-Reflective Theory
   e. Health Belief Model
   f. Social Cognitive Theory
   g. Socioecological Model
   h. Behavior Change Techniques
3. Perceived Benefits and Barriers to Exercise With Cancer Survivors
   a. Perceived Benefits of Exercise
   b. Commonly Reported Perceived Barriers to Exercise
   c. Cancer Treatment-Related Barriers
   d. Other Reported Physiological and Psychosocial Barriers to Behavior Change
4. Strategies for Increasing Cancer Survivors' Physical Activity Levels
   a. Self-Efficacy
   b. Self-Monitoring
   c. Goal Setting
   d. Reinforcement/Rewards
   e. Social Support
   f. Motivational Interview Techniques
5. Physical Activity Preferences by Cancer Survivors
   a. Type of Exercise
   b. Where to Exercise
   c. Provision of Advice
   d. When to Start an Exercise Program
   e. With Whom to Exercise
6. Summary
7. Case Study
8. Meet the Expert
9. Study Questions
10. References

OBJECTIVES

After completing review of this chapter, students will be able to:

1. Comprehend the theories and behavior-change techniques used to guide behavior change in cancer survivors.
2. Analyze perceived barriers and facilitators to being active with cancer survivors at different stages of treatment and different types of cancer.
3. Identify the roles that self-efficacy, self-monitoring, goal setting, and social support have in changing behavior in cancer survivors.
4. Understand cancer survivors' preferences on when, how, and with whom they like to exercise.

INTRODUCTION

Despite the convincing evidence on the many benefits of being active after a cancer diagnosis, as described in Chapters 10 to 14 studies, different countries show that only a low percentage of cancer survivors stay active at the levels recommended to gain these health benefits. In the US, it is estimated that <10% of cancer patients will be active during treatment (1) and <20% to 30% after treatment (2). In Japan, less than half of gynecological cancer survivors engage in any physical activities in their leisure time (3). Even in countries such as Denmark, where exercise-based rehabilitation is an integral part of cancer care, uptake of programs is less than the estimated number needing rehabilitation. Regarding underserved populations' access to cancer rehabilitation services, inequality for ethnic minority patients was observed in 41 Danish (46%). A total of 25 municipalities (28%) perceived younger patients with cancer to be less likely to participate than older adult patients with cancer, and 8 municipalities (9%) observed lower referral rates for male patients with cancer than female patients with cancer (4). This chapter will describe the theories and behavior-change techniques that have been used to promote behavior change and maintenance in cancer survivors, the observed challenges and barriers that need to be considered when working with this clinical population, and some validated techniques that can be used to help promote physical activity adoption and maintenance.

A cancer diagnosis can be a teachable moment (5) when cancer patients may be more receptive to advice and assistance to changing some of their negative lifestyle behaviors. The spontaneity and unpredictability of teachable moments, however, highlight the need for prepared unique support and resources to effectively exploit this moment. If this is not readily available, then the teachable moment may not lead to a successful behavior change outcome (6).

BEHAVIOR CHANGE THEORIES

Lifestyle interventions have been shown to be more effective when they are based on a theoretical model; therefore, different theory-based approaches are used to increase the levels of physical activity undertaken in exercise interventions with cancer survivors (Box 15.1).

Box 15.1 The Most Common Theoretical Approaches Used in Exercise Oncology Studies

The following are the most common theoretical approaches used in exercise oncology studies:

- Transtheoretical Model (TTM)
- Self-Determination Theory (SDT)
- Affective-Reflective Theory (ART)
- Theory of Planned Behavior (TPB)
- Health Belief Model (HBM)
- Social Cognitive Theory (SCT)
- Socioecological Model (SEM)

The Transtheoretical Model

The transtheoretical model (TTM) (7) is one of the most predominant approaches to promote exercise behavior (Figure 15.1). It theorizes that individuals are at different stages of readiness to make a behavior change, which may require different strategies to help them progress through the 5 stages of change (Box 15.2).

In this behavior-change theory, there are 10 processes of change that describe the various strategies used by individuals in attempting to change their behavior (each process of change is seen in each stage of change), a decisional balance component that looks at weighing the pros and cons of changing the exercise behavior, and a **self-efficacy** component. It is theorized that self-efficacy is lowest in the earliest stages of change and highest in the later stages.

A large number of studies in exercise oncology have successfully used TTM alone or in conjunction with other theories to guide physical activity behavior (8).

Self-Determination Theory

The self-determination theory (SDT) (9) focuses on an individual's motivational determinants. This theory assumes that individuals have 3 primary psychosocial needs they wish to satisfy: **autonomy**, **competency** (or mastery), and the ability to experience meaningful social interactions with others (or **relatedness**). The SDT proposes that motivation exists on a continuum from amotivation, extrinsic motivation, and intrinsic motivation sources. The use of extrinsic motivation sources to engage in exercise, e.g., to feel more attractive to others, out of a sense of duty, to get rewards, or out of fear of punishment if they do not exercise, does not promote exercise adherence over time. Individuals using intrinsic motivation sources have the highest level of self-determination and

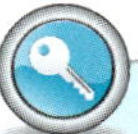

Self-efficacy. A person's belief in their capacity to execute behaviors necessary to produce specific performance attainments.

Autonomy. Being free and independent to live one's life according to reasons and motives that are taken as one's own.

Competency. The experience of mastery and being effective in one's activity.

Relatedness. To the need to feel connected and a sense of belongingness with others.

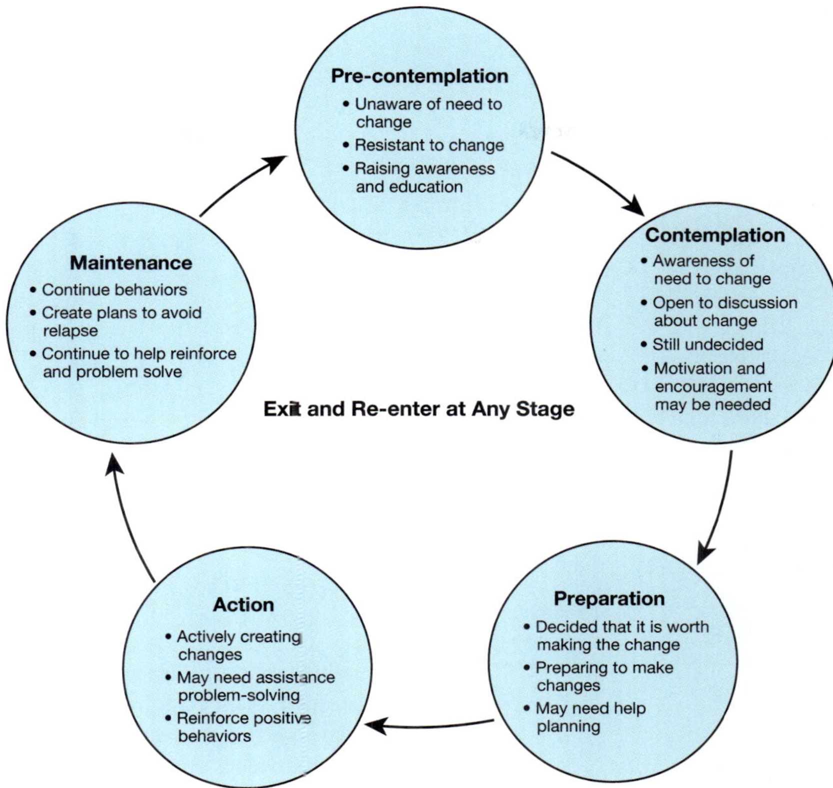

FIGURE 15.1. Transtheoretical model: stages of behavior change.

Box 15.2 Example Strategies to Facilitate Stage Transitions

Precontemplation → Contemplation

- Provide information about the benefits of regular physical activity.
- Discuss how some of the barriers they perceive may be misconceived, such as "It can be done in shorter and accumulated bouts if they don't have the time."
- Have them visualize what they would feel like if they were physically active with an emphasis on short-term, easily achievable benefits of activity, such as sleeping better, reducing stress, and having more energy.
- Explore how their inactivity impacts individuals other than themselves, such as their spouse and children.

Contemplation → Preparation

- Explore potential solutions to their physical activity barriers.
- Assess the level of self-efficacy and begin techniques to build efficacy.
- Emphasize the importance of even small steps in progressing toward being regularly active.
- Encourage viewing oneself as a healthy, physically active individual.

Preparation → Action

- Help develop an appropriate plan of activity to meet their physical activity goals and use a goal-setting worksheet or contract to make it a formal commitment.
- Use reinforcement to reward steps toward being active.
- Teach self-monitoring techniques such as tracking time and distance.
- Continue the discussion of how to overcome any obstacles they feel are in their way of being active.
- Encourage them to help create an environment that helps remind them to be active.
- Encourage ways to substitute sedentary behavior with activity.

Action → Maintenance

- Provide positive and contingent feedback on goal progress.
- Explore different types of activities they can do to avoid burnout.
- Encourage them to work with and even help others become more active.
- Discuss relapse prevention strategies.
- Discuss potential rewards that can be used to maintain motivation.

From American College of Sports Medicine®. *ACSM's® Guidelines for Exercise Testing and Prescription.* 11th ed. Indianapolis (IN): American College of Sports Medicine®; 2021, Box 12.2.

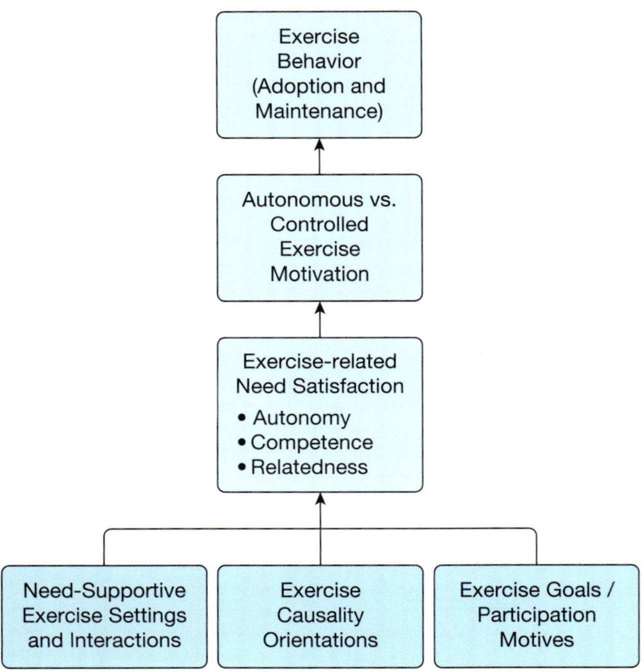

FIGURE 15.2. Self-determination theory.

engage in exercise simply for the satisfaction or pleasure that it brings. The SDT suggests that using rewards may have limited long-term effectiveness because they promote extrinsic motivation sources that are not sustainable and that exercise interventions should be designed to enhance autonomy by promoting choice and incorporating simple, easy exercises to enhance feelings of competence and enjoyment (Figure 15.2).

Theory of Planned Behavior

According to the theory of planned behavior, the intention to perform a behavior is the main determinant of the actual behavior (Figure 15.3). Intentions reflect an individual's perceived probability that they will exercise. However, this does not necessarily directly result in the behavior because of issues related to behavioral control and attitudes. Subjective norms are the social component, that is, whether an individual believes that the important people in their life value this behavior change in exercise. Perceived behavioral control is the perceived ease or difficulty in engaging in a behavior. So, if a person believes that exercise leads to positive outcomes, that this change is valued by someone important in their life, and that it is within their control, then she or he will have a strong intention to be active. In this theory, intention is the primary predictor of behavioral change.

Affective-Reflective Theory

Affective-Reflective Theory (ART) (10) is a default-interventionist dual-process theory that emphasizes the importance of automatic positive and negative associations for subsequent physical inactivity or exercise. It suggests that the automatic

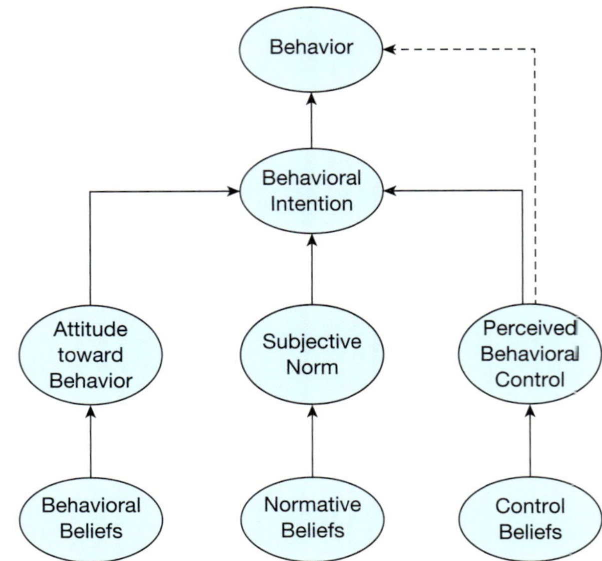

FIGURE 15.3. Theory of planned behavior.

valuation (an immediate action impulse) of exercise and physical inactivity is the basis from which subsequent, more complex **affective** and **cognitive** operations (eg, evaluating a person's beliefs and values and action planning) can arise. In this way, the ART attempts to incorporate findings from exercise motivation studies that emphasize the role of rational thinking in behavioral choices. The ART offers an explanation, other than the lack of motivation to change, why many people remain in a state of physical inactivity. It proposes that the core attractiveness associated with the current state of physical inactivity is more positive than the pleasure associated with exercise.

Health Belief Model

The health belief model (HBM) postulates that health-related practice, especially related to disease such as cancer, is influenced by several factors, including susceptibility and seriousness of the disease, perceived benefits, and barriers toward the behavior, cues to action, and self-efficacy (Table 15.1, Figure 15.4). An individual needs to believe that the benefits of taking action outweigh the perceived barriers. The 6 constructs of the HBM provide strategies for motivating individuals to change their exercise behavior.

The HBM was used to develop a model by Elshahat et al (11) that illustrates the main findings in terms of factors that influence cancer patients' performance and maintenance of physical activity as a healthy behavior (Figure 15.5).

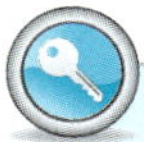

Affective. The experience of feeling the underlying emotional state.

Cognitive. The mental process used to comprehend information and turn it into knowledge.

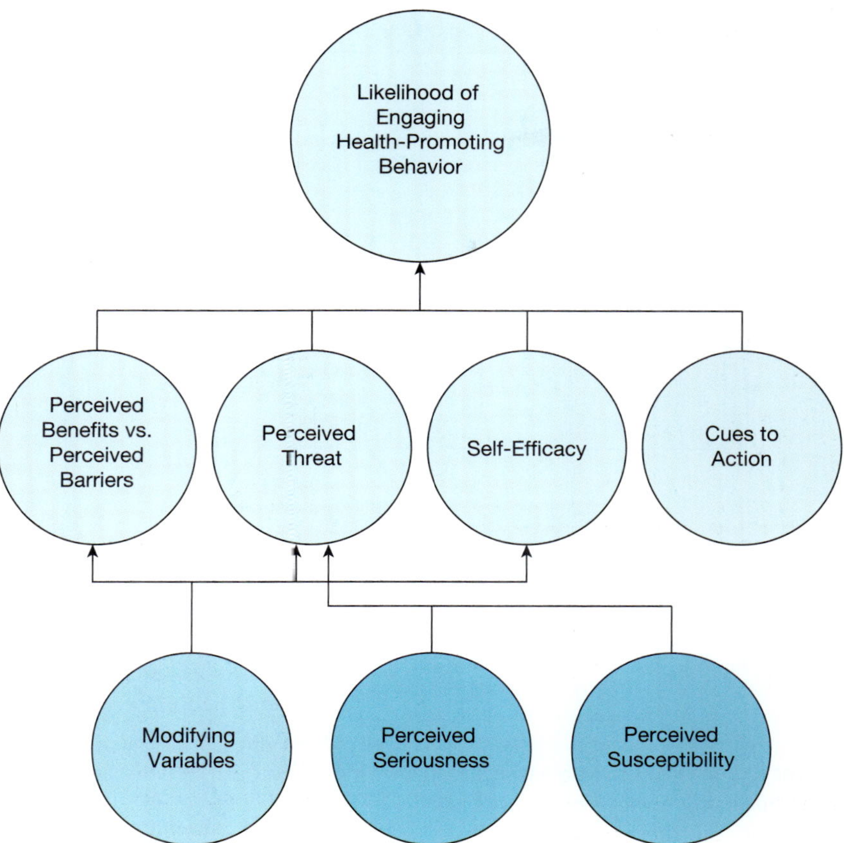

FIGURE 15.4. Health belief model.

Table 15.1 Health Belief Model Constructs and Strategies

CONSTRUCT	EXERCISE-SPECIFIC DEFINITION	CHANGE STRATEGY
Perceived susceptibility	Beliefs about the chances of getting a disease/condition if do not exercise	• Explain risk information based on current activity, family history, other behaviors, etc.
Perceived severity	Beliefs about the seriousness/consequences of disease/condition as a result of inactivity	• Refer individual to medically valid information about disease. • Discuss different treatment options, outcomes, and costs.
Perceived benefits	Beliefs about the effectiveness of exercising to reduce susceptibility and/or severity	• Provide information on benefits of exercise to preventing/treating condition or disease. • Provide information regarding all of the other potential benefits of exercise (eg, quality of life, mental health).
Perceived barriers	Beliefs about the direct and indirect costs associated with exercise	• Discuss Ex R_x options to minimize burden. • Provide information on different low-cost activity choices.
Cues to action	Factors that activate the change process and get someone to start exercising	• Help individual look for potential cues. • Ask the individual what it would take for him or her to get started.
Self-efficacy	Confidence in ability to exercise	• Assess level of confidence for different types of activity. • Use self-efficacy building techniques to enhance exercise confidence.

Ex R_x, exercise prescription.
Data from Rosenstock IM, Strecher VJ, Becker MH. Social learning theory and the health belief model. *Health Educ Q.* 1988;15(2):175–83, Table 12.3.

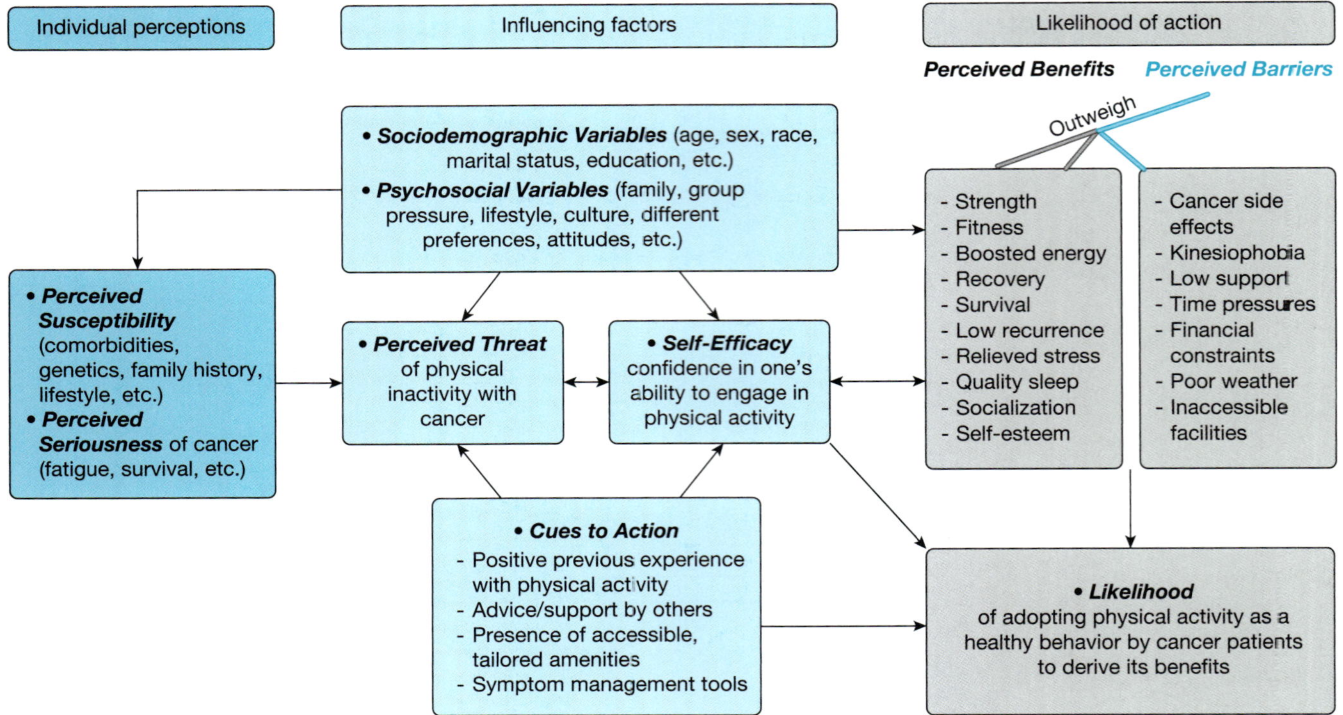

FIGURE 15.5. Health belief model-based conceptual model showing what predicts physical activity performance as a healthy behavior by cancer patients. (From Elshahat S, Treanor C, Donnelly M. Factors influencing physical activity participation among people living with or beyond cancer: a systematic scoping review. *Int J Behav Nutr Phys Act.* 2021;18(1):50, Figure 2.)

Social Cognitive Theory

Social cognitive theory (SCT) is based on the principle that the individual, behavior, and environment all interact to influence behavior (12). Central to SCT are task and barrier self-efficacy, outcome expectations, and **self-regulation**. The last is an individual's ability to set goals and, when faced with barriers, to be able to problem solve, monitor progress, and self-reward. A meta-analysis of 11 studies (13) that used SCT-based physical activity behavior-change interventions with cancer survivors reveals a significant intervention effect for physical activity (SMD = 0.33; $P < .01$).

Socioecological Model

The socioecological model (SEM) is defined by the recognition of a strong relationship between an individual's ability to change behavior and their environment (14). It identifies environmental and policy influences on 4 domains of active living: recreation, transport, occupation, and household.

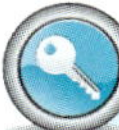

Self-regulation. The ability of an individual to be aware of and understand their thoughts, feelings and behaviors, and flexibly manage their reactions to these, according to their values and goals no matter what is happening around them.

Behavior Change Techniques

In a recent review (15) of 24 behavior-change interventions with breast cancer survivors, only 15 studies (62%) were theoretically based: 11 studies (46%) were based on a single theory and 4 studies used multiple theories (16%). behavior-change theories help to identify potentially effective content for the interventions and the processes by which that content will positively change behavior. The link between the theoretical constructs and the intervention content is based on a set of behavior-change techniques. A behavior-change technique is defined as "an observable, replicable and irreducible component of an intervention designed to alter or redirect causal processes that regulate behavior" (16). Michie et al (16) developed a classification of 93 different behavior-change techniques to accurately classify and specify which strategies are utilized and effective in different interventions. This chapter will concentrate on the specific application of some of these theory-based techniques in helping people affected by any type of cancer, both during and after treatment, to become or remain active. One theory may resonate with how one thinks about exercise and working with people with cancer, or several theories could work in combination in different situations. Table 15.2 outlines the theoretical constructs derived from the various theories and the specific behavior-change strategies/techniques that are appropriate to target each concept.

Table 15.2 Overarching Theoretical Constructs, Associated Theories, and Change Strategies

THEORETICAL CONSTRUCT	THEORIES	BEHAVIOR CHANGE STRATEGY
Intentions	• TPB: intentions • TTM: stages of change	• Goal setting • Implementation intentions
Knowledge	• SCT • TTM • HBM • SDT • TPB • SEM	• Brief counseling/motivational interviewing • Stage of change tailored counseling
Self-regulation	• SCT • ART	• Self-monitoring • Reinforcement • Relapse prevention • Problem solving • Affect regulation • Social support
Social influences and subjective norms	• SCT • SDT • TPB • SEM	• Social support • Reinforcement • Vicarious experience • Brief counseling/motivational interviewing • Stage of change tailored counseling
Environmental context and resources	• SCT • SEM	• Brief counseling/motivational interviewing • Stage of change tailored counseling • Problem solving
Beliefs about consequences (ie, outcome expectancies, and decisional balance)	• SCT • TTM • TPB • HBM	• Brief counseling/motivational interviewing • Stage of change tailored counseling • Vicarious experience • Physiological feedback • Problem solving
Beliefs about capabilities (ie, self-efficacy and perceived behavioral control)	• SCT • TTM • TPB • HBM	• Mastery experience • Vicarious experience • Verbal persuasion • Physiological feedback • Problem solving • Relapse prevention
Skills	• SCT • SDT	• Mastery Experience
Reinforcement	• SCT • SDT • TTM • ART	• Reinforcement • Social Support • Affect Regulation

HBM, health belief model; SCT, social cognitive theory; SDT, self-determination theory; SEM, social ecological model; TPB, theory of planned behavior; TTM, transtheoretical model.
Reprinted from *ACSM's® Guidelines for Exercise Testing and Prescription*. 11th ed. Indianapolis (IN): American College of Sports Medicine®; 2021, Table 12.1.

PERCEIVED BENEFITS AND BARRIERS TO EXERCISE WITH CANCER SURVIVORS

Perceived Benefits of Exercise

The most commonly perceived benefits reported by PLWC across cancer types and treatment stages in different studies are that being active promotes health, well-being, and cancer recovery (8). The main perceived benefit for many cancer patients is that exercise can prevent or reduce cancer-related fatigue (17, 18). Additional perceived benefits include improving cardiorespiratory fitness, increasing energy levels, building up muscular strength, and managing body weight. Many cancer survivors also believe that physical activity can enhance their resilience, reduce stress levels, enhance their

Table 15.3 Most Common Exercise Barriers, Relevant Theories, and Potential Strategies

COMMON PROBLEM	APPLICABLE THEORIES	EXAMPLE STRATEGIES
"I don't have enough time."	SCT, TPB, SEM	• Discuss modifications to FITT principles • Examine priorities/goals • Brief counseling/motivational interviewing
"I don't have enough energy."	SCT, HBM, SEM, TPB	• Discuss modifications to FITT principles • Brief counseling/motivational interviewing • Discuss affect regulation techniques for setting exercise intensity
"I'm just not motivated."	SCT, HBM, TPB, TTM, SEM, SDT	• Discuss attitudes and outcome expectations • Determine the stage of change and provide stage-tailored counseling • Examine perceived susceptibility and severity • Discuss potentially effective reinforcements
"It costs too much."	HBM, TTM, SEM	• Examine exercise alternatives to meet goals • Evaluate exercise opportunities in the environment
"I'm sick or hurt."	TTM	• Discuss maintenance/relapse prevention • Discuss alternative exercises to keep progressing toward goals
"There's nowhere for me to exercise."	SEM	• Evaluate exercise opportunities in the environment • Discuss different types of activities for which there are resources
"I feel awkward when I exercise."	SCT, TPB	• Discuss how to deal with task self-efficacy issues • Discuss alternative settings/options
"I don't know how to do it."	SCT, HBM, TTM, TPB	• Build task self-efficacy using appropriate strategies
"I might get hurt."	SCT, HBM, TPB	• Evaluate exercise prescription • Determine task-specific self-efficacy
"It's not safe."	M	• Evaluate exercise opportunities in the environment
"No one will watch my child if I exercised."	SCT, SEM	• Develop social support structures • Examine opportunities for exercise in which child care may be provided
"There is no one to exercise with me."	SCT, TPB, TTM	• Develop social support and exercise buddy system • Identify different types of activities one can do on his or her own

FITT, *F*requency, *I*ntensity, *T*ime, and *T*ype of exercise; HBM, health belief model; SCT, social cognitive theory; SDT, self-determination theory; SEM, social ecological model; TPB, theory of planned behavior; TTM, transtheoretical model.
Reprinted from *ACSM's® Guidelines for Exercise Testing and Prescription.* 11th ed. Indianapolis (IN): American College of Sports Medicine®; 2021, Table 12.5.

quality of the sleep, improve self-esteem, and help them to focus on the positive aspects of life (19, 20). Across many cancer types, group exercising is perceived as beneficial at reducing loneliness and isolation by providing socialization opportunities.

Commonly Reported Perceived Barriers to Exercise

Many cancer survivors, similar to people without cancer, may face a variety of personal, social, and environment-related challenges in the adoption and maintenance of physical activity. Common psychological barriers include lack of motivation, fear, dislike of the gym, not being *the exercise type*, and contextual and environmental barriers such as employment status, caregiving roles, proximity/access to facilities, and the weather. Task self-efficacy refers to an individual's confidence in his or her ability to perform the elemental aspects of a task (eg, confidence in the ability to walk for 30 min at a prescribed intensity). Table 15.3 lists common noncancer-related barriers and potential strategies to overcome these barriers.

Cancer Treatment-Related Barriers

As mentioned in previous chapters, cancer treatments can have a negative impact on a patient's physical, functional, social, and emotional QoL. A list of potential side effects that can act as barriers to exercise are shown in Box 15.3.

CRF is one of the most common barriers to exercise (11, 17, 21, 22). Treatments such as surgery can temporarily or permanently limit active daily living and chronic

Box 15.3 Acute/Chronic/Late Side Effects of Treatment for Cancer

Physical

- Fatigue
- Weight changes
- Reduced fitness—C/V and MSE
- Endocrine problems
- Osteoporosis
- Cardiotoxicity
- Lymphoedema
- Limited range of movement
- Pain and arthralgia
- Sexual dysfunction

Psychological

- Lack of confidence
- Changes in body image
- Anxiety
- Depression
- Cognitive dysfunction
- Social isolation
- Loneliness
- Loss of control
- Self-esteem
- Helplessness

treatment-related side effects, such as joint stiffness (arthralgia), peripheral neuropathy, gastrointestinal issues, and lymphoedema, which have all been cited as barriers to becoming active (11). Some treatment toxicities even persist as barriers 5 years following breast cancer treatment (23). Risk for pain has been reported as a barrier to exercise by ~30% lung cancer patients (24) and breast cancer patients (18). Another common barrier to exercising is weight gain during cancer treatment, which has been shown to impact body image and confidence (23, 25, 26).

Other Reported Physiological and Psychosocial Barriers to Behavior Change

It is worth remembering that cancer is a disease of older adults, and more than 70% of people with cancer are also living with one or more other potentially serious long-term health condition. Almost half (47%) have 2 or more conditions as well as cancer, and more than 1 in 4 (29%) have 3 or more conditions as well as cancer, leading to low levels of physical activity. The most prevalent comorbidities reported by cancer patients are arthritis, diabetes, and heart disease (27), and the presence of these chronic conditions alongside a cancer diagnosis negatively predicts engagement in physical activity behavior change (28). In addition, it is worth noting that many older adult cancer survivors may be frail and have a fear of falling when exercising or being active or a fear that some exercises may result in injury (29-31).

A patient's history of physical activity prior to diagnosis can also play a role in an individual's willingness to become and remain physically active during cancer treatment. In a review of levels of exercise and physical activity participation after a lung cancer diagnosis, survivors who were active prior to diagnosis were more motivated to begin exercising following diagnosis than those who were not. Patients sometimes describe themselves as being exercisers or nonexercisers, and the nonexercisers usually prefer to perform usual activities such as walking rather than structured exercise (32). Cancer patients also report feelings of embarrassment and concerns about their appearance post surgery, during, and after treatments when exercising in public (33).

STRATEGIES FOR INCREASING CANCER SURVIVORS' PHYSICAL ACTIVITY LEVELS

Self-Efficacy

Self-efficacy is defined as "having the confidence in one's ability to carry out actions necessary to maintain or increase exercise behavior" (34). There are 2 types of self-efficacy when considering exercise behavior. *Task self-efficacy* is an individual's belief that they can actually do the exercise, whereas *barrier self-efficacy* refers to whether they believe that they can exercise in the face of common barriers, such as lack of time and a bad weather. A review by Stacey et al (13) of 18 RCTs that used SCT to help cancer survivors become more active found that, in these studies, increases in self-efficacy were associated with increased physical activity, and those with higher self-efficacy tended to increase their physical activity levels faster than those with lower self-efficacy. Therefore, with cancer patients who are preparing or just beginning to become active, participating in light everyday activities (such as casual walking and light gardening) may be a feasible way to start. The sense of achieving light-intensity physical activity goals will enhance task and barrier self-efficacy, ensure adherence to the activity, and serve as a launch to future higher intensity activities.

Self-Monitoring

The review by Stacey et al (13) found that the most common way to increase self-efficacy is to provide cancer survivors with a means of monitoring their progress. Currently, the use of wearables (pedometers or accelerometers in smartphones, watches, etc) to track physical activity levels has become quite commonplace, and trackers such as Fitbit™ are relatively inexpensive and allow data to be downloaded and stored onto a computer or mobile phone. A review of 41 trials where pedometers or accelerometers were worn by patients receiving or after cancer treatments showed that those undergoing treatment, on average, take 2,885 to 8,300 steps per day, and post treatment, survivors typically take 4,660 to 11,000 steps per day (35). Therefore, monitoring and gradually increasing step counts can be an effective tool in promoting changes in physical activity during and after cancer treatments (36), particularly when working with cancer survivors living in rural areas for whom the cost burden of traveling for face-to-face sessions is not feasible.

Goal Setting

Setting, monitoring, and adjusting appropriate individualized goals can lead to positive changes in exercise behavior. Short-, medium-, and long-term goals should be set using the SMARTS principle:

- **S**pecific
- **M**easurable
- **A**ction
- **R**ealistic
- **T**imely
- **S**elf-determined

In a review of 27 studies that used various behavior-change techniques to increase physical activity levels in breast cancer survivors, goal setting was found to be effective in all the high-quality studies (15). A Cochrane review of 23 behavior-change studies with 1,372 patients with breast, prostate, colorectal, and lung cancers also showed that interventions characterized by goal setting, graded tasks (eg, increasing frequency/duration/intensity of physical activity), and instruction on how to perform the exercises achieved the adherence of >75% to the physical activity guidelines (37).

Reinforcement/Rewards

A review of 30 studies with cancer survivors by Finne et al (38) found that the provision of prompts or cues to be active acting as reinforcements/rewards can be very effective. Significant increases in physical activity levels are observed when different kinds of nonspecific or social rewards are provided for efforts (eg, immediate reinforcement via positive automated text messages and praise for participants who attain their personal exercise goal or progress toward goals). As mentioned earlier, physical activity apps and wearable devices can provide rewards and reinforcement through praise either automatic, user-generated, or through various social networking features, for example, Strava (San Francisco, CA). For example:

- Intermittent phone calls as reinforcements that can gradually decrease over time as the cancer survivor becomes more independent.
- Providing tasks that gradually increase in difficulty (eg, increasing the frequency and/or duration of exercise sessions from week to week or progressing to more demanding exercises) and rewarding the participant's progress.

Social Support

For many individuals, social support is a powerful motivator to exercise. This support provided in many ways—instrumental, emotional, informational, companionship, and validation—can be particularly important at the start of the behavior change when there are some challenging times or when the exercise plan is perceived as challenging. Social support comes in many forms: participating alongside the cancer survivor, acting as a sounding board, demonstrating proper technique, etc. Cancer survivors perceive social support for physical activity as providing companionship (shared experience), motivation (encouragement to participate), and health promotion (benefits such as less fatigue) (39). Peer support, that is, exercising with other cancer survivors appears to be particularly important and beneficial (26). Participants in a group exercise program during breast cancer treatment strongly emphasized the importance of exercising in a group because they valued the empathy they received from others "who were in the same boat," and it stopped them from feeling isolated but made them feel recognized and accepted (26). Face-to-face peer support, however, can be difficult for survivors who work full time or live in a rural community or have limited access to transport options. Fortunately, with advances in technology, social support can include live or recorded online exercise sessions, exercise consultations, discussion boards, and social media networks.

Motivational Interview Techniques

Motivational interviewing is a form of collaborative conversation for strengthening a person's own motivation and commitment to change that is increasingly being used to promote and support physical activity interventions in cancer survivors (Figure 15.6) (40). This type of consultation is person-centered, helping the individual to explorie their own barriers, goals, motivation and confidence and commitment to making a change that they are ambivalent about. The practitioner uses open questions that focus on desire, ability, reasons and needs related to the desired behaviour, e.g. being more active, and reflective listening that deliberately tunes into the individuals' strengths and what they say in the direction of their desired change. The approach invites practitioners to step out of the expert, directive role into one

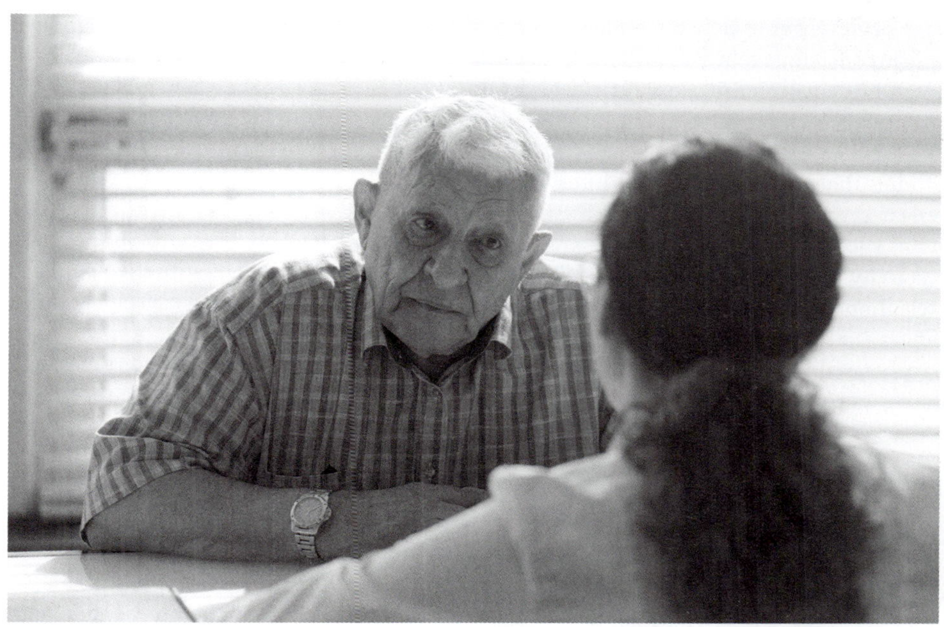

FIGURE 15.6. Motivational interviewing to promote physical activity interventions among patients with cancer. (Stock Photo ID: 2245991105, PeopleImages.com, Yuri A.)

characterized more by guiding. This way of relating is captured by partnership (work together as equals), acceptance (honour their worth and autonomy with accurate empathy and affirmation), compassion (work in the person's interest), and empowerment (help people realise and utilise their own strengths and abilities and to call it forth in them). The counseling approach should be empathic, nonjudgmental, and respectful of the individual's autonomy and that the individual is fully responsible for any change, rather than trying to persuade the person to change or proving that they should exercise. As an exercise professional you will want to provide advice and a suggested exercise plan, however, it should always be offered, not provided, and only after allowing the person to think about and verbalize what they already understand about exercise and its benefits, what exercise they feel they want to do, what they are capable of, and what they are confident with. All of this should be acknowledged before asking for permission to share your exercise advice/suggestions. Ambivalence about behavior change occurs when someone has conflicting opinions, for example, "I know I

Table 15.4 Change Talk

APPROACH	EXAMPLE
Ask evocative questions	What are some of the benefits of becoming active after a cancer diagnosis?
Use the readiness ruler	Start with: How ready are you to start a physical activity program?
Use the important ruler	Start with: How important is it for you to be physically active?
Use the confidence ruler	Start with: How confident are you that you can engage in some regular activities at this time?
Explore pros and cons	What are the disadvantages of being physically active at this time? What are the advantages of being physical active at this time?
Elaborate	You said exercise might give you more energy. Can you tell me more about that?
Query extremes	What would you imagine would be the best results imaginable if you made a change and started to get active?
Look back	You mentioned that you used to go out on your bike every week. What was that like?
Look forward	You say that because of your fatigue, you worry about the future. How would you like things to be different?
Explore values and goals	What is most important to you in your life?

should exercise to stay healthy, but I really don't like the way I feel when I'm exercising." Change talk includes the discussion of desire, ability, confidence, and reasons and needs for change. There are a number of approaches that can be used to evoke change talk (Table 15.4).

A review of 6 studies that used motivational interviewing to assist in physical activity behavior change in cancer patients and survivors showed small-to-moderate positive effects on physical activity levels (41). In 1 study (42) that conducted weekly telephone motivational interviewing sessions with breast cancer survivors, after 16 weeks, the average physical activity increased from a baseline of 39 minutes per week to 252 minutes per week.

PHYSICAL ACTIVITY PREFERENCES BY CANCER SURVIVORS

A recent review of 34 studies looking at physical activity preferences in people living with and beyond cancer (11) found that these preferences can be put into 6 categories (Box 15.4).

Type of Exercise

Cancer patients' preferences for the type of physical activity and exercise programs can be as varied and individual as their cancer treatment side effects after diagnosis. However, most studies show that walking is the most preferred type of physical activity across cancer types both during the treatment and post-treatment, with swimming, cycling, and yoga also being popular (11). Preferences are also influenced by the survivor's culture, ethnicity, and geographic location. For example, Dutch breast cancer survivors enjoy Nordic walking (43), and aerobic activities such as dancing are more appealing to some Latin breast cancer survivors (44). Other preferences include exercising at a moderate intensity (as opposed to high intensity) and an access to a variety of programs in order to prevent boredom (32).

Box 15.4 Physical Activity Preferences of Cancer Survivors

Following are physical activity preferences of cancer survivors:

- Type of exercise
- Where to exercise
- Who should provide the advice/exercise
- When after a cancer diagnosis to start exercising
- With whom to exercise
- What time of the day to exercise

Where to Exercise

The most preferred place for exercise among mixed cancer patients at different treatment stages is either home or at a fitness center. About 80% to 90% of participants in 3 separate qualitative and quantitative studies reported that they would prefer performing exercise at home. This is because it reduces the burden and cost of travel, allows the activity to be fit into a flexible schedule, and thus can be more convenient. However, home-based exercise programs require self-motivation and are more effective for cancer survivors who have a history of regular physical activity (45). Hospital setting is preferred by a significant number of cancer patients (particularly during treatment stages) as they consider hospitals the safest place to exercise. The benefit of community-based fitness centers or hospital programs is that they often offer personalized exercise demonstration and/or supervision—a safe and encouraging environment and an opportunity for social interaction (46-48).

Provision of Advice

Studies show that oncologists are the most preferable source of exercise information among patients across cancer types, followed by physical therapists and nurses. A recommendation and/or referral from an oncologist to an exercise program has been shown to be effective in encouraging exercise behavior change (49, 50). To help health care professionals to routinely provide physical activity behavior-change counseling to patients, the Moving Through Cancer Initiative provides a referral pathway to make assessment of physical activity a vital sign in health care (51). Preferences show that cancer patients want physical activity interventions to be undertaken by licensed rehabilitation professionals and clinical exercise physiologists. These 2 professionals possess complementary skillsets that when integrated can optimize the adherence and effectiveness of an exercise intervention for all cancer survivors of different cancers and stages (52).

When to Start an Exercise Program

Overall, cancer patients state that they would prefer to start a physical activity program after finishing their cancer treatment. However, 20% of the patients said that they preferred immediately after cancer diagnosis and during treatment. Recent studies with prehabilitation exercise interventions show various health benefits by starting immediately after diagnosis and before surgery (Chapter 10) and that, with the appropriate support, the majority of cancer patients are willing to start and engage with the program at this stage (53).

With Whom to Exercise

Around half of mixed cancer participants in 4 cross-sectional studies admitted that they preferred exercising alone. Conversely, about half of the cancer patients preferred group exercising with family members or other cancer patients who face similar challenges. Therefore, it is important when planning any intervention to help increase physical activity levels to take these preferences into consideration (17, 54).

SUMMARY

Most cancer survivors have a positive attitude toward physical activity participation and perceive physical activity to be beneficial for their health and well-being. However, the main barriers to engagement among cancer patients include treatment-related side effects, low motivation, fear of injury through activity, low social support, time pressures, and inaccessible fitness facilities. Effective behavior-change strategies that should be employed include perceived health benefits, social support and guidance, and the availability of appropriately trained cancer exercise specialists and facilities. Physical activity and exercise preferences vary from individual to individual in terms of when, what, and by whom, highlighting the need for personalized safe physical activity programs that are tailored to meet a patient's needs.

Case Study

Jeff is a 57-year-old postal delivery worker who has just completed his radiotherapy treatment for prostate cancer. He had severe side effects during his radiotherapy treatment, including having to pass urine frequently (eg, during the night), bouts of diarrhea, and redness and soreness of his skin in the pubic region. The diarrhea has now passed, but Jeff is still suffering from incontinence and is utterly exhausted. Up until 2 years ago, Jeff was a smoker, but he quitted smoking when his general practitioner diagnosed the beginnings of chronic bronchitis; he quitted smoking "for the good of his health." Jeff has since then gained 15-kilogram weight and now feels too embarrassed to go to a gym. Jeff used to love do-it-yourself projects around the house and bowling regularly, but he is now feeling very out of condition. In fact, he feels that he has no longer muscular strength. He even had to ask a neighbor to help him move some furniture a few weeks ago, something that appalled him and made him feel quite depressed. Jeff went to his doctor recently telling her that he is really scared of the cancer coming back and requesting antidepressants, but he agreed that prior to any further drug treatment, he would chat with an exercise professional with the aim of trying to improve his physical activity levels. Jeff also has high BP and a high cholesterol level. Jeff is divorced and lives alone. He is still in contact with his 2 teenage boys who live with their mother about 2 miles away from his apartment. Both of Jeff's sons love playing all sports but are particularly keen soccer players.

Questions

1. What are Jeff's perceived barriers?
   a. Cancer treatments' side effects
   b. Comorbidities
   c. Fear
   d. Low body image
   e. All of the above
2. What tools can be used to improve Jeff's self-efficacy?
   a. Light-to-moderate activities, for example, walking to build his confidence
   b. Monitoring using a wearable device
   c. Reinforcements using the app
   d. All of the above
3. How can we improve Jeff's social support?
   a. Qualified cancer exercise instructor
   b. Peer support
   c. Family and friends
   d. All of the above
4. What type of exercise, when, and with whom?
   a. Walking
   b. Initially at home and then group exercise in gym with other cancer survivors
   c. Cancer exercise expert and sons
   d. All of the above

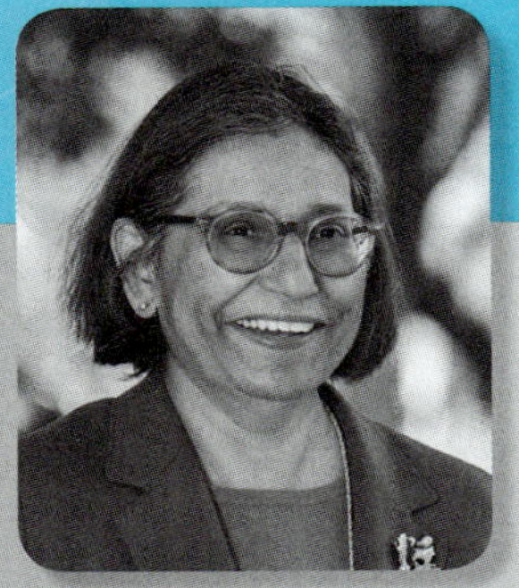

Meet the Expert

FEATURED PROFESSIONAL

Bernadine Pinto, PhD

Associate Dean for Research, Inaugural Health Science Endowed Professor, and Co-Director Cancer Survivorship Center
College of Nursing
University of South Carolina
Columbia, SC, USA
Behavioral Scientist

Q: "Where did you grow up?"

Middle East and India.

Q: "Where did you train? What is your training?"

PhD in Clinical Psychology from Western Michigan University, Postdoctoral Fellowship at Alpert School of Medicine, Brown University, Providence, RI.

Q: "What are you best known for?"

Behavioral science expertise, community-based interventions for cancer survivors.

Q: "What are you currently working on?"

Scaling up an evidence-based program into dissemination and implementation to reach more survivors.

Q: "Anything else you want to include?"

Making a positive impact on patients' lives is key.

Favorite Quote:

"It's not a disgrace not to reach for the stars but it is a disgrace to have no stars to reach for. Not failure, but low aim is sin."
—*Dr. Benjamin Mays*

STUDY QUESTIONS

1. According to Ottenbacher's study in 2015, approximately what percentage of cancer survivors are active in the US after treatment?
   a. 10
   b. 30
   c. 50
   d. 70
2. What is the definition of the "Teachable Moment" with reference to cancer patients and physical activity?
3. Which behavior-change theory is abbreviated to SCT?
4. Which of the following perceived benefits of exercise is most commonly reported by cancer survivors?
   a. Increased resilience
   b. Improved muscular strength
   c. Reduced fatigue
   d. Reduced anxiety
5. List some of the physiological cancer treatment-related side effects most commonly cited as barriers to becoming active by most cancer survivors.
6. What percentage of people with cancer are also living with 1 or more other potentially serious long-term health conditions?
   a. 30
   b. 50
   c. 70
   d. 90
7. What is self-efficacy?
8. Describe tools that can help a cancer survivor to self-monitor progress in increasing physical activity levels.
9. List what SMARTS stands for when goal setting.
10. Cancer survivors state that social support helps to increase physical activity levels in what ways?
11. Which of the following is the most popular type of exercise preferred by cancer survivors?
    a. Gardening
    b. Weight training
    c. Badminton
    d. Walking
12. Where do most cancer survivors prefer to exercise?
    a. At home or in hospital
    b. At hospital or in a gym
    c. At home or in a gym
    d. None of the above

REFERENCES

1. Garcia DO, Thomson CA. Physical activity and cancer survivorship. *Nutr Clin Pract*. 2014;29(6):768–79.
2. Ottenbacher A, Yu M, Moser RP, Phillips SM, Alfano C, Perna FM. Population estimates of meeting strength training and aerobic guidelines, by gender and cancer survivorship status: findings from the Health Information National Trends Survey (HINTS). *J Phys Act Health*. 2015;12(5):675–9.
3. Shimizu Y, Tsuji K, Ochi E, et al. Study protocol for a nationwide questionnaire survey of physical activity among breast cancer survivors in Japan. *BMJ Open*. 2020;10(1):e032871.
4. Kristiansen M, Adamsen L, Piil K, Halvorsen I, Nyholm N, Hendriksen C. A three-year national follow-up study on the development of community-level cancer rehabilitation in Denmark. *Scand J Public Health*. 2019;47(5):511–18.
5. Demark-Wahnefried W, Aziz NM, Rowland JH, Pinto BM. Riding the crest of the teachable moment: promoting long-term health after the diagnosis of cancer. *J Clin Oncol*. 2005;23(24):5814–30.
6. Lawson PJ, Flocke SA. Teachable moments for health behavior change: a concept analysis. *Patient Educ Couns*. 2009;76(1):25–30.
7. Prochaska JO, DiClemente CC. Self change processes, self efficacy and decisional balance across five stages of smoking cessation. *Prog Clin Biol Res*. 1984;156:131–40.
8. Pinto BM, Kindred MM, Grimmett C. Cancer survivors becoming and staying physically active: challenges of behavior change. In: Schimtz K, editor. *Exercise Oncology*. Cham: Springer; 2020, pp. 351–68
9. Deci EL, Ryan RM. *Intrinsic Motivation and Self-Determination in Human Behavior*. New York (NY): Plenum; 1985.
10. Brand R, Ekkekakis P. Affective–Reflective Theory of physical inactivity and exercise. *Ger J Exerc Sport Res*. 2017;48(1):48–58.
11. Elshahat S, Treanor C, Donnelly M. Factors influencing physical activity participation among people living with or beyond cancer: a systematic scoping review. *Int J Behav Nutr Phys Act*. 2021;18(1):50.
12. Bandura A. *Social Foundations of Thought and Action: A Social Cognitive Theory*. Englewood Cliffs (NJ): Prentice Hall; 1985, p. 544.
13. Stacey FG, James EL, Chapman K, Courneya KS, Lubans DR. A systematic review and meta-analysis of social cognitive theory-based physical activity and/or nutrition behavior change interventions for cancer survivors. *J Cancer Surviv*. 2015;9(2):305–38.
14. Sallis JF, Cervero RB, Ascher W, Henderson KA, Kraft MK, Kerr J. An ecological approach to creating active living communities. *Annu Rev Public Health*. 2006;27:297–322.
15. Hailey V, Rojas-Garcia A, Kassianos AP. A systematic review of behaviour change techniques used in interventions to increase physical activity among breast cancer survivors. *Breast Cancer*. 2022; 29(2):193–208.
16. Michie S, Richardson M, Johnston M, et al. The behavior change technique taxonomy (v1) of 93 hierarchically clustered techniques: building an international consensus for the reporting of behavior change interventions. *Ann Behav Med*. 2013;46(1):81–95.
17. Blaney JM, Lowe-Strong A, Rankin-Watt J, Campbell A, Gracey JH. Cancer survivors' exercise barriers, facilitators and preferences in the context of fatigue, quality of life and physical activity participation: a questionnaire–survey. *Psychooncology*. 2013;22(1):186–94.
18. Rogers LQ, Courneya KS, Shah P, Dunnington G, Hopkins-Price P. Exercise stage of change, barriers, expectations, values and preferences among breast cancer patients during treatment: a pilot study. *Eur J Cancer Care*. 2007;16(1):55–66.
19. Hennessy EM, Stevinson C, Fox KR. Preliminary study of the lived experience of exercise for cancer survivors. *Eur J Oncol Nurs*. 2005; 9(2):155–66.
20. Husebo AM, Karlsen B, Allan H, Soreide JA, Bru E. Factors perceived to influence exercise adherence in women with breast cancer participating in an exercise programme during adjuvant chemotherapy: a focus group study. *J Clin Nurs*. 2015;24(3–4):500–10.
21. Keogh JW, Patel A, MacLeod RD, Masters J. Perceived barriers and facilitators to physical activity in men with prostate cancer: possible influence of androgen deprivation therapy. *Eur J Cancer Care (Engl)*. 2014;23(2):263–73.
22. Lynch BM, Owen N, Hawkes AL, Aitken JF. Perceived barriers to physical activity for colorectal cancer survivors. *Support Care Cancer*. 2010;18(6):729–34.
23. Hefferon K, Murphy H, McLeod J, Mutrie N, Campbell A. Understanding barriers to exercise implementation 5-year post-breast cancer diagnosis: a large-scale qualitative study. *Health Educ Res*. 2013; 28(5):843–56.
24. Karvinen KH, Vallance J, Walker PR. Newly diagnosed lung cancer patients' preferences for and beliefs about physical activity prior to chemotherapy. *Psychol Health Med*. 2016;21(5):593–600.
25. Latka R, Alvarez-Reeves M, Cadmus L, Irwin M. Adherence to a randomized controlled trial of aerobic exercise in breast cancer survivors: the Yale exercise and survivorship study. *J Cancer Surviv*. 2009; 3(3):148–57.
26. Emslie C, Whyte F, Campbell A, et al. "I wouldn't have been interested in just sitting round a table talking about cancer"; exploring the experiences of women with breast cancer in a group exercise trial. *Health Educ Res*. 2007;22(6):827–38.
27. Bluethmann SM, Foo W, Winkels RM, Mama SK, Schmitz KH. Physical activity in older cancer survivors: what role do multimorbidity and perceived disability play? *J Aging Phys Act*. 2020;28(2): 311–19.
28. Frikkel J, Gotte M, Beckmann M, et al. Fatigue, barriers to physical activity and predictors for motivation to exercise in advanced cancer patients. *BMC Palliat Care*. 2020;19(1):43.
29. Santa Mina D, Petrella A, Currie KL, et al. Enablers and barriers in delivery of a cancer exercise program: the Canadian experience. *Curr Oncol*. 2015;22(6):374–84.
30. Smith SA, Ansa BE, Yoo W, Whitehead MS, Coughlin SS. Determinants of adherence to physical activity guidelines among overweight and obese African American breast cancer survivors: implications for an intervention approach. *Ethn Health*. 2018;23(2):194–206.
31. Rogers LQ, McAuley E, Courneya KS, Verhulst SJ. Correlates of physical activity self-efficacy among breast cancer survivors. *Am J Health Behav*. 2008;32(6):594–603.
32. Granger CL, Connolly B, Denehy L, et al. Understanding factors influencing physical activity and exercise in lung cancer: a systematic review. *Support Care Cancer*. 2017;25(3):983–99.
33. Romero SAD, Brown JC, Bauml JM, et al. Barriers to physical activity: a study of academic and community cancer survivors with pain. *J Cancer Surviv*. 2018;12(6):744–52.
34. Resnick B. Reliability and validity of the outcome expectations for exercise scale-2. *J Aging Phys Act*. 2005;13(4):382–94.
35. Gresham G, Schrack J, Gresham LM, et al. Wearable activity monitors in oncology trials: current use of an emerging technology. *Contemp Clin Trials*. 2018;64:13–21.
36. Purswani JM, Ohri N, Champ C. Tracking steps in oncology: the time is now. *Cancer Manag Res*. 2018;10:2439–47.
37. Turner RR, Steed L, Quirk H, et al. Interventions for promoting habitual exercise in people living with and beyond cancer. *Cochrane Database Syst Rev*. 2018;9:CD010192.
38. Finne E, Glausch M, Exner AK, Sauzet O, Stolzel F, Seidel N. Behavior change techniques for increasing physical activity in cancer survivors: a systematic review and meta-analysis of randomized controlled trials. *Cancer Manag Res*. 2018;10:5125–43.
39. Barber FD. Effects of social support on physical activity, self-efficacy, and quality of life in adult cancer survivors and their caregivers. *Oncol Nurs Forum*. 2013;40(5):481–9.
40. Miller WR, Rollnick S. *Motivational Interviewing: Helping People Change and Grow*. New York, NY: The Guilford Press; 2023.

41. Spencer JC, Wheeler SB. A systematic review of Motivational Interviewing interventions in cancer patients and survivors. *Patient Educ Couns*. 2016;99(7):1099–105.
42. Spector D, Deal AM, Amos KD, Yang H, Battaglini CL. A pilot study of a home-based motivational exercise program for African American breast cancer survivors: clinical and quality-of-life outcomes. *Integr Cancer Ther*. 2014;13(2):121–32.
43. Fischer MJ, Krol-Warmerdam EM, Ranke GM, et al. Stick together: a Nordic Walking Group intervention for breast cancer survivors. *J Psychosoc Oncol*. 2015;33(3):278–96.
44. Spector D, Battaglini CL, Groff D. Perceived exercise barriers and facilitators among ethnically diverse breast cancer survivors. *Oncol Nurs Forum*. 2013;40(5):472–80.
45. Adamsen L, Stage M, Laursen J, Rorth M, Quist M. Exercise and relaxation intervention for patients with advanced lung cancer: a qualitative feasibility study. *Scand J Med Sci Sports*. 2012;22(6):804–15.
46. Bock C, Jarczok MN, Litaker D. Community-based efforts to promote physical activity: a systematic review of interventions considering mode of delivery, study quality and population subgroups. *J Sci Med Sport*. 2014;17(3);276–82.
47. Buffart LM, Kalter J, Sweegers MG, et al. Effects and moderators of exercise on quality of life and physical function in patients with cancer: an individual patient data meta-analysis of 34 RCTs. *Cancer Treat Rev*. 2017;52:91–104.
48. Brown JC, Huedo-Medina TB, Pescatello LS, et al. The efficacy of exercise in reducing depressive symptoms among cancer survivors: a meta-analysis. *PLoS One*. 2012;7(1):e30955.
49. Jones LW, Courneya KS, Fairey AS, Mackey JR. Effects of an oncologist's recommendation to exercise on self-reported exercise behaviour in newly diagnosed breast cancer survivors: a single-blind, randomized controlled trial. *Ann Behav Med*. 2004;28(2):105–13.
50. Kirkham AA, Van Patten CL, Gelmon KA, et al. Effectiveness of oncologist-referred exercise and healthy eating programming as a part of supportive adjuvant care for early breast cancer. *Oncologist*. 2018; 23(1):105–15.
51. Schmitz KH, Campbell AM, Stuiver MM, et al. Exercise is medicine in oncology: engaging clinicians to help patients move through cancer. *CA: Cancer J Clin*. 2019;69(6):468–84.
52. Coletta AM, Campbell A, Morris GS, Schmitz KH. Synergy between licensed rehabilitation professionals and clinical exercise physiologists: optimizing patient care for cancer rehabilitation. *Semin Oncol Nurs*. 2020;36(1):150975.
53. Chapman O, Taylor RM. Barriers and facilitators for healthcare professionals to implementing a prehabilitation programme: review of the literature. *J Cancer Rehabil*. 2021;4:86–90.
54. Owusu C, Antognoli E, Nock N, et al. Perspective of older African-American and non-Hispanic white breast cancer survivors from diverse socioeconomic backgrounds toward physical activity: a qualitative study. *J Geriatr Oncol*. 2018;9(3):235–42.

CHAPTER

16

Logistical Challenges Unique in Exercise Oncology

OUTLINE

1. Introduction
2. Problems Introducing Exercise Programs Into Oncology Settings
3. Barriers to Implementation in Exercise Oncology
   a. Organizational Issues
   b. Individual Professional Issues
   c. Innovation Issues: Embedding Into Clinical Practice
   d. Accessibility
   e. Patient Barriers: Knowledge
   f. Economic/Political Barriers
   g. Social Context Issues: Collaboration and Leadership
4. Implementation Science
5. Implementation Pathway
   a. Generating Referrals for Exercise Programs
   b. Medical Screening and Risk Stratification
   c. Workforce Issues in an Exercise Oncology Program Pathway
   d. Evaluation
6. Summary
7. Case Study
8. Meet the Expert
9. Study Questions
10. References

OBJECTIVES

After completing review of this chapter, students will be able to:

1. Recognize barriers to implementation at different levels of a health care system.
2. Understand implementation science and how to evaluate implementation.
3. Understand exercise oncology implementation pathways.
4. Comprehend the importance of screening triage and workforce development in implementation.

INTRODUCTION

One of the main issues in exercise oncology is the gap between clinical research and the implementation of these findings into cancer care. This chapter will provide an insight into the challenges of moving from theory to practice by looking at the potential barriers to implementation. Evaluated program pathways for people affected by cancer will be explored and potential solutions to authentic barriers located at different stages of the pathway will be discussed. Finally, some tools for evaluating the success of an implemented exercise oncology program will be provided.

PROBLEMS INTRODUCING EXERCISE PROGRAMS INTO ONCOLOGY SETTINGS

Introducing exercise programs in an oncology setting can be challenging. It has been calculated that it takes approximately 17 years to move health research findings into clinical practice (1, 2). Despite the overwhelming evidence of the physical and psychological benefits to individuals affected by cancer, interventions to help cancer patients become or stay active are not typically part of a standard cancer care package. One reason is that most clinical trials do not take into consideration the messiness of the real world. Research studies that aim to establish the efficacy of exercise oncology interventions have been conducted in controlled research settings. Thus, in an attempt to recruit a homogeneous sample, studies often recruit a specific subset of cancer patients. This itself is not an issue unique to exercise oncology; often patients participating in any clinical trials are already intending to make a change and, as a result, are already a selected group of individuals. In addition, the exercise interventions in such research settings tend to be very precise and rigid in their prescription detail, extensively monitored and heavily supervised. In this book, we present *what* to do (using FITT principles and behavior-change techniques) and *why* (engaging all patients at any time post diagnosis to improve their health and well-being) through exercise and active living. We are still learning *how* to do it in the real world, that is, *who* does *what*, *where*, and *when*.

BARRIERS TO IMPLEMENTATION IN EXERCISE ONCOLOGY

When planning complex changes in practice, all the potential barriers need to be identified and addressed. Planning needs to consider the structure of the intervention; the characteristics of the professionals and patients involved; and the social, organizational, economic, and political environment. Using Grol and Wensing's framework (3), the potential barriers - across 6 distinct levels within a health care system - to the implementation of exercise programs can be examined (Table 16.1).

Table 16.1 Barriers to Implementation at Different Levels of Health Care

LEVEL	BARRIERS/INCENTIVES
Innovation	Advantages in practice, feasibility, credibility, accessibility, attractiveness
Individual professional	Awareness, knowledge, attitude, motivation to change, behavioral routines
Patient	Knowledge, skills, attitude, adherence
Social context	Opinion of colleagues, culture of the network, collaboration, leadership
Organizational context	Organization of an established pathway, staff, capacities, resources, structures
Economic and political context	Financial arrangements, regulations, policies

A recent review by Kennedy et al (4) extracted 243 implementation barriers to implementing exercise oncology into a cancer care setting from 50 studies. The most common barriers in each level of Grol and Wensing's framework (3).

Organizational Issues

Capacity Within Current Health Care Systems

A major issue is that in the time allotted during a patient visit, members of the oncology team are unable to advise, prescribe, and/or refer patients to an appropriate exercise intervention. In a survey of oncologists, 66% of 540 respondents (5) stated that the lack of time for counseling or setting up a referral amid other clinical activities is a barrier to providing any kind of exercise rehabilitation program to patients. The oncology health care professionals (HCPs) stated that they did not have the capacity within their current workload to add extra time and work in a clinic to provide exercise counseling and referrals.

Staff and Resources

A lack of staff with the expertise in exercise counseling and exercise oncology prescription is often reported as a barrier to implementation both in hospital and community settings. Linked to this, funding to support the hiring of qualified staff, providing appropriate facilities for counseling or exercise programs, and purchasing equipment are also noted as organizational issues.

Established Structure/Pathway Within the Cancer Care Setting to Appropriate Programs

Currently in many clinical oncology settings, there is no standard or effective direct referral pathway to an appropriate exercise program, and indeed there have been reports of community exercise programs for people with cancer to which none of the participants were referred by their oncology team (6). The availability of inaccessible fitness facilities is a major issue that hinders physical activity engagement among people with disabilities, including cancer-related side effects (7). Other structural issues include the lack of a system to collate and review medical information, current fitness status, and physical activities in order to screen, triage, and refer or signpost to the most appropriate exercise program.

Individual Professional Issues

Knowledge

One of the main issues with HCPs working in the oncology setting is the lack of knowledge on how to advise patients about exercise. Specifically, studies show that many HCPs know that exercise is beneficial for cancer patients and survivors but have a lack of understanding of the guidelines, particularly during cancer treatment, and also a lack of skill and confidence around motivational interviewing and behavior-change techniques (4). This can result in vague advice for patients, such as "do whatever you want, but not too much." In a survey of 120 oncology HCPs, 77% rated their knowledge as poor regarding how to counsel on the basis of exercise guidelines and knowing when, how, and which patients to refer to a supervised exercise program (8).

Attitude

In many cases, HCPs believe that cancer patients are not interested in receiving exercise information. They also tend to judge and decide which specific patients would be most willing to accept the offer of exercise and thus hesitate to discuss opportunities to get active/exercise with patients who are inactive, are older adults, have multiple comorbidities, or are undergoing complex treatments. In addition, many HCPs report that they are uncertain about the safety and quality of the exercise intervention. In a sample of 167 oncologists, only 40% agreed that exercise is safe for cancer patients, and only 7.2% believed that cancer patients would manage to exercise during cancer treatment (9). There can be a reluctance of oncologists and nurses to refer patients to an exercise program because they are concerned about their patients' safety. Finally, as mentioned in organizational issues, for many HCPs, offering advice or a referral to an exercise program is not perceived as a high priority in clinical appointments. They believe that their job is to provide an expert opinion on the management of the cancer, and exercise is an auxiliary issue that should be someone else's responsibility.

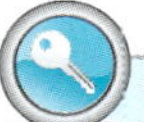

Signposting. Where health professionals, navigators, and advisors assist patients to be aware of and access community-based services that are provided to improve their health.

Innovation Issues: Embedding Into Clinical Practice

Many clinicians are still unaware of or are skeptical about the benefits of exercise for cancer patients, resulting in a noncommitment or disinterest in providing an exercise service in cancer care. The following barriers are often cited.

Accessibility

Cost

In times of austerity, the cost of establishing and running an exercise program may be considered prohibitive (see organizational issues). From the patient's perspective, the direct cost to attend an unsubsidized exercise program and the indirect costs such as transportation to the location of the program can be a barrier.

Location

The location and accessibility of the program can deter participation if it requires long travel times or if there are issues such as the lack of public transport, parking, and changing facilities.

Availability

Many exercise oncology programs offer fixed schedules that can be incompatible with a patient's personal and clinical schedules. In addition, some supervised programs, which limit numbers to small groups or individual sessions, can quickly become fully booked.

Patient Barriers: Knowledge

Many patients admit that they do not know what they should or could do in terms of staying active and exercising and are unaware of the provision of any programs to support them. Cancer survivors also state that the advice from medical professionals is sometimes unhelpful because of the ambiguity and generality of the recommendations. One study reported that 20% of 834 patients found that inconsistent information about being physically active made them hesitant about exercising (10).

Economic/Political Barriers

A lack of standard policies within public health and oncology health care settings for directing and regulating the inclusion of exercise into cancer care is a main barrier to implementation. In addition, in some countries, the lack of structured financial reimbursement policies is also an issue (11).

Social Context Issues: Collaboration and Leadership

Poor interprofessional communication and collaboration, specifically between the oncology teams, other HCPs (eg, secondary and primary HCPs), and the exercise program coordinators are some of the common concerns. Some studies specified lack of leadership support as an issue impeding the integration of exercise into oncology care where exercise initiatives were perceived as either unsafe or too expensive to coordinate (12).

As you may have noticed, all the barriers stated are interrelated; therefore, concentrating on solving one level will probably not be sufficient for a successful program implementation. Implementation in exercise oncology is complex, and solutions require input from many different stakeholders across every level of the health care system. Clinical managers are often the gatekeepers for system change and are responsible for the cultural shifts within an organization that are necessary to adopt new practices; yet their perspective is largely absent. Their engagement is critical in working toward actionable solutions to integrate exercise into cancer care.

As we are at the very early stages of understanding the field of implementation and exercise oncology, sharing experiences of how programs are designed, created, and implemented can help others overcome barriers and begin the process of identifying best practice. Examples of pathways describing the development and implementation of an integrated cancer program are discussed later in Section 5 of this chapter.

IMPLEMENTATION SCIENCE

Implementation science is the study of *how* to help people and places adopt an evidence-based practice. It can be defined as "the scientific study of methods to promote the systematic uptake of research findings and other evidence-based practices into routine practice, and, hence, to improve the quality and effectiveness of health services" (13).

Implementation science uses theories and frameworks to help design solutions to overcome barriers to action and focuses on different outcomes to traditional research. A popular implementation framework is RE-AIM (**R**each, **E**ffectiveness, **A**doption, **I**mplementation, **M**aintenance). RE-AIM was originally developed to encourage consistent reporting of evidence-based practice and is now used extensively in research translation (14). PRISM (**P**ractical, **R**obust **I**mplementation and **S**ustainability **M**odel) identifies key factors—such as policies, implementation infrastructure, and multilevel organizational perspectives (15)—and has been successfully used to guide planning, make midcourse adjustments to implementation, and evaluating interventions (see Box 16.1).

An example of how the RE-AIM framework can be used is in the evaluation of a nationwide community program for cancer survivors called Livestrong at the YMCAs throughout the US (16). This study examined the data from all the YMCAs that delivered the Livestrong program (a free 12-week exercise program for cancer patients and survivors) from 2010 to 2018. The program had a reach of 62,044 survivors (0.004% of all US cancer survivors), and by 2018, 29.2% of all YMCA associations had adopted the program. As mentioned in Box 16.1, implementation fidelity is the degree to which an intervention is delivered as intended and is critical to a successful translation of evidence-based interventions into practice. Diminished fidelity is one reason why interventions that work well in highly controlled trials may fail to yield the same outcomes when applied in real-life contexts (17). Indeed, of all YMCAs offering Livestrong, only 40% implemented the 3 fidelity checklists (observational assessment, goal setting, and functional assessment). In terms of the maintenance of the program, most YMCAs offered at least 1 program per year. Measuring maintenance with participants was quantified by member conversion percentage, with 46.9% of the participants purchasing a YMCA fitness membership to continue to exercise at the end of the 12-week program. However, Faro et al (16) found that the household area income was associated with the membership

Box 16.1 RE-AIM Framework

The RE-AIM framework evaluates a program on 5 individual components:

- Ability to **REACH** the target population. The absolute number, proportion, and representativeness of individuals who are able to participate in a given program and reasons why or why not.
- **EFFECT** on key outcomes (eg, QoL and economic outcomes; variability across subgroups).
- Willingness to be **ADOPTED** by those responsible for its delivery. The absolute number, proportion, and representativeness of settings and people who are willing to initiate and deliver a program, and why. Note that adoption can have many levels, for example, staff in a hospital or clinic, community setting.
- Success of **IMPLEMENTATION** refers to the intervention agents' fidelity to the various elements of an intervention's key functions or components, including the consistency of delivery as intended and the time and cost of the intervention.
- Potential for it to be **MAINTAINED** is the extent to which a program becomes institutionalized or part of the routine organizational practices and policies. Within the RE-AIM framework, maintenance also applies at the individual level. At the individual level, maintenance has been defined as the long-term effects of a program on outcomes after a program is completed. The specific time frame for the assessment of maintenance or sustainment varies across projects.

conversion rate, and those participants facing financial stress were less likely to buy a membership and continue to exercise at the YMCA. Therefore, to improve the Livestrong service, it was identified that pathways to screen and refer survivors to this program need to be integrated into the standard of cancer care, and efforts to identify strategies and tools to enhance program maintenance need to be developed.

IMPLEMENTATION PATHWAY

To address how to overcome some of the barriers and logistical challenges discussed earlier, it is helpful to examine some current exercise oncology implementation pathways and how they have addressed these issues at different stages of the pathway. Figure 16.1 shows a pathway (18) devised to create accessibility and engagement from clinical to community in rural and urban areas in Ontario, Canada. Also, MoveMore, a nationwide behavior-change program in the United Kingdom (UK), has a pathway that aims to deliver tailored behavior-change support to help PLWC to exercise or become more active at a level that is right for them, depending on their stage of the cancer journey (19). Both pathways consider the need for:

- a team approach to exercise messaging and referrals to reduce the burden on the primary oncology specialists;
- direct access to local programs;
- behavior-change skills for long-term sustainability and participation in independent exercise/active living.

Generating Referrals for Exercise Programs

The role of oncology HCPs in exercise promotion with cancer patients cannot be overemphasized; they represent the starting point for access to appropriate resources and exercise interventions. As mentioned in Section 3, counseling and generating referrals from hospital-based oncology teams to exercise programs can be perceived as time consuming, difficult, and not part of any of the oncology team's job. Webb et al (20) found that only 9% of nurses in the UK talk to all of their cancer patients about the benefits not sure why this is scored through staying active because of time restrictions and difficulty. One way of overcoming this barrier is to help the whole oncology team to understand that increasing accessibility to exercise options for cancer patients is the responsibility of the whole team and not the task of just 1 or a few HCPs. In 2007, the Exercise is Medicine® (EIM) initiative was developed with the goal of incorporating physical activity assessment, advice, and referral as a standard part of patient health care (21). To date, very few studies have used EIM in the oncology care setting (22). The ASCO recommends "the 5 As" process that is the basis of the EIM approach (5), and this is clearly detailed in the paper by Schmitz et al (23) and Figure 11.3.

Step 1: Assess

The HCP should assess physical activity as a vital sign using the questions in Figure 16.2. Asking about physical activity

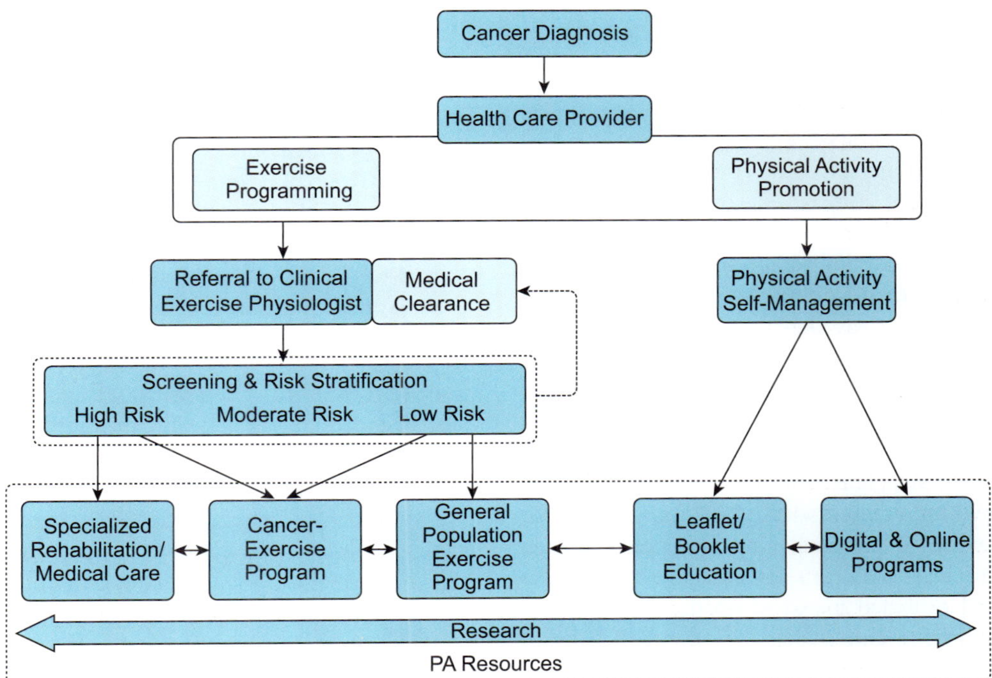

FIGURE 16.1. Ontario cancer pathway. Cancer survivors can enter the pathway at any point after diagnosis. In addition, for those receiving palliative care or living with advanced cancer, the pathway could be instrumental for well-being and overall quality of life. Abbreviation: PA, physical activity. (From Santa Mina D, Sabiston CM, Au D, et al. Connecting people with cancer to physical activity and exercise programs: a pathway to create accessibility and engagement. *Curr Oncol.* 2018;25(2):149–62. https://doi.org/10.3747/co.25.3977.)

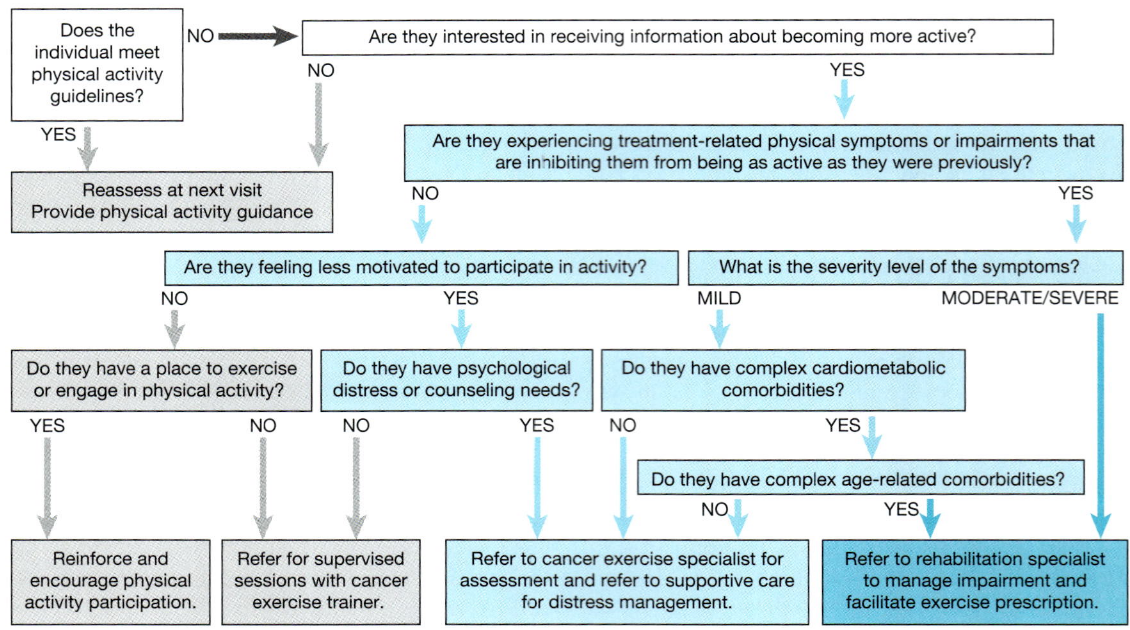

FIGURE 16.2. Referral triage pathway. (From Stout NL, Brown JC, Schwartz AL, et al. An exercise oncology clinical pathway: screening and referral for personalized interventions. *Cancer.* 2020;126(12):2750–8, Figure 2, Part A.)

behavior conveys to the patient that their HCP believes exercise is important to their functioning and recovery.

Step 2: Advise

Clinicians can then advise patients to increase physical activity if they are not currently reaching recommended activity levels. The HCP's willingness to discuss exercise during patient visits serves as a key transition point to change a patient's behavior.

Step 3: Refer

Patients should then be referred to appropriate exercise programs on the basis of their current activity levels, medical status, and preferences. It is also key that all the clinical team repeat these 3 steps (assess, advise, and refer) and reinforce patients' efforts to increase exercise at regular intervals. Webb et al (24) developed a face-to-face/online training for oncology nurses on the delivery of *very brief advice* on staying active to cancer patients. This advice takes 30 seconds to 2 minutes to deliver following an ask, advise, assist (or act) framework. The training was found to be acceptable and practical, improved the delivery of very brief advice on staying active by nurses to cancer patients and ultimately increased referrals (20).

Successful programs also manage to gain the trust of the referring HCPs by providing a referral pathway that is quick and easy to administrate, for example, an electronic record system linking health care databases to local social/community services and establishing an ongoing 2-way communication concerning referred participants. An example of a successful referral pathway is outlined in the evaluation of a nationwide industry-led community exercise program for men with prostate cancer receiving the androgen deprivation treatment called Lucrin (25). From 2014 to 2020, 1,515 eligible prostate cancer patients were referred into the program across Australia by the HCP responsible for prescribing the Lucrin. The Man Plan provides a program with 3 potential forms of delivery: (A) supervised group exercise, (B) home-based exercise, and (C) a support program for those patients unable to exercise. Group allocation is based on patient preference (in consultation with their HCP), presence of comorbidities, and individual fitness levels. Medical consent was provided at referral to the exercise program via a dedicated website. The Ontario and UK cancer program pathways also try to address the issue of providing options for the **hard-to-reach group** of

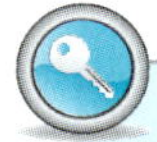

Hard-to-reach group. Sometimes used to describe those populations in a community that face obstacles and challenges to participation in health care services. It can also be used to refer to racial and ethnic minority groups, the LGBTQ+ population, and homeless people, or to refer to groups of people who do not wish to be found or contacted, such as illegal substance users or gang members. In the context of exercise oncology services, it refers to the people underserved by this service, namely, all of the above, including older adults, young people, and people with disabilities, those slipping through the net, and the service-resistant.

PLWC who, for a number of reasons (eg, financial, travel, cancer type, or stage) do not participate in clinical exercise trials.

Cancer patients and survivors have diverse exercise needs and preferences, and one type of exercise intervention will not fit all. Therefore, the pathways to the appropriate exercise offer should include an initial behavior-change intervention and health promotion component delivered by an HCP, preferably with motivational interviewing training. The MoveMore evaluation shows that when high quality motivational interviewing is provided by a competent trainer who completes the process thoroughly, patients find it to be a positive and useful experience that improves adherence to their exercise/activity preferences. Rather than prescribing one standard gym or circuit session, the pathway should offer access to a wide range of physical activities. The MoveMore evaluation demonstrates that the most effective referrals are based on the wishes of the patient, consider local facilities and services, and provide activities at a variety of times and locations easily accessed by public transport.

Medical Screening and Risk Stratification

In order to increase promotion and recruitment by the oncology team to a variety of exercise offers, triage and risk stratification should be an integral part of an implementation pathway. This screening and stratifying into high, moderate, and low risk reassure the oncology team that their patients will be referred to an appropriate and safe program (Box 16.2). Triage provides an understanding of the complexity of a patient's health status, guides clinical decision-making on individual exercise recommendations, and defines the risk for exercise-related complications. Stout et al (26) set out 5 domains that provide a perspective on the complexity of a cancer survivor's condition to guide clinical decision-making for individualized recommendations. The domains include cardiometabolic status, oncologic factors, aging considerations, behavioral characteristics, and environmental elements.

Box 16.2 Patients Requiring Specialist Assessments and Interventions

Patients requiring specialist assessments and interventions:

- Complex acute/chronic cancer treatment side effects, for example, bone metastases.
- Severe physical impairment and/or disability, for example, complex comorbidities.
- Very low functioning levels, for example, frailty.
- Unstable or stable cardiac/respiratory issues, for example, unstable blood pressure.
- Severe psychological disabilities, that is, clinically depressed/high level of anxiety.

Guidance for when to obtain medical clearance is provided in Table 16.2 (27).

Workforce Issues in an Exercise Oncology Program Pathway

It is obvious that one challenge is the development of the appropriate workforce for the implementation of an exercise oncology pathway and program. It is clear that in most situations, no one group of professionals should or could triage, assess, provide advice/behavior change, design, and deliver active living and exercise interventions to every person living with and beyond a cancer diagnosis. On the basis of triage and baseline assessments undertaken by appropriately trained HCPs or clinical exercise professionals, cancer patients can be categorized into 3 groups—high risk, moderate risk, or low risk—and consequently provided with different programs (eg, specialist rehabilitation, targeted support, or universal) run by different professionals.

Table 16.2 Adapted National Comprehensive Cancer Network Triage Approach Based on the Risk of Exercise-Induced Adverse Events

DESCRIPTION OF PATIENTS	EVALUATION, PRESCRIPTION, AND PROGRAMMING RECOMMENDATIONS
No comorbidities	No further medical evaluation[a] Follow general exercise recommendations
Peripheral neuropathy, arthritis/musculoskeletal issues, poor bone health (eg, osteopenia or osteoporosis), lymphedema	Recommend pre-exercise medical evaluation[a] Modify general exercise recommendations based on assessments Consider referral to trained personnel[b]
Lung or abdominal surgery, ostomy, cardiopulmonary disease, ataxia, extreme fatigue, severe nutritional deficiencies, worsening/changing physical condition (ie, lymphedema exacerbation), bone metastases	Pre-exercise medical evaluation[a] and clearance by physician prior to exercise Referral to trained personnel[b]

[a]Medical evaluation as NCCN guidelines for specific symptoms and side effects.
[b]Physical and occupational therapists, certified exercise professionals and rehabilitation specialists.
From Campbell KL, Winters-Stone KM, Wiskemann J, et al. Exercise guidelines for cancer survivors: consensus statement from international multidisciplinary roundtable. *Med Sci Sports Exerc.* 2019;51(11):2375–90. doi:10.1249/MSS.0000000000002116.

Models and settings can vary, but trained cancer exercise professionals play the central role in program design and delivery in clinical, community, and home-based virtual settings.

The specialist and targeted interventions are often delivered by clinical exercise physiologists and physical therapists; targeted interventions are also able to be delivered by trained cancer exercise fitness instructors; and volunteers, support workers, fitness instructors/personal trainers, and rehabilitation/therapy assistants often support people in the universal category. In Australia and some European countries, academic institutions contain a training pathway for undergraduate and/or graduate clinical exercise physiologists to be considered as allied health professionals and work in oncology settings (Exercise and Sport Science Australia and Clinical Exercise Physiologists, UK). Examples of these institutions in the US include the University of Utah, University of Northern Colorado, and Saint Francis University (in Loretto, PA). ACSM® and CanRehab now provide an accredited exercise oncology training programs that are available through ACSM® (https://www.acsm.org/). It is estimated that there are close to 15,000 certified exercise oncology specialists in the US and internationally. More training opportunities through universities or quality-assured commercial training companies are needed to build the workforce and lead to sustained operation in hospitals and communities.

Another validated triage tool is the EXCEEDs tool (28). This approach has been incorporated into the Moving Through Cancer Exercise Directory, which includes over 1,800 programs around the globe. Patients, their caregivers, or HCPs can complete the EXCEEDs tool to receive a report that documents whether the recommendation is for self-directed exercise, community-based exercise, supervised clinical exercise, or cancer rehabilitation. The hope is that by providing this triage tool, free of charge, on the Moving Through Cancer website, it will facilitate one of the most difficult steps in exercise oncology referrals: triage (https://www.exerciseismedicine.org/eim-in-action/moving-through-cancer/).

Evaluation

One of the key components of implementation science is to evaluate the program under real-world conditions. Czosnek et al (29) reviewed 31 real-world programs and showed that the most common outcomes evaluated were feasibility

Box 16.3 Guidelines for a Successful Exercise Oncology Program

1. Ensure that the appropriate workforce is trained and available for the various tasks of the service.
2. Develop a business case ensuring that there is sponsorship and support from the executive/senior-level health care teams.
3. Work with these leaders and clinical academics to develop and undertake an implementation evaluation to justify sustainability of the service.

Tools to Help When Considering Implementation

- RE-AIM: The RE-AIM website provides reflection questions for each factor for planning (link embedded).
- Implementation outcomes: Implementation Outcomes Taxonomy developed by Proctor E, Silmere H, Raghavan R, et al. Outcomes for implementation research: conceptual distinctions, measurement challenges, and research agenda. *Adm Policy Ment Health.* 2011;38(2):65–76. https://doi.org/10.1007%2Fs10488-010-0319-7.
- Business plan template (see the following).

Business plan template:

Executive summary: Briefly summarize your entire proposal so the funder can easily see what your service proposes to do with respect to cost and patient benefits.

Background: Set the scene by giving a background of the issue you are trying to address and how it affects the desired population, and how much it costs/impacts the health care system.

Current service provision (if any): Describe what is currently being done to tackle the issue (if anything).

Proposed service provision: Provide an outline of your proposed service including projected patient benefit as well as financial information, that is, staff costs, equipment costs, venue costs, and travel costs.

Drivers for sustainability: Link how your proposed service will impact on local and national policies and objectives, other advantages to the patient, and organizational advantages.

Deliverables: Include an estimated minimum and maximum number of the patients your service is likely to assist in a specific timescale.

Additional components: Include references and appendices as well as any case studies' examples or patient quotes you have to compliment your proposed service. This helps strengthen your business case and brings it to life.

From Adamson J, Stutz A, Richards N, et al. *Physical Activity Behavior Change Care Pathway.* (Internet). June 2016. Available from https://www.macmillan.org.uk/_images/physical-activity-behaviour-change-care-pathway_tcm9-298138.pdf.

(54.8%) and adoption (45.2%). Interventions were typically delivered in the community (58.6%), in groups (48.3%), and supervised by a qualified health professional (48.3%). Implementation outcomes infrequently evaluated were penetration (3.2%) and sustainability (3.2%). However, very few programs have provided the following valuable information that the RE-AIM framework suggests; these pieces of information should also be collected:

- how many providers are adopting exercise interventions, for example how many clinics within a specific region;
- what portion of total eligible patient population are being referred to interventions;
- the total cost of setting up and running the program implementation;
- how is the program being sustained over time.

Measuring, evaluating, and reporting implementation outcomes from exercise oncology programs offer enormous potential to help conceptualize what is implementation success to pave the way to develop causal relationships between the strategies or tools used during implementation, the exercise offers, and the outcome achieved. Only then do we begin to unpack the implementation process and explain *how* and *why* implementation was successful. See Box 16.3 for guidelines for a successful exercise oncology program.

SUMMARY

This chapter discusses the challenges of implementing exercise programs into oncology settings. Exercise is not included in standard care owing to challenges at organizational, professional, innovation, patient, economic/political, and social levels. Frameworks like RE-AIM, which help evaluate real-world programs, have shown that successful pathways involve referrals from the oncology team, screening for risk stratification, direct community program access, behavior-change support, and the employment of appropriately trained exercise professionals.

Initiatives like *Exercise is Medicine*® promote integrating activity assessment, advice, and referral into patient care. Screening and triaging patients into low-, medium-, or high-risk levels of complexity help to ensure the provision of safe and suitable programs. In conclusion, a successful exercise oncology program requires a multilevel health care system support, communication between stakeholders, workforce training, and evaluation focused on translation into practice.

Case Study

This case study is based on the paper by Kennedy et al (20) "If you build it, will they come? Evaluation of a co-located exercise clinic and cancer treatment centre using the RE-AIM framework. A partnership between radiation oncologists and an international private oncology treatment center and a research team led to the creation of a colocated exercise clinic in an unused space in a newly built cancer treatment center (30). The RE-AIM framework was then used to find if this program increased access to exercise for people receiving treatment and whether it offered an organizational fit and was suitable for continued investment and dissemination by the private international oncology company.

Reach: Over a 50-month period, overall reach was 12%. The majority were female (66%) and 57.2% self-reported as "currently active." When surveying the participants who did not use the service, the common reason was a lack of awareness of its availability.

Effectiveness: The program provided a positive source of connection and socialization, and a chance for connection with people going through a similar experience. The participants felt the program improved their treatment experience, either attributing their participation with a lack of treatment-related side effects or improved ability to recover from treatment. The quality of the program staff was a key aspect of the program. Patients trusted the knowledge and experience of the staff, who were an integral part of the program success.

Adoption: Referrals were mostly from either the center's oncologists (21%) or nurses (20%), with additional pathways including self-referral and social media. All oncologists stated that they were aware of the benefits of exercise and discussed this with their patients when they remembered or had the time to do so.

Implementation: The program started in 2013, but it had to change its availability hours from 6 hours per week to 2 hours per week caused by a reduction in funding. Although the majority of clinicians reported that they were actively referring patients for exercise programs, it is not clear whether there was ever a standard referral structure in place.

Maintenance: No financial model exists for the program. The original aim was to ensure that the program was free to participants so that there would be no financial barrier. The authors stated that there was no ongoing income stream and discretionary funding was volatile.

So, to answer the question "if you build it, will they come?" colocating an exercise clinic into a treatment facility did not overcome the logistical challenges of providing integrated exercise services to patients during cancer treatment. Three important findings from this implementation study are: (A) effective integration requires planning and linking with all stakeholders, (B) a robust model of implementation needs adequate continuous funding, and (C) despite many challenges, an exercise clinic appears to be a good organizational fit for some oncology treatment centers and can assist in the promotion and provision of exercise programs during cancer, specifically to overcome the identified issues, and create a service that is effective, feasible, and sustainable and could inform the development of future hospital-located models of patient care.

Questions

1. Did the exercise program reach those who would most benefit for it?
2. Was it effective?
3. What was the main barrier to sustainability?

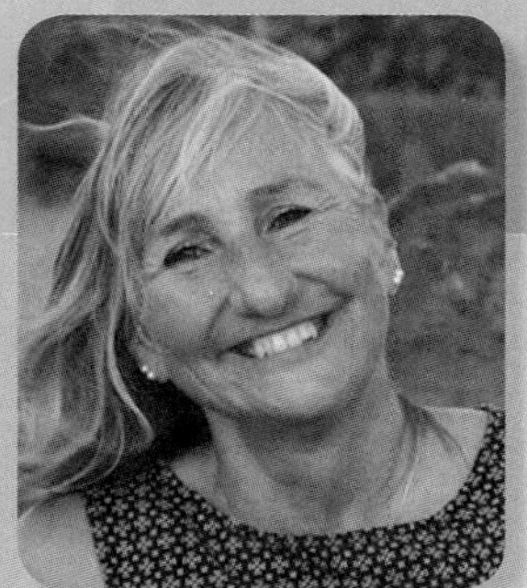

Meet the Expert

FEATURED PROFESSIONAL

Anna Campbell, BSc, PhD

Professor, Clinical Exercise Science
School of Applied Science
Edinburgh Napier University
Edinburgh, Scotland, UK

Q: "Where did you grow up?"

Glasgow, Scotland, United Kingdom.

Q: "Where did you train? What is your training?"

I have a BSc in Immunology from University of Glasgow, Scotland. I then worked as a lab technician at Scripps Clinic, La Jolla, San Diego, CA, USA for 2 years before returning to UK to undertake a PhD in Biochemistry. I completed 1 year of my thesis at University College London, then 3 years at St. Andrews University in Scotland. Subsequently, I worked in the biotechnology industry in Scotland and The Netherlands for 10 years before returning to postgrad school to do a MSc in Sport and Exercise Science at the University of Glasgow.

Q: "What are you best known for?"

I am probably best known for focusing my research on the implementation of exercise oncology evidence into practice with an emphasis on the development of the appropriate workforce, clear referral pathways, and the design and evaluation of pragmatic interventions.

Q: "What are you currently working on?"

I am currently working on developing appropriate training and qualifications for a standard international exercise oncology workforce. In addition, I am researching the effectiveness of virtual supervised exercise programs in terms of cancer-specific outcomes, reach, and cost-effectiveness.

Q: "Anything else you want to include?"

It took me many years to find the ideal job (exercise oncology) that fits with my skills, knowledge, and passion. So remember that your career pathway doesn't need to be clear or straightforward. Personally, I have found supporting people with cancer to become or stay active has been the most fulfilling part of my work.

Favorite Quote:

"It always seems impossible until it is done."
—*Nelson Mandela*

STUDY QUESTIONS

1. Why do clinical trials not translate effectively in the real world?
2. Which of the following is NOT an organizational barrier?
   a. Attitude
   b. Staff
   c. Resources
   d. Capacity
3. In a survey of oncology health care professionals, what % rated their knowledge on counseling based on exercise guidelines as "poor"?
   a. 17
   b. 37
   c. 57
   d. 77
4. From the patient's perspective, what barriers are there with accessibility linked to cost?
5. What do the initials RE-AIM stand for?
   a. Reach, Effectiveness, Application, Implementation, Maintenance
   b. Reach, Effectiveness, Adoption, Implementation, Maintenance
   c. Reach, Effectiveness, Adoption, Innovation, Maintenance
   d. Reach, Effectiveness, Adoption, Implementation, Motion
6. When the Livestrong at the YMCA program was evaluated? Approximately what percentage of the YMCAs had adopted the program?
   a. 10
   b. 30
   c. 50
   d. 70
7. How long does the "very brief advice" take to deliver using the "ask, advise, assist" framework?
8. When undertaking a medical screening, which of these patients would NOT require specialist assessments and interventions?
   a. Complex cancer side effects, for example, bone metastases
   b. Frailty
   c. Cancer-related fatigue
   d. Unstable cardiac issues
9. When Czosnek et al (29) evaluated exercise oncology programs in the real world, which outcome was often NOT collected?
   a. Sustainability
   b. Feasibility
   c. Adoption
   d. Setting
10. When developing the workforce to screen, stratify, assess, design, and deliver an exercise oncology program, which professionals could be involved?

REFERENCES

1. Morris ZS, Wooding S, Grant J. The answer is 17 years, what is the question: understanding time lags in translational research. *J R Soc Med.* 2011;104(12):510–20.
2. Ijsbrandy C, Hermens R, Boerboom LWM, Gerritsen WR, van Harten WH, Ottevanger PB. Implementing physical activity programs for patients with cancer in current practice: patients' experienced barriers and facilitators. *J Cancer Surviv.* 2019;13(5):703–12.
3. Grol R, Wensing M. What drives change? Barriers to and incentives for achieving evidence-based practice. *Med J Aust.* 2004;180(suppl 6):S57–60.
4. Kennedy MA, Bayes S, Newton RU, et al. Implementation barriers to integrating exercise as medicine in oncology: an ecological scoping review. *J Cancer Surviv.* 2022;16(4):865–81.
5. Ligibel JA, Jones LW, Brewster AM, et al. Oncologists' attitudes and practice of addressing diet, physical activity, and weight management with patients with cancer: findings of an ASCO survey of the oncology workforce. *J Oncol Pract.* 2019;15(6):e520–e8.
6. Hardcastle SJ, Maxwell-Smith C, Kamarova S, Lamb S, Millar L, Cohen PA. Factors influencing non-participation in an exercise program and attitudes towards physical activity amongst cancer survivors. *Support Care Cancer.* 2018;26(4):1289–95.
7. Elshahat S, Treanor C, Donnelly M. Factors influencing physical activity participation among people living with or beyond cancer: a systematic scoping review. *Int J Behav Nutr Phys Act.* 2021;18(1):50.
8. Nadler M, Bainbridge D, Tomasone J, Cheifetz O, Juergens RA, Sussman J. Oncology care provider perspectives on exercise promotion in people with cancer: an examination of knowledge, practices, barriers, and facilitators. *Support Care Cancer.* 2017;25(7):2297–304.
9. Park JH, Oh M, Yoon YJ, et al. Characteristics of attitude and recommendation of oncologists toward exercise in South Korea: a cross sectional survey study. *BMC Cancer.* 2015;15:249.
10. Höh JC, Schmidt T, Hubner J. Physical activity among cancer survivors—what is their perception and experience? *Support Care Cancer.* 2018;26(5):1471–8.
11. Haussmann A, Ungar N, Gabrian M, et al. Are healthcare professionals being left in the lurch? The role of structural barriers and information resources to promote physical activity to cancer patients. *Support Care Cancer.* 2018;26(12):4087–96.
12. Fong AJ, Faulkner G, Jones JM, Sabiston CM. A qualitative analysis of oncology clinicians' perceptions and barriers for physical activity counseling in breast cancer survivors. *Support Care Cancer.* 2018;26(9):3117–26.
13. Bauer MS, Damschroder L, Hagedorn H, Smith J, Kilbourne AM. An introduction to implementation science for the non-specialist. *BMC Psychol.* 2015;3:32.
14. Glasgow RE, Harden SM, Gaglio B, et al. RE-AIM planning and evaluation framework: adapting to new science and practice with a 20-year review. *Front Public Health.* 2019;7:64.

15. McCreight MS, Rabin BA, Glasgow RE, et al. Using the Practical, Robust Implementation and Sustainability Model (PRISM) to qualitatively assess multilevel contextual factors to help plan, implement, evaluate, and disseminate health services programs. *Transl Behav Med.* 2019;9(6):1002–11.
16. Faro JM, Arem H, Heston AH, et al. A longitudinal implementation evaluation of a physical activity program for cancer survivors: LIVESTRONG® at the YMCA. *Implement Sci Commun.* 2020;1:63.
17. Breitenstein SM, Gross D, Garvey CA, Hill C, Fogg L, Resnick B. Implementation fidelity in community-based interventions. *Res Nurs Health.* 2010;33(2):164–73.
18. Santa Mina D, Sabiston CM, Au D, et al. Connecting people with cancer to physical activity and exercise programs: a pathway to create accessibility and engagement. *Curr Oncol.* 2018;25(2):149–62.
19. Adamson J, Stutz A, Richards N, et al. *Physical Activity Behavior Change Care Pathway.* [Internet]. June 2016. Available from https://www.macmillan.org.uk/_images/physical-activity-behaviour-change-care-pathway_tcm9-298138.pdf
20. Webb J, Hall J, Hall K, Fabunmi-Alade R. Increasing the frequency of physical activity very brief advice by nurses to cancer patients: a mixed methods feasibility study of a training intervention. *Public Health.* 2016;139:121–33.
21. Lobelo F, Stoutenberg M, Hutber A. The exercise is medicine global health initiative: a 2014 update. *Br J Sports Med.* 2014;48(22):1627–33.
22. Kirkham AA, Van Patten CL, Gelmon KA, et al. Effectiveness of oncologist-referred exercise and healthy eating programming as a part of supportive adjuvant care for early breast cancer. *Oncologist.* 2018;23(1):105–15.
23. Schmitz KH, Campbell AM, Stuiver MM, et al. Exercise is medicine in oncology: engaging clinicians to help patients move through cancer. *CA Cancer J Clin.* 2019;69(6):468–84.
24. Webb J, Foster J, Poulter E. Increasing the frequency of physical activity very brief advice for cancer patients: development of an intervention using the behaviour change wheel. *Public Health.* 2016;133:45–56.
25. Schumacher O, Galvao DA, Taaffe DR, et al. Nationwide industry-led community exercise program for men with locally advanced, relapsed, or metastatic prostate cancer on androgen-deprivation therapy. *JCO Oncol Pract.* 2022;18(8):e1334–e41.
26. Stout NL, Brown JC, Schwartz AL, et al. An exercise oncology clinical pathway: screening and referral for personalized interventions. *Cancer.* 2020;126(12):2750–8.
27. Campbell KL, Winters-Stone KM, Wiskemann J, et al. Exercise guidelines for cancer survivors: consensus statement from international multidisciplinary roundtable. *Med Sci Sports Exerc.* 2019;51(11):2375–90.
28. Covington KR, Marshall T, Campbell G, et al. Development of the Exercise in Cancer Evaluation and Decision Support (EXCEEDS) algorithm. *Support Care Cancer.* 2021;29(11):6469–80.
29. Czosnek L, Richards J, Zopf E, Cormie P, Rosenbaum S, Rankin NM. Exercise interventions for people diagnosed with cancer: a systematic review of implementation outcomes. *BMC Cancer.* 2021;21(1):643.
30. Kennedy MA, Bayes S, Galvao DA, et al. If you build it, will they come? Evaluation of a co-located exercise clinic and cancer treatment centre using the RE-AIM framework. *Eur J Cancer Care (Engl).* 2020;29(4):e13251.

CHAPTER

17

Other Common Types of Exercise

OUTLINE

1. Introduction
2. Other Forms of Exercise
    a. Tai Chi
    b. Yoga
    c. Pilates
    d. Dragon Boat Racing
    e. Other Types of Activities
3. Appropriateness of Other Forms of Exercise
4. Modifying Different Forms of Exercise
5. Summary
6. Case Study
7. Meet the Expert
8. Study Questions
9. References

OBJECTIVES

After completing review of this chapter, students will be able to:

1. Describe the benefits of different types of exercise.
2. Explain why exercise that has not been studied among people living with and beyond cancer may still be beneficial.
3. Comprehend the basics of exercise modification during cancer treatment.
4. Demonstrate how to modify other forms of exercise for individuals to help them meet their goals.

INTRODUCTION

We now discuss the different forms of exercise that have been presented in previous chapters (eg, walking and resistance exercise). Exercises that are discussed here do not have the same volume of research as walking and resistance exercises, yet they are commonly engaged in by people living with and beyond cancer. The threshold used by the 2019 ACSM roundtable authors for evaluating the benefits of aerobic and resistance exercise for people living with and beyond cancer is that there need to be at least 5 RCTs, with a relatively consistent effect of the intervention across studies. In addition, the effect from the studies needs to be greater than zero. For these various different forms of exercise, this level of methodologic rigor for research review is not yet possible, although the body of research for tai chi and yoga is rapidly growing. We include the data that are available, but with the caveat that currently there is neither the volume of studies nor the level of rigor that was required to be included in the ACSM roundtable review (1). Forms of exercise that will be discussed include tai chi, yoga, Pilates, and dragon boat racing. Also reviewed are safety concerns about other forms of activity and sport and ways to modify exercise and an exercise prescription to individualize an exercise program for the person living with or beyond cancer.

OTHER FORMS OF EXERCISE

Many people living with and beyond cancer engage in other forms of exercise than those described in the *ACSM® Exercise Guidelines for Cancer Survivors* (1). Although these other exercises are not formally recommended, they provide many benefits. We review different types of exercises that have a growing body of research to support their recommendations. Other sports and activities should not be discouraged because of a lack of research, but the exercise professional should be thoughtful of how those activities may need to be adapted or the exercise prescription modified for their patients.

Tai Chi

Tai chi, also called *tai chi chuan* or *taiji*, is a form of *qigong*. It is an ancient form of exercise that originated in China. It is a light-to-moderate intensity mind/body form of exercise. There are limited data to support the benefits of tai chi. Some studies used a form of tai chi where the person was either seated or stationary or was a standing qigong meditation. These types of tai chi are not beneficial from an exercise perspective. When tai chi is performed with the intention of obtaining the benefits of physical activity and performed 3 times a week for 40 to 60 minutes over an 8- to 12-week period, there is evidence to support that it improves fatigue and sleep quality in cancer survivors (2). Improvements in hand strength, physical fitness, and physical well-being are also observed with tai chi (3). Self-esteem has also been noted to increase among breast cancer survivors, and QoL improved among a mixed group of cancer survivors (4, 5). Studies of tai chi have been limited by small sample sizes but have suggested that there may be a beneficial effect on cognitive function; however, this finding needs further study (2, 6, 7). Tai chi is an attractive exercise option for people living with and beyond cancer because it does not require special equipment or facilities to practice and does not put undue stress on joints. It also helps to build one's balance. Further rigorous studies are needed to confirm the findings from these studies. A systematic review and meta-analysis of qigong among women with breast cancer demonstrated improved QoL and reduced depression and anxiety when practiced for 60 minutes 5 days a week for 3 months. This study found no effect on fatigue or sleep disturbance compared with women living with breast cancer in the control group (8). In contrast, a systematic review that examined the interventions of Baduanjin qigong found that moderate-to-severe fatigue was reduced and sleep quality was improved for a mixed group of cancer patients (9). Among lung cancer patients qigong appears to improve fatigue, anxiety, and dyspnea (10) when practiced for at least 6 weeks (11). An observational study of 340 participants (N = 184 patients and 120 caregivers) who engaged in tai chi and qigong found significant improvement in well-being among patients in the tai chi class and caregivers in the qigong class. Fatigue significantly decreased for both patients and caregivers in the qigong class, and global distress decreased for both patients and caregivers in the tai chi and qigong groups (12).

Yoga

Yoga is another popular exercise among people living with and beyond cancer. It is a gentle mind/body approach to exercise that includes holding a variety of physical poses, breathing exercises, and mindfulness exercises. A growing body of research demonstrates that this integrative, nonpharmacological activity can reduce the following treatment-related symptoms: sleep disruption, CRF, cognitive impairment, psychological distress (anxiety and depression), musculoskeletal pains, aches, and general discomfort (13, 14). However, a different systematic review noted that pain was not reduced with yoga (7). The differing findings of meta-analyses suggest that more research is needed in the area of pain to determine the effects of yoga. A meta-analysis of 29 RCTs observed that yoga decreased fatigue and depression (15). The type and duration of yoga (gentle hatha, restorative, Iyengar yoga, or Tibetan yoga) varied by study, and some studies did not note an effect until after the intervention ended. Table 17.1 shows a proposed yoga exercise prescription to manage cancer treatment-related toxicities by type of yoga (13, 16-27).

The effect of yoga on the immune system is of great interest for people living with and beyond cancer, but the research on the impact of yoga on biomarkers of stress, inflammation, and immune function is mixed and limited in number.

Table 17.1 Possible Yoga Prescription Cancer-Related Toxicities During and Following Treatment

SIDE EFFECT	TYPE YOGA	TIME (MIN)	INTENSITY	# DAYS	DURATION
Cancer-related fatigue	Anusara Hatha, Iyengar, restorative with breathing exercises and meditation	75-120	Low to moderate	2 days	4-12 weeks
Cognitive impairment	Gentle Hatha, restorative, Iyengar	75-90	Low to moderate	2 days	4-12 weeks
Anxiety, depression, psychological distress	Hatha, Iyengar with weekly counseling	60-90	Low to moderate	1-7 days	3-12 weeks
Insomnia	Gentle Hatha, restorative with breathing exercises and meditations	75-120	Low to moderate	2 days	4-8 weeks
Musculoskeletal symptoms	Gentle Hatha, restorative	75	Low to moderate	2 days	4 weeks

Although there have only been a few studies, the results demonstrated beneficial effects on inflammatory markers of pro-inflammatory cytokines and cortisol levels (CRP, IL-1β, IL-6, IL-8, TNF-α, CD56, and IgA) in RCTs during cancer treatment (23, 28-31). In contrast, other studies found no effect on IL-6, IL-8, TNF-α, or CRP (32, 33). There is a growing interest in the effects of yoga practice on the immune system, specifically on the levels of circulating cortisol and inflammatory markers, such as CRP (32) and cytokines (eg, IL-1β and IL-1α), IL-6, TNF-α, and INF-γ. In the future, biobehavioral research will unveil new understanding about the relationship of physical activity, stress, inflammation, and immune function.

A hypothesized mechanism by which yoga affects cancer-treatment-related toxicities or side effects is shown in Figure 17.1. This theory proposes that cancer and cancer treatment negatively impact the body's normal circadian rhythm and physical function (cardiopulmonary and muscular), heighten the stress response (the HPA axis and cortisol), and impair immune function (32). This in turn leads to fatigue, cognitive impairment, psychological distress, and musculoskeletal symptoms. The theory proposes that yoga may be an intervention to change these biologic mechanisms and improve cancer-treatment-related toxicities. However, few clinical trials have been well designed to test whether these mechanisms explain the benefits of yoga.

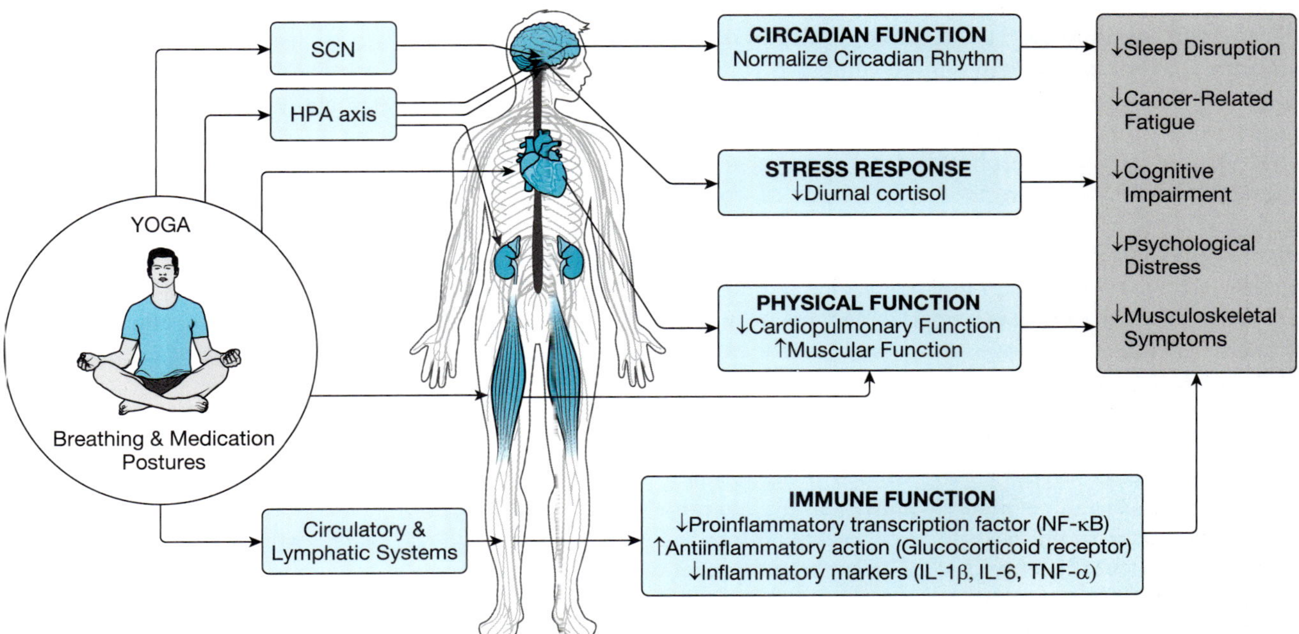

FIGURE 17.1. Theoretical model of behavioral and biological systems affected by yoga on cancer treatment-related toxicities. Denotations and abbreviations: ↑, increased; ↓, decreased; HPA, Hypothalamic-pituitary-adrenal; IL-6, interleukin 6; TNF-α, tumor necrosis factor-alpha. (From Lin PJ, Peppone LJ, Janelsins MC, et al. Yoga for the management of cancer treatment-related toxicities. *Curr Oncol Rep.* 2018;20(1):5.)

Studies of the theory have used Iyengar yoga to demonstrate reduced inflammatory activity in the yoga group compared with the control group that had either stable or increased inflammatory markers (23, 33, 34). Other studies have found no changes in inflammatory markers over a 6-month yoga program (32). The theory and data are promising, but more research is needed to understand the biologic mechanisms involved in the relationship of yoga and the management of cancer-related side effects.

Although there are many promising results from tai chi, qigong, and yoga studies, there is still much to be learned—for example, the optimal style or type of each activity to yield the optimal results for an individual patient. There are also questions about what exercise or exercises are best for cancer patients at different phases of survivorship.

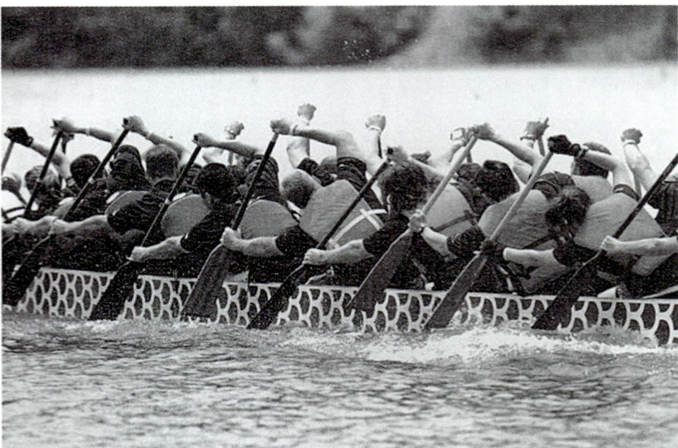

FIGURE 17.2. Dragon boat racing. (From iStock/Serega, August 14, 2007. Available at: https://www.istockphoto.com/photo/dragon-boat-race-crew-gm172212835-3965807?phrase=dragon+boat+racing.)

Pilates

Pilates is a form of exercise that is focused on strengthening specific muscle groups and developing flexibility. A systematic review of 4 studies of women living beyond breast cancer demonstrated that the Pilates exercise group had significant improvements in shoulder ROM, QoL, pain, upper extremity function, mood, physical fitness, and upper extremity circumference compared with the control group (35). Other studies of mat Pilates in women living beyond breast cancer have demonstrated consistent results with significant increases in upper and lower body strength and flexibility (36). A study of 60 women with arthralgia from hormone therapy for breast cancer was randomly assigned to Pilates, a circuit-based exercise program or a control group (37). The exercise groups followed this regimen 2 days a week for 75 minutes, and the control group was asked to continue their usual activities. Pain was significantly reduced in the Pilates group compared with the circuit exercise group. Although the outcomes of these studies show promising results, more research is needed to develop an exercise prescription for Pilates related to different treatment side effects. Another study of women on hormone therapy found that Pilates exercises improved balance and postural alignment (38). Both of these findings are important because improving balance and posture may reduce the risk of falls in a population who are at risk of fracture because of the age and possible osteopenia or osteoporosis (bone thinning and bone loss) associated with aging and cancer treatment.

Only 1 study examined the effect of Pilates exercise at least 1 year post surgery among women living beyond breast cancer with shoulder mobility limitations (39). In this study, 44 participants engaged in twice weekly 60-minute Pilates sessions over 12 weeks. Significant improvement was observed in functional capacity, pain, and QoL measured using the DASH Questionnaire (39) and the Shoulder Pain and Disability Index (39). Significantly fewer women had physical function disabilities, such as difficulty placing objects on a shelf overhead or changing a lightbulb than before the Pilates intervention. The results of this study suggest that an intervention applied during the late postoperative phase can have beneficial effects on functional capacity, QoL, pain, and disability.

Dragon Boat Racing

Dragon boat racing (Figure 17.2) is a way for women living with and beyond breast cancer to engage in a combination of physical, psychological, community, and social support without the focus on cancer (40). The opportunity to participate in dragon boat racing is a means to connect with a community in a health-focused way that fosters camaraderie, fitness, and improved QoL (40-43). An observational study of 100 women living beyond breast cancer found that dragon boat racers reported higher QoL and lower incidence of lymphedema than women engaged in other sports (44). Dragon boat racing has also been observed to reduce CRF (45, 46). A longitudinal study of 60 dragon boat racers followed from 2006 to 2018 noted that only 5 participants developed mild lymphedema (circumference difference about 0.5 cm) (47). This study supports the growing body of research that physical activity improves outcomes of upper limb lymphedema in women living beyond breast cancer. Although there is limited research on this activity, it is a popular activity for women living beyond breast cancer. Men with prostate cancer have begun to discover the benefits of the social support and reframing that come from the dragon boat racing team experience (48).

Other Types of Activities

This chapter has limited the presentation of exercises to activities and exercises that are most commonly engaged in by people living with and beyond cancer. It is important to recognize that there are many other ways to engage in physical activity and exercise that are healthy and beneficial, even if there is no research to support the activity. Any sustained activity will have an aerobic benefit. Therefore, if an individual enjoys hiking, backpacking, mountaineering, cross-country skiing, triathlon, paddle boarding, or any other form of aerobic sport they will reap cardiovascular benefits from these activities. The same is true for resistance exercise. If one is moving a weight in a gym or moving a bale of hay or lifting their body in an activity, such as rock climbing, they are benefiting from resistance exercise. The mechanism may be purer and precisely focused on 1 muscle with free weights or in a gym setting, but the physical act of stacking hay or moving landscaping material is a form of resistance exercise stacking hay or moving landscaping materials is a form of functional resistance exercise which will make one's muscles stronger. At this point, even if there is no research to support a specific form of activity or exercise, there is no reason to say that it is not good or could not have a beneficial effect, as long as it does not cause injury or harm.

APPROPRIATENESS OF OTHER FORMS OF EXERCISE

The appropriateness of other forms of exercise depends on an individual with whom you are working or counseling. Is the individual at risk of falling, drowning, or bleeding? Do they have bone metastasis or CIPN? These are examples of 2 conditions that you must consider and guide an individual to perform an activity that decreases their risk for falls and facture. For example, horseback riding may not be safe for an individual with CIPN that is severe enough to compromise the feeling in their feet and effects their balance. It also may not be appropriate or safe for someone with bone metastasis who could be at risk of a fall and fracture. Another area of concern is risk of infection. Individuals who have access lines, such as a PICC line, are at risk of infection if they swim. Swimming is absolutely contraindicated. It is important to get medical clearance before recommending water sports to such people. Besides the obvious trauma and bleeding associated with a fall, many people receiving cancer treatment may be at increased risk of bleeding because of low platelet counts (thrombocytopenia). Thrombocytopenia puts the individual at risk for a life-threatening bleeding if they hit their head. Therefore, the awareness of where a person is in their treatment cycle and cancer journey is important when counseling people about different activities. Review the side effects of cancer in Chapter 4 and the exercise programming considerations in Chapter 13. Table 17.2 provides examples of some activities people enjoy engaging in and potential risks associated with them.

MODIFYING DIFFERENT FORMS OF EXERCISE

People living with and beyond cancer want to engage in all types of activities and sports without limitations, but this is not always possible. Therefore, it is incumbent upon the exercise professional to determine how to adapt exercise to make these different types of activities possible. Sometimes the modifications may simply be developing the strength to engage in an activity or sport. In this case, an exercise program will be focused on specific resistance exercises to build the strength and power to safely engage in an activity or sport. In another situation, it may involve finding equipment that fits a new prosthesis or a brace to support a recovering limb.

Table 17.2 Examples of Risks and Considerations for Certain Activities

ACTIVITY ↓ RISK →	FALLING	DROWNING	BLEEDING	INFECTION RISK
Skating (ice, roller, skiing)	x		x	
Rock climbing	x		x	
Bicycling, ATV motocross	x		x	
Boating (speed, canoe, raft, kayak, etc)	x	x	x	x
Swimming		x		x
Diving/scuba	x	x	x	x
Skiing (xc skiing, water, downhill)	x	x	x	x
Ranch & agricultural work	x		x	x
Parachute, hang gliding, skydiving	x		x	
Hiking, backpacking, mountaineering	x	x	x	x

ATV, all-terrain vehicle; xc skiing, cross-country skiing.

Table 17.3 Key Concepts Exercise Prescription

Specificity	Exercises, both aerobic and resistance, that are specific to one's success in being able to engage in a specific activity or sport.
Periodicity	Exercise training strategy to increase strength and aerobic capacity. Exercise programs are broken into training periods that consist of cycles of varying lengths. Goal is to increase volume and intensity without causing overtraining, injury, and fatigue.
Microcycle	A variety of exercises planned over a week with different volume and intensity.
Mesocycle	A 2- to 4-week period of exercise training including rest. The 2-week cycle would be more appropriate for someone who is debilitated or just beginning an exercise program. Longer bicycling is more appropriate for fit individuals and athletes. Each mesocycle should conclude with a period of rest or recovery prior to the start of another cycle.
Macrocycle	Cycles of training over an extended period of time (eg, 1- to 4-year period).

If a person living with or beyond cancer wants to resume rock climbing and has been inactive for a year, the exercise program may need to focus on aerobic and resistance conditioning and should include some flexibility exercises so that the individual does not get injured overreaching for a hold or straining and scrambling to maintain their position on a rock wall.

Many people living with and beyond cancer will have a "bucket-list" goal, such as to backpack the Grand Canyon, climb Kilimanjaro, run the Paris marathon, or some other lofty ambitions. Whatever it may be, the exercise professional is key in leading the individual to successfully reach their dream. Slow, methodical exercise programs that carefully consider periodicity, specificity (Table 17.3), and, of course, where the person is at the start of the exercise program (eg, newly diagnosed, learning to adapt to cancer treatment, long-term survivor, and exercise history) will bring them to peak fitness if the principles of exercise physiology are thoughtfully applied. Crafting an exercise prescription requires thought and creativity and some imagination and knowledge of what a person wants to achieve and in what time frame. Exercise programs need to be developed to promote optimal improvement while minimizing the risks of worsening cancer-related side effects (eg, fatigue) or causing injury by prescribing an exercise program that is too demanding and physically overloads the individual. When exercise programs are developed using periodization, there are specific times of higher volume and intensity and rest. The exercise program builds over the course of 2 to 3 weeks and then backs off for active recovery. Within each week (microcycle) rest or recovery is also incorporated into the program. Each microcycle builds on the next with a gradual increase in volume and intensity (Figure 17.3). After 2 to 3 microcycles, the volume and intensity of the next microcycle is reduced to promote active recovery (Figure 17.4). When mesocycles are planned over an extended period, they become a macrocycle. A macrocycle has a wave-like pattern of increasing workload intensity and volume, followed by a period of active recovery (lower workload and intensity). As the individual gets stronger and fitter, the recovery weeks begin to look more like the higher workloads were a few weeks earlier in the exercise plan (Figure 17.5).

SUMMARY

People living with and beyond cancer engage in a wide variety of activities. Tai chi, yoga, Pilates, and dragon boat racing all have some research to demonstrate the benefits for people living with and beyond cancer. Getting people to become more active is key. Therefore, any activity is good, even if there is no research to support it, as long as it does not pose a risk for serious injuries. Exercise programs need to be modified and adapted for individuals based on where they are along the cancer trajectory, their fitness level and exercise experience, and their goals. It is critical to use the principles of exercise physiology when developing an exercise prescription that can be modified when an individual becomes too tired, stressed with work or life events or other factors to help the person living with and beyond cancer meet their individual goals.

Monday	Tuesday	Wednesday	Thursday	Friday	Saturday	Sunday
20 min Aerobic Exercise (AE)	Resistance Exercise (RE) 2 lower body, 3 supper body/core, 8–12 reps x 3 sets	REST	20 min AE	RE	30 min AE	REST

FIGURE 17.3. Microcycle over 7 days includes specificity and recovery.

Monday	Tuesday	Wednesday	Thursday	Friday	Saturday	Sunday
20 min AE walk, jog, bike steady	RE	REST	20 min AE	RE	30 min AE	REST

Monday	Tuesday	Wednesday	Thursday	Friday	Saturday	Sunday
22 min AE	RE	REST	22 min AE 10 min warm-up, 2 min fast pace, 2 min slow, repeat intervals (3 Xs), cool down, easy pace	RE	30 min AE 10 min steady warm-up, 5 min faster pace, 5 min slower, 10 min steady	REST

Monday	Tuesday	Wednesday	Thursday	Friday	Saturday	Sunday
20 min AE steady pace	RE	REST	20 min AE 10 min warm-up, 2 min fast, 2 min slow, 2 min faster pace, 4 min slow to cool down	RE	30 min AE steady	REST

FIGURE 17.4. Three-week mesocycle of increasing intensity followed by an active recovery week. Abbreviations: AE, aerobic exercise; RE, resistance exercise.

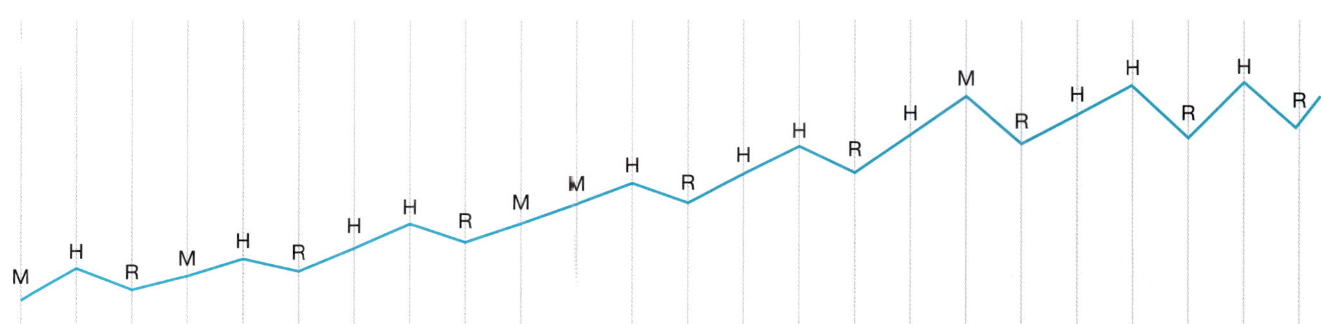

FIGURE 17.5. Macrocycle over a year shows the stair-step pattern and the gradual increase in workload volume followed by recovery. Abbreviations: M, moderate intensity and volume workload; H, high intensity and volume workload; R, active recovery; W, week.

Case Study

Jack is 72 years old with Stage III prostate cancer. His treatment included prostatectomy surgery, radiation therapy, and now ADT with leuprolide to keep the disease under control. He is a hiker and backpacker. Jack worked for the United States National Park Service and was stationed for most of his life at the Grand Canyon. He often hiked to the bottom of the canyon and back to the rim in a day—a hike of at least 16 to 18-miles round trip and an approximately 7,000-feet elevation change. Today he hikes 5 to 7 miles 3 to 4 days a week. He wants to continue his activities despite the severe side effects from his therapy (eg, fatigue, muscle weakness, loss of muscle mass from ADT, depression, and weight gain). Jack has a reunion backpacking trip in the Grand Canyon planned with old friends from his National Park Service days. They will be in the backcountry for 5 days, covering 8 to 10 miles per day with 3,000 to 5,000-foot elevation changes each day. He will be carrying approximately 30 pounds in his backpack.

Questions

1. Is it safe for Jack to backpack? Why?
2. What is an exercise prescription for Jack to prepare for his backpacking trip?
3. How do you modify exercise for an individual who is interested in going backpacking but has been sedentary for 6 months?

Meet the Expert

FEATURED PROFESSIONAL

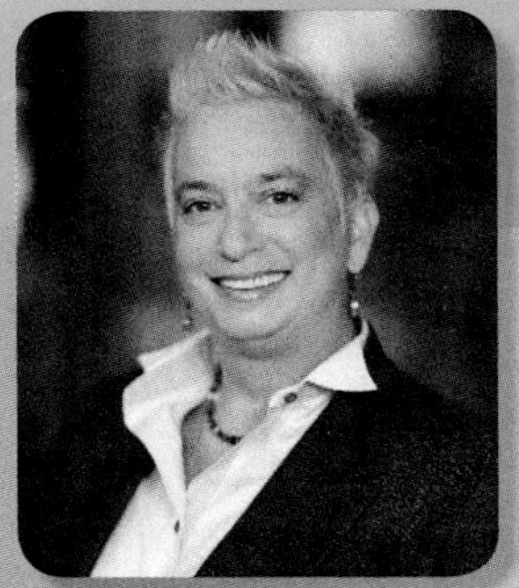

Karen Mustian, PhD, MPH

Professor
Dean's Professorship, Department of Surgery
University of Rochester
Rochester, New York

Q: "Where did you grow up?"

I was born in Henderson, NC, and I grew up moving up and down the East Coast between Florida and New Jersey.

Q: "Where did you train? What is your training?"

I earned my BS in Exercise Science (with a specialization in athletic medicine) and MA in Biomechanics from Eastern Carolina University. My PhD in Exercise Science was earned at the University of North Carolina at Greensboro, where I also specialized in exercise physiology and exercise psychology. I earned 2 additional graduate certifications in Gerontology and Women and Gender Studies. Finally, my MPH in Epidemiology and Clinical Investigation is from the University of Rochester.

Q: "What are you best known for?"

Being the investigator who inserted exercise, yoga, and other mindfulness modes of exercise into clinical trials into the national clinical trial structure.

Q: "What are you currently working on?"

I am currently developing exercise interventions for cancer patients, including interventions to improve function and mobility. I am focusing on translating yoga interventions for underserved populations, including developing a yoga application using evidence-based protocols in an online platform. My goal is to be able to prescribe yoga through the electronic medical record.

Q: "Anything else you want to include?"

When I began my education in exercise science, there was no field of exercise oncology. We thought exercising for cancer patients was harmful and that yoga was a dirty word. I could have never imagined the possibility of a career doing what I do that I love so much and feel so passionate about, and making such a huge difference. I would say to students: be willing to take a risk, be willing to go where others won't go, be willing to do things others tell you are impossible, and never leave your imagination behind.

Favorite Quote:

"There really isn't a better honor in this lifetime than to be able to help good people through lousy times in the work that you do. That's what exercise oncology gives me."
—*Karen Mustian*

STUDY QUESTIONS

1. Tai chi may be indicated to improve for which of the following cancer side effects?
   a. Fatigue, quality of life, sleep, anxiety, and dyspnea
   b. Quality of life, sleep, anxiety, dyspnea, and depression
   c. Sleep, anxiety, dyspnea, and body composition
   d. Anxiety, dyspnea, and body composition
   e. Dyspnea, anxiety, body composition, fatigue, sleep, and quality of life
2. Yoga can reduce which cancer's side effects?
   a. Fatigue
   b. Musculoskeletal discomfort
   c. Cognitive impairment
   d. Psychological distress
   e. All of the above
3. Pilates has been studied mostly with which group of people living with and beyond cancer?
4. True or false. Dragon boat racing increases the risk of lymphedema.
5. Explain why other forms of activities can be safe and acceptable to engage in.
6. Give 3 examples of risks associated with common activities and how to assess if an individual is at risk for them.

REFERENCES

1. Campbell KL, Winters-Stone KM, Wiskemann J, et al. Exercise guidelines for cancer survivors: consensus statement from international multidisciplinary roundtable. *Med Sci Sports Exerc.* 2019;51(11):2375–90.
2. Yang L, Winters-Stone K, Rana B, et al. Tai chi for cancer survivors: a systematic review toward consensus-based guidelines. *Cancer Med.* 2021;10(21):7447–56.
3. Pan Y, Yang K, Shi X, Liang H, Zhang F, Lv Q. Tai chi chuan exercise for patients with breast cancer: a systematic review and meta-analysis. *Evid Based Complement Alternat Med.* 2015;2015:535237.
4. Mustian KM, Katula JA, Gill DL, Roscoe JA, Lang D, Murphy K. Tai chi chuan, health-related quality of life and self-esteem: a randomized trial with breast cancer survivors. *Support Care Cancer.* 2004;12(12):871–6.
5. Mustian KM, Katula JA, Zhao H. A pilot study to assess the influence of tai chi chuan on functional capacity among breast cancer survivors. *J Support Oncol.* 2006;4(3):139–45.
6. Reid-Arndt SA, Matsuda S, Cox CR. Tai chi effects on neuropsychological, emotional, and physical functioning following cancer treatment: a pilot study. *Complement Ther Clin Pract.* 2012;18(1):26–30.
7. Ruano A, Garcia-Torres F, Galvez-Lara M, Moriana JA. Psychological and non-pharmacologic treatments for pain in cancer patients: a systematic review and meta-analysis. *J Pain Symptom Manage.* 2022;63(5):e505–e20.
8. Meng T, Hu SF, Cheng YQ, et al. Qigong for women with breast cancer: an updated systematic review and meta-analysis. *Complement Ther Med.* 2021;60:102743.
9. Kuo CC, Wang CC, Chang WL, Liao TC, Chen PE, Tung TH. Clinical effects of Baduanjin qigong exercise on cancer patients: a systematic review and meta-analysis on randomized controlled trials. *Evid Based Complement Alternat Med.* 2021;2021:6651238.
10. Albrecht TA, Taylor AG. Physical activity in patients with advanced-stage cancer: a systematic review of the literature. *Clin J Oncol Nurs.* 2012;16(3):293–300.
11. Molassiotis A, Vu DV, Ching SSY. The effectiveness of qigong in managing a cluster of symptoms (breathlessness-fatigue-anxiety) in patients with lung cancer: a randomized controlled trial. *Integr Cancer Ther.* 2021;20:15347354211008253.
12. Lopez G, Narayanan S, Christie A, et al. Effects of center-based delivery of tai chi and qi gong group classes on self-reported symptoms in cancer patients and caregivers. *Integr Cancer Ther.* 2020;19:1534735420941605.
13. Lin PJ, Peppone LJ, Janelsins MC, et al. Yoga for the management of cancer treatment-related toxicities. *Curr Oncol Rep.* 2018;20(1):5.
14. Danhauer SC, Addington EL, Cohen L, et al. Yoga for symptom management in oncology: a review of the evidence base and future directions for research. *Cancer.* 2019;125(12):1979–89.
15. Armer JS, Lutgendorf SK. The impact of yoga on fatigue in cancer survivorship: a meta-analysis. *JNCI Cancer Spectr.* 2020;4(2):pkz098.
16. Kleckner IR, Dunne RF, Asare M, et al. Exercise for toxicity management in cancer: a narrative review. *Oncol Hematol Rev.* 2018;14(1):28–37.
17. Banasik J, Williams H, Haberman M, Blank SE, Bendel R. Effect of Iyengar yoga practice on fatigue and diurnal salivary cortisol concentration in breast cancer survivors. *J Am Acad Nurse Pract.* 2011;23(3):135–42.
18. Bower JE, Garet D, Sternlieb B, et al. Yoga for persistent fatigue in breast cancer survivors: a randomized controlled trial. *Cancer.* 2012;118(15):3766–75.
19. Carson JW, Carson KM, Olsen MK, Sanders L, Porter LS. Mindful yoga for women with metastatic breast cancer: design of a randomized controlled trial. *BMC Complement Altern Med.* 2017;17(1):153.
20. Carson JW, Carson KM, Porter LS, Keefe FJ, Seewaldt VL. Yoga of awareness program for menopausal symptoms in breast cancer survivors: results from a randomized trial. *Support Care Cancer.* 2009;17(10):1301–9.
21. Derry HM, Jaremka LM, Bennett JM, et al. Yoga and self-reported cognitive problems in breast cancer survivors: a randomized controlled trial. *Psychooncology.* 2015;24(8):958–66.
22. Janelsins MC, Peppone LJ, Heckler CE, et al. YOCAS©® Yoga reduces self-reported memory difficulty in cancer survivors in a nationwide randomized clinical trial: investigating relationships between memory and sleep. *Integr Cancer Ther.* 2016;15(3):263–71.
23. Kiecolt-Glaser JK, Bennett JM, Andridge R, et al. Yoga's impact on inflammation, mood, and fatigue in breast cancer survivors: a randomized controlled trial. *J Clin Oncol.* 2014;32(10):1040–9.
24. Kovačič T, Kovačič M. Impact of relaxation training according to Yoga In Daily Life® system on perceived stress after breast cancer surgery. *Integr Cancer Ther.* 2011;10(1):16–26.
25. Mustian KM, Sprod LK, Janelsins M, et al. Multicenter, randomized controlled trial of yoga for sleep quality among cancer survivors. *J Clin Oncol.* 2013;31(26):3233–41.
26. Peppone LJ, Janelsins MC, Kamen C, et al. The effect of YOCAS©® yoga for musculoskeletal symptoms among breast cancer survivors on hormonal therapy. *Breast Cancer Res Treat.* 2015;150(3):597–604.

27. Yagli NV, Ulger O. The effects of yoga on the quality of life and depression in elderly breast cancer patients. *Complement Ther Clin Pract.* 2015;21(1):7–10.
28. Witek-Janusek L, Albuquerque K, Chroniak KR, Chroniak C, Durazo-Arvizu R, Mathews HL. Effect of mindfulness based stress reduction on immune function, quality of life and coping in women newly diagnosed with early stage breast cancer. *Brain Behav Immun.* 2008;22(6):969–81.
29. Yadav RK, Magan D, Mehta N, Sharma R, Mahapatra SC. Efficacy of a short-term yoga-based lifestyle intervention in reducing stress and inflammation: preliminary results. *J Altern Complement Med.* 2012;18(7):662–7.
30. Rao RM, Vadiraja HS, Nagaratna R, et al. Effect of yoga on sleep quality and neuroendocrine immune response in metastatic breast cancer patients. *Indian J Palliat Care.* 2017;23(3):253–60.
31. Van Acker HH, Capsomidis A, Smits EL, Van Tendeloo VF. CD56 in the immune system: more than a marker for cytotoxicity? *Front Immunol.* 2017;8:892.
32. Long Parma D, Hughes DC, Ghosh S, et al. Effects of six months of yoga on inflammatory serum markers prognostic of recurrence risk in breast cancer survivors. *Springerplus.* 2015;4:143.
33. Bower JE, Ganz PA, Desmond KA, et al. Fatigue in long-term breast carcinoma survivors: a longitudinal investigation. *Cancer.* 2006; 106(4):751–8.
34. Rao RM, Nagendra HR, Raghuram N, et al. Influence of yoga on postoperative outcomes and wound healing in early operable breast cancer patients undergoing surgery. *Int J Yoga.* 2008;1(1):33–41.
35. Pinto-Carral A, Molina AJ, de Pedro Á, Ayán C. Pilates for women with breast cancer: a systematic review and meta-analysis. *Complement Ther Med.* 2018;41:130–40.
36. Bertoli J, Bezerra ES, Winters-Stone KM, Alberto Gobbo L, Freitas IFJ. Mat Pilates improves lower and upper body strength and flexibility in breast cancer survivors undergoing hormone therapy: a randomized controlled trial (HAPiMat study). *Disabil Rehabil.* 2022;45(3):494–503.
37. Barbosa KP, da Silva LGT, Garcia PA, et al. Effectiveness of Pilates and circuit-based exercise in reducing arthralgia in women during hormone therapy for breast cancer: a randomized, controlled trial. *Support Care Cancer.* 2021;29(10):6051–9.
38. Fretta TB, Boing L, Baffa ADP, Borgatto AF, Coutinho de Azevedo Guimarães A. Mat pilates method improve postural alignment women undergoing hormone therapy adjunct to breast cancer treatment. Clinical trial. *Complement Ther Clin Pract.* 2021;44:101424.
39. Ferreira de Rezende L, Thesolim BL, Dias de Souza S, Bellotto Leme Nagib A, Fonseca Vilas Boas V. The effects of a pilates exercise program on pain, functional capacity, and quality of life in breast cancer survivors one year postsurgery. *Oncol Nurs Forum.* 2022;49(2):125–31.
40. McDonough MH, Patterson MC, Weisenbach BB, Ullrich-French S, Sabiston CM. The difference is more than floating: factors affecting breast cancer survivors' decisions to join and maintain participation in dragon boat teams and support groups. *Disabil Rehabil.* 2019;41(15):1788–96.
41. Sabiston CM, McDonough MH, Crocker PR. Psychosocial experiences of breast cancer survivors involved in a dragon boat program: exploring links to positive psychological growth. *J Sport Exerc Psychol.* 2007;29(4):419–38.
42. Guinto-Adviento ML, Zavala MA. "I am a complete woman": dragon boat and breast cancer survival. *J Sport Psychol.* 2017;26(Suppl 3): 12–16.
43. Harris SR. "We're All in the Same Boat": a review of the benefits of dragon boat racing for women living with breast cancer. *Evid Based Complement Alternat Med.* 2012;2012:167651.
44. Iacorossi L, Gambalunga F, Molinaro S, De Domenico R, Giannarelli D, Fabi A. The effectiveness of the sport "Dragon Boat Racing" in reducing the risk of lymphedema incidence: an observational study. *Cancer Nurs.* 2019;42(4):323–31.
45. Denieffe S, Castineira C, Denny M. The impact of dragon boating for fatigue in cancer survivors. *J Nurse Pract.* 2021;17(8):1019–22.
46. Koehler L, Rosenberg S, Cater J, et al. Quality of life in breast cancer survivors: an assessment of international breast cancer dragon boat racers. *Lymphology.* 2020;53(4):195–203.
47. Mirandola D, Miccinesi G, Grazie Muraca M, et al. Long-term follow up of the impact of dragon boat racing on lymphedema in breast cancer survivors: the Florence Dragon Lady experiment. *Ital J Anat Embryol.* 2018;123(1 suppl):150.
48. Cinà IV, Di Sebastiano KM, Faulkner GE. "One stroke, with twenty-two people": exploring prostate cancer survivors' participation in dragon boating. *J Psychosoc Oncol.* 2020;38(4):375–88.

CHAPTER

18

Models of Exercise Oncology Practice

OUTLINE

1. Introduction
2. Optimal Exercise Oncology Practice Model
3. Models of Exercise Oncology Practice
   a. United States
   b. Beyond the United States
4. Summary
5. Case Study
6. Meet the Expert
7. Study Questions
8. References

OBJECTIVES

After completing review of this chapter, students will be able to:

1. Explain the ideal exercise oncology practice model.
2. Describe multiple current models of exercise oncology practice.
3. Compare models of exercise oncology practice with regard to advantages and disadvantages.
4. Review potential new models that may be possible in the future.

INTRODUCTION

Exercise oncology programs exist in many settings, including hospitals, clinics, rehabilitation centers, the community, and online. The purpose of this chapter is to describe examples of multiple exercise oncology practice models, provide an overview of the reasons multiple models are needed, and compare the types of programs that currently exist. Exercise oncology practice is not a "one-size-fits-all" proposition. After reading this chapter, students will be prepared to propose programming that is appropriate to the population they propose to serve.

OPTIMAL EXERCISE ONCOLOGY PRACTICE MODEL

PLWBC will be connected to exercise programming at specific times in their cancer journey (see Figure 10.1), and may be experiencing a variety of symptoms and challenges based on their health prior to cancer diagnosis and their current treatment regimen (if any).

As an example of extremes, consider Amy, an otherwise healthy 35-year-old woman who plays tennis 4 times a week, and who could be diagnosed with ductal carcinoma in situ (DCIS) (for which treatment may be limited to the excision of the tumor). At the other extreme, consider Fred, a 75-year-old obese, diabetic, sedentary man with osteoarthritis, who could be diagnosed with Stage III colon cancer (for which treatment would be expected to include major abdominal surgery and chemotherapy, with the possibility of an ostomy). The effects of cancer treatment are vastly different for these 2 patients, and potential risk for complications of treatment and potential side effects from exercise for these individuals are distinctly different. What they will need with regard to initial evaluation, instruction, and supervision will be distinct as well. Figure 18.1 depicts proposed steps of an exercise oncology clinical pathway.

The process starts with asking whether the patient meets current physical activity guidelines, followed by identifying and triaging patients according to current symptoms to receive specialized evaluation (eg, from a physical therapist) versus patients requiring no such special evaluation. An example of a symptom requiring additional special evaluation might be recent falls or dizziness. Symptom severity and motivation can be assessed, in addition to logistical and cardiometabolic comorbidities. Taken together, this triage system can lead to 4 possible outcomes:

- Reinforce and encourage physical activity participation.
- Refer to a cancer exercise professional for supervised sessions.
- Refer to a cancer exercise professional for assessment and refer to supportive care for symptom management.
- Refer to outpatient rehabilitation to manage impairments and facilitate exercise prescription.

Regardless of triage outcome, all patients require education regarding the value of exercise for the risk reduction of treatment-related comorbidities, evaluation of current health and fitness and symptoms, and ongoing surveillance for changes in symptoms that might require medical intervention (eg, lymphedema). Finally, after a baseline assessment, all patients should receive an exercise prescription on the basis of their baseline assessment data.

Figure 18.1B denotes appropriate training of professionals, setting, and timing of these activities according to time since diagnosis and current physical status. For example, the person who has recently been diagnosed will require more education, might benefit from a more medicalized evaluation with a physical therapist, and could start with more supervised exercise (high complexity). The cancer survivor who is 5 years out and has returned to normal daily activities requires less evaluation and supervision to start exercise (low complexity or independent).

Amy, a 35-year-old woman with DCIS, would progress through the model with minimal evaluation and education, proceeding to unsupervised exercise soon after evaluation.

Fred, a 75-year-old sedentary, obese, diabetic man with Stage III colon cancer, would progress through the model with more medicalized evaluation and prospective surveillance for the multitude of symptoms and cancer-related outcomes that may arise from the cancer or ongoing comorbid conditions (osteoarthritis).

There is a need to consider the underlying health of the patient, including current and previous comorbid conditions. The more complex the patient's medical condition, the more likely they would benefit from a more medicalized setting, working with an outpatient cancer rehabilitation health care professional. The challenge is that in the vast majority of cancer care delivery settings, no one plays the role with the required educational skills to risk stratify, assess, design, and deliver the optimal program for a patient. Efforts are in development to educate the workforce in courses, such as this text, to be prepared to fill these roles. For example, nurses and physicians and clinical exercise physiologists need to be able to triage and assess patients to refer them to the proper exercise rehabilitation programs, and exercise oncology professionals need to be certified, skilled, and available to welcome them into their practices.

This is an example of a clinical pathway that the field of exercise oncology can aspire to, in collaboration with our interprofessional colleagues in outpatient rehabilitation/health promotion. Licensed health care professionals in outpatient cancer rehabilitation include physical therapists, occupational therapists, speech and language pathologists, dieticians, and psychologists. There are impairments and side effects that might be typically addressed by an outpatient cancer rehabilitation health care professional (eg, lymphedema) or an exercise oncology professional (eg, fatigue). However, it is not useful to make a list of impairments that belong to one versus the other type of professional for several reasons. First, the "right" type of professional may not be available in the

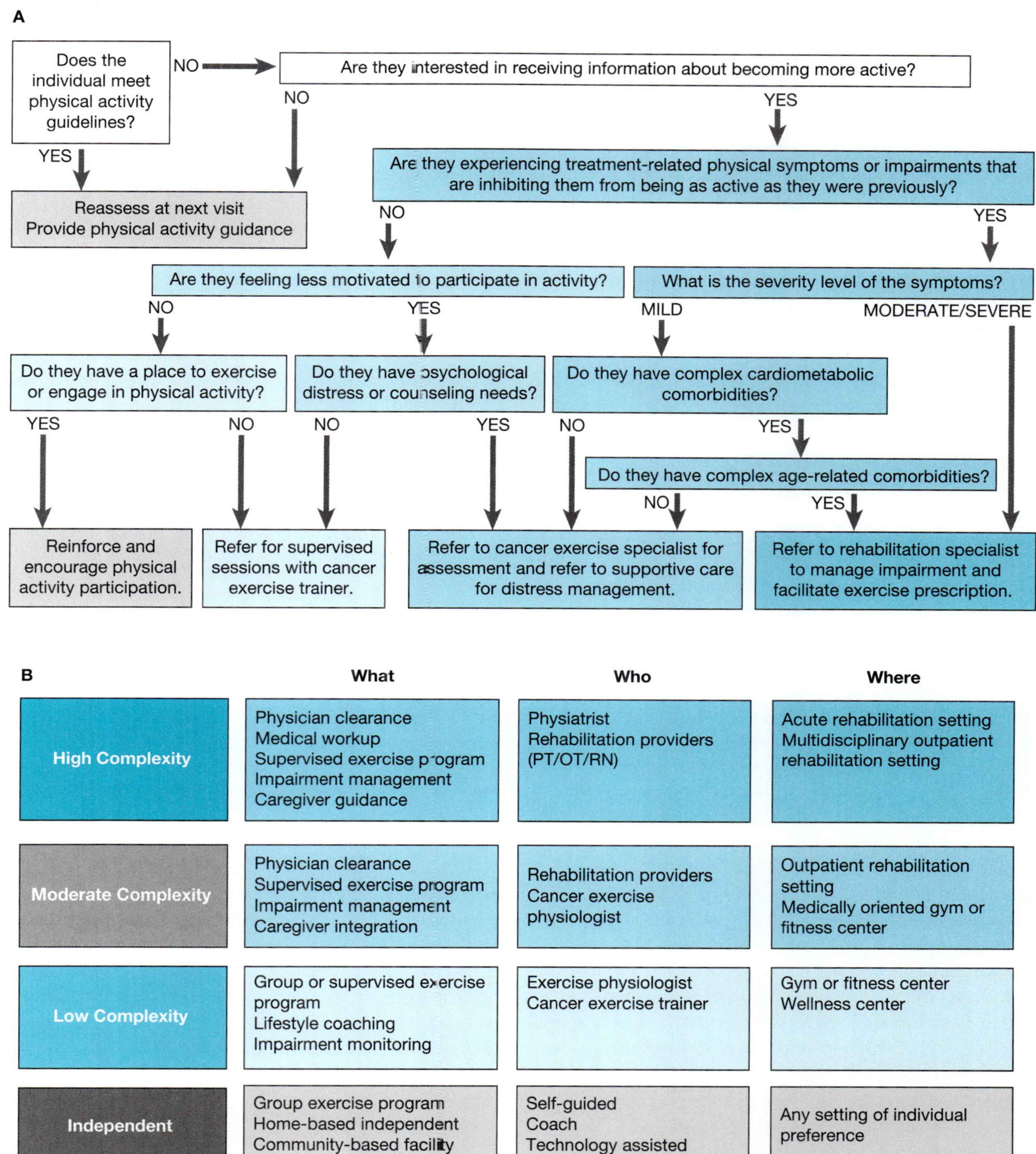

FIGURE 18.1. (A) Algorithm for an exercise referral clinical pathway. The pathway is intended to stratify individuals to higher (red) or lower (green) condition complexity, which provides an insight into the level of supervision and guidance that they may need to successfully engage in exercise and informs referrals to the settings outlined in panel B. (B) Suggested exercise settings and supervision based on individual condition complexity and risk for decline. Abbreviations: OT, occupational therapist; PT, physical therapist; RN, registered nurse. (From Nicole L. Stout DPT, Justin C. Brown PhD, et al. An exercise oncology clinical pathway: screening and referral for personalized interventions. *Cancer*. 2020;126(12):2750–8.)

setting where the patient needs help. If an exercise oncology professional is local but there is no licensed cancer rehabilitation health care professional available, the exercise oncology professional should approach the impairment to the best of their ability and seek consultation from rehabilitation professionals. For this to be an effective approach, exercise oncology professionals need to be adequately trained, including certifications from organizations such as ACSM® or CanRehab. The same is true if there is an outpatient oncology rehabilitation health care professional able to work on specific side effects but no exercise oncology professional available to help the person to become and remain active in an appropriate and enjoyable way. Either way, there are ACSM® resources available to refer patients to an appropriate professional on the Moving Through Cancer website, including a robust, valid triage tool (https://www.exerciseismedicine.org/eimin-action/moving-through-cancer/). Second, patient preferences must be acknowledged. Some patients may feel safer being active in a more medicalized setting, whereas others will prefer a local community or home setting. Third, there is a continuum of impairment or symptom severity that impacts the decision regarding the best setting of care for a given patient. More severe impairments and symptoms may be managed more appropriately and safely in a medical setting with the appropriate equipment and facility.

In short, there are few places around the world practicing exercise oncology or cancer rehabilitation. Challenges to making this standard of practice include that there is currently no funding for exercise oncology professionals in many countries. Cancer rehabilitation is reimbursed in most countries, although inadequately. Exercise oncology professionals do not routinely receive third-party reimbursement for their professional services. Exceptions include the UK and Australia where sessions with qualified exercise professionals are covered by the national health care scheme and several European countries in which physiotherapists provide screening, assessment, and exercise programs in a manner similar to exercise professionals (Netherlands, Germany). Although it is rare, there are examples of this model in the US as well (1). Unfortunately, there is often no staff person in the current cancer care delivery setting to carry out the actions (eg, oncology training physical therapist or oncology exercise professional). When there is a staff member available, it will often be an outpatient rehabilitation professional a licensed health care professional. Connecting that staff member with patients often requires that oncology clinicians make referrals. This requires a shift in clinician behavior in a setting already experiencing time pressures. In short, the incorporation of the approach depicted in Figure 18.1 into cancer care will require a shift in cancer care delivery approaches. There is ongoing research to attempt such changes, but it may be years before this approach is available to the average cancer patient treated in the community oncology setting. At present, for most PLWBC, there is no systematic manner to refer patients into exercise oncology practice.

This situation could contribute to the health disparities seen in cancer survivorship (2). It could be hypothesized that patients with more resources and ability to be flexible with their time (more likely to be both White and higher income) are more likely to find their way to exercise oncology programs than those with fewer resources who are often racial/ethnic minority, have lower income, and live in rural or medically underserved areas. Lower income, rural, and racial/ethnic minority patients are more likely to report the symptoms addressed by an exercise oncology program (3-5). Making exercise oncology standard of care may address inequalities of health care across race, ethnicity, income, and geography. Exercise oncology professionals are urged to share this perspective with the leadership of the oncology settings with whom they partner, toward the goal of making progress on this health equity challenge.

MODELS OF EXERCISE ONCOLOGY PRACTICE

United States

In the US, there is no third-party coverage for exercise oncology programs unless it is delivered by a licensed health care professional, such as a physical therapist. As such, the models that have developed can be described as covered or not covered by insurance.

Exercise oncology as delivered by licensed health care professionals may also be called cancer rehabilitation services (1). These services are offered by licensed physical therapists or occupational therapists and, with rare exception, will be impairment driven. This means that the patient is referred to the therapist on the basis of an impairment identified by an oncology clinician as needing medical attention. The impairments for which oncology clinicians may make this referral include many of the symptoms for which exercise is documented to be an effective intervention, such as BCRL, fatigue, or physical function impairments. If a patient is referred to a physical or occupational therapist for fatigue or physical function impairments, the patient will receive a treatment plan that includes exercise training, which may be supervised by an exercise professional who may or may not be an oncology-certified exercise professional.

Exercise oncology is also practiced in the US by exercise professionals with specialty training in how to safely and effectively deliver exercise to PLWBC (6). The format of these programs varies broadly, including group fitness programs; structured one-on-one supervised programs; consultation programs that evaluate the patient, prescribe an exercise program, and send the patient home to exercise on their own; synchronous online group fitness classes; and asynchronous online exercise videos that patients and survivors can follow along on their own timing. There have

Table 18.1 Models of Exercise Oncology Practice in the US Model

	ADVANTAGES	DISADVANTAGES
Dragon boat racing teams	• Evidence shows that the activity is safe with regard to lymphedema risk • Camaraderie • Social support • Structured activity	• Only available in select cities • Requires time commitment • Training of coaches may not include standard exercise oncology training
Charity-based team training	• Social support • Structured activity	• Training of coaches may not include standard exercise oncology training
Group fitness programs	• Some of these programs are free • Social support • Sometimes training of coaches is standardized	• Only available in select cities • Restricted to times and places when the classes are offered
Structured one-on-one programs	• Convenience • One-on-one attention • Highly trained staff	• Cost • Only available where there are trained staff
Consultation programs	• Convenience • One-on-one attention • Highly trained staff	• Cost • Only available in settings where consultation programs exist
Personal training	• Convenience • One-on-one attention • Highly trained staff	• Cost • Only available where there are trained staff
Synchronous online exercise classes	• Convenience • Highly trained staff • Social support	• Requires technology and Wi-Fi connectivity
Asynchronous online exercise for people living with and beyond cancer	• Convenience	• No supervision • Requires technology and Wi-Fi connectivity

been prior reviews of community-based exercise oncology research; however, these reviews have primarily focused on the results of research studies performed in a community setting, rather than community-based programs outside of the realm of research (7). Identified community-based programs that exist separate from research include multiple models of practice, such as dragon boat racing teams, charity-based team training, group fitness programs, structured one-on-one training programs, personal training, and consultation approaches. Examples of each of these models of practice are described in the following sections and in Table 18.1.

Dragon Boat Racing Teams

Dragon boat racing started originally in China. It is a water sport in which 16 people sit astride in a long boat, with a drummer guiding the cadence of oar strokes. In 1995, a sports medicine physician named Don McKenzie at the University of British Columbia started a dragon boat racing team of breast cancer survivors. Not long thereafter, he and his colleagues published case-study evidence that the activity was safe with regard to lymphedema risk (8). The sport has grown in popularity for breast cancer survivors, with thousands participating competitively annually around the world (9). Training of the dragon boat racing coaches in exercise oncology is not currently standardized.

Charity-Based Team Training

Several cancer charities have developed programs to train people to compete in running, cycling, and other types of athletic events. Participation requires raising a specific amount of money for the charity, in return for coaching and support to get ready for the event. An example of this is the "Team in Training" program of the Leukemia & Lymphoma Society® (10). These charity-based team training programs are not specifically designed to address the needs of PLWBC, but they are inclusive. The training of charity team coaches is general to the sport being coached, not specific to exercise oncology.

Group Fitness Programs

Group fitness programs bring PLWBC together at a fitness facility, once a week or more, for a specified number of weeks (eg, a 12-week program). Some programs focus on patients currently receiving treatment, others focus on those who have completed treatment, whereas some include both. The staff will have specialty training to work with PLWBC. The program may include time for social activities in addition to exercise, exercise evaluations, and some individualized attention to participants from staff. Generally, the focus will be on aerobic and resistance exercise as well as flexibility training, although there may be specific sessions during which yoga and other forms of exercise are introduced. To participate, it is often required that there be a written referral from an oncology professional. There are usually screening procedures as well to ensure the safety of participation. (Details of common screening processes are covered in Chapters 9, 11-13.) An example of this type of program is the Livestrong at the YMCA, which has been in place since 2008 and has served around 62,000 survivors (11). Advantages of this type of program include that (A) it is free to the participants and (B) the social aspect of the program. The benefits of social support for promoting exercise adherence are well documented (12). Disadvantages include that the program is usually offered 2 or 3 times a year by the participating YMCAs, and if a patient's cancer timing does not match up with the start of a new class, then there can be delays in starting the class. Further, despite being free, there are concerns about the potential for inequities in access to this program, given it is offered at a specific time of day, requiring that participants have the freedom to make their calendar and transportation availability fit with the program. It has been estimated that the program costs the YMCAs approximately $500 per participant (13). There is a specific training standard operating procedure and certification required of all YMCA staff who participate in leading the Livestrong program.

Structured One-on-One Programs

Structured one-on-one programs can be offered onsite at an oncology clinic or at a separate location, such as a fitness facility. Such programs can be offered before, during, and after neoadjuvant and adjuvant therapies. The most convenient option is to offer the program onsite at times when the patient is coming into the clinic for treatment. This enables patients in active treatment to complete an exercise session the same day as a clinical oncology appointment. These structured programs generally require permission to participate from a treating oncologist and include baseline evaluations to discern the appropriate exercise prescription. Some of these programs work in phases, like cardiac rehabilitation, including a phase for pretreatment (prehabilitation), during active treatment, immediately post treatment, and in long-term survivorship. These programs may supervise the exercise onsite once weekly and encourage patients to perform some activities on their own at other times during the week. The focus of these programs is individualized according to the baseline evaluation and may include aerobic exercise, resistance exercise, balance activities, or flexibility training. It has been estimated that a 12-week program of exercise one-on-one onsite at a clinical setting would cost a hospital or health system about $610 per patient, but the program is provided without any cost to the patient (14, 15). Advantages of this approach include the convenience for the patient, as well as access to and support from trained staff. Disadvantages include the need for space in a setting where space is at a premium: the oncology clinic. One such approach was taken by Maple Tree Cancer Alliance®, which has 54 locations across the US and beyond (16). Maple Tree Cancer Alliance® has served over 11,000 patients in its 10 years of existence, underscoring the convenience for patients. To begin working with cancer patients and survivors, Maple Tree Cancer Alliance® requires a minimum of a bachelor's degree, a nationally recognized personal training certification, and completion of a specific 12-week training program from Maple Tree University.

Consultation Programs

Consultation programs can also be offered on site at an oncology clinic, or at a separate location, such as a fitness facility. As with the other examples, this approach starts with a referral from an oncology clinician and a baseline evaluation. After that, there is a personalized exercise prescription developed and written materials are provided to the patient. There may be a few supervised sessions to teach the participant how to do the exercises mentioned in the prescription. Equipment such as resistance bands might be provided to the participant for home use. As soon as the exercise oncology professional feels the patient can safely perform the exercise program independently, the participant is released to continue the program at home. The option always exists to come back with further questions or to adjust the prescription as the patient proceeds through their cancer journey. The advantages of this model include that it can be done on site with minimal space, and (in theory) a greater number of patients can be served by a single exercise oncology staff person than with the one-on-one supervised program. Disadvantages include that there may be patients who are not ready to safely exercise on their own. An example of this program is the Cancer Wellness for Life program at 7 hospitals in Kansas, developed by Sami Mansfield (17). It has been estimated that consultation programs cost hospitals/health systems $193 per patient, but the programs are often provided to patients without cost (17, 18). Cancer Wellness for Life trainers work in tandem with physical therapists and must have at least a bachelor's degree, a national personal training certification, and specialty training and certification in exercise oncology.

Personal Training

In addition to structured one-on-one programs with specific protocols, those living with and beyond cancer may choose to work with a personal trainer for a brief time or for ongoing help over a period of weeks, months, or years. This structure is determined by mutual agreement of the survivor and the personal trainer, as opposed to following a particular structured program as discussed earlier. According to the ACSM®, it is estimated that there are over 15,000 certified exercise oncology professionals in the US. Most of them have a national certification as a fitness professional in addition to specialty training appropriate for delivering the program. There are multiple organizations that offer training programs to prepare exercise professionals to carry out exercise programs with PLWBC, including the Cancer Exercise Training Institute (www.thecancerspecialist.com) or CanRehab (www.canrehab.com). These professionals can carry out much of what is described in the ideal exercise oncology practice in Figure 18.1. They should partner appropriately with licensed outpatient rehabilitation professionals when there is a medical issue to address beyond the scope of practice for exercise oncology professionals (eg, onset or worsening of lymphedema), as discussed in Chapters 10 to 13. Advantages and disadvantages of working with a personal trainer with oncology specialty training are similar to the advantages of the structured one-on-one onsite programs, though these services are fee for service and typically not colocated with oncology treatment centers (Table 18.2).

Synchronous Online Exercise Classes

Partly as a result of the COVID-19 pandemic, there has recently been a rise of available online classes for cancer patients and survivors. Two examples of organizations that offer these classes are 2Unstoppable (www.2unstoppable.org) and FitSteps for Life (www.cancerfoundationforlife.org/fitsteps-live-zoom-exercise-class-schedule/). These classes can be specifically designed for a variety of fitness levels (chair exercise vs standing whole body workouts) or specific disease groups (metastatic breast). FitSteps and 2Unstoppable both offer their classes on a drop-in basis, and patients can join online for any class they choose. In addition, 2Unstoppable offers a structured 6- and 10-week group class that includes cardiovascular and resistance training activities. Advantages of synchronous online classes include that they are generally offered without cost to the patient, they are convenient, and the instructors usually have specialty training in exercise oncology. Disadvantages include limited personalization, the need to be available when the classes are offered, and limitations of what is offered compared to what might be needed or preferred by patients. Finally, there is an assumption of access to technology and internet connectivity.

Asynchronous Online Exercise for People Living With and Beyond Cancer

Finally, there are options for those impacted by cancer to log on and use a preloaded video to help them exercise. Examples include the library from FitSteps for Life (www.cancerfoundationforlife.org/exercise-videos/), the videos at www.MovingThroughCancer.org, and a subscription service called MyVictory.com that charges $5 a month for access to a library of thousands of videos ranging from a mild exercise like chair exercise to vigorous aerobic and resistance exercise sessions.

Cancer Exercise is an app developed by Dr. Anna Schwartz, which she developed on the basis of more than 20 years of her research. It uses the principles of exercise physiology and has built-in periodicity that varies according to the fitness and strength testing done at baseline and 6-week intervals. The app constantly adapts to each user to create an individualized exercise program depending on where the person living with or beyond cancer is in their cancer journey, their previous experience with exercise, and their goals. On a daily basis, the app adapts to the individual's level of fatigue to deliver a personalized exercise prescription for a beginner just starting to exercise to an advanced athlete learning to balance exercise during treatment or returning to exercise. The *Cancer Exercise* app is available for iPhone and android users at no charge for PLWBC, and there is a data collection version available for research.

Asynchronous online exercise options are perhaps the most convenient possibilities, as they can be accessed when and where the patient prefers. They are generally developed by experts; however, there is obviously limited personalization or supervision with these options. Some of the asynchronous options are free, whereas some cost a nominal amount. They all assume access to technology and internet connectivity.

Beyond the United States

The US-based models discussed in the aforementioned sections exist in many places around the globe. However, there are some specific exercise program-related and organizational implementation differences in specific international locations that are worth noting. Some of these are reviewed in the following sections.

United Kingdom

In the UK, a large cancer charity called Macmillan Cancer Care took on the issue of trying to support people affected by cancer to become or stay active in a large behavior-change initiative called Move More (19). Move More is an evidence-based service providing tailored, behavior-change support to help PLWC to become more active or maintain a level of physical activity, depending on their stage of the cancer journey. It comprises 5 elements: raising awareness, referral pathway, behavior-change intervention, physical activity offer, and ongoing behavior-change support. All services offer access to a wide range of physical activities that consider local facilities and services and provide activities at a variety of times and locations that can be accessed by public transport, based on the needs of PLWC. Services based in

Table 18.2 Qualified Exercise Professionals Appropriate to Work With People Living With and Beyond Cancer: Credentials and Oncology Training in North America

	PREREQUISITES	CONTINUING ED	CERTIFICATION RECOGNITION	LIABILITY INSURANCE
QEP EXERCISE OCCUPATIONAL CERTIFICATIONS				
Canadian Society for Exercise Physiology				
Certified Exercise Physiologist	• Minimum of 100 h of practical experience • Qualifying theory exam • Qualifying practical exam	Required	Canada	Required
American College of Sports Medicine®				
Exercise physiologist	• Qualifying theory exam	N/A	US	Recommended
Certified clinical exercise physiologist	• Bachelor's degree with 1,200 h experience or master's with 600 h practical experience • Qualifying theory exam	Required	US	Recommended
American Council on Exercise				
Medical exercise specialist	• Bachelor's degree with 500 h of practical experience • Qualifying theory exam	Required	US	Recommended
SPECIALIZED CANCER EDUCATION/TRAINING				
American College of Sports Medicine®				
ACSM®/American Cancer Society Cancer Exercise Specialist	• Completion of a 12-module course • Summative assessment • Qualifying practical exam • Bachelor's degree in exercise physiology	Required	US	Recommended
University of Northern Colorado Cancer Rehabilitation Institute				
Clinical cancer exercise specialist workshop	• Exercise physiologists, physical therapists, nurses, nurse practitioners, rehabilitation specialists, personal trainers, and other medical professionals	N/A	US	N/A
Thrive Health Services				
Thrive health services	• No prerequisites noted on website • Qualifying theory exam	Required	Canada	N/A
Cancer Exercise Training Institute				
Cancer exercise specialist	• No prerequisites noted on website • Qualifying theory exam	N/A	US	N/A

leisure settings benefit from easier access to a wider range of classes and facilities, which makes the transition from free sessions to continued activity more straightforward than in a health care setting. A key factor to success in any delivery model is ensuring that instructors are knowledgeable concerning physical activities and the needs of PLWC.

Current services include signposting (educating patients on benefits of and opportunities to stay active), provision of information booklets, asynchronous online classes, in-person group exercise sessions, and volunteers who organize physical activity opportunities, such as walking groups and gentle movement sessions in libraries. The scheme is intended to provide a full year of support to become physically active and maintain a physically active lifestyle. Patients can self-refer to the program or can be referred to the program by a cancer charity or a medical professional. The advanced exercise professionals who are employed by the UK's National Health System or council-run community centers and work with the Move More program are largely trained by CanRehab, led by Dr. Anna Campbell.

The Netherlands

In the Netherlands, exercise for patients with cancer is often supervised by physiotherapists. Physiotherapists can obtain a master's degree in oncology. The majority of oncology physiotherapists is registered at Onconet (www.onconet.nu). This is a foundation that aims to provide accessible and high-quality supervision of exercise programs in patients with cancer. Being registered at Onconet ensures training according to the most recent standards and regular education is obligatory. Another possibility for patients is to exercise under the supervision of a fitness trainer. Fitness trainers can acquire the status oncological fitness trainer by taking the ACSM®-certified exercise-oncology course, which is offered regularly in the Netherlands. Physiotherapists and fitness trainers are listed at the website www.kanker.nl, which is an initiative of the Dutch Cancer Society (KWF), Dutch Federation of Cancer Patient Organisations (NFK) and the Netherlands Comprehensive Cancer Organisation (IKNL). Through this website, healthcare professionals and patients can search for a qualified exercise professional close to their home. Both physiotherapists and oncological fitness trainer have their own training facility to accommodate exercise training. In addition, there are some local initiatives that, for example, provide running training to patients with breast cancer.

Generally, exercise for patients with cancer is not reimbursed as part of the standard health insurance. There are certain conditions under which (part of) the exercise program is reimbursed. Reimbursement conditions of insurers can change every year.

Spain

In Spain, access to health care is "universal," that is, guaranteed by the government for everyone (eg, including recent, unemployed immigrants) and thus based on a public system solely supported by citizens' taxes—although there is also the option of private health care. Thus, all patients with cancer of all ages, ethnicities, or socioeconomic status receive the best possible cancer treatment available irrespective of the associated cost. Obviously, this setting makes it difficult to implement large-scale exercise interventions for patients with cancer in public centers as there are other priorities.

In fact, as opposed to clinicians, nurses, physical therapists or even some basic researchers working in hospitals with public contracts, fitness specialists (ie, those with an academic background in exercise sciences/physiology) are not yet considered health professionals per se that must be paid by the government. As such, professionally supervised, structured exercise interventions are seldom included in public hospitals, unless in a research setting with funding and staff's salaries coming from grants or patients' foundations. In this effect, arguably the only exception for systematic exercise implementation in public hospitals is the project led by Dr. Carmen Fiuza-Luces (https://paherg.com/), where all the children and adolescents with cancer treated in the 4 main reference public hospitals of the capital of Spain, Madrid (Niño Jesús University Children's Hospital, the La Paz University Hospital, Hospital 12 de Octubre, and Hospital Gregorio Marañón, all prestigious university hospitals) are offered the possibility of performing supervised exercise programs during (including hematopoietic stem cell transplantation) and/or shortly after treatment with well-trained fitness specialists whose salaries come from national/international research grants or private foundations. These 4 hospitals are well equipped with gymnasia ad hoc (that include modern training machines, treadmills or cycle-ergometers; see examples https://aceleradoraunoentrecienmil.org/; https://aladina.org/apoyo-emocional/programa-de-ejercicio-fisico/) and clinical exercise physiology laboratories funded by the aforementioned grants (from Spain, the UK [https://www.wcrf.org/researchwefund/exercise-lifestyle-intervention-adolescents-cancer/], and the European Union [https://fortee-project.eu/]), as well as patients' foundations.

There are currently 4 possibilities through which patients can participate in physical exercise programs:

1. Research in the public health setting, as mentioned in the prior paragraph.
2. Foundations or patients' associations: different nonprofit institutions are developing exercise programs for cancer patients in public hospitals, such as "Unoentrecienmil Foundation," "Aladina Foundation," "Spanish Association Against Cancer (AECC)," "UAPO Foundation," "Amiga Foundation"; "ICAPEM Association," and "VEnCE Program" (20-22).
3. Private centers specialized in exercise and cancer, with exercise programs prescribed by well-trained fitness or personal trainers.
4. Public programs developed in community sports centers, with patients referred by the public health services. This possibility is rare and only offered in certain locations of the country (city of Murcia or Basque country).

Germany

In Germany, professionals with a sports science background or other movement-associated education can qualify for a variety of exercise oncology licenses. Most comprehensive qualifications are offered though the German Union for Health Exercise and Exercise Therapy (DVGS) addressing professionals mostly with an academic background, including physiotherapists. Professionals educated through the DVGS are qualified to work in in- and outpatient cancer rehabilitation, as well as in local physiotherapy facilities. Every cancer patient in Germany has the opportunity to participate in a 3- to 4-week in- or outpatient interdisciplinary cancer rehabilitation covered by the pension or health care insurance. Rehabilitation includes exercise/movement therapy-based interventions, as well as psychosocial, nutritional, and other supportive measures. Exercise/movement therapy-based interventions represent more than a half of the administered sessions during rehabilitation. After going through this rehab process, patients in Germany have the option to participate in a close-to-home exercise program offers for up to the 6 months to transfer lessons-learned on exercise behavior into their daily routine. According to the needs of patients and based on availability, there are a variety of offerings available from community-based exercise groups (up to 12-15 participants) led by qualified sport club trainers to exercise therapy-based offers in smaller groups (up to 5 participants). The education for trainers in sports clubs is led and organized by the National Paralympic Committee.

Even with having a comprehensive rehabilitation offering for cancer patients (even for those who are in advanced stages), the main challenge in Germany is that only about a third of all cancer patients are participating in such a program and that there is no coverage for exercise therapy before or during cancer treatment. Qualified exercise programs and counseling offers in Germany can be found through the OnkoAktiv network (https://netzwerk-onkoaktiv.de) and through the German Olympic Organization and National Paralympic Committee (https://bewegungslandkarte.de/).

Australia

In Australia, exercise professionals can acquire the status of Accredited Exercise Physiologist or AEP. AEPs are university-trained practitioners who have accumulated at least 500 hours of supervised, practical experience, including at least 360 hours working with clients with chronic conditions such as cancer during their training. Once in practice, AEPs must meet yearly professional development standards and maintain at least 1,000 hours of practice every 5 years. AEPs can receive reimbursement for working with PLWC through the Medicare General Practitioner Management Plan (GPMP) program (23). This program provides people living with a chronic condition access to comprehensive care from a range of 13 allied health professionals under a Team Care Arrangement. Up to 5 allied health appointments are available each year. The 5 appointments are shared across all professionals. Only general practitioners can prescribe these plans; oncologists cannot. This has posed a barrier for some patients to access funded exercise services during and after cancer treatment.

Similar to the US, there are large specialty centers in urban centers of Australia with charity-funded exercise oncology programs that practice using many of the same models described as occurring in the US. Additionally, there are pharmaceutical-funded exercise programs available nationally for people with prostate cancer who receive a referral from their oncology care team.

SUMMARY

The field of exercise oncology practice is changing rapidly. A major ongoing challenge is the standardization of referrals to an exercise oncology program and the patchwork of available programs to meet the needs of individual patients, as evidenced by the directory of over 2,000 programs across the US at exerciseismedicine.org/eim-in-action/moving-through-cancer/. Exercise oncology professionals will need to continue to advocate for the standardization of an exercise oncology program to ensure that all patients are able to benefit from exercise during and after their cancer treatment.

Case Study

Rather than providing a single case study, for this chapter, we provide a list of patients with varying diagnoses, treatments, and underlying medical conditions, as well as timing since diagnosis. The goal is for students to match the patient with the least restrictive model of practice described in the chapter.

Patient A. A 40-year-old man, obese, diabetic, sedentary, smoker, had bladder cancer last year, has an external bladder, and is currently undergoing biological therapy every few months to prevent recurrence.

Patient B. An 80-year-old woman walked 15 miles a week, normal weight, elevated BP, no diabetes, Stage I breast cancer, lumpectomy completed, and no further treatment planned. Flexible schedule.

Patient C. An 18-year-old woman, runs track, generally healthy, Stage III melanoma, just diagnosed, will undergo immunotherapy for several months.

Patient D. A 55-year-old man, sedentary, high BP, overweight, not diabetic, former football player, diagnosed with colon cancer 2 years ago, no ostomy, small amount of ongoing neuropathy, otherwise no morbidities. Very busy at work.

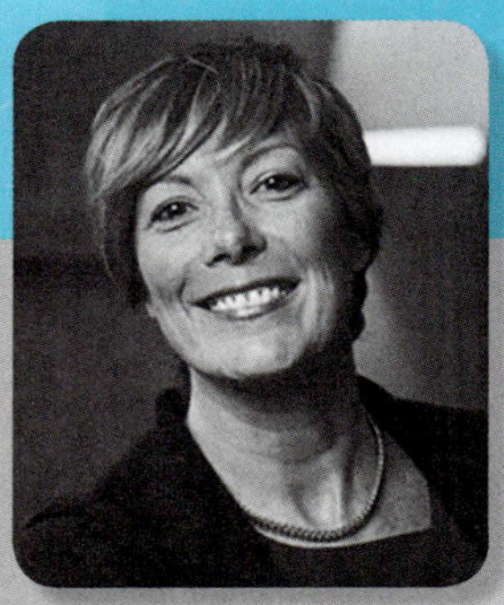

Meet the Expert

FEATURED PROFESSIONAL

Kathryn H. Schmitz, PhD, MPH

Professor of Hematology and Oncology
Associate Director of Population Sciences
Director, UPMC Moving Through Cancer Program
Co-leader, Biobehavioral Cancer Control Program
Hillman Cancer Center
University of Pittsburgh
Pittsburgh, PA, USA

Q: "Where did you grow up?"

Gaithersburg, MD

Q: "Where did you train? What is your training?"

I completed my bachelor's degree in Economics at the University of North Carolina at Greensboro; masters in Exercise Science from Queens College at the City University of New York; and PhD in Kinesiology, masters of public health in Epidemiology, and post doc in Cardiovascular Epidemiology at the University of Minnesota.

Q: "What are you best known for?"

I conducted the seminal research that demonstrated that resistance training is safe and effective for breast cancer survivors with and at risk for breast-cancer-related lymphedema. I have also led the American College of Sports Medicine® Guidelines for Exercise for Cancer Survivors.

Q: "What are you currently working on?"

Large clinical exercise trials ranging from primary prevention to addressing the supportive care needs of advanced cancer patients.

Q: "Anything else you want to include?"

Expanding the workforce in exercise oncology is crucial to making exercise standard of care for people living with and beyond cancer.

Favorite Quote:

"Play is the highest form of research."
—*Albert Einstein*

STUDY QUESTIONS

1. Name 3 exercise oncology delivery models in the US.
2. In what 2 countries is 3 reimbursement for exercise oncology professionals to work with cancer patients?
3. The key missing element in current oncology practice to connect patients to exercise is:
4. The ideal exercise oncology practice model includes which 3 primary elements?
5. Exercise prescription for PLWBC will need to vary according to what elements?

REFERENCES

1. Leach HJ, Covington KR, Pergolotti M, et al. Translating research to practice using a team-based approach to cancer rehabilitation: a physical therapy and exercise-based cancer rehabilitation program reduces fatigue and improves aerobic capacity. *Rehabil Oncol*. 2018;36(4):206–13.
2. American Association for Cancer Research. *Congress Briefing: AACR Cancer Disparities Progress Report 2022*. [Internet]. 2023. Available from http://www.cancerdisparitiesprogressreport.org/
3. Hu X, Chehal PK, Kaplan C, et al. Characterization of clinical symptoms by race among women with early-stage, hormone receptor-positive breast cancer before starting chemotherapy. *JAMA Netw Open*. 2021;4(6):e2112076. doi:10.1001/jamanetworkopen.2021.12076
4. Bubis LD, Davis L, Mahar A, et al. Symptom burden in the first year after cancer diagnosis: an analysis of patient-reported outcomes. *J Clin Oncol*. 2018;36(11):1103–11. doi:10.1200/JCO.2017.76.0876

5. Gilbertson-White S, Perkhounkova Y, Saeidzadeh S, Hein M, Dahl R, Simons-Burnett A. Understanding symptom burden in patients with advanced cancer living in rural areas. *Oncol Nurs Forum.* 2019;46(4): 428–41. doi:10.1188/19.ONF.428–41
6. Wonders KY, Wise R, Ondreka D, Seitz T. Supervised, individualized exercise mitigates symptom severity during cancer treatment. *J Adenocarcinoma Osteosarcoma.* 2018;3(1):1–5.
7. Covington KR, Hidde MC, Pergolotti M, Leach HJ. Community-based exercise programs for cancer survivors: a scoping review of practice-based evidence. *Support Care Cancer.* 2019;27(12):4435–50. doi:10.1007/s00520-019-05022-6
8. McKenzie DC. Abreast in a boat: a race against breast cancer. *CMAJ.* 1998;159(4):376–8.
9. United States Dragon Boat Federation. [Internet]. 2023. Available from www.usdbf.org
10. The Leukemia & Lymphoma Society. *Team in Training.* [Internet]. 2023. Available from www.teamintraining.org
11. Faro JM, Arem H, Heston AH, et al. A longitudinal implementation evaluation of a physical activity program for cancer survivors: LIVESTRONG® at the YMCA. *Implement Sci Commun.* 2020;1:63. doi:10.1186/s43058-020-00051-3
12. McDonough MH, Beselt LJ, Kronlund LJ, et al. Social support and physical activity for cancer survivors: a qualitative review and meta-study. *J Cancer Surviv.* 2021;15(5):713–28. doi:10.1007/s11764-020-00963-y
13. Rogers A. Livestrong® at YMCA helps cancer patients move toward fitness. *The Spokesman-Review.* 2014, April 15. Available from https://www.spokesman.com/stories/2014/apr/15/livestrong-at-ymca-helps-cancer-patients-move/
14. Wonders K. Supervised, individualized exercise programs help mitigate costs during cancer treatment. *J Palliat Care Med.* 2018;8(4):338. doi:10.4172/2165-7386.1000338
15. Wonders KY, Schmitz K, Wise R, Hale R. Cost-savings analysis of an individualized exercise oncology program in early-stage breast cancer survivors: a randomized clinical control trial. *JCO Oncol Pract.* 2022;18(7):e1170–e80. doi:10.1200/OP.21.00690
16. Wonders KY. *Maple Tree Cancer Alliance®.* [Internet]. 2023. Available from www.mapletreecanceralliance.org
17. Mansfield S. *Cancer Wellness for Life.* [Internet]. 2023. Available from www.cancerwellnessforlife.com
18. Schmitz KH, Potiaumpai M, Schleicher EA, et al. The exercise in all chemotherapy trial. *Cancer.* 2021;127(9):1507–16. doi:10.1002/cncr.33390
19. Move More. *Physical Activity the Underrated "Wonder Drug."* [Internet]. 2023. Available from https://www.macmillan.org.uk/documents/aboutus/commissioners/movemorereport.pdf
20. Unidad de Apoyo al Paciente Oncologico. [Internet]. 2023. Available from https://www.fundacionuapo.org/
21. ICAPEM Association for Lung Cancer Research in Women. *ACTÍVATE 2023 Program.* [Internet]. 2023. Available from https://icapem.es/programa-activate-2023/
22. European University. *VEnCE Program.* [Internet]. 2023. Available from https://fundacion.universidadeuropea.es/?page_id=552
23. Services Australia. *Chronic Disease GP Management Plans and Team Care Arrangements.* [Internet]. September 18, 2023. Available from https://www.servicesaustralia.gov.au/chronic-disease-gp-management-plans-and-team-care-arrangements?context=20

Case Study Answers

Chapter 1, Case Study

1. This case study is used for the purpose of explaining that exercise does not prevent cancer; it reduces the risk of cancer and decreases the (still nonzero) chance that cancer will occur. Highly active people can still develop cancer.
2. Mary has a strong family history of cancer, as her mother and sister had the same cancer. It seems likely that the oncology providers who will treat her will recommend testing for the *BRCA1* and *BRCA2* genes that, when mutated, increase the risk of developing breast cancer in more than 50% of patients.
3. Exercise may have played a role in making the tumor smaller, making it grow slower, and improving the profile of the tumor in a way that would make it easier to treat. We review many of these factors in Chapter 2.

Chapter 3, Case Study

1. Obesity, poor diet, alcohol, smoking history, sedentary lifestyle, and history of injecting drugs.
2. Reduce weight to a BMI < 25.
3. George should focus on intake of fruits and vegetables and avoid fast food.
4. Breast (men do get breast cancer), colorectal, liver, stomach, head and neck, and esophageal cancers.
5. Continue to avoid smoking.
6. The goal is to get to 150 minutes per week of aerobic exercise per week and twice weekly strength training. Perhaps he could start by going on a few walks per week.
7. On the basis of George's age and health history, it is recommended that he undergo 2 cancer screening tests: low-dose CT for lung cancer and colorectal cancer screening (either FIT and stool DNA every 1-3 years or direct visualization methods, such as colonoscopy every 5-10 years). It would be recommended that George get tested for hepatitis C infection and treated if he is infected.

Chapter 4, Case Study

1. The diagnosis of cancer must be accurate and precise to determine the optimal treatment. Biopsies must be reviewed by a pathologist; diagnostic scans and tests must be read by radiologists; and some lab tests take a week or more to get results. There are some cancers (eg, leukemias) that can be diagnosed more quickly.
2. Acute side effects occur during active treatment. Some common side effects are: nausea, fatigue, alopecia, chemotherapy-induced peripheral neuropathy, diarrhea, myelosuppression.
3. *Doxorubicin side effects*: alopecia, stomatitis, bone marrow suppression, myelosuppression, nausea, vomiting, fatigue, weakness, and cardiac toxicity.
   Paclitaxel side effects: chemotherapy-induced peripheral neuropathy, nausea, diarrhea, myelosuppression, pulmonary inflammation, fatigue, and weakness.
   Differences between the two: they are different because they target different phases in the cell cycle and cause different side effects, especially the long-term and late effects (eg, cardiac toxicity with doxorubicin and chemotherapy-induced peripheral neuropathy with paclitaxel).
4. Fatigue, weakness, nausea, diarrhea, alopecia, stomatitis, bone marrow suppression, and myelosuppression.
5. Begin an exercise program that starts slowly and gradually increases over time.

Chapter 5, Case Study #1

1. He has cancer-related fatigue from his treatment (interferon-α) and is weaker because he does not exercise.
2. Sarcopenia is a condition that includes loss of muscle mass, strength, and function. This is debilitation from inactivity.
3. Jim has cancer-related fatigue and he suffers lack of exercise.

Chapter 5, Case Study #2

1. Risk of bleeding. If someone falls, there is a risk of head injury from bleeding.
2. Chemotherapy-induced peripheral neuropathy can cause numbness in the toes and feet which may cause problems with balance and increases her risk for a fall.

3. She obtained clearance from her medical team to train and go backpacking. Metastasis to the femur increases the risk of fracture, but she is on denosumab, a bisphosphonate used to manage bone metastasis, and her medical team deemed it safe and important to exercise.

Chapter 6, Case Study

1. Darnell would benefit from a weight loss program that includes an exercise component. Identify nutrition or weight loss experts to maximize the help that Darnell can receive. Allow the nutrition or weight loss experts to lead the dietary portion of the program.
2. For the exercise part of the program, possibly start with walking exercise that Darnell can do while pushing a stroller with his twins. Given his prior lack of exercise and current BMI, that is likely to be moderate-intensity aerobic exercise. Start with short bouts that are easy to fit into a busy day (15 min) and build the time to 60 minutes per day for 6 days a week. This is sufficient exercise to contribute to meaningful fat loss, translating to reduced colon cancer risk. If Darnell is open to more, add twice weekly progressive resistance exercise.
3. If there is time and resources, resistance exercise may allow Darnell to feel particularly successful, since those with higher BMI typically have greater muscle mass. Further, resistance exercise during weight loss will minimize the loss of muscle mass as he loses weight. If there is time and capacity to do 1-repetition maximum (1-RM) testing, start exercises at 40% 1-RM and build to 60% to 70% 1-RM over 12 weeks. If there is not the option for testing, start with weights that feel comfortable to Darnell and increase every 3 to 4 sessions. Ensure that there is at least 1 exercise for each major muscle group. Start with 1 set and build to 2 to 3 sets over the first month.

Chapter 7, Case Study

1. Boosts anti-inflammatory response and switches immune cells from immunosuppression to immunosurveillance
2. Rituximab is a monoclonal antibody that targets a cell receptor protein called CD20, found on the surface of B cells. Rituximab locks on to the CD20 receptor on the malignant B cells, and then triggers the body's immune system to attack the cells and destroys them. Rituximab destroys both abnormal and normal B cells. Once treatment is over, the body can replace the normal B cells.
3. Clinically, neutropenia is defined as an absolute neutrophil count in the blood below 1.5×10^9 cells L^{-1}, and it may only be manifested as fatigue. Febrile neutropenia is described as an absolute neutrophil count in the blood below 0.5×10^9 cells L^{-1} with an oral temperature of >38.5 °C or 2 readings of >38°C for 2 hours.
4. - A fever with a temperature of 100.5 °F (38 °C) or higher
   - Chills or sweating
   - Sore throat, sores in the mouth, or a toothache
   - Abdominal pain
   - Pain near the anus
   - Pain or burning when urinating or often urinating
   - Diarrhoea or sores around the anus
   - A cough or shortness of breath
   - Any redness, swelling, or pain (especially around a cut, wound, or catheter)
5. Yes, back to doing as much as in the active surveillance stage, obviously being aware of reporting any changes in fatigue, bone pain, etc.

Chapter 8, Case Study

1. Exercise will help to reduce feelings of fatigue, improve and reduce depression and anxiety, and improve physical function and quality of life. There is moderate evidence that exercise will also improve bone health and sleep. We do not know yet if it will help cognitive function or sexual health, but healthy people who exercise often feel better in these areas.
2. No. Although some research studies indicate that exercise will reduce nausea, if the patient is using antiemetic medications, it is unlikely that they will see additional benefits related to nausea. There are no studies that show exercise is superior to current medications.
3. The exercise guidelines were developed for the weakest and sickest people living with cancer. She will benefit from and be successful with an exercise program.

Chapter 9, Case Study

1. Dorothy is in a risk category that requires a physician's clearance prior to initiating an exercise program. This is because of chronic disease diagnoses and her age. The first step for the exercise oncology professional is to obtain written clearance to proceed with initiating an exercise program.
2. Assuming permission is obtained from her physician, note that she is already doing 60 minutes of aerobic activity a week, walking her dog. This is likely being done at the 2 to 3 MET intensity levels. The goal is to get Dorothy to the recommended physical activity levels in 12 weeks, followed by the application of the behavioral approaches to maintenance outlined in the chapter. The following table is an example of progression that might be appropriate for this case.

Plan for Dorothy to Adhere to Physical Activity Recommendations for Cancer Risk Reduction (After 12 Weeks)

Exercise	Wk 1	Wk 2	Wk 3	Wk 4	Wk 5	Wk 6	Wk 7	Wk 8	Wk 9	Wk 10	Wk 11	Wk 12
Aerobic	10 min 5× weekly 15 min 2× MET levels 2-3 (walking dog)	10 min 3× weekly 15 min 4× MET levels 2-3	15 min 7× weekly MET levels 2-3	20 min 7× weekly MET levels 2-3	20-25 min 7× weekly MET levels 2-3	20-25 min 7× weekly MET levels 3-4 (walking faster)	20-25 min 7× weekly MET levels 3-4	20-25 min 7× weekly MET levels 3-4	20-25 min 7× weekly MET levels 3-4	20-25 min 7× weekly MET levels 3-4	20-25 min 7× weekly MET levels 3-4	20-25 min 7× weekly MET levels 3-4
Resistance	Nothing	Nothing	Nothing	Nothing	Nothing	Nothing	2 sessions 1 exercise per 9 muscle groups[a]: 1× each 10 repetitions, initial resistance set low to allow learning biomechanics	2 sessions 1 exercise per 9 muscle groups[a]: 2× each 10 repetitions, no increase in resistance	2 sessions 1 exercise per 9 muscle groups[a]: 2× each 10 repetitions, 10%-20% increase in resistance	2 sessions 1 exercise per 9 muscle groups[a]: 2× each 10 repetitions, no increase in resistance	2 sessions 1 exercise per 9 muscle groups[a]: 2× each 10 repetitions, 10%-20% increase in resistance	2 sessions 1 exercise per 9 muscle groups[a]: 2× each 10 repetitions, no increase in resistance
Sitting time	Advice to sit less throughout the day and, in particular, to watch for and avoid increases in sitting time as physical activity goes up.											

[a]chest, back, deltoids, biceps, triceps, quadriceps, hamstrings, qluteus maximus, calves.

Chapter 10, Case Study

1. This is a simple submaximal field test that is often used with lung cancer patients to assess baseline aerobic capacity and endurance. The 6MWT is useful in the assessment of operative risk in patients undergoing a lobectomy for lung cancer. It also provided a baseline value on which to develop Sylvia's aerobic exercise endurance program.
2. Functional strengthening exercises included sit to stand, heel raises, and toe raises, and balance training included heel-to-toe stand, one-leg stand, and heel-to-toe walking.
3. Sylvia's 6MWT distance increased by 53%, which means that she walked 490 meters at the end of the 6-week prehabilitation program.
4. This is double the time Sylvia spent in the hospital as she was home after only 3 days in hospital.

Chapter 11, Case Study

1. a. The exercise recommendation for cancer-related side effects includes moderate-intensity aerobic exercise at least 3 days a week for at least 30 minutes, for 8 to 12 weeks. Combining resistance training with aerobic training, at least 2 days per week, using at least 2 sets of 8 to 15 repetitions, with at least 60% of 1 repetition.
   b. Caution is needed with the ostomy with weight lifting. Chemotherapy-induced peripheral neuropathy will require attention to balance and use of weight equipment.
2. Empty the ostomy bag before engaging in exercise. Weight lifting/resistance exercises should start with low resistance and progress slowly under the guidance of trained exercise professionals. Focus on breathing.
3. All of the following:
   a. Safety is most important.
   b. Stability, balance, and gait should be assessed before engaging in exercise; consider balance training as indicated.
   c. Consider alternative aerobic exercise (stationary biking and water exercise) rather than walking if neuropathy affects stability or use treadmill with safety hand rails
   d. Resistance training recommendations:
      i. Monitor discomfort in hands when using handheld weights
      ii. Consider using dumbbells with soft/rubber coating and/or wearing padded gloves
      iii. Consider resistance machines over free weights
4. Exercise should reduce his fatigue as indicated by strong and moderate pieces of evidence.
5. True

Chapter 12, Case Study

1. a. Full lymph node clearance
   b. Radiotherapy to axilla region
   c. BMI >30.0 kg/m^2
   d. Poor range of movement
2. a. In order to be safe when providing a resistance program for cancer survivors with or at risk of lymphedema, it is important to focus on the large muscle group and progress with the principle "start low, progress slow." Include shoulder range of movement exercises
   b. Monitor for any swelling on affected arm or hand
   c. Avoid static contractions
3. a. High blood pressure
   b. High cholesterol levels
   c. High BMI
4. Current guidelines suggest that to reduce fatigue, a training program of at least 12 weeks of moderate to vigorous aerobic training plus resistance training sessions (with or without stretching) 3 times per week will reduce cancer-related fatigue after treatment. Aerobic activity should be 40% to 60% of the heart rate reserve (brisk walking, aerobic machine, stair climbing, cycle, swimming), for at least 30 minutes. Resistance training 2 to 3 per week with a minimum of 48 hours between workouts. One to 3 sets of repetitions between 6 and 15. Increase weight as tolerated once 15 or more repetitions have been achieved on all sets. Stretching can be done every day but at least 2 to 3 times per week. Stretches should be held for 10 to 30 seconds and repeated 3 to 4 times.
5.
   - Program to help with weight loss
   - Possible fear of recurrence increasing her anxiety levels
   - Possible unreported side effects of hormone treatment

Chapter 13, Case Study

1. His abdomen is distended because he is recovering from major abdominal surgery. He may also have more extensive disease in the abdominal cavity that could not be removed with surgery.
2. False.

3. Abdominal distention can impinge on the diaphragm and make breathing difficult. He also may have lung metastasis. The trainer should ask about this.

Chapter 14, Case Study

1. Paffenbarger Physical Activity Questionnaire (PPAQ)
2. True
3. True
4. a. Increases body fat, decreases muscle mass, and causes loss of balance

Chapter 15, Case Study

1. e. All of the above
2. d. All of the above
3. d. All of the above
4. d. All of the above

Chapter 16, Case Study

1. Probably not. with up to 88% of potential clients not aware of the program and 60% of the participants already reporting that they were "currently active."
2. For those who attended the program, it did appear to reduce or prevent treatment-related side effects, helped with recovery, and provided a very positive social experience.
3. This appears to be a lack of a continued income stream or a source of stable financial support.

Chapter 17, Case Study

1. Yes. Jack does not have bone metastasis, which might put him at risk for carrying the extra weight of the backpack. There is a risk of falling, but that is the usual risk that all hikers and backpackers face. It is not an elevated risk because of the stage of his disease or treatment. His treatment does make him lose muscle mass, so it will be important for him to do resistance exercises to maximize his leg and core strength.
2. Discuss how resistance exercise would be used to increase strength to carry backpack, what exercises would be recommended, and how aerobic exercises and intervals can increase cardiovascular fitness to prepare for carrying the backpack load on the ascents and descents over unstable ground and long distances.
3. Develop an exercise prescription with periodization (periods of rest and stress) to get them stronger without increasing risk for injury and worsening cancer-related side effects. Consider the person's previous experience with exercise. Assess their current condition and readiness to exercise.

Chapter 18, Case Study

Patient A. The best-fit model is one-on-one training with an exercise oncology professional
Patient B. The best-fit model is Livestrong
Patient C. The best-fit model is consultation
Patient D. The best-fit model is consultation

Study Questions Answers

Chapter 1

1. c. Apoptosis
2. a. Hippocrates
3. d. Spread beyond the original tissue where it developed
4. c. Carcinoma, sarcoma, melanoma, lymphoma, leukemia, and central nervous system
5. d. Denominators
6. 1 and 6
7. c. Prostate and lung
8. d. 80
9. a. Breast, endometrial, kidney, bladder, esophageal, stomach, and colon
10. b. Active surveillance

Chapter 2

1. apoptosis
2. b. Initiation, promotion, and progression
3. Possible answers:
   a. Enter the cell cycle without a growth factor
   b. Evade growth suppressors
   c. Divide indefinitely
   d. Show increased genetic instability
   e. Resist programmed cell death
   f. Sustain angiogenesis
   g. Exhibit deregulated metabolism
   h. Exhibit the capacity for invasion and metastasis
   i. Ability to evade immune clearance stimulate tumor promoting inflammation
4. a. A gene that has not yet been mutated in a way that causes cancer
5. c. Encode proteins that regulate cell proliferation
6. c. 27 to 83 days
7. b. The ecosystem that surrounds the tumor in the body
8. True
9. d. Exercise increases mitochondrial function and lactate clearance capacity
10. False
11. d. All of the above
12. b. Gene mutations and genetic instability
13. d. 10,000
14. Possible answers:
    a. Mismatch repair
    b. Base excision repair,
    c. Nucleotide excision repair
    d. Direct reversal
    e. Two types of response to double strand breaks: homologous recombination and nonhomologous end-joining
15. a. Preventing the growth of blood vessels
16. Growth, immune surveillance, and cancer prevention
17. b. The process by which cells know when to grow and when to stop
18. a. Loss of contact inhibition
19. c. Elimination, equilibrium, and escape
20. d. 20
21. d. a and b

Chapter 3

1. Avoid/quit smoking
2. A body mass index (BMI) between 18 and 25 kg/m^2
3. 150 to 300 minutes per week of moderate-intensity aerobic physical activity or 75 to 150 minutes of vigorous-intensity aerobic physical activity and 2 to 3 times weekly progressive resistance exercise.
4. d. Fruits, vegetables, avoiding alcohol, and limiting red meat
5. Breast and ovarian cancers
6. In the home
7. Possible answers:
   a. Use sunscreen
   b. Wear a hat with a brim
   c. Wear sunglasses
   d. Wear long-sleeve shirts and pants
   e. Sit in the shade
   f. Avoid tanning beds

8. Possible answers:
   a. Cervical
   b. Back of the throat
   c. Anus
   d. Vulva
   e. Penis
   f. Vagina
9. b. Infants to 18 years
10. b. Because it is treatable in most people in 8 to 12 weeks
11. d. All of the above
12. Possible answers:
    a. The test is inexpensive (as it will be used in large populations)
    b. The test is easy to administer
    c. The screening test is acceptable to the population to be screened
    d. The test is reliable (gives the same results on repeated tests)
    e. The test is valid (distinguishes between diseased and healthy people)
    f. Cancers caught earlier, because of screening, can be treated in a way that results in a more favorable symptom burden and mortality outcome
    g. The test has low false positives (tests that indicate there is cancer when there is no cancer)
    h. The test has low false negatives (tests that indicate there is no cancer when there is a cancer).
13. The US Preventive Services Task Force (USPSTF)
14. False
15. d. 21 to 65 years
16. f. a–c
17. e. b and c only
18. Reduced exposure to estrogen
19. Possible answers:
    a. Insulin and glucose metabolism
    b. Immune function
    c. Inflammation
    d. Sex hormones
    e. Oxidative stress
    f. Genomic instability
20. Possible answers:
    a. Chronic inflammation
    b. Excess estrogen
    c. High levels of insulin and other hormones that can then contribute to the growth of cancer cells

Chapter 4

1. Determine the type of cancer and cell lines
2. Tumor markers are released by cancer cells into the blood or urine and are a reflection of tumor and disease activity. They can be used in diagnosis, staging disease, determining prognosis, predicting response to treatment, determining optimal targeted treatment, and monitoring response to treatment.
3. Prostate-specific antigen and carcinoembryonic antigen.
4. To determine the extent of disease, including how large the tumor is and if it has spread.
5. Port-a-Cath, Broviac, Groshong, and Hickman.
6. It affects as many as 90% of patients during treatment and 60% after treatment ends.
7. The point where blood counts (white blood cells, red blood cells, and platelets) are at the lowest.
8. Increased risk of infection (low white blood cells, anemia [low red blood cells], and bleeding [low platelets]).
9. Trastuzumab is used to treat breast cancer and Imatinib is used to treat chronic myelogenous leukemia. They are both targeted therapies.
10. Aromatase inhibitors block estrogen. Androgen ablation drugs block male androgens (testosterone). Examples are anastrozole, exemestane, bicalutamide, flutamide.
11. An engineered treatment used to treat relapsed acute lymphoblastic leukemia, non-Hodgkin lymphoma, and multiple myeloma. It is made from the person's own white blood cells and is given in a hospital setting. Side effects include cytokine release syndrome (eg, difficulty breathing, fever, chills, shaking, severe nausea, vomiting or diarrhea, severe muscle and joint pain, and dizziness or lightheadedness). It also causes neurologic toxicities, such as altered consciousness, delirium, confusion, agitation, seizures, difficulty speaking and understanding, and loss of balance. Like other cancer treatments, CAR-T therapy can cause serious infections, prolonged low blood cell counts, hypogammaglobulinemia (low immunoglobulins), and risk for developing secondary cancers.

Chapter 5

1. National Comprehensive Cancer Network and Commission on Cancer
2. Cancer-related fatigue
3. Inactivity, debilitation, some treatments
4. b. Flexibility exercise
   d. Yoga exercise
5. Tingling, pain, pins and needles, fullness sensitivity to vibration in fingers, and toes.
6. Amount of bone loss or T score >-2.5 = osteoporosis
7. False
8. Control the disease and treat the cancer more like a chronic disease.
9. Symptom management
10. Relieving symptoms and providing support at the end of life; not extending life.

Chapter 6

1 Possible answers:
   a. Breast
   b. Colorectal
   c. Endometrial
   d. Esophageal
   e. Gallbladder
   f. Kidney
   g. Liver
   h. Oral
   i. Ovarian
   j. Pancreatic
   k. Prostate
   l. Certain types of brain cancers
   m. Stomach cancers
2. b. DXA, CT scan, and D_3-creatine dilution
3. True
4. a. Up
5. c. Higher
6. d. A ring of macrophages surrounding a dead fat cell
7. Possible answers:
   a. Tells the brain that the fat cells are full
   b. Regulates blood pressure
   c. Regulates thyroid function
   d. Regulates insulin secretion
   e. Regulates heart rate
   f. Regulates bone mass
   g. Regulates the menstrual cycle
8. d. 37
9. False
10. True

Chapter 7

1. c. Caused by trauma
2. d. Natural killer cells and cytokines
3. b. 15 to 20
4. a. C-reactive protein
5. a. By immunosuppression
6. b. CRP and TNF-α
7. c. Causes bone marrow suppression
8. c. Engineered T-cell receptors
9. c. HBV vaccine
10. a. Avoiding infection exposures

Chapter 8

1. c. The sickest and weakest
2. Possible answers:
   a. Weight gain
   b. Health-related quality of life
   c. Fatigue
   d. Cardiotoxicity
   e. Lymphedema
   f. Sexual function
3. An accumulation of lymphatic fluid in the affected extremity (arm or leg) that is unable to be removed into the central circulation.
4. A compression sleeve has higher pressure at the fingers and arm to help move the lymphatic fluid back up the arm toward the body.
5. False. Fatigue affects up to 90% of people receiving treatment.
6. Health-related quality of life concerns physical and mental health, social support, and functional status. It examines the impact of cancer on quality of life.
7. CIPN is a treatment-related side effect associated with taxanes-, platinum-, and vinca alkaloid-based chemotherapy. It causes numbness, tingling, pain, cold sensitivity, and impaired function in hands and feet.
8. Treatment tolerance is the ability of a person actively receiving treatment to get the full treatment done on schedule.
9. Multidimensional is something that has many different parts or aspects.

10. Possible answers:
    a. Swelling in an arm or leg
    b. Limb feels heavy
    c. Skin feels tight
    d. Swelling may interfere with movement (eg, fingers, hand, arm, toes, and leg)
    e. Skin may become thick
    f. Affected area my itch or burn
    g. Difficult to wear rings, watch, bracelet, and socks

Chapter 9

1. a. 150 to 300 minutes per week of moderate-intensity aerobic physical activity or 75 to 150 minutes per week of vigorous-intensity aerobic physical activity, as well as twice weekly strengthening exercises.
2. Possible answers:
    a. Bladder
    b. Breast
    c. Colon
    d. Endometrium
    e. Esophagus
    f. Stomach
    g. Kidney
    h. Lung
    i. Ovary
    j. Pancreas
3. c. To triage participants into risk levels
4. d. Assess physical activity, assess signs and symptoms, and assess known diseases/diagnoses and histories.
5. True
6. a. Frequency, intensity, time, and type of exercise
7. True
8. Possible answers:
    a. Walking 2 to 2.9 miles per hour
    b. Stationary cycling at 50 Watts
    c. Leisurely canoeing
    d. Croquet
    e. Bowling
    f. Slow ballroom dancing
    g. Golf with a cart
    h. Playing catch
    i. Playing piano
    j. Stretching exercises or yoga
9. f. All of the above
10. True
11. True
12. a. Greater than

Chapter 10

1. d. Immediately after diagnosis
2. b. Financial support
3. c. Cardiopulmonary exercise test
4. d. All of the above
5. True
6. b. Abdominal and lung: these surgical procedures are challenging, complex, and normally entail a significant time period under general anesthetic.
7. a. Pelvic floor exercises
8. b. Shorter hospital stay
9. c. Screen

Chapter 11

1. Exercise includes moderate-intensity aerobic exercise at least 3 days a week for at least 30 minutes, for 8 to 12 weeks plus resistance training 2 days per week, using at least 2 sets of 8 to 15 repetitions at least 50% of 1 repetition maximum.
2. Each person has different side effects of cancer and its treatment. This is a good time to propose different scenarios with lymphedema, ostomy, and amputation, and let the class discuss how they might adapt a FITT prescription for each person.
3. True
4. Not enough high-quality research studies with quantifiable exercise dose with other forms of exercise.
5. False. They are not within the scope of the ACSM® guidelines because there has not been enough research to determine their safety and efficacy
6.

Frequency	Intensity	Time	Type
3 days	Moderate	30 min	Aerobic
2 days	Moderate	30 min	Resistance
2-3 days	Moderate	30 min	Aerobic + resistance

7. To avoid causing lymphedema or a lymphedema flare.
8. False. Cancer symptoms tend to occur in clusters.
9. True
10. Assess, advise, and refer

11. Possible answers:
    a. Swelling in an arm or leg
    b. Limb feels heavy
    c. Skin feels tight
    d. Swelling may interfere with movement (eg, fingers, hand, arm, toes, and leg)
    e. Skin may become thick
    f. Affected area my itch or burn
    g. Difficult to wear rings, watch, bracelet, or socks

Chapter 12

1. False
2. Increase
3. False
4. Depressive symptoms in cancer survivors after treatment can be reduced with moderate-intensity aerobic training 3 times per week for at least 12 weeks or twice weekly combined aerobic plus resistance training lasting 6 to 12 weeks.
5. Sarcopenia is characterized by a progressive and generalized loss of skeletal muscle mass and loss of muscle strength or physical functioning.
6. A supervised progressive resistance training program for a period of at least 12 weeks is effective for improving muscle strength, muscle mass, and physical performance.
7. b. Limited range of movement
8. c. Hot flashes
9. Combined moderate-to-vigorous intensity of resistance training plus high impact training (ie, exercise that generates ground reaction forces above 3-4 times body weight) performed 2 to 3 days per week is the best mode of exercise to improve bone health (eg, slow loss or slightly improve bone mineral density at the hip and lumbar spine).
10. Diet and exercise interventions for breast cancer survivors result in significant improvements in body weight, waist circumference, hip circumference, BMI, systolic BP, blood glucose levels, body fat, fat mass, and lean body mass.

Chapter 13

1. Metastatic disease
2. True
3. Consider using weight machines, stationary bicycle, rowing machine, and wrist/ankle weights.
4. Rated Perceived Exertion after warm-up exercise at the intensity level of 5 to 6.
5. Daily and adapt exercise according to his pain level like he would for fatigue. He should be told to take his pain medication.
6. Clinical care team, oncology physical therapy
7. Tumor pressing nerves and organs and CIPN from treatment.
8. Tumor might be causing abdominal distension and some ascites.
9. See Box 13.1

Chapter 14

1. Palliative care often starts earlier when a patient may be beginning treatment. Hospice starts when life expectancy is less than 6 months.
2. Potential for fracture. This should be discussed with the medical team even if the patient is at end of life. Additional modifications can be found in Chapter 15.
3. Yes, pulmonary function can be increased. However, if fluid is quickly accumulating in the lung, exercise may not be effective.
4. Assess the person's condition and develop an individualized exercise program that combines aerobic and resistance exercises to improve function.
5. False
6. False
7. False

Chapter 15

1. b. 30
2. After a cancer diagnosis, some people may be ready to change some of their negative lifestyle behaviors and receptive to advice and assistance to become more physically active.
3. Social cognitive theory
4. c. Reduced fatigue
5. Fatigue, pain, arthralgia, peripheral neuropathy, gastrointestinal issues, lymphoedema, and weight gain.
6. c. 70
7. Self-efficacy is about having the strong, positive belief that you have the capacity and the skills to achieve your goals.
8. Wearables such as accelerometers in smartphones, watches, etc to track physical activity levels are relatively inexpensive and allow data to be downloaded and stored onto a computer or mobile phone.

9. Specific, Measurable, Action, Realistic, Timely, Self-determined.
10. Providing companionship (shared experience) motivation (encouragement to participate) and health promotion (discussed benefits such as less fatigue).
11. d. Walking
12. c. At home or in a gym

Chapter 16

1. Efficacy exercise oncology trials are conducted in controlled way and do not consider the variability of implementation in the real world.
2. a. Attitude
3. d. 77
4. Direct cost to attend an unsubsidized exercise program and indirect costs such as travel to venue, that is, transportation or parking cost.
5. b. Reach, Effectiveness, Adoption, Implementation, Maintenance.
6. b. 30
7. 30 seconds to 2 minutes
8. c. Cancer-related fatigue
9. a. Sustainability
10. Physical therapists, clinical exercise physiologists, and qualified cancer exercise specialists.

Chapter 17

1. a. Fatigue, quality of life, sleep, anxiety, and dyspnea
2. e. All of the above
3. People living with and beyond breast cancer
4. False
5. There may not be research to support them, but if they increase aerobic capacity and muscle strength, there are benefits if the activity does not pose a risk of injury.
6. Refer to Table 17.2: skating, rock climbing, cycling, parachuting, paragliding, skydiving (falling and bleeding); boating, diving/scuba, skiing, hiking, backpacking, mountaineering (falling, drowning, bleeding, and infection); swimming (drowning and infection); ranch/agricultural work (falling, bleeding, and infection risk).

Chapter 18

1. Possible answers:
   a. One-on-one supervised
   b. Consultation model
   c. Group fitness
   d. Synchronous online
   e. Asynchronous online
2. UK and Australia
3. Triage
4. Education, surveillance, and exercise prescription
5. Background health status, current diagnosis, and treatments (if any), patient preference, and severity of impairments/symptoms.

Index

Note: Page numbers followed by "*f*" indicate figures. Page numbers followed by "*t*" indicate tables. Page numbers followed by "*b*" indicate boxes.

C

F

Q

R

U

V

W

Y

Z